The Urinary Tract

Donna E. Hansel · Jesse K. McKenney
Andrew J. Stephenson · Sam S. Chang
Editors

The Urinary Tract

A Comprehensive Guide to Patient Diagnosis and Management

Springer

Editors
Donna E. Hansel, MD, Ph.D
Department of Pathology
Cleveland Clinic
Cleveland, Ohio, USA

Jesse K. McKenney, MD
Department of Pathology
Stanford University Medical Center
Stanford, California, USA

Andrew J. Stephenson, MD
Section of Urologic Oncology
Glickman Urologic and Kidney Institute
Cleveland Clinic
Cleveland, Ohio, USA

Sam S. Chang, MD
Department of Urologic Surgery
Vanderbilt University Medical Center
Nashville, Tennessee, USA

ISBN 978-1-4614-5319-2 ISBN 978-1-4614-5320-8 (eBook)
DOI 10.1007/978-1-4614-5320-8
Springer New York Heidelberg Dordrecht London

Library of Congress Control Number: 2012952106

Printed on acid-free paper

Springer is part of Springer Science+Business Media (www.springer.com)

Our thanks to our families for their support and patience during the making of this book.

Foreword

As cofounder and president of the Bladder Cancer Advocacy Network, I am so pleased to see this comprehensive guide to the diagnosis and management of urinary tract diseases. As a "below the belt" condition, bladder cancer, and more benign bladder conditions, suffers from a lack of awareness and understanding—both from the medical community as well as the general population.

Drawing on the expertise of specialists across the country from multiple disciplines, this thorough and practical textbook is an essential tool for all physicians and physicians-in-training for understanding the specific issues and complexities that arise in the treatment of bladder cancer, as well as other urinary tract diseases. Early and correct diagnosis, along with the most appropriate treatment for the specific stage and grade of the patient's disease, is keys to survival in bladder cancer. I believe that when utilized, this Guide will improve patients' lives.

On behalf of bladder cancer patients and their families, along with family members who have lost loved ones to this disease, I applaud the work and effort of the editors and contributors to this valuable treatise.

Bethesda, MA, USA — Diane Zipursky Quale

Preface

Diseases of the urinary tract—whether benign or malignant—can present challenges in diagnosis and patient management. Increasing awareness of the complexity of urinary tract disease has prompted the formation of several national and international working groups focused on this anatomic region to better address outstanding questions in the field.

It is clear that one factor contributing to delayed progress in understanding and treating urinary tract disease is the sometimes limited communication between pathologist and treating physician. With the expansion of subspecialty publications, new diagnostic pathology entities in bladder cancer may be limited to a pathology-only audience; similarly, new treatment methods and their impact in clinical care may be viewed primarily by an urologist and oncologist audience. The lack of crosstalk and collaborative communication in such situations can lead to missed opportunities in disease understanding and management. In light of this, we took a novel approach to designing this textbook: each chapter is written by a pathologist and treating physician, often assigned from different institutions. We deliberately structured our text in this manner to not only highlight challenging areas that arise in the "cross-talk" arena but also address potential institutional differences in the management of urinary tract patients.

This book covers urethral, bladder, and upper tract disease, with emphasis on selected benign conditions—such as polypoid lesions, diverticular disease, and inflammatory processes—and most neoplastic processes. Neoplasia is addressed from a clinical and pathological perspective, with chapters addressing urothelial carcinoma and variant histology, as well as a chapter describing mesenchymal lesions. Additional chapters address anatomy and histology of the urinary tract, the role of urine cytology, pathology-endoscopy correlates, chemotherapy for neoplasia, and the molecular pathogenesis of bladder cancer.

Our primary goal in designing this text is to provide a comprehensive guide to the diagnosis and management of urinary tract disease for physicians and other health-care providers who diagnose and treat patients with urinary tract disease. We hope that by emphasizing potentially problematic areas for each disease entity, we can not only draw attention to areas of needed improvement but also stimulate the necessary discussions to solve these outstanding problems.

Cleveland, Ohio, USA — Donna E. Hansel, MD, PhD
Stanford, California, USA — Jesse K. McKenney, MD
Cleveland, Ohio, USA — Andrew J. Stephenson, MD
Nashville, Tennessee, USA — Sam S. Chang, MD

Contents

Contributors

Hikmat Al-Ahmadie, MD Department of Pathology, Memorial Sloan-Kettering Cancer Center, New York, NY, USA

Mahul B. Amin, MD Department of Pathology and Laboratory Medicine, Cedars-Sinai Medical Center, Los Angeles, CA, USA

Kenneth Angermeier, MD Center for Genitourinary Reconstruction, Cleveland Clinic, Glickman Urological and Kidney Institute, Cleveland, OH, USA

Bernard Bochner, MD Department of Surgery, Memorial Sloan Kettering Cancer Center, Kimmel Center for Prostate and Urologic Cancers, New York, NY, USA

Donald R. Bodner, MD Department of Urology, UH Case Western Medical Center, Case Western Reserve University, Cleveland, OH, USA

Christine N. Booth, MD Pathology and Laboratory Medicine Institute, Cleveland Clinic, Cleveland, OH, USA

Sam S. Chang, MD Department of Urologic Surgery, Vanderbilt University Medical Center, Nashville, TN, USA

Liang Cheng, MD Indiana University School of Medicine, Indianapolis, IN, USA

Edward E. Cherullo, MD Department of Urology, UH Case Western Medical Center, Cleveland, OH, USA

Michael S. Cookson, MD Department of Urologic Surgery, Vanderbilt University Medical Center, Vanderbilt University, Nashville, TN, USA

Colin Dinney, MD Department of Urology, The University of Texas M.D. Anderson Cancer Center, Houston, TX, USA

Renee Dintzis, PhD Department of Cell Biology, Johns Hopkins University School of Medicine, Baltimore, MD, USA

Robert Dreicer, MS, MD, FACP Department of Solid Tumor Oncology, Taussig Cancer Institute, Cleveland Clinic Lerner College of Medicine, Cleveland Clinic, Cleveland, OH, USA

Jonathan I. Epstein, MD Department of Pathology, Urology, Oncology, The Johns Hopkins Medical Institutions, Baltimore, MD, USA

Amr Fergany, MD, PhD Sections of Oncology, Laparoscopy and Robotics, Cleveland Clinic, Glickman Urological and Kidney Institute, Cleveland Clinic, Cleveland, OH, USA

Jorge A. Garcia, MD, FACP Departments of Solid Tumor Oncology and Urology, Taussig Cancer Institute, Glickman Urological & Kidney Institute, Cleveland Clinic Lerner College of Medicine of CWRU, Cleveland, OH, USA

Howard B. Goldman, MD Glickman Urological Kidney Institute, Cleveland Clinic, Cleveland, OH, USA

Mark L. Gonzalgo, MD, PhD Department of Pathology, Stanford University Medical Center, Stanford, CA, USA

Charles C. Guo, MD, MSc Department of Pathology, University of Texas MD, Anderson Cancer Center, Houston, TX, USA

Omar Hameed, MBChB Departments of Pathology and Surgery, The Comprehensive Cancer Center, University of Alabama at Birmingham, Birmingham, AL, USA

Donna E. Hansel, MD, PhD Department of Pathology, Cleveland Clinic, Cleveland, OH, USA

Brent M. Hardin, MD University of Tennessee Graduate School of Medicine, Knoxville, TN, USA

Jeff Holzbeierlein, MD, FACS Department of Urology, University of Kansas Hospital, Kansas City, KS, USA

Robert Jackson, MD Department of Urology, University of Michigan, Ann Arbor, MI, USA

Thomas W. Jarrett, MD Department of Urology, George Washington University, Washington, DC, USA

Rafael E. Jimenez, MD Department of Laboratory Medicine and Pathology, Mayo Clinic, Rochester, MN, USA

J. Stephen Jones, MD, FACS Department of Regional Urology, Cleveland Clinic, Glickman Urological Kidney Institute, Lerner College of Medicine at CWRU, Cleveland, OH, USA

Joseph C. Klink, MD Section of Urologic Oncology, Glickman Urologic and Kidney Institute, Cleveland Clinic, Cleveland, OH, USA

William A. Larchian, MD Department of Urology, Case Western Reserve University School of Medicine, Cleveland, OH, USA

Cheryl T. Lee, MD Department of Urology, University of Michigan, Ann Arbor, MI, USA

Gregory T. MacLennan, MD Department of Pathology, University Hospitals Case Medical Center, Case Western Reserve University, Cleveland, OH, USA

Luigi Marchionni, MD, PhD Department of Oncology, Johns Hopkins University School of Medicine, Baltimore, MD, USA

Jennifer McBride, PhD Cleveland Clinic Lerner College of Medicine, Cleveland, OH, USA

Jesse K. McKenney, MD Department of Pathology, Stanford University Medical Center, Stanford, CA, USA

Courteney K. Moore, MD Department of Surgery, Glickman Urological and Kidney Institute and Obstetrics and Gynecology, Cleveland Clinic Lerner College of Medicine of Case Western Reserve University, Cleveland, OH, USA

Todd M. Morgan, MD Department of Urology, University of Michigan, Ann Arbor, MI, USA

George J. Netto, MD Department of Pathology, Johns Hopkins University, Baltimore, MD, USA

Adeboye O. Osunkoya, MD, FCAP Department of Pathology and Urology, Emory School of Medicine, Atlanta, GA, USA

Gladell P. Paner MD Department of Pathology and Section of Urology, Department of Surgery, The University of Chicago, Chicago, IL, USA

Anil Parwani, MD, PhD University of Pittsburgh Medical Center Shadyside, Pittsburgh, PA, USA

Lee E. Ponsky, MD, FACS Urologic Oncology and Minimally Invasive Therapies Center, Urology Institute, University Hospitals Case Medical Center, Cleveland, OH, USA

Diane Zipursky Quale Bladder Cancer Advocacy Network (BCAN), Bethesda, MD, USA

Stephen S. Raab, MD Department of Pathology, University of Washington School of Medicine, Seattle, WA, USA

Victor E. Reuter, MD Department of Pathology, Memorial Sloan-Kettering Cancer Center, New York, NY, USA

W. Stuart Reynolds, MD, MPH Department of Urologic Surgery, Vanderbilt University Medical Center, Nashville, TN, USA

Jonathan J. Rhee, MD Department of Urology, George Washington University, Washington, DC, USA

Harriette M. Scarpero, MD Associated Urologists of Nashville, Nashville, TN, USA

Wade J. Sexton, MD Moffitt Cancer Center, Genitourinary Oncology Program, Tampa, FL, USA

Dale R. Shepard, MD, PhD Department of Solid Tumor Oncology, Taussig Cancer Institute, Cleveland Clinic Lerner College of Medicine, Cleveland Clinic, Cleveland, OH, USA

Arlene Siefker-Radtke, MD Department of Genitourinary Medical Oncology, The University of Texas M.D. Anderson Cancer Center, Houston, TX, USA

Andrew J. Stephenson, MD, FRCSC Section of Urologic Oncology, Glickman Urologic and Kidney Institute, Cleveland Clinic, Cleveland, OH, USA

Jennifer M. Taylor, MD University of Pittsburgh Medical Center, Pittsburgh, PA, USA

Dan Theodorescu, MD, PhD University of Colorado Cancer Center, Consortium Comprehensive Cancer Center, Aurora, CO, USA

Theodorus H. van der Kwast, MD, PhD, FRCPC Department of Pathology and Laboratory Medicine, Princess Margaret Hospital, University Health Network, Toronto, ON, Canada

Hadley Wood, MD Cleveland Clinic, Glickman Urological and Kidney Institute, Cleveland, OH, USA

Part I

The Urinary Tract

Anatomy, Embryology, and Histology

1

Renee Dintzis and Jennifer McBride

Embryonic Origin of the Urinary Tract

Although the urinary and genital systems function as two separate systems, they are intimately related anatomically and embryologically. Both develop from a longitudinal elevation of intermediate mesoderm along the posterior aspect of the body wall identified as the urogenital ridge. The urogenital ridge is divided into the nephrogenic cord that gives rise to the urinary system and the gonadal ridge that gives rise to the genital system. The following sections will focus on the development of the urinary system structures including the kidneys, ureters, urinary bladder, and urethra.

Kidneys

In the developing human embryo, three successive sets of kidneys form along the posterior body wall. The initial set—the pronephroi—appears early in the fourth week as rudimentary nonfunctional structures (Fig. 1.1). These initial structures are localized in the cervical region and are composed of a small cluster of cells with tubular ducts that open caudally into the cloaca, the terminal part of the hindgut. While the collective mass of the pronephroi degenerates by the end of the fourth week, a length of the pronephric ducts endures as a precursor to the next set of kidneys.

The second set of kidneys appears late in the fourth week as the mesonephroi immediately caudal to the initial pronephroi (Fig. 1.1a). This second set is well developed and continues to function until approximately the ninth week of fetal development when the permanent kidneys become fully developed. As the mesonephric tubules grow medially they surround a cluster of capillaries to form a glomerulus and the surrounding Bowman's capsule; collectively, these structures are referred to as a renal corpuscle. Laterally, the mesonephric tubules enter the mesonephric (Wolffian) ducts, originally the pronephric ducts, and continue caudally to open into the cloaca (Fig. 1.1a). While the mesonephroi degenerate near the end of the first trimester, the mesonephric ducts persist in the male and contribute to the formation of the genital system including the seminal vesicles, ejaculatory ducts, epididymis, and vas deferens.

The third and permanent set of kidneys—the metanephroi—begins to develop early in the fifth week and to become functional in approximately the ninth week. The metanephroi develop from two sources: the metanephric diverticulum (ureteric bud), an outgrowth of the mesonephric

R. Dintzis (✉)
Department of Cell Biology, Johns Hopkins University School of Medicine, 725 North Wolfe Street, Hunterian G12, Baltimore, MD 21205-2196, USA
e-mail: rdintzis@jhmi.edu

J. McBride
Cleveland Clinic Lerner College of Medicine, 9500 Euclid Avenue, NA/24, Cleveland, OH 44195, USA
e-mail: mcbridj@ccf.org

D.E. Hansel et al. (eds.), *The Urinary Tract: A Comprehensive Guide to Patient Diagnosis and Management*, DOI 10.1007/978-1-4614-5320-8_1, © Springer Science+Business Media New York 2012

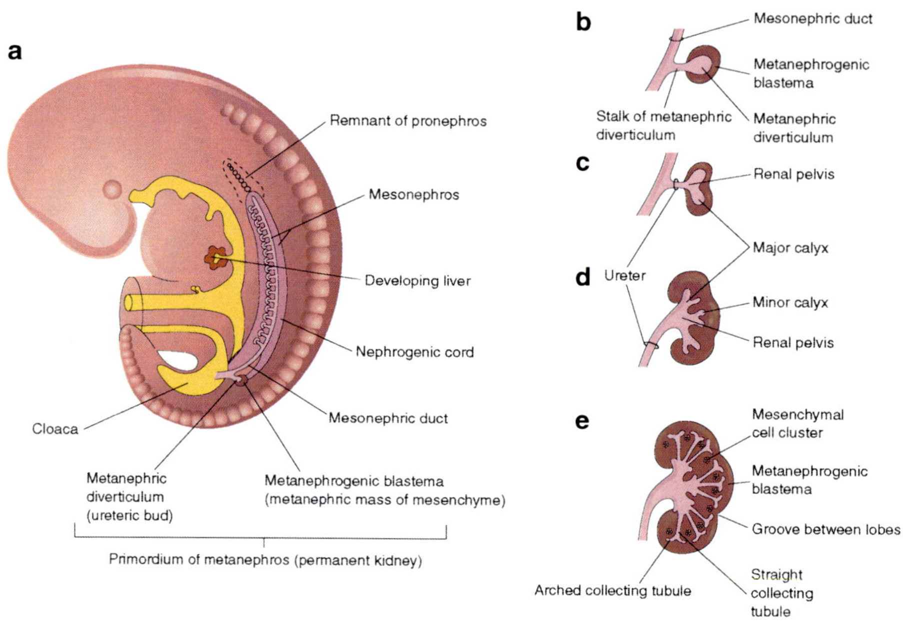

Fig. 1.1 Lateral view of the developing metanephros in a 5-week embryo (reprinted with permission from Moore and Persaud [4])

duct adjacent to its entrance into the cloaca, and the metanephrogenic blastema (metanephric mass of mesenchyme) that arises from the caudal aspect of the nephrogenic cord (Fig. 1.1a). The connecting stalk of the metanephric diverticulum develops into the ureters, and the cranial portion infiltrates the metanephrogenic blastema, subsequently causing the bulb of the diverticulum to subdivide repetitively into several branches. This branching pattern will form the primitive renal pelvis, major and minor calyces, and the collecting tubules (Fig. 1.1b–e). After penetrating the metanephrogenic blastema, the distal end of each collecting tubule induces the cells in the blastema to form metanephric vesicles that develop into S-shaped metanephric tubules with the proximal end invaginated by a glomeruli (Fig. 1.2). These tubules become distal convoluted tubules, proximal convoluted tubules, and the nephron loop (of Henle). Along with the glomeruli and its capsule, these tubules comprise a nephron or excretory unit. At its "distal" end each distal convoluted tubule is confluent with a collecting tubule, thus establishing a confluence between Bowman's capsule and the collecting unit.

Continuing up until the 32nd week of gestation the number of kidney glomeruli steadily increases. Nephrons also continue to form until birth when nephron development and formation is completed, with approximately 1–2 million nephrons in each kidney. At birth, the kidney has a lobulated appearance that diminishes during infancy as the nephrons and surrounding tissues continue to grow.

Initially, the metanephric kidneys are located in the pelvis just ventral to the sacrum. By the ninth week of development, the kidneys have ascended from the pelvis into the abdomen to reach their adult position along the posterior abdominal wall. Increased growth of the lumbar and sacral regions induces kidney ascent. As they ascend, the kidneys receive arterial branches from surrounding blood vessels. While in the pelvis, the kidneys receive arterial blood supply from the common iliac arteries. During their ascent, the kidneys are supplied by the aortic arterial branches until they reach the abdominal aorta, at which point they receive blood supply from the permanent renal arteries. The more caudal arterial branches from the common iliac

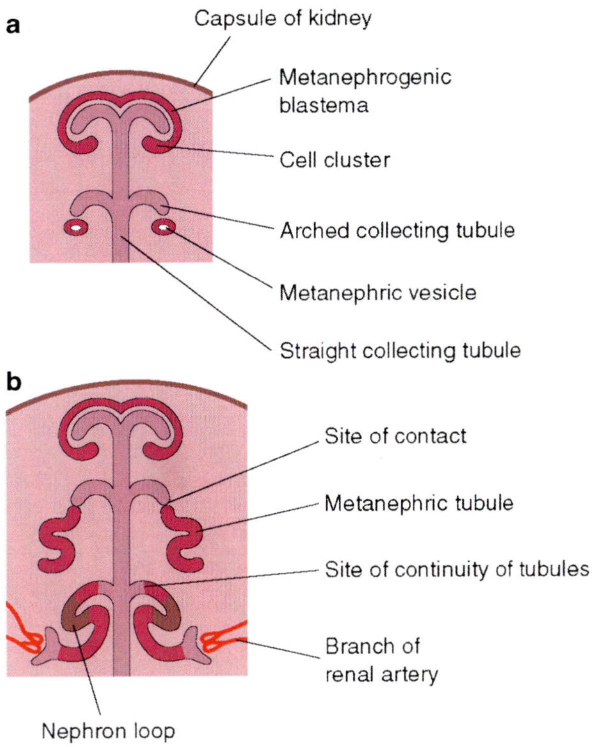

Fig. 1.2 Nephron development from the metanephric tubules. (**a**) Initiation of nephrogenesis, week 8. (**b**) Uriniferous tubules are formed by continuity of the collecting tubules with the metanephric tubules (reprinted with permission from Moore and Persaud [4])

and distal aorta degenerate as the kidneys migrate rostrally; however, some vessels may remain as accessory renal arteries. These accessory arteries directly reflect the changing blood supply to the kidneys during development. Typically, these arteries branch off the aorta near the renal artery to enter the hilum of the kidney. Branches that course anterior to the ureter to enter the inferior pole of the kidney may lead to obstruction of the ureter resulting in obstructive hydronephrosis.

Bladder and Ureters

The bladder and urethra develop from the urogenital sinus that is formed during the fourth to seventh week of gestation, when the cloaca is divided by the urorectal septum into an anal canal posteriorly and urogenital sinus anteriorly (Fig. 1.3a). Three divisions of the urogenital sinus are identified: an upper or cranial part that forms the majority of the bladder, a middle pelvic section that will become the entire urethra in females as well as the bladder neck and prostatic urethra in males, and a caudal phallic part that extends towards the genital tubercle. Early during bladder development, the bladder is continuous with the allantois, a sac-like structure that collects liquid waste and exchanges gases used by the embryo. Eventually, the allantois constricts and forms a fibrous cord—the urachus—that connects the apex of the bladder to the umbilicus and that subsequently forms the median umbilical ligament in the adult (Fig. 1.3b, c).

As the bladder develops, the caudal aspects of the mesonephric ducts are absorbed into the bladder wall and contribute to the formation of the trigone. As a result, the ureters that initially developed from the mesonephric ducts enter the bladder separately. During kidney ascent, the ureteral openings migrate superolaterally to enter the base of the bladder at an oblique angle, whereas the mesonephric duct openings move

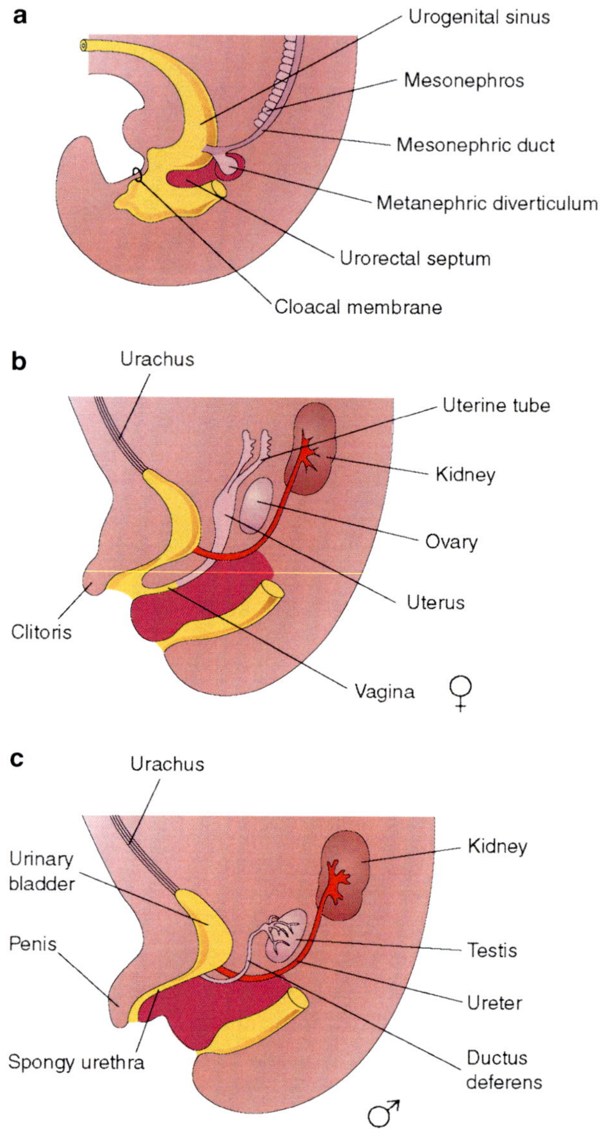

Fig. 1.3 Lateral view of the 5-week embryo. (**a**) Development of the urogenital sinus and rectum formed by division of the cloaca. (**b**) Male urogenital sinus and rectum at 12 weeks. (**c**) Female urogenital sinus and rectum at 12 weeks (reprinted with permission from Moore and Persaud [4]

close together to form the ejaculatory ducts in the prostatic urethra. In females, the distal ends of the mesonephric ducts degenerate.

Urethra

In both sexes, the majority of epithelium lining the urethra is derived from the urogenital sinus endoderm, while surrounding smooth muscle and connective tissues originate from splanchnic mesenchyme. The distal epithelium of the male urethra is derived from the glandular plate ectoderm that migrates from the glans penis to line the navicular fossa and join the spongy urethra. Near the end of the third month, the epithelium lining the prostatic urethra develops outgrowths that infiltrate the surrounding mesenchyme to form the prostate gland in males and urethral and paraurethral glands in females.

Anatomy of the Urinary Tract

Kidney

Structure

The kidneys function primarily to maintain fluid volume and composition and secondarily to regulate homeostatic functions such as acid–base balance and blood pressure. The kidneys are retroperitoneal organs positioned lateral to the vertebral column at the T12–L3 level in the supine position. The right kidney sits slightly lower due to its relationship with the liver above, while the left kidney sits closer to the midline, is somewhat narrower and generally 1 cm longer. Blood vessels, nerves, lymphatics, and the ureters enter and exit the bean-shaped organs through the concave hilum on the medial surface.

In the living tissue, the parenchyma of the kidney appears reddish brown and is divided into an outer cortex and inner medulla, the organization of which can be seen clearly in longitudinal section. The cortex contains a filtration apparatus that consists of an extensive vascular supply, collecting tubules and ducts, convoluted and straight tubules, and renal corpuscles. As the cortex arches over the medullary pyramids it sends intervening projections called renal columns into the medulla towards the renal sinus, a cavity within the kidney containing, nerves, vessels, calyces, and the renal pelvis. These renal columns are considered structures of the renal medulla. The inner medulla contains 6–12 pale conical-shaped medullary pyramids with the base of each pyramid oriented towards the cortex and an apex, or renal papilla oriented towards the renal sinus. Each renal papilla drains urine into a cup-like minor calyx, with 2–3 minor calyces combining to form a major calyx. Within the renal sinus the major calyces then converge to drain into the renal pelvis, the dilated proximal portion of the ureters.

Fascia and Relationships

Surrounding the kidneys are alternating layers of fascia and adipose tissue. The fascial layer in immediate contact with the kidney is the renal capsule—a histological component of the kidney itself. Encompassing the renal capsule is a mass of extraperitoneal fat referred to as perinephric fat (Fig. 1.4). Anterolateral to the kidney, two membranous layers split from the surrounding transversalis fascia and course medially enclosing the perinephric fat as renal (Gerota's) fascia. The anterior layer continues medially and fuses with the connective tissue of the inferior vena cava and aorta or may join with the anterior layer from the opposing side. The posterior layer also continues medially to fuse with fascia of the psoas major muscle. Inferiorly, both layers surround the ureter. Superiorly, these layers cover the adjacent adrenal gland with an intervening septum separating the gland from the kidney. The final layer, paranephric fat, is positioned along the posterolateral aspect of the kidney between the posterior layer of renal fascia and transversalis fascia.

Blood Vessels and Lymphatic Drainage

The kidneys receive blood from the left and right renal arteries that arise from the abdominal aorta just inferior to the superior mesenteric artery at the L1-L2 vertebral level (Fig. 1.5). Both arteries are positioned posterior to the renal veins as they project laterally towards the renal hilum. Due to the location of the abdominal aorta slightly left of midline, the right renal artery is longer than the left renal artery and passes posterior to the inferior vena cava. As the renal arteries approach the hilum they split into anterior and posterior branches that divide into multiple segmental arteries perfusing the parenchyma of the kidneys. Extrahilar or accessory arteries are common and usually branch off the abdominal aorta superior or inferior to the main renal artery trunk.

The renal veins leave the renal hilum to drain into the inferior vena cava at the L1 vertebral level. Due to the location of the inferior vena cava to the right of midline, the left renal vein is longer than the right renal vein and passes posterior to the superior mesenteric artery as it crosses the midline to join the inferior vena cava (Fig. 1.6).

Lymphatic vessels from the kidneys follow the renal veins to drain into the left and right lateral lumbar (caval or aortic) nodes near the origin of the renal arteries.

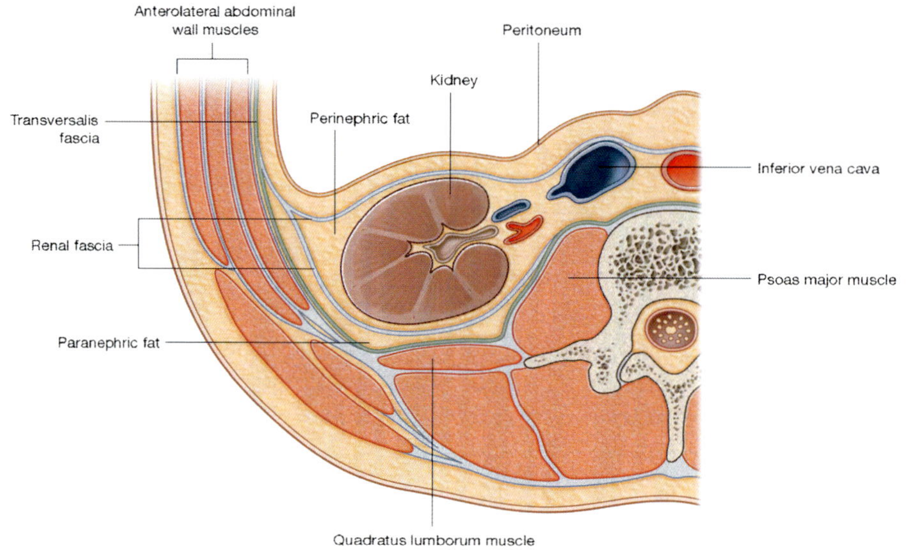

Fig. 1.4 Relationship of the surrounding fat and fascia to the kidney (reprinted with permission from Drake et al. [1, 2])

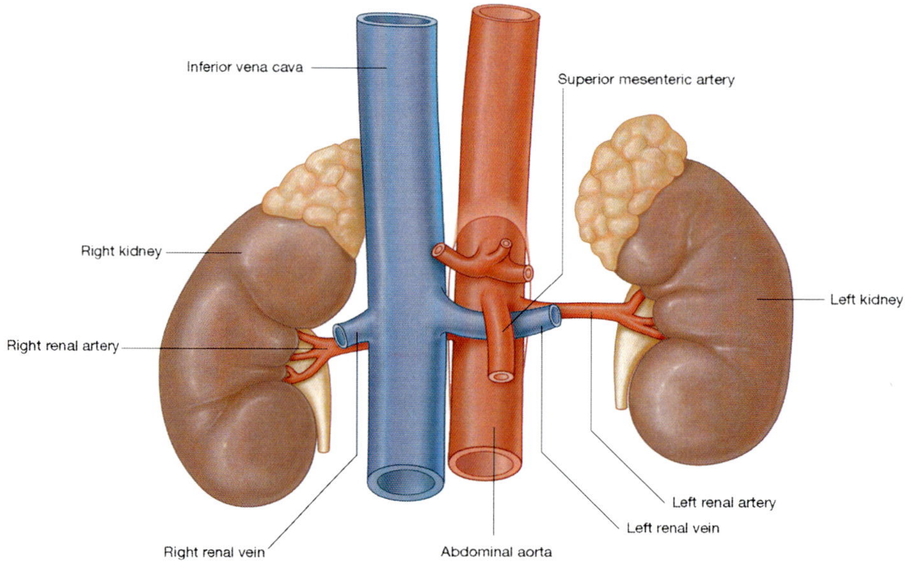

Fig. 1.5 Arterial and venous blood supply to the kidney (reprinted with permission from Drake et al. [1, 2])

Innervation

Innervation of the kidneys originates from sympathetic nerve fibers from T1-L1 spinal cord levels traveling in the renal plexus along the surface of the renal artery. This plexus receives postganglionic fibers from the celiac plexus and preganglionic fibers from the least splanchnic and first lumbar splanchnic nerves. Nerves from the renal plexus travel along the renal arteries to enter the hilum of the kidney for innervation of the tubules, glomeruli, and blood vessels. While parasympathetic fibers are present in this plexus, these fibers do not appear to play a role in kidney function.

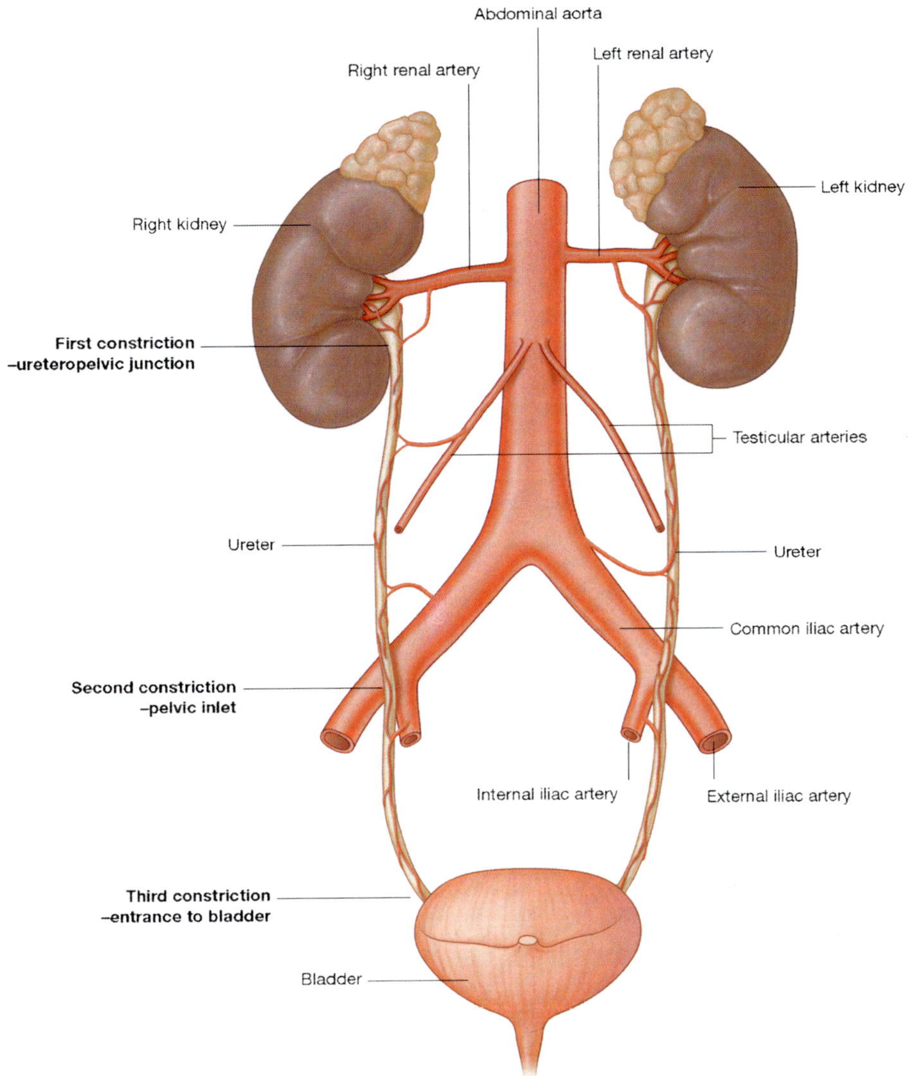

Fig. 1.6 Areas of constriction along the course of the ureter (reprinted with permission from Drake et al. [1, 2])

Ureters

Pathway and Relationships

The ureters are muscular ducts that transmit urine from the kidneys to the urinary bladder. In adults, the ureters are approximately 3–4 mm in diameter, 25–30 cm long and course retroperitoneally between the renal pelvis of the kidneys and base of the urinary bladder. As the renal pelvis projects inferiorly from the hilum of the kidneys, it narrows to connect with the ureters at the ureteropelvic junction (Fig. 1.6). This is the first of three constriction points along the path of the ureter where renal calculi or other debris may become lodged. Other areas where the ureters may be anatomically constricted include the pelvic inlet as the ureters pass anterior to either the distal common iliac artery or proximal external iliac artery and the ureterovesical junction as the ureters pass through the bladder wall.

Along their course towards the pelvic cavity the ureters are related to several different struc-

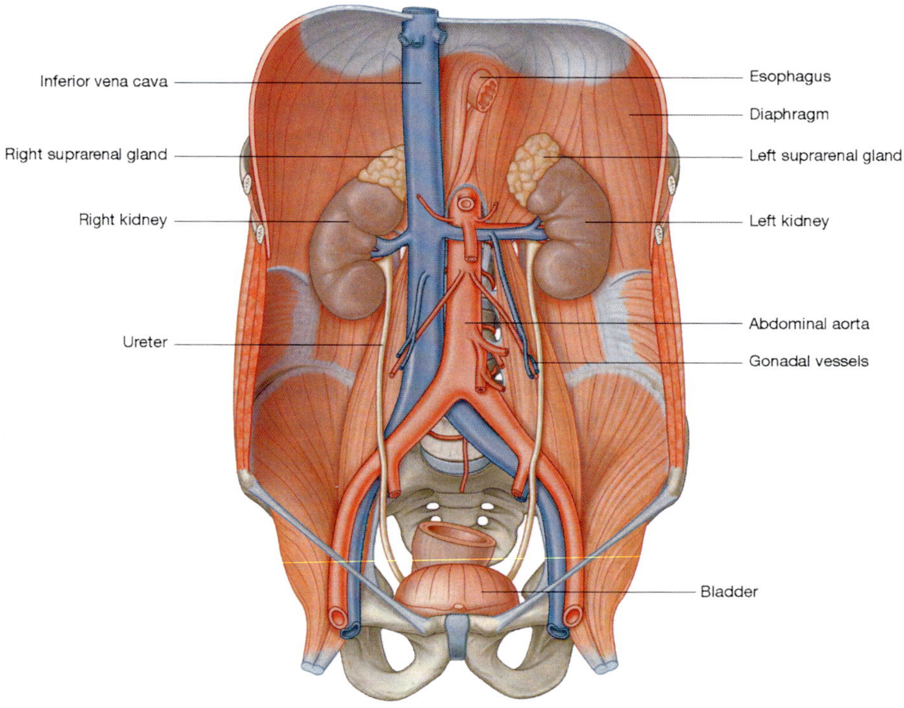

Fig. 1.7 Relationship of the ureters to posterior abdominal wall structures (reprinted with permission from Drake et al. [1, 2])

tures. At the ureteropelvic junction, the left ureter is lateral to the aorta whereas the right ureter is lateral to the inferior vena cava (Fig. 1.7). In the abdomen, both ureters pass anterior to the psoas major muscle, genitofemoral nerve, and are crossed obliquely on their anterior surface by the gonadal vessels. Continuing inferiorly, the left ureter is positioned lateral to the inferior mesenteric vein through much of its path and courses posterior to the jejunal and sigmoid portions of the small and large bowel. From its point of origin the right ureter is situated posterior to the descending duodenum and is crossed anteriorly by the right colic and ileocolic arteries inferiorly. Near its entrance into the pelvic cavity it is located posterior to the terminal portion of the ileum.

After passing through the pelvic inlet, the ureters are positioned along the posterior aspect of the lateral pelvic wall, anterior to the internal iliac artery and initial segment of the anterior trunk of the internal iliac. Upon reaching the ischial spine the ureters turn anteromedially to enter the outer wall of the bladder. Along their course in the pelvis, the ureters pass over the fascia of the obturator internus, levator ani muscles, and are located medial to the umbilical artery, inferior vesical artery, uterine artery (in the female), and obturator nerve, artery, and vein.

In addition to the previously mentioned relationships, the ureters are associated with different structures present in the male and female pelvic cavity. In females, once the ureters have crossed the pelvic brim they are located posterior to the ovaries and travel anteriorly and medially in the uterosacral folds (Fig. 1.8a). Near the base of the broad ligament they pass inferior to the uterine arteries and continue on to the base of the bladder. After crossing the pelvic brim in males, the ureters pass anteriorly and medially in the sacrogenital folds (Fig. 1.8b). As they travel towards the base of the urinary bladder they lie inferior to the ductus deferens and anterior to the seminal vesicles.

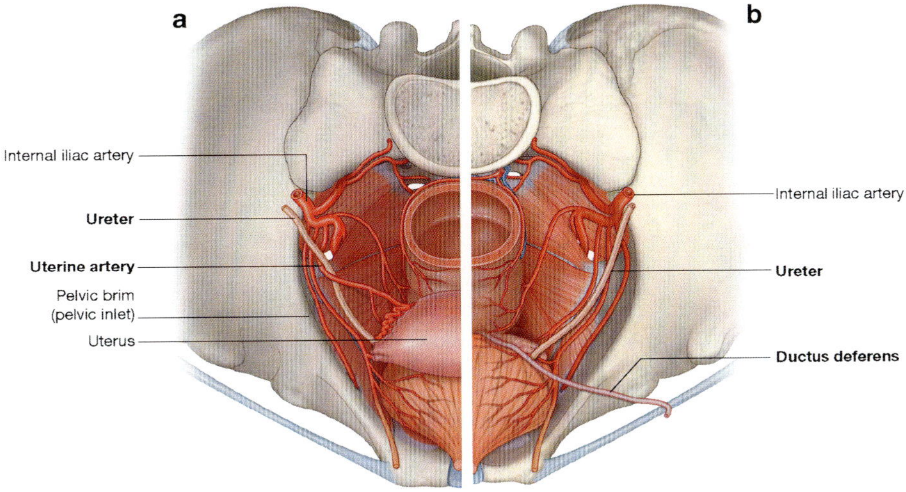

Fig. 1.8 Relationship of the ureters to the pelvic cavity. (**a**) In the female. (**b**) In the male. (reprinted with permission from Drake et al. [1, 2])

Blood Vessels and Lymphatics

Arterial branches perfusing the ureters arise directly from the aorta as well as the renal, gonadal, common iliac, internal iliac, vesical, and uterine arteries (Fig. 1.6). While the distribution of these anastomosing vessels to the ureters is variable, branches from the renal arteries and inferior vesical arteries appear to be the most consistent. Venous drainage from the ureters follows a pattern similar to the arterial supply.

Lymphatic fluid from superior regions of the ureters may follow lymphatic vessels from the kidneys or drain into lateral aortic nodes next to the lumbar vertebrae. Vessels from the mid-region of the ureters coalesce in common iliac nodes and inferior portions drain into nodes related to the common, external, and internal iliac vessels.

Innervation

Nerve fibers innervating the ureters arise from sympathetic fibers from T12 to L1 and parasympathetic fibers from S2 to S4 spinal cord levels. These fibers reach the superior, intermediate, and inferior regions of the ureter by passing through the renal, abdominal aortic, superior hypogastric, and inferior hypogastric plexuses. The functional role of these fibers is to modulate contractile events. Initiation of contraction is believed to occur through possible pacemaker sites in the minor calyces. Contraction initiated in the minor calyces is then propagated through the adjacent major calyces to maintain flow of urine away from the kidney parenchyma.

Pain associated with extreme distention or spasm of the ureter is primarily referred to cutaneous areas innervated by the T11-L2 spinal cord levels. Areas affected would most likely include the lateral and posterior abdominal wall, pubic region, scrotum, labia majora, and anterior aspect of the proximal thigh.

Bladder

Structure

The hollow urinary bladder is a reservoir for temporary storage of urine conveyed by the ureters from the kidneys. When empty, the bladder is located entirely in the pelvic cavity and takes on a pyramidal shape with a superior surface, two inferolateral surfaces, an apex, and a base. As it fills, the bladder extends anteriorly and superiorly into the abdominal cavity and has a dome-like appearance (Fig. 1.9). In children, the bladder is mostly in the abdominal cavity and continues descending to reach the pelvic cavity after puberty. The bladder wall has several layers

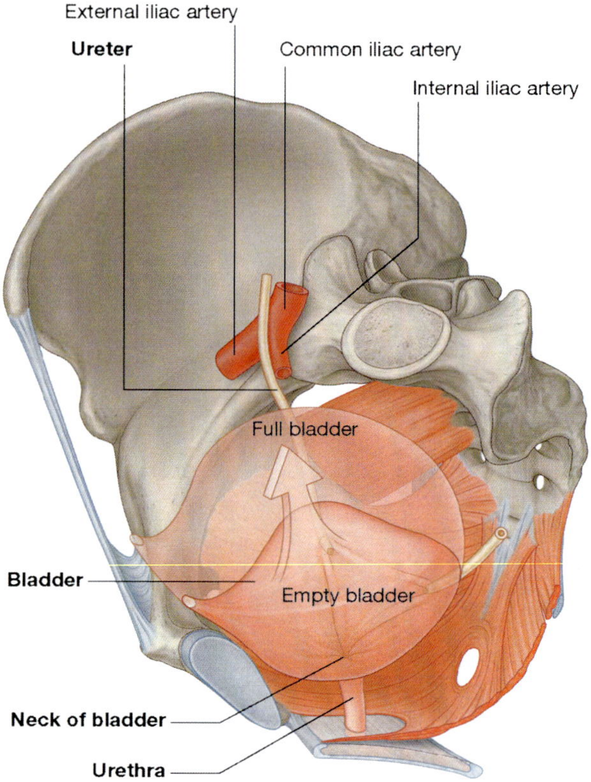

Fig. 1.9 Shape and orientation of the urinary bladder when full and empty (reprinted with permission from Drake et al. [1, 2])

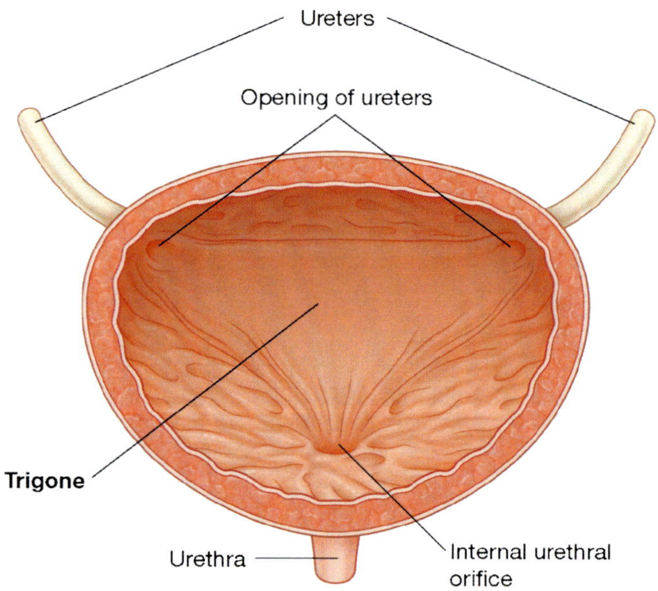

Fig. 1.10 Interior surface of the urinary bladder base showing the trigone (reprinted with permission from Drake et al. [1, 2])

of smooth muscle that allows it to distend for accommodation of urine and to contract for voiding when the bladder becomes full. Internally, along the base of the bladder is a smooth area known as the trigone. This is a triangular-shaped region that connects the openings of the two ureters superiorly and urethra inferiorly (Fig. 1.10).

Fascia, Relationships, and Ligaments

The entire superior surface of the bladder in males and majority of the superior surface in females is covered by peritoneum that is continuous with the median and medial umbilical folds on the anterior abdominal wall. This reflection of peritoneum creates the supravesical fossa. Posteriorly in the male, the peritoneum extends to the base of the bladder, forms the lining of the rectovesical pouch (Fig. 1.11a), and terminates laterally as the sacrogenital folds. In females, the peritoneum extends posteriorly without reaching the base of the bladder and reflects onto the body and isthmus of the uterus to form the lining of the vesico-uterine pouch (Fig. 1.11b). In both males and females, the inferolateral surface of the bladder is devoid of peritoneum and is separated from the pubis and puboprostatic ligament in males, or pubovesical ligament in females, by the retropubic space (of Retzius).

The bladder is bordered by several different structures in the male and female pelvic cavity. The anterior surface is in contact with the pubic symphysis, retropubic fat pad, and anterior abdominal wall. Laterally, it is related to the obturator internus superiorly and levator ani muscles inferiorly. The remaining surfaces of the bladder are associated with different structures depending on location in the male or female. In the male, the neck of the bladder is in contact with the superior aspect of the prostate gland. Posteriorly are the rectovesical pouch, ductus deferens, and seminal vesicles. The superior aspect is related to the peritoneal cavity, ileum, and sigmoid colon. In the female, the neck of the bladder rests on the urogenital diaphragm. Immediately posterior to the bladder is the vagina

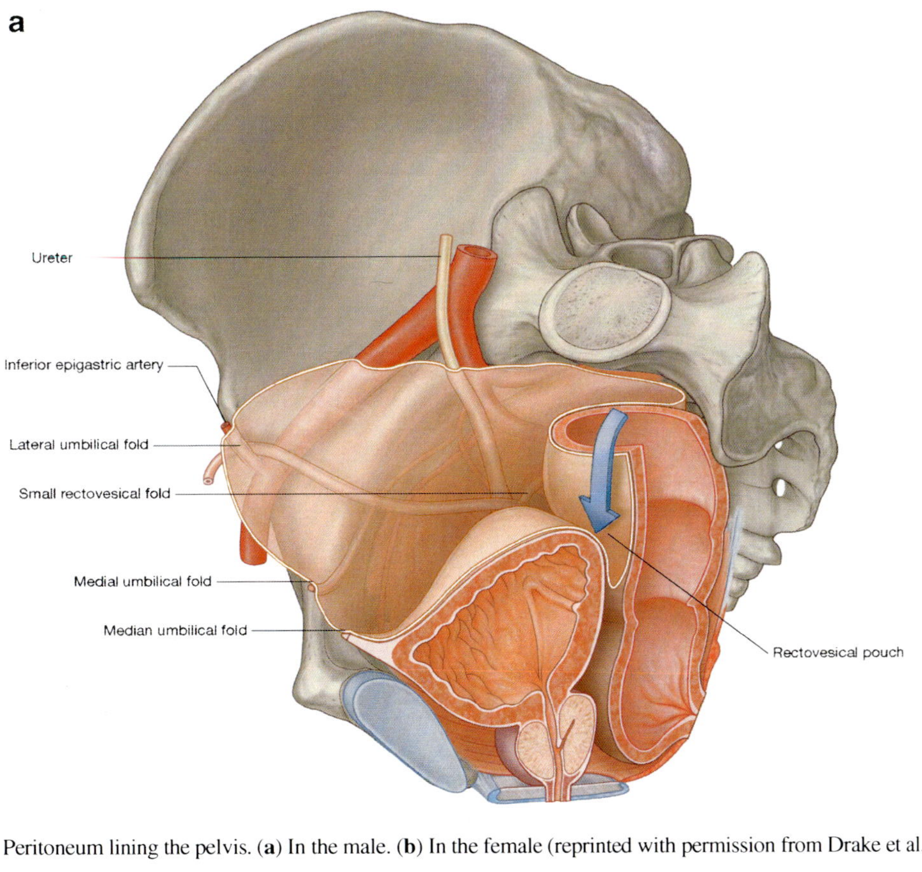

Fig. 1.11 Peritoneum lining the pelvis. (**a**) In the male. (**b**) In the female (reprinted with permission from Drake et al. [1, 2])

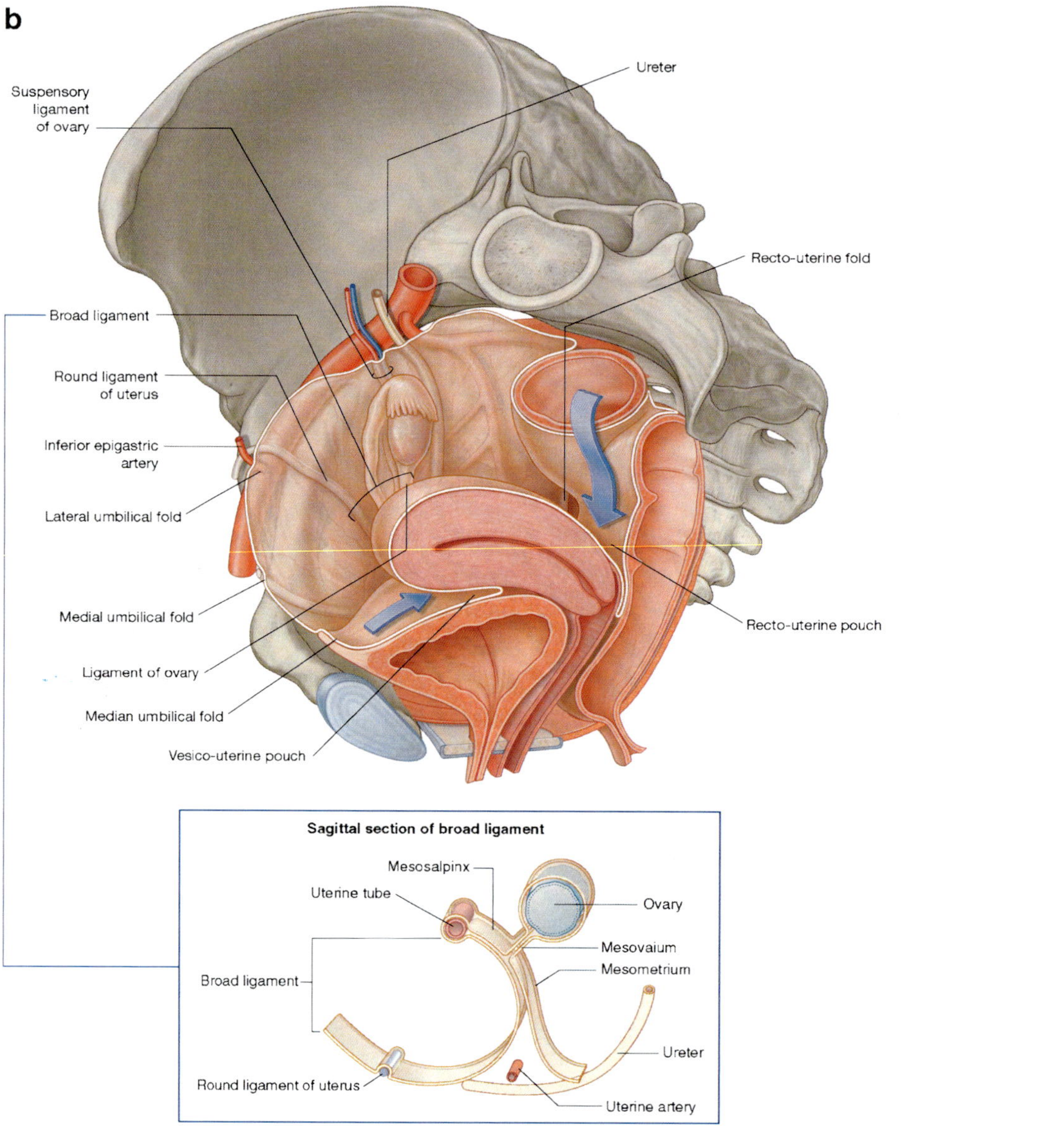

Fig. 1.11 (continued)

and lower portion of the uterus. The superior aspect is related to the peritoneal cavity, vesicouterine pouch, and body of the uterus.

Stabilization of bladder position is achieved by condensations of pelvic fascia and peritoneum that connect the bladder to the anterior abdominal wall, pubis, lateral pelvis, and rectum. Anteriorly, the obliterated urachus or median umbilical ligament connects the apex of the bladder to the umbilicus on the anterior abdominal wall. Rarely, extravasation of urine into the patent urachal remnant can result in urachal cyst or fistula. In the female pelvis, anterior extensions of the tendinous arch of pelvic fascia connect the bladder to the pubis as the pubovesical ligaments (Fig. 1.12a). Inferiorly the tendinous arch connects with the visceral fascia of the vagina as the paracolpium to assist the vagina in bearing the weight of the bladder. The male counterpart to the pubovesical ligament is the puboprostatic

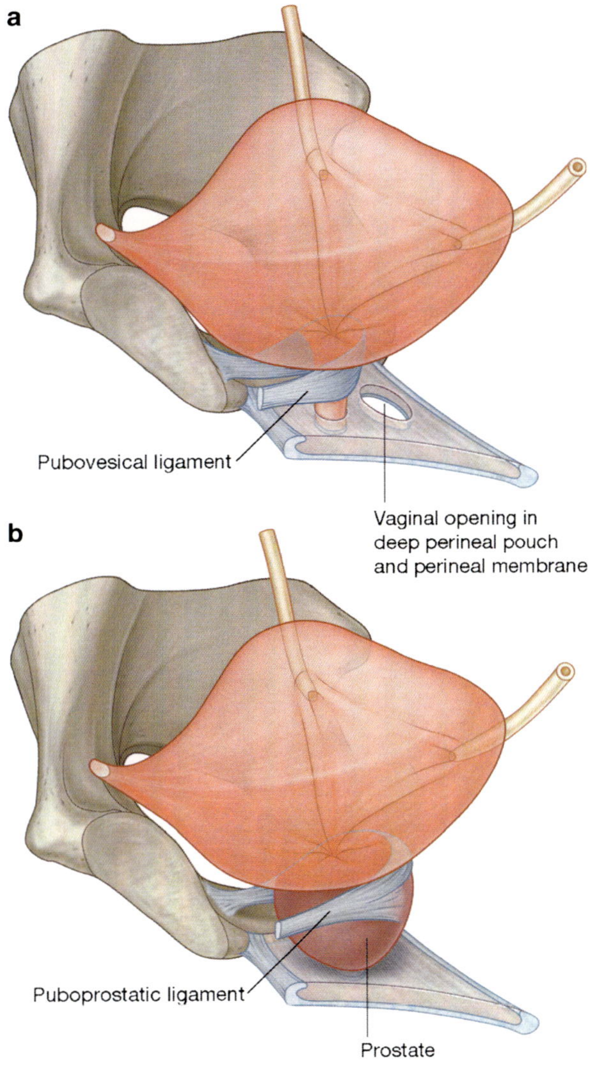

Fig. 1.12 Ligament surrounding the neck of the bladder and pelvic urethra in (**a**) the female and (**b**) the male (from Drake et al. [1, 2])

ligament that connects the prostate to the pubis (Fig. 1.12b). From the side wall of the pelvis, a condensation of pelvic fascia referred to as the hypogastric sheath sends a layer medially, which connects with the lateral aspect of the bladder as the lateral ligaments. These ligamentous structures convey the superior vesical arteries and veins. A second layer of the hypogastric sheath—the rectovesical septum—forms a partition between the posterior surface of the prostate and bladder and anterior surface of the rectum in males. In the female this layer is considerably thicker and is referred to as the cardinal or transverse cervical ligaments, passing medial to the cervix and vagina.

Blood Vessels and Lymphatics

The main blood supply to the bladder is through the superior and inferior vesical arteries. Both arteries are branches off the anterior trunk of the internal iliac (Fig. 1.13). After branching off the umbilical artery, the superior vesical artery turns medially and courses inferior to supply the fundus of the bladder and distal ureter. The inferior vesical artery is present in the male and distributes to the base of the bladder, distal ureter, pros-

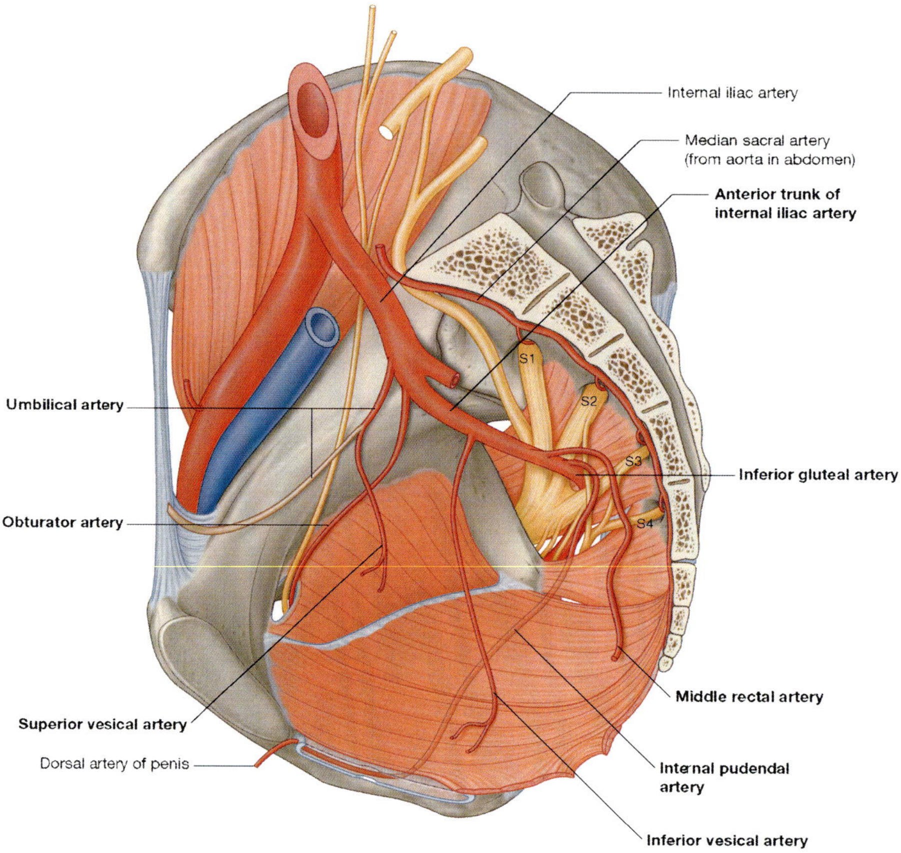

Fig. 1.13 Arterial branches from the anterior trunk of the internal iliac artery (from Drake et al. [1, 2])

tate, and seminal vesicles. In the female, the vaginal artery is equivalent to the inferior vesical artery and supplies the vagina as well as neighboring portions of the bladder and rectum.

Venous drainage from the bladder follows a network of vessels referred to as the vesical venous plexus near the neck of the bladder. These vessels then travel posteriorly through the lateral ligaments of the bladder to reach the internal iliac veins. Lymphatic drainage from the bladder coalesces in nodes related to the common, internal, and external iliac arteries; however, the external iliac receives the vast majority of lymphatic drainage.

Innervation

Visceral efferent nerve fibers to the bladder arise from the pelvic plexus, a collection of autonomic nervous system fibers and ganglia along the lateral aspect of the bladder, rectum, and internal genitalia. Parasympathetic nerves in this plexus arise from spinal cord levels S2-S4 as the pelvic splanchnics and inferior hypogastric plexus. These fibers supply motor innervation to the detrusor muscle of the bladder wall for urine voidance. Sympathetic fibers arise from the spinal cord levels T10-L2 as well as the hypogastric plexuses and nerves. These fibers facilitate contraction of the internal urethral sphincter to discontinue urine voidance. Afferent information regarding pain and distention from the inferior aspect of the bladder travels with parasympathetic nerves. Because the superior surface of the bladder is covered by peritoneum, it is above the pelvic pain line so afferent fibers from this region travel with sympathetic fibers to T11-L3 spinal ganglia.

Urethra

The urethra extends from the internal urethral orifice of the bladder to the external urethra

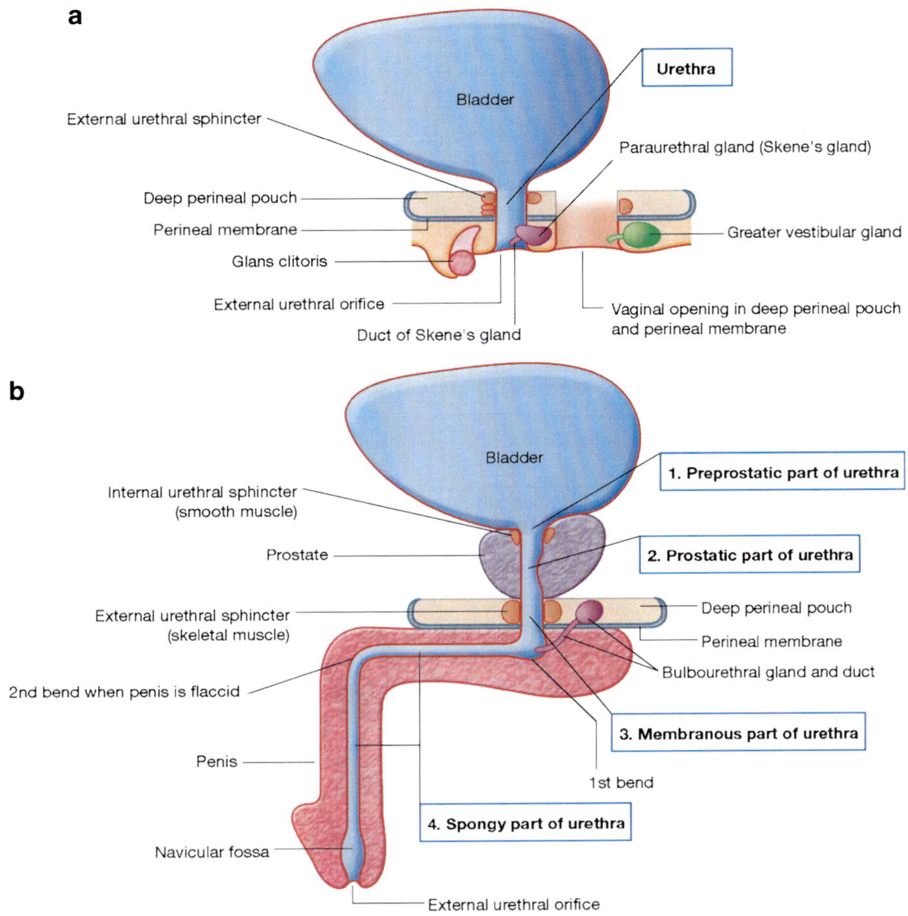

Fig. 1.14 (**a**) The female urethra. (**b**) Divisions of the male urethra (from Drake et al. [1, 2])

orifice in the perineum. The pathways of the female and male urethra are vastly different and will be described separately. In females, the urethra is generally 4 cm long and is located posterior to the pubic symphysis and anterior to the vaginal wall (Fig. 1.14a). As the urethra courses anteriorly and inferiorly, it passes through the deep perineal pouch where it is surrounded by the external urethral sphincter. Inferiorly, the urethra passes through the perineal membrane to end in the vestibule as the external urethral orifice, immediately posterior to the vaginal orifice. Multiple mucous glands are located along the length of the urethra. Near the distal portion of the urethra a collection of these glands group together as the paraurethral or Skene's glands and drain into the paraurethral duct to reach the lateral wall of the external urethral orifice.

The male urethra is approximately 20 cm in length and is divided into a bulbar and pendulous component based on its location within and distal to the perineum (Fig. 1.14b). Along its course it is further subdivided into a preprostatic, prostatic, membranous, and spongy division. Extending from the internal urethral orifice of the bladder to the prostate is the preprostatic portion. Coursing through the prostate gland is the prostatic urethra, which has a longitudinal fold of mucosa along its inner posterior wall referred to as the urethral crest. Along the urethral crest is a prominent crescent-shaped bulge identified as the seminal colliculus, a landmark used in surgery for localizing the internal urethral sphincter superiorly. On the surface of the seminal colliculus are openings for the prostatic utricle and ejaculatory ducts for passage of seminal fluid. Lateral to the colliculus on either side are the prostatic sinuses with several small openings for the prostatic ducts. The 2-cm segment inferior to the prostatic urethra is the membranous urethra, which passes through the deep perineal pouch to reach the bulb of the penis as the spongy urethra. Surrounding the epithelial lining of the membranous urethra inferiorly is a striated muscle layer that forms the external urethral sphincter. Embedded in this muscular structure in the deep perineal pouch are the bulbourethral glands that secrete into the spongy urethra during sexual arousal. The longest and most distal section of the urethra is referred to as the spongy urethra that travels through the corpus spongiosum to reach the glans of the penis. Within the glans, the spongy urethra enlarges as the navicular fossa prior to its termination has the external urethral orifice at the distal end of the glans. Along its course the spongy urethra makes two turns, the first is within the bulb of the penis as the urethra turns anteriorly and the second is at the transition point between the bulb and the pendulous portion as the urethra turns inferiorly in the flaccid penis.

Blood Supply and Lymphatics

The internal pudendal artery, a branch from the anterior trunk of the internal iliac, supplies the majority of blood to the urethra. In the female, the urethra also receives contributions from the vaginal artery. In the male, the dorsal artery of the penis as well as the abundant vascular network of the corpus spongiosum perfuses the urethra.

Venous drainage is via a large venous plexus within the pelvic cavity that coalesces into the internal and finally common iliac vessels. Lymphatic drainage from the urethra passes primarily to the internal and external iliac nodes. In the male, lymphatics from the mid urethra and distal urethra can drain into the deep and superficial inguinal nodes.

Innervation

The urethra is innervated by parasympathetic fibers from the pelvic splanchnics (S2-S4) and sympathetic fibers from the lumbar splanchnics (L1-L2). These nerve fibers travel in the vesical plexus in females or prostatic plexus in males for contraction of the urethral walls and relaxation of the internal urethral sphincter. Skeletal muscle structures surrounding the urethra, such as the external urethral sphincter, are innervated by the branches of the pudendal nerve (S2-S4). Afferent fibers from the urethra travel back to the spinal cord with the parasympathetic fibers of the pelvic splanchnic nerves.

Histology of the Urinary Tract

Urothelium

The hallmark of the urinary tract—including the renal pelvis, ureter, bladder, and urethra—is the presence of distinctive urothelium (formerly "transitional epithelium") that lines these structures. The urothelium functions to maintain an impermeable barrier to urine, while still allowing expansion and contraction of the urinary tract lining. Urothelial cells contain thickened cell membranes, with surface plaques and plasmalemma infoldings. This surface modification allows for additional plasma membrane to be inserted or removed, thus allowing marked changes in the surface area during cycles of expansion or contraction. There are also numerous junctional complexes between urothelial cells, allowing the passage and storage of toxic and concentrated urine without damage to the underlying tissues.

The urothelium generally consists of 3–7 layers of urothelial cells capped by a layer of umbrella cells (Fig. 1.15a). Under normal circumstances, benign urothelium demonstrates nuclear orientation towards the luminal surface, longitudinal nuclear grooves, and a relatively uniform appearance. Variation in urothelial thickness can occur and often the result of the expanded/contracted state of the lining during specimen fixation. However, certain pathological conditions may also result in a thickened appearance to the urothelium, termed "hyperplasia." Although the urothelial cells maintain relative uniformity, umbrella cells have a notorious reputation for displaying marked atypia under normal conditions, which may periodically lead to confusion with neoplastic conditions. At all sites, the urothelium is sepa-

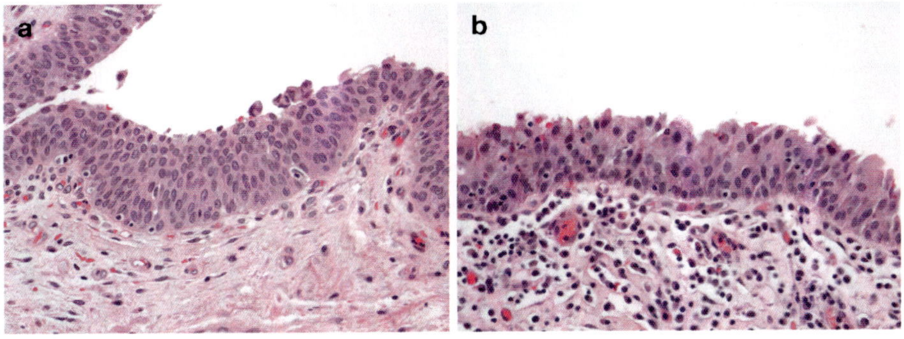

Fig. 1.15 (**a**) Normal urothelium is approximately 4–7cell layers thick and demonstrates open chromatin with occasional nuclear grooves. (**b**) Reactive urothelium is often associated with inflammation and may show disorganization and pinpoint nucleoli

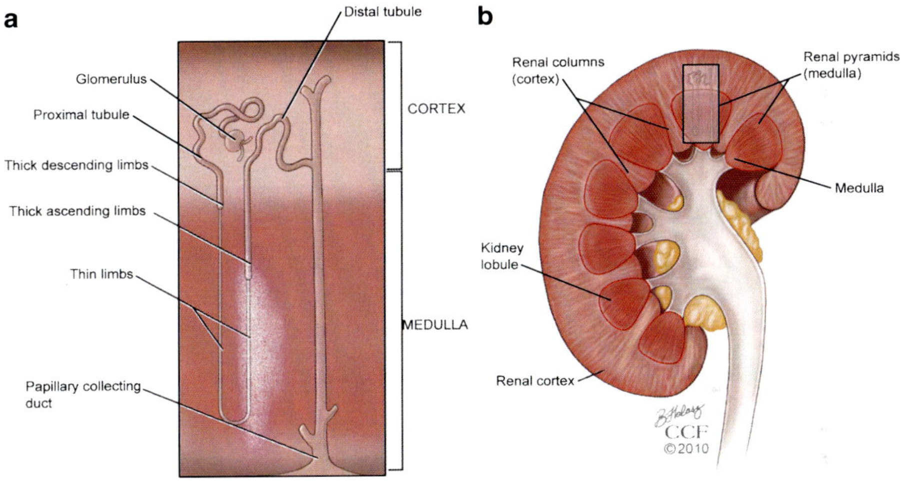

Fig. 1.16 Kidney structure. *Inset* shows cortical and medullary segments of the kidney nephron. © CCF 2010

rated from underlying structures by the presence of a thin basement membrane.

Under reactive conditions, the urothelium may acquire "atypical" features, including nuclear enlargement, variation in nuclear orientation, and small nucleoli (Fig. 1.15b). However, reactive urothelium maintains the open chromatin and smooth nuclear contours that define benign urothelial cells, thus aiding in the correct diagnosis. The presence of acute and chronic inflammatory cells within the urothelium is also a helpful indicator of a reactive process, although it is not exclusive to benign conditions.

As the kidney is responsible for urine formation and may represent the source of a subset of urothelial carcinomas within the urinary tract, a brief discussion of kidney histology is presented, followed by a histological overview of the ureter, bladder, and urethra.

Kidney

Organization

Each kidney is divided into an outer cortex and an inner medulla (Fig. 1.16). The medulla consists of 10–18 cone-shaped structures termed pyramids. Each pyramid contains a cap of cortical tissue and is collectively termed a kidney lobe. The functional unit of the kidney is the nephron, with approximately one million nephrons housed within each kidney. The nephron consists of a

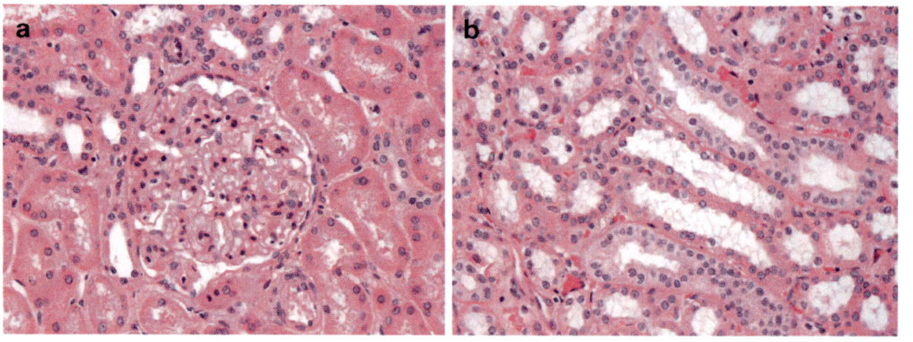

Fig. 1.17 Normal kidney histology can be readily distinguished. (**a**) The cortex contains glomeruli and an abundance of proximal tubules. (**b**) The medulla consists primarily of distal tubules and collecting ducts

dilated portion—the glomerulus or "renal corpuscle"—connected to a long, elaborate renal tubule containing distinct regions, each of which has a different function and histological appearance. The nephron arises in the cortex, loops down into the medulla, returns to the cortex, and then drains into collecting ducts that descend again into the medulla. Collecting ducts converge into large papillary ducts that empty urine into the minor renal calyces through small holes on the surface of the tips of the papillae.

The Glomerulus

The glomerulus consists of a tuft of capillaries that is surrounded by Bowman's capsule (Fig. 1.17a). The ultrafiltrate of blood—containing mainly water and salts—is formed here and collected within the surrounding space. The glomerulus consists of a number of distinct components, including the capillaries, podocytes, and mesangial cells. The glomerular capillaries are lined by a simple layer of fenestrated endothelium. The fenestrae at this site have a larger (50–100 nm) diameter than that found in fenestrated endothelium elsewhere in the body, which allows for increased permeability of the capillary wall. Podocytes rest on top of the glomerular capillaries and contain spider-like processes that interdigitate with one another, resulting in some of the most complex epithelial–epithelial interactions in the body. Mesangial cells are modified pericytes that are situated between the capillary tufts of the glomerulus. They have properties distinct from pericytes elsewhere in the body: they can contract and relax, thus modifying glomerular filtration; they respond to local injury by proliferating; and they aid in the production and breakdown of the basement membrane lying between the capillary endothelial cells and the podocytes.

Substances filtered from the blood in the glomerulus must pass through three morphological structures: (1) the fenestrated endothelium, (2) the glomerular basement membrane, and (3) the filtration slits between the pedicels of the podocytes. The glomerular basement membrane is synthesized by both the podocytes and the capillary endothelial cells and measures 320–340 nm in thickness. Three layers constitute the basement membrane: a central, electron dense layer (lamina densa) and two less dense layers (lamina rara) on either side. The membrane acts as a selective size and charge barrier.

Renal Tubules and Collecting Ducts

The ultrafiltrate formed at the level of the glomerulus drains from Bowman's capsule into a series of tubules: (1) the proximal convoluted tubule, (2) the loop of Henle, (3) the distal convoluted tubule, and (4) the collecting ducts (Fig. 1.17b).

The *proximal tubule* is the longest tubule in the cortex and is the tubule most frequently seen in a section of the cortex. It has a wide lumen, lined by eosinophilic, cuboidal epithelium with abundant apical microvilli that serve to increase the absorptive surface area of these cells. In this section of the tubule, 80% of water and salts are reabsorbed and all glucose is reabsorbed. Amino acids and small proteins that may have leaked through are also reabsorbed. Certain organic acids and bases are secreted into the tubule here as well. To provide the energy for their salt-pumping functions, proximal tubule cells have abundant mitochondria, which result in the striking eosinophilic appearance of these cells. Proteins of molecular mass less than 60 kD that may have leaked through the filtration barrier are removed by endocytosis and subsequent lysosomal digestion within the proximal tubule cells.

The *loop of Henle* is the U-shaped structure of the nephron and consists of the thick descending limb, the thin descending and ascending limbs, and the thick ascending limb. The thick descending limb is similar in structure to the proximal tubule, while the thick ascending is similar in structure to the distal tubule. The thick ascending limb is one of the most important loop structures that maintain the salt gradient in the medulla; it performs this function by actively pumping NaCl out of the tubule and into the medullary interstitium. The cells in the wall of the ascending thick limb are impermeable to water, so the contents become hypotonic as salt is pumped out of the tubule. As in the proximal tubule cells, mitochondria in the thick ascending limb cells are abundant to supply energy for ion pumping.

As the thick ascending limb returns to the cortex, it makes contact with the vascular pole of the "parent" renal corpuscle from which the tubules originated, to form the *macula densa*. Macula densa cells sense the ionic content and water volume of the tubular fluid and influence the glomerular filtration rate as well as blood pressure via stimulating renin secretion and nitric oxide synthesis.

The *distal convoluted tubule* is the convoluted continuation of the thick ascending limb of the loop of Henle after it enters the cortex. It is lined by cuboidal epithelium, similar in appearance to that of the thick ascending limb. The cells of the distal convoluted tubule are responsive to aldosterone, resulting in ion exchange; Na^+ is absorbed and K^+ is excreted. This section of the nephron helps to maintain the acid–base balance of blood by secreting hydrogen and ammonium ions into the urine.

Finally, the *collecting tubules* are continuous with the distal convoluted tubules and empty into cortical collecting ducts. The cells of the cortical collecting tubules and ducts are columnar and pale staining, with no brush borders and sparse mitochondria (Fig. 1.17b). When a number of them course together, they appear as pale medullary rays. The larger papillary collecting ducts course through the medulla and empty the formed urine into the minor and then major calyces. Ultimately, the urine passes through the renal pelvis and into the ureter.

Renal Pelvis

The renal pelvis represents the outflow tract from the kidney and transitions to the ureter at the ureteropelvic junction, which demonstrates no defined distinction at the histological level. The renal pelvis consists of several layers that range in order from superficial to deep of urothelium, subepithelial connective tissue, muscularis, peripelvic fat, and ultimately renal parenchyma (Fig. 1.18). Although staging of urothelial carcinomas at this location is performed relative to these histological structures, the distinction of these layers is not always clearly apparent, with discontinuous or absent muscularis in sections taken from various locations.

Ureter

The ureter allows the passage of urine from the kidney to bladder via peristaltic action of the surrounding muscle. The ureter itself consists of several layers that include the urothelium, subepithelial connective tissue, muscularis, periureteral fat, and either adventitia or serosa, depending upon the location of ureter (Fig. 1.19a, b). The muscularis is arranged into inner longitudinal and outer cir-

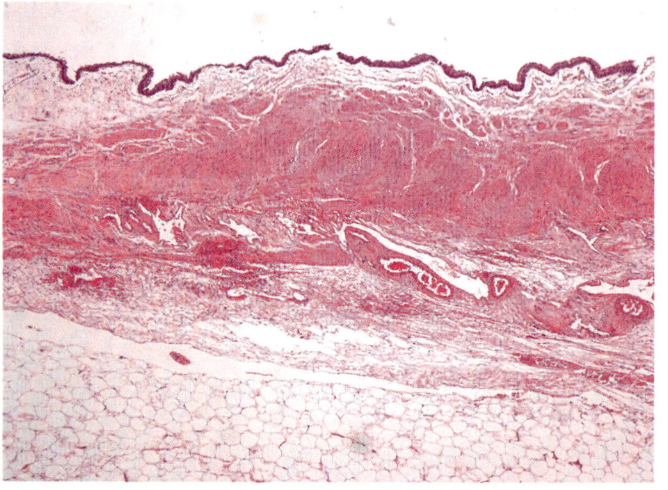

Fig. 1.18 Low magnification of the renal pelvis shows several layers, including the urothelium, subepithelial connective tissue, muscularis, and renal pelvic fat

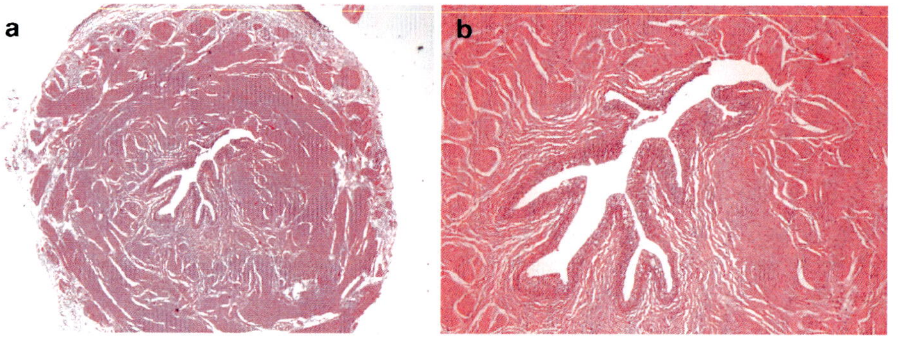

Fig. 1.19 (**a**) Low magnification cross section through the ureter demonstrating the ureteral lumen surrounded by urothelium and ureteral wall. (**b**) The transition between the subepithelial connective tissue and muscularis is often irregular and relatively abrupt

cular layers that can be readily distinguished by light microscopy; a third, outermost longitudinal layer is present at the distal end of the ureter. Under normal conditions, the ureter demonstrates a star-shaped lumen due to the surrounding musculature, but has the capacity to expand to permit the passage of urine.

Bladder

The bladder is the main site for urine storage and consists of an expansile structure whose shape is mediated by the surrounding bladder muscle. At the histological level, the bladder consists of the urothelium, lamina propria, muscularis propria (detrusor muscle), perivesical fat, and either a serosa at the superior surface or adventitia at other locations (Fig. 1.20). The urothelium is often thrown up into folds in the contracted state, but may appear flattened and thinned when the bladder expands. The lamina propria is relatively similar to the subepithelial connective tissue of the urinary tract at other sites and consists of connective tissue, blood vessels, lymphatics, nerve fibers, fat, and thin, wispy muscle fibers called muscularis mucosae. The muscularis mucosae represent small smooth muscle fibers that are often discontinuous and frequently arranged in a haphazard pattern (Fig. 1.21a). Occasionally, the muscularis mucosae may appear hyperplastic or thickened, resulting in diagnostic challenges when attempting to distinguish these structures from the muscularis propria (Fig. 1.21b).

Beneath the lamina propria lies the muscularis propria—or detrusor muscle. This smooth muscle layer provides overall structure to the bladder and consists of three large indistinguishable layers of muscle. Also present within this layer of the bladder wall are blood vessels, lymphatics, nerve fibers, and fat cells. Due to the slightly irregular boundaries of the muscularis propria, the transition to the perivesical fat is often poorly defined, with low magnification assessment often required to distinguish carcinomas invading beyond this plane. In males, the muscularis propria merges with the prostatic fibromuscular tissue. Finally, the outermost layer of the bladder wall consists of either a serosa or adventitia, depending upon the location as described previously.

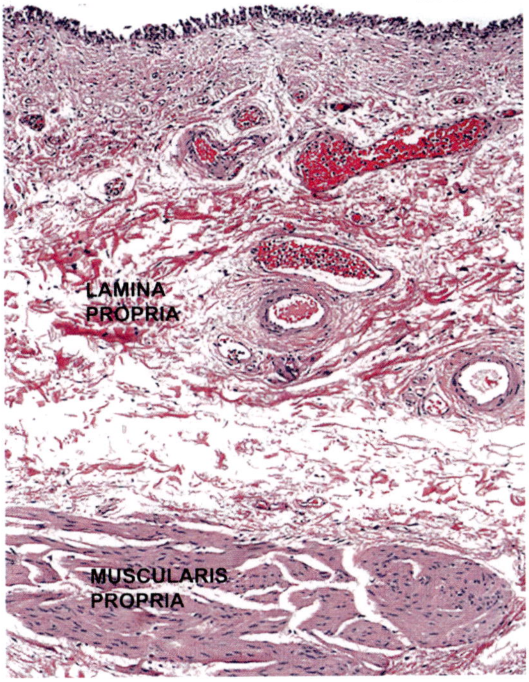

Fig. 1.20 Section of urinary bladder wall, showing surface urothelium with underlying lamina propria and muscularis propria (detrusor muscle)

The urethra emerges from the lower end of the bladder with the surrounding layers of smooth muscle forming the internal urethral sphincter.

Urethra

The urethra represents the final structure in the excretion of urine. In the male, the urethra is long (approximately 20 cm) and has a dual function, allowing passage of urine and also allowing passage of semen during ejaculation. The male urethra contains three segments that include the prostatic, membranous, and spongy urethra. The prostatic portion is lined by urothelium, extends through the prostate gland and receives as many as twenty small prostatic ducts (Fig. 1.22). The membranous portion extends from the prostate apex to the bulb of the penis corpus cavernosus, and the spongy portion extends through the bulb, body, and glans of the

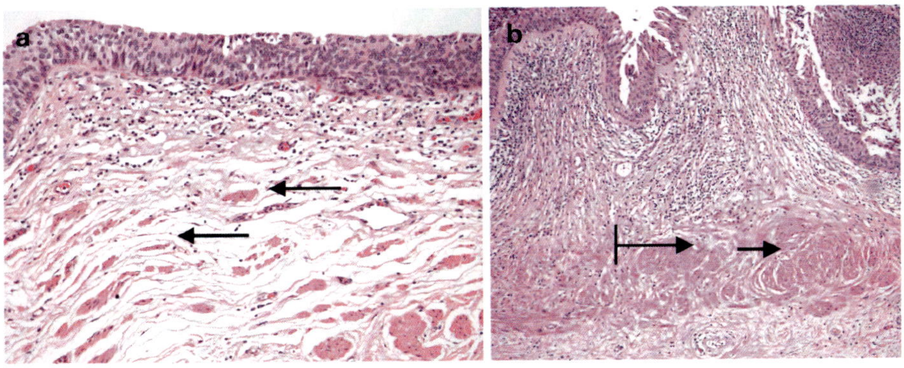

Fig. 1.21 Muscularis mucosae of the lamina propria may have a variable appearance, including (**a**) thin, wispy, discontinuous muscle bundles (*arrow*); (**b**) larger, hypertrophic muscle bundles (*arrow*)

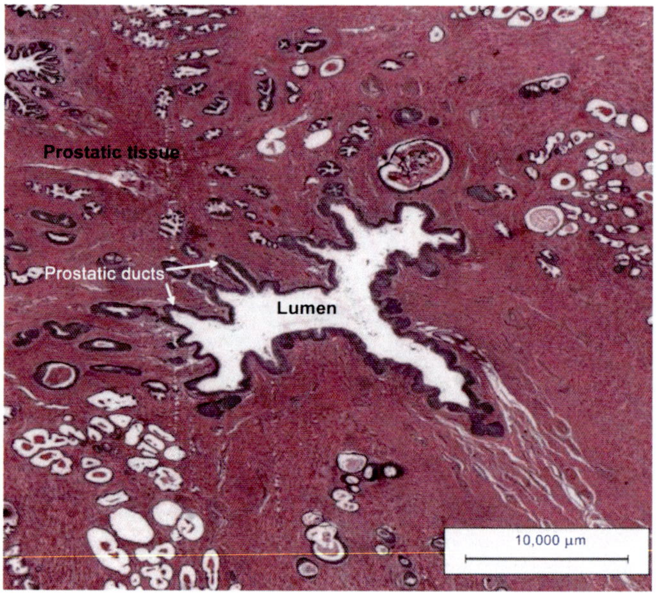

Fig. 1.22 The prostatic urethra with numerous prostatic glands (*arrows*) opening into the urethral lumen

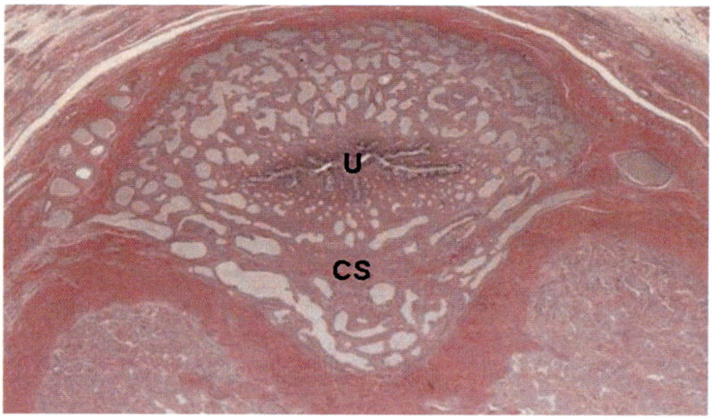

Fig. 1.23 The distal section of the male urethra (*U*; spongy section) courses through the corpus spongiosa of the penis (*CS*)

penis and is surrounded by the corpus spongiosum (Fig. 1.23). The length of the urethra is primarily lined by urothelium, although squamous epithelium may be prevalent at the distal end of the urethra. Mucus-secreting glands of Littre empty into the male urethra, mainly in the spongy portion.

The female urethra is short (3–5 cm long), with most of its crescent-shaped lumen lined by stratified squamous epithelium (Fig. 1.24). The subepithelial connective tissue is vascular and is surrounded by two layers of muscle: a thick inner circular smooth muscle and an outer longitudinally arranged layer.

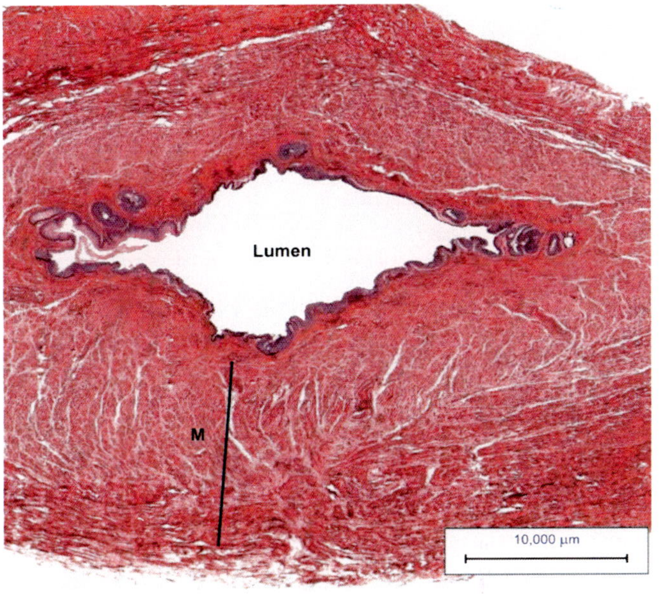

Fig. 1.24 Wall of the female urethra that includes the urothelium, subepithelial connective tissue, and extensive muscularis (*M*)

References

1. Drake RL, Vogl AW, Mitchell AWM. Abdomen. In: Drake RL, Vogl AW, Mitchell AWM, editors. Gray's anatomy for students. 2nd ed. Philadelphia, PA: Churchill Livingstone; 2010. p. 249–403.
2. Drake RL, Vogl AW, Mitchell AWM. Pelvis. In: Drake RL, Vogl AW, Mitchell AWM, editors. Gray's anatomy for students. 2nd ed. Philadelphia, PA: Churchill Livingstone; 2010. p. 406–509.
3. Koeppen BM, Stanton BA. Structure and function of the kidneys. In: Koeppen BM, Stanton BA, editors. Renal physiology. 4th ed. Philadelphia, PA: Mosby; 2007. p. 19–30.
4. Moore KL, Persaud TVN. The urogenital system. In: Moore KL, Persaud TVN, editors. The developing human clinically oriented embryology. 8th ed. Philadelphia, PA: Saunders; 2008. p. 243–84.
5. Sadler TW. Urogenital systems. In: Sadler TW, editor. Langman's medical embryology. 11th ed. Baltimore, MD: Lippincott Williams & Wilkins; 2010. p. 235–64.
6. Standring S. Bladder, prostate and urethra. In: Standring S, editor. Gray's anatomy the anatomical basis of clinical practice. 40th ed. Spain: Churchill Livingstone; 2008. p. 1245–60.
7. Standring S. Kidney and ureter. In: Standring S, editor. Gray's anatomy the anatomical basis of clinical practice. 40th ed. Spain: Churchill Livingstone; 2008. p. 1225–44.
8. Paner GP, Ro JY, Wojcik EM, Venkataraman G, Datta MW, Amin MB. Further characterization of the muscle layers and lamina propria of the urinary bladder by systematic histologic mapping: implications for pathologic staging of invasive urothelial carcinoma. Am J Surg Pathol. 2007;31(9):1420–9.

Part II

Non-neoplastic Diseases of the Bladder

Benign Polypoid and Papillary Lesions

2

Rafael E. Jimenez and Jeff Holzbeierlein

Introduction

Currently cystoscopic evaluation of the bladder is performed for indications such as hematuria, either gross or microscopic, irritative voiding symptoms, and abnormalities found on computed tomograph (CT) scan. Depending on the clinical scenario, urologists, and pathologists may be confronted with a series of lesions that are not clearly recognizable as malignant tumors. Many of these lesions, which grow in a polypoid or papillary pattern, are identified cystoscopically, but after pathologic evaluation are determined to be benign entities unrelated to urothelial neoplasia. The importance of the accurate recognition of these lesions is twofold: First, they may explain the clinical symptomatology of the patient, and second, they must be properly diagnosed so that they are not confused with a urothelial neoplasm leading to unnecessary therapy. These lesions frequently range from small, incidental, and clinically irrelevant lesions to cystoscopically evident or symptomatic processes. Close communication between urologists and pathologists may help facilitate the distinction between these scenarios.

The most common benign conditions that are cystoscopically described as polypoid or papillary are florid von Brunn nests proliferations, cystitis cystica et glandularis, polypoid/papillary cystitis, and nephrogenic adenoma. Other less common conditions include the prostatic-type and the fibroepithelial polyp and mulleraniosis of the bladder. These entities will be discussed individually, but common features, such as their clinical presentation and surgical management, will be discussed jointly.

Like many malignant tumors of the bladder, most benign polypoid or papillary lesions of the bladder present with either irritative voiding symptoms or hematuria (either gross or microscopic). Irritative voiding symptoms commonly include frequency of urination, urgency, nocturia, and occasionally painful urination. Hematuria may or may not be present and may be either microscopic or gross hematuria. In patients with these symptoms, a careful history and physical examination should be performed including a prostate examination. For those with microscopic hematuria (>5 red blood cells per high powered field) or gross hematuria an in-office flexible cystoscopy is mandatory. For those with mainly irritative symptoms who fail to respond to medical therapy, such as antibiotics and anticholinergics, further evaluation with cystoscopy is recommended. Depending on the clinical scenario, a cup biopsy in the office or a formal biopsy of the

R.E. Jimenez (✉)
Department of Laboratory Medicine and Pathology, Mayo Clinic, 200 First Street SW, Rochester, MN 55902, USA
e-mail: Jimenez.Rafael@mayo.edu

J. Holzbeierlein
Department of Urology, University of Kansas Hospital, 3901 Rainbow Boulevard., mail stop 3016, Kansas City, KS 66160, USA
e-mail: jholzbeierlein@kumc.edu

D.E. Hansel et al. (eds.), *The Urinary Tract: A Comprehensive Guide to Patient Diagnosis and Management*, DOI 10.1007/978-1-4614-5320-8_2, © Springer Science+Business Media New York 2012

lesion under anesthesia should be performed if the clinical suspicion for a urothelial neoplasm is sufficiently high. All biopsies must then be examined by a pathologist for diagnosis. It is also critical that the urologist communicate the clinical scenario with the pathologist, as the pathologic diagnosis can occasionally be challenging and clinical information may help in diagnosis.

Von Brunn Nests and Cystitis Cystica et Glandularis

von Brunn nests are islands of normal-appearing urothelial cells that are embedded in the lamina propria, beneath the basement membrane of the surface urothelium. They arise due to invagination of the urothelium into the lamina propria and may be detached from the overlying mucosa. von Brunn nests are usually asymptomatic and are considered a normal anatomical variant. However, in some patients, von Brunn nests may become quite prominent such that they are cystoscopically evident and clinically symptomatic [1, 2]. In addition, they may also be associated with previous treatment of lesions that have required resection or intravesical therapy.

Cystitis glandularis represents a process of glandular metaplasia of the urothelium. This metaplasia may consist of the development of a central lumen within von Brunn nests, surrounded by a layer of columnar-type epithelium and variable degrees of residual urothelium, or the more evident development of intestinal metaplasia with presence of goblet cells and other cellular elements of the intestinal mucosa. The first scenario is usually referred to as cystitis glandularis typical type, while the second one is commonly known as cystitis glandularis intestinal type [3, 4]. The cystic dilatation of von Brunn nests with cystitis glandularis is usually referred to as cystitis cystica. Both processes may coexist.

Pathogenesis

As stated, von Brunn nests are a normal histologic finding of the urothelial tract. In a study of 100 grossly normal bladders examined on autopsy, von Brunn nests were observed in 89% [5]. While the cause for the invagination of the urothelium is unknown, they are found most commonly in the bladder trigone, followed by the renal pelvis and ureter. Proliferation of von Brunn nests is usually associated with inflammatory processes.

Cystitis glandularis refers to the development of columnar-type glandular epithelium within von Brunn nests. It is also associated with inflammatory processes, although it may be seen in otherwise normal bladders. Cystitis cystica is also seen in association with inflammation or irritation, but has been shown to be present in 60% of patients with grossly normal bladders on autopsy [5]. Prominent von Brunn nests, cystitis cystica, and cystitis glandularis usually occur simultaneously and are considered a spectrum of a common reactive process.

Intestinal metaplasia (i.e., cystitis glandularis of intestinal type) is characterized by the appearance of morphologic features typical of intestinal-type mucosa. This altered phenotype is also evident at the molecular level, as intestinal metaplasia also expresses proteins associated with intestinal differentiation, such as 7E12 H12 [6] and CDX-2, and, unlike typical cystitis glandularis, expresses CK20 and is negative for CK 7 expression [7]. Intestinal metaplasia may occur with increased frequency in bladder exstrophy, neurogenic bladder, or in association with pelvic lipomatosis [8]. However, the biological significance of these associations, and their magnitude, are incompletely defined.

Of the lesions discussed in this chapter, intestinal metaplasia is the one that has been suspected to have a premalignant potential [9]. The coexistence of intestinal metaplasia with adenocarcinoma has been historically recognized. The increased risk for adenocarcinoma in patients with bladder exstrophy has always been thought to be secondary to the extensive intestinal metaplasia observed in these bladders [10]. Morphologically, intestinal metaplasia is similar to Barrett's esophagus, and accumulation of beta-catenin in the nucleus, a phenomenon known to occur in Barrett's, has also been demonstrated

[11]. However, long-term follow-up studies have not been able to document an increased risk of developing adenocarcinoma for patients with a diagnosis of cystitis glandularis, whether typical or intestinal type [3, 12].

Clinical Presentation

As a normal anatomic variant, von Brunn nests are usually asymptomatic. However, hyperplastic or florid von Brunn nests, cystitis cystica, and cystitis glandularis may be associated with hematuria and irritative voiding symptoms such as dysuria, urgency, and frequency [1, 2, 13]. These symptoms are nonspecific and should serve only as indicators for the need for further evaluation. Several case reports have documented obstructive voiding symptoms in association with these lesions. In these rare cases, if large enough, the mass-like lesion may act in a ball-valve fashion to occlude the bladder outlet [14]. Similarly, the presence of such a lesion at or near the ureteral orifice may cause ureteral obstruction and, therefore, hydroureteronephrosis and/or flank pain [15].

The lesions should be biopsied to rule out malignancy and then resected or fulgurated. If symptomatic, the lesions are best treated by eradicating any chronic irritants to the bladder, and if the urine culture is positive, a 2–4-week course of antibiotics may be necessary to clear the lesions. Periodic cystoscopy should be performed to rule out recurrence. If a recurrence is found, then this should be resected or fulgurated to remove the lesions. There is no evidence that treatment with antibiotics or intravesical agents is helpful in preventing recurrence, but any known irritants should be treated or removed.

Cystoscopic Findings

von Brunn nests are usually only demonstrated on microscopic evaluation, as they are often undetectable by cystoscopy. Thus, they are often identified incidentally while a biopsy of the bladder is performed for another reason. When prominent, von Brunn nests may be cystoscopically evident as submucosal blebs that are pink to white and slightly raised. Due to their common flat-like abnormal appearance, the cystoscopic findings of these lesions may be confused with CIS or other forms of urothelial carcinoma. Further, since these lesions comprise urothelium, the potential exists for CIS to involve cystitis cystica or von Brunn nests (see later) [16]. On the other hand, von Brunn nests associated with cystitis cystica often have a distinct cystoscopic appearance. In contrast to the variable distribution and morphology of urothelial carcinoma, they tend to be regularly distributed and appear as large, well-circumscribed lobular lesions with flat bases [17]. Unlike typical urothelial carcinoma, these lesions appear more like papular lesions rather than the frondular lesions of urothelial carcinoma. They are typically white to light pink although they may appear red, further mimicking CIS. The most common locations are the bladder neck and trigone [5]. In cystitis glandularis the lesions may have a more yellow appearance and also may look slightly oily. These lesions range from small papules to larger bleb-type lesions. They may be associated with or next to adjacent areas of abnormal mucosa such as those of chronic irritation.

Pathologic Findings

Microscopically, von Brunn nests are solid nests of urothelial cells. They are usually immediately underneath the surface urothelium, but they may appear detached from it, particularly the deeper nests. The urothelial cells show no cytologic atypia and similar organization as the surface urothelium, or they may display reactive changes. When prominent, a polypoid growth may be observed on low power (Fig. 2.1). The separation of "normal" von Brunn nests from "proliferative" or "prominent" von Brunn nests is arbitrary, and should probably be based on whether the lesion was cystoscopically evident or symptomatic.

The main clinical significance of von Brunn nests is their potential to be confused with a particularly deceptively bland variant of urothelial

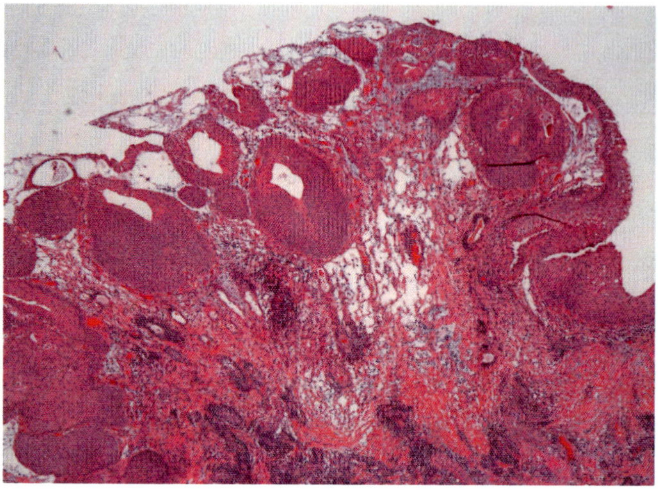

Fig. 2.1 Prominent von Brunn nests associated with edema and inflammatory changes of the submucosa, forming a vaguely polypoid elevation which may be detected cystoscopically

carcinoma referred to as "nested variant." [2, 17–20]. As its name implies, nested urothelial carcinoma grows in a nested architecture, which contrary to von Brunn nests, has a very infiltrative growth pattern. It is usually a larger lesion, but its true size may not be easily appreciated on small biopsies. If superficially sampled, nested urothelial carcinoma may be impossible to distinguish from von Brunn nests. Keys to its recognition include a very distorted, disorganized, and nonlobular architecture. Infiltration into deep structures of the lamina propria, and particularly into the muscularis propria, is a diagnostic feature. Confluence of nests is seen at least focally in most cases. A stromal reaction may or may not be associated. On the contrary, von Brunn nests, even when proliferative, tend to be superficial to an imaginary line within the lamina propria, beyond which no nests are seen. Volmar et al. [2]. studied a series of florid von Brunn nests cases and compared them to cases of nested urothelial carcinoma. No significant differences in the expression of p53, p27, or cytokeratin 20 could be found to differentiate between the two entities. Although nested urothelial carcinomas had a higher MIB-1 expression, no specific cutoff value could be determined for diagnostic purposes. The authors concluded that morphologic assessment was the only reliable way of differentiating between the two processes. In a recent study, Oberg et al. [21]. found a significant difference in polysomy detected by FISH (fluorescent in situ hybridization) within cells of von Brunn nests and those of nested urothelial carcinoma, suggesting that genomic differences may help distinguish between both entities.

Another potential pitfall in diagnosis associated with von Brunn nests is when they are associated with carcinoma in situ (CIS) of the urothelium. Because of their connection to the surface urothelium, CIS may extend to von Brunn nests and because of their lamina propria location, they may be confused with lamina propria invasion, leading to over staging of the disease [22]. Attention should be paid to the rounded regular contours of von Brunn nests, and the absence of a stromal reaction, in order to avoid this relatively common misinterpretation.

Inverted urothelial papilloma may also be confused with von Brunn nest proliferation. In these, the urothelial nests present in the lamina propria tend to be more crowded and numerous, and a more trabecular, architecture can be observed. Distinction may sometimes be arbitrary, particularly in small biopsies. Correlation with cystoscopic findings is usually helpful where a gross lesion is typically present in inverted papilloma while not often present in von Brunn nests.

Cystitis glandularis of the typical type is characterized by a central lumen surrounded by

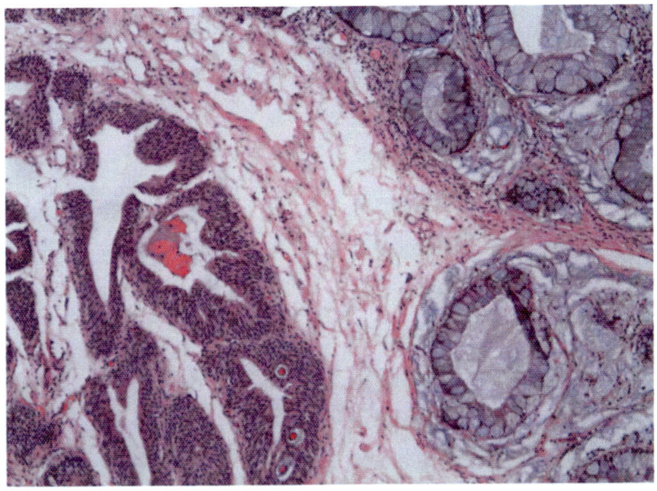

Fig. 2.2 Cystitis glandularis of both the typical and intestinal types. Usually both variants coexist, the difference between them being the presence of goblet cells in the latter

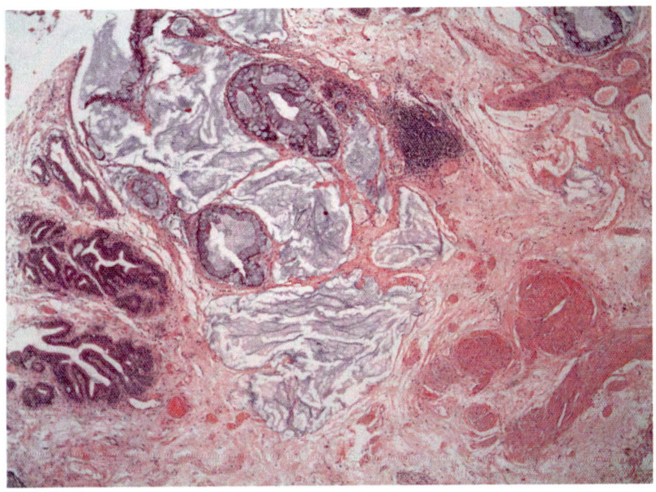

Fig. 2.3 Mucinous extravasation from cystitis glandularis of intestinal type. The pools of mucin that extravasate into the stroma may resemble the ones seen in mucinous adenocarcinoma. Contrary to this, however, the pools in cystitis glandularis are acellular and no cytologic atypia is identified in the glandular elements

columnar-or cuboidal-type epithelium. These, in turn, are surrounded by urothelium of various degrees of thickness. The lumen is variably dilated, and when prominently so, the lesion is referred to as cystitis cystica [1]. Many pathologists choose to diagnose these lesions as *cystitis cystica et glandularis* to underscore the common occurrence of both entities and the irrelevance of their strict separation. If clustered and voluminous, areas of cystitis glandularis or cystica may have a polypoid configuration on low power.

The presence of goblet cells defines a lesion as cystitis glandularis of intestinal type or intestinal metaplasia. Aside from goblet cells, Paneth cells and intestinal-type epithelial cells may also be identified [23]. The intestinal metaplasia may be limited to von Brunn nests or may involve the surface epithelium. It usually coexists with areas of typical cystitis glandularis (Fig. 2.2).

A common phenomenon in cases of intestinal metaplasia is the extravasation of intraluminal mucin into the surrounding lamina propria, creating acellular mucin pools that may dissect even into submucosa or superficial muscularis propria, and which can be easily confused with invasive adenocarcinoma of mucinous type (Fig. 2.3)

[1, 23]. The mucin pools associated with cystitis cystica glandularis may contain intact glands that display at most reactive-type atypia, but they do not contain malignant cells or irregular cellular aggregates that are typical of mucinous carcinoma. While the mucin pools may dissect quite deeply, the glandular elements remain confined to the lamina propria. This differential diagnosis may be quite challenging in small endoscopic biopsies, resulting sometimes in equivocal diagnoses that may need to be followed by a more generous sample.

Nephrogenic Adenoma

Another lesion that may be confused with urothelial carcinoma of the bladder is nephrogenic adenoma (NA). This lesion was first described by Davis in 1949 and was originally called a hamartoma of the bladder [24]. Just 1 year later, Friedman and Kuhlenbeck gave the lesion its current name, nephrogenic adenoma, due to its histological similarity to kidney tubules [25].

Pathogenesis

The pathogenesis of NA has been a source of controversy for many years. The traditional opinion is that NA represents a benign metaplastic process of the urothelium. While the exact etiology is unclear, it is thought that the metaplastic process is induced by local trauma or irritation such as infection, calculi, previous endourologic procedures, and intravesical chemotherapy [1, 26, 27]. This concept was significantly challenged with the findings of Mazal et al.28]. These authors reported a series of NA occurring in kidney transplant recipients of the opposite sex to the donor in which the nephrogenic adenoma showed the chromosomal sex of the donor, suggesting that the lesion results from the implantation of shedding tubular epithelial cells in an inflamed urothelial mucosa [28, 29]. The fact that there are reported cases of NA occurring in the intestinal mucosa of ileal conduits also challenges the idea that they are of urothelial origin 30]. NA is very frequent in renal transplant patients, suggesting that their immunocompromised status facilitates the implantation of these shedding cells [31]. The expression of PAX-2 and PAX-8 in NA, a protein usually expressed in renal epithelium, also suggests the possibility of a renal tubular origin of this lesion [32].

Clinical Presentation

The clinical presentation of NA often varies. Any age may be affected, but the majority of cases are seen during the fourth decade of life. The male-to-female ratio is approximately 3-to-1 in patients over the age of 20 years, though the reverse is true for those younger than 20 years [26, 33]. Approximately 10% of reported cases are found in children, while 10% of these lesions are seen in patients with renal transplants [1]. The presenting symptoms of NA are generally nonspecific. Approximately 70% of patients present with irritative voiding symptoms [33, 34]. Hematuria, microscopic or gross, may be seen in up to 40% of patients. They typically occur in a multifocal fashion and are most often found in the bladder (70%), but may also be in the urethra (15%), ureter (15%), and renal pelvis (5%) [31, 35].

Cystoscopic Findings

On cystoscopy, NA may often be confused with a papillary urothelial carcinoma as they often have a pink polypoid appearance very similar to that of a low-grade urothelial carcinoma and grossly are often indistinguishable from carcinomas. The typical size of the lesion varies from 1 to 7 cm, although they can also be smaller 26]. NA occurring in the bladder are most likely to be located in the trigone (40%), though they may also occur on the side walls (30%) and bladder dome (20%) and even rarely in the prostatic urethra [34].

Pathologic Findings

NA has several growth patterns that can result in a morphologic wide spectrum. The most common

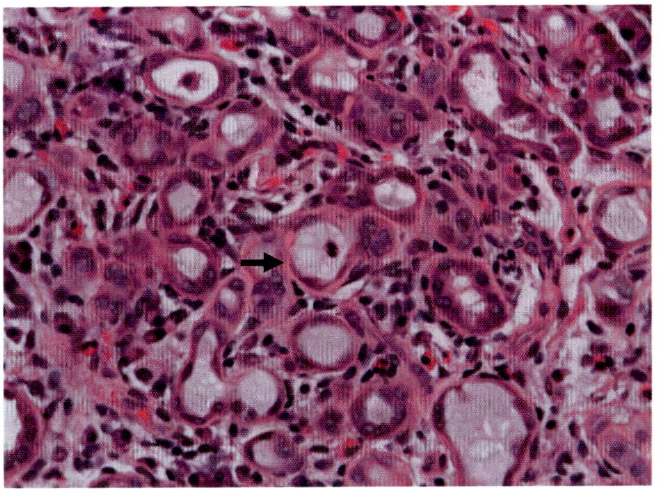

Fig. 2.4 Nephrogenic adenoma of tubular type. The small, compact tubules are lined by cytologically bland cells with focal hobnailing. A thick basement membrane visible on light microscopy surrounds most of the tubular elements (*arrow*)

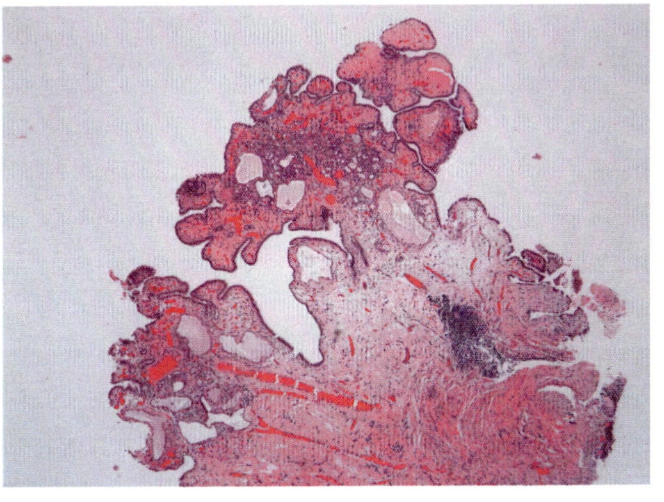

Fig. 2.5 Nephrogenic adenoma of papillary type. Notice the papillary exophytic growth. A focus of tubular pattern is seen in the center of the larger papilla

pattern is the tubular/glandular pattern, which may appear quite infiltrative. The tubules are lined by cuboidal cells with a hobnail appearance, with clear to eosinophilic cytoplasm, and may have relatively prominent nucleoli. Some of these tubules may cystically dilate, while others appear to be formed by single cells. They are usually surrounded by a thick hyalinized basement membrane, easily visible on routine light microscopy (Fig. 2.4). Other growth patterns include an exophytic papillary pattern, in which the papillae are lined by a single layer of cells, a feature that aids in the distinction from papillary urothelial neoplasia that has a stratified urothelial lining. A solid pattern may also be seen. Frequently two or more of these patterns coexist (Fig. 2.5) [36, 37].

By immunohistochemistry, the epithelial cells express cytokeratin 7 and pancytokeratin [38]. They also express several proteins associated with prostatic adenocarcinoma, such as AMACR, PAP, and occasionally PSA [39] (Fig. 2.6). This overlapping immunophenotype, particularly when faced with the tubular/glandular growth pattern, may potentially result in a misdiagnosis

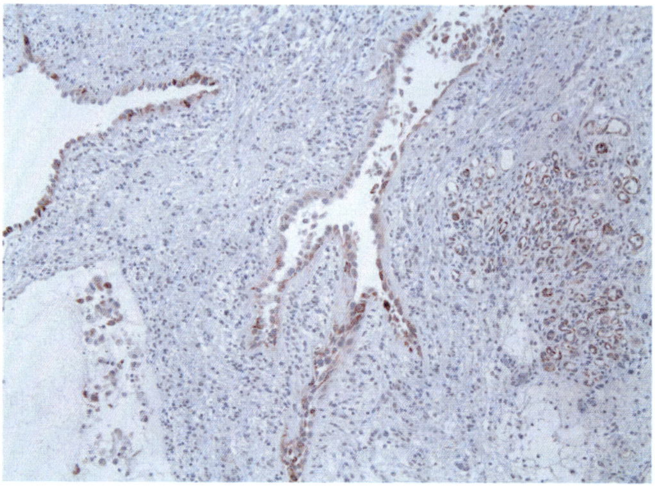

Fig. 2.6 Expression of prostatic-specific acid phosphatase in epithelial elements of nephrogenic adenoma. When faced with a tubular pattern, the expression of this and other prostatic markers may lead to an incorrect diagnosis of prostatic adenocarcinoma

of prostatic adenocarcinoma [40]. Other markers commonly present in NA include PAX-2 and PAX-8, which can help out in distinguishing this entity from prostatic adenocarcinoma [32, 41].

The main differential diagnosis of NA is clear cell adenocarcinoma of the urinary tract 37]. This tumor may grow in a cystic tubular and papillary pattern, and shares some histologic features of NA, including hobnailing of the lining cells. However, the degree of hyperchromasia and pleomorphism is much higher, and the lesion is usually mitotically active. It is usually more infiltrative, although this may not be appreciated in a small biopsy.

Other tumors that may grow in a tubulocystic pattern include some variants of urothelial carcinoma and prostatic adenocarcinoma. The latter may be particularly challenging, as stated previously, due to overlapping morphology and immunophenotype [40]. However, prostatic adenocarcinoma involving urinary bladder is usually high grade, and only infrequently grows in a tubular pattern. Morphologic features not seen in prostatic adenocarcinoma include the prominent hobnailing and the thick hyalinized basement membrane. As mentioned, PAX-2 and PAX-8 should be negative in prostatic adenocarcinoma. Urothelial carcinoma, particularly if of the microcystic variant, can mimic NA. Immunohistochemistry for p63 and high molecular weight keratins may help in identifying unusual patterns of urothelial carcinoma.

Polypoid/Papillary Cystitis

The clinical entity of polypoid/papillary cystitis represents a spectrum of mucosal changes seen secondarily to local irritation. Polypoid cystitis refers to lesions that are edematous and broad based, whereas the term papillary cystitis is thought to represent the more chronic phase of the process, in which better-formed papillae are usually appreciated [42]. There is obvious overlap between the two phases [1, 42]; they may be clinically referred to as bullous cystitis or bullous edema.

Clinical Presentation

As these lesions are frequently associated with chronic irritation, patients typically present with symptoms of frequency, urgency, hematuria, and often recurrent urinary tract infections/colonization. Bullous edema is commonly associated with indwelling catheter or suprapubic tubes, and may be found in these patients even several weeks after removal of a catheter. Patients who have fistulas either vesicovaginal or entero-or colovesical fistulas may also have associated bullous edema and hence may present with symptoms of pneumaturia, vaginal drainage, or fecaluria.

Pathogenesis

Essentially any type of chronic irritation of the bladder can result in polypoid cystitis. Patients with chronic indwelling catheters are most likely to present with polypoid cystitis, and the location of the lesions usually corresponds to that of the catheter tip, namely the posterior bladder wall and bladder dome. Another clinical entity associated with polypoid/papillary cystitis is colovesical fistula. Diverticular disease is by far the most common cause of colovesical fistulas, though they may also be found in patients with inflammatory bowel disease, colon cancer, or in those who have received radiation therapy [43, 44]. Radiation therapy is also a common cause of polypoid cystitis. Other associated causes include transurethral resection and other instrumentations for concomitant urothelial carcinoma.

Cystoscopic Findings

Like other benign lesions of the bladder, polypoid/papillary cystitis is often confused with papillary urothelial carcinoma [1, 42]. The urologist often has an advantage over the pathologist in the diagnosis of this condition as several key findings in the patient's clinical history will often point towards an inflammatory rather than a malignant condition. Also, the fronds seen in polypoid cystitis will typically appear more broad than those in papillary urothelial carcinoma, while the thinner papilla of papillary cystitis are more difficult to distinguish from carcinoma. Despite these descriptions it may be very difficult to distinguish cystoscopically between these entities and urothelial carcinoma and the diagnosis is ultimately made histologically. In patients with chronic polypoid cystitis the lesions often have less erythema and smooth polypoid appearance.

Pathologic Findings

Polypoid cystitis is characterized by the presence of exophytic projections of the urothelial mucosa predominantly due to edema of the lamina propria (Fig. 2.7). The papillae are typically broad-based, and lack complex secondary or tertiary branching. They contrast to the thin delicate papillae of urothelial carcinoma, which are usually thick enough only to harbor a thin fibrovascular core. The process is usually associated with inflammatory changes. The urothelium may show reactive-type changes, but no evidence of neoplastic-type cytologic atypia. Mitotic figures are commonly seen. In more chronic lesions, the papillae become more fibrotic and less edematous, giving them a thinner appearance, and the lesion in this stage is referred to as "papillary cystitis." The fibrotic papillae are still thicker than those in urothelial neoplasia, and are associated with chronic inflammation. Both stages of polypoid and papillary cystitis usually coexist, and the distinction is usually arbitrary and clinically irrelevant.

The main differential diagnosis is papillary urothelial neoplasia, particularly urothelial papilloma or papillary urothelial neoplasm of low malignant potential; however, when reactive urothelial atypia is present, papillary urothelial carcinomas may also be included in the differential. Lane and Epstein [42] reported a series of 41 cases misdiagnosed as papillary urothelial neoplasms. In urothelial neoplasia, the fibrovascular cores are thin and delicate. Branching of the papillae is commonly seen. Immunohistochemistry is generally not useful in this differential diagnosis, as more frequently the consideration is lower grade lesions, which share a similar phenotype with reactive urothelium. In those rare cases where high-grade papillary carcinoma is being considered, CD44, CD20, and p53 staining would show a reactive staining pattern [45].

While probably of no clinical significance, as both entities are benign, polypoid cystitis may be confused with papillary-type nephrogenic adenoma. Both lesions usually arise in a background of inflammation of the bladder wall. NA is lined by a single layer of cuboidal cells, while polypoid

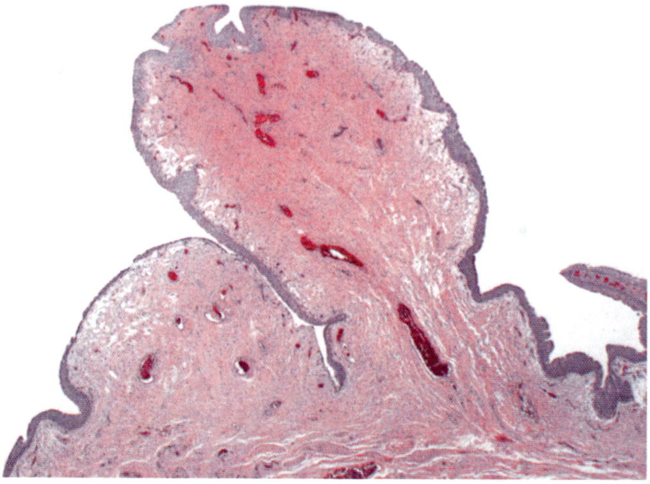

Fig. 2.7 Polypoid/papillary cystitis. The broad based papillae are formed not by a proliferation of the epithelium, but by an edematous/fibrotic submucosa with variable degrees of inflammation. This lesion may be misinterpreted as a papillary urothelial neoplasm, both cystoscopically and histologically

cystitis displays a multilayered urothelium. NA commonly shows two or more patterns of growth, including the solid or tubular patterns, which would be incompatible with polypoid cystitis.

Other Benign Papillary/Polypoid Lesions

Fibroepithelial Polyp

This is a benign, probably hamartomatous, polypoid lesion, which commonly presents in children and adolescents, mostly males. It is usually present within the verumontanum or bladder neck, and may present with acute urinary retention, hematuria, or bladder outlet obstruction [46]. Grossly, these lesions are typically indistinguishable from a low-grade transitional cell carcinoma of the bladder or urethra. Histologically, it consists of polypoid or papillary projections lined by unremarkable or, at most, reactive urothelium. They are commonly associated with cystitis glandularis in the stalk, and the stroma appears fibrotic, occasionally with atypical stromal cells. The lesion shares some features with polypoid/papillary cystitis, and some suggest it may represent the end stage of this entity. Because of its occurrence in children, a botryoid type rhabdomyosarcoma needs to be excluded by morphologic and immunohistochemical features. The treatment is usually conservative transurethral resection.

Prostatic Type Polyp

Prostatic-type polyp is a true polyp within the urothelial tract comprised of benign prostatic glands and stroma. Its pathogenesis is controversial, and it may represent a metaplastic process or developmentally ectopic prostatic tissue [47]. It occurs in a wide age range, from young adults to patients in their eighth or ninth decade [48]. Clinical presentation is usually hematuria or hematospermia. It is typically located in the bladder neck, trigone, or around the ureteral orifices and again is typically grossly indistinguishable from a low-grade TCC. Histologically it is characterized by the presence of columnar prostatic-type secretory epithelium, whether in submucosal glands or in the surface epithelium, variably admixed with urothelium. Columnar cells are positive for PSA and PSAP. The lesion has to be differentiated from a ductal type prostatic adenocarcinoma, papillary urothelial neoplasms, and nephrogenic adenoma. They can be resected transurethrally and show no tendency to recurrence.

Mullerianosis

Mullerianosis refers to the occurrence of endometriosis, endocervicosis, endosalpingiosis, or a mixture of these entities within the bladder wall [49]. Involvement of the urinary tract by endometriosis is not uncommon, and it occurs most frequently within the bladder [50]. The presenting symptoms of mullerianosis are often variable and include urinary urgency (78%), frequency (71%), and suprapubic pain/dysuria (43%) [51]. Cyclic hematuria may occur and is considered the hallmark symptom of mullerianosis; however, this occurs in only 20% of cases [52]. Cystoscopically, mullerianosis lesions may present as blunt polypoid elevations of the mucosa, but usually appear as blue or red-brown submucosal masses and range in size from 2 to 4 cm [53, 54]. Cold cup biopsy is recommended, but may not render diagnostic tissue given the submucosal location of the lesions [51]. Histologically, the lesion is characterized by a mixture of endometrial glands and stroma, endocervical, or tubal-like glandular inclusions, with variable hemorrhage. It should be differentiated from invasive adenocarcinoma. Unlike other benign bladder lesions such as cystitis glandularis, mullerianosis involves the muscularis propria, thus making it a transmural lesion. Given this, when complete resection is attempted, patients are at an increased risk of bladder perforation or incomplete resection. With this in mind, many advocate the use of oral contraceptives, danazol, or gonadotropin-releasing hormone agonists [51]. However, complete resection is often possible either through transurethral resection or partial cystectomy.

Surgical Management

The cornerstone treatment for these benign lesions is transurethral resection of all visible abnormalities. This not only provides tissue for correct pathologic characterization but may also cure the patient's symptoms. For most of the described lesions the potential for recurrence is very low, but the identification and removal of offending agents is critical in reducing recurrence. In patients in whom it is not possible to remove the etiologic agent (i.e., those with chronic catheters or radiation therapy) an initial biopsy is mandatory as is further cystoscopic surveillance. However, repeat biopsy should only be used when a significant change in the appearance has occurred.

Technique

The patient should be placed in a dorsal lithotomy position after the induction of anesthesia. Following the sterile prep and drape, the bladder should be entered with the aid of a visual obturator. Once the resectoscope has entered the bladder, a careful and thorough inspection of the entire mucosa should be performed. For optimal visualization, both 30° and 70° lens should be used. A bladder washing should be performed using saline to obtain cells for cytological examination.

Once the suspected lesion has been identified, consideration should be given to perform biopsies using the cold cup biopsy forceps for smaller lesions as cautery artifact may limit the pathologist's ability to accurately diagnose the lesion and/or coexisting carcinoma. Resection may then proceed with a partially distended bladder to reduce the risk of bladder perforation. This may be facilitated with a continuous-flow sheath that allows a continual flow of irrigation improving visibility. If multiple lesions are present, one should consider resecting those in more difficult or poorly accessible locations (bladder dome, lateral walls) first while visualization is optimal. Tumors located at the dome and anteriorly may be reached with the use of suprapubic pressure and a nearly empty bladder [55].

The cutting current is used with the resecting loop to begin resection. Care should be taken to follow the natural curvature of the bladder lumen as the loop is manipulated to avoid perforation. Depending on the size of the lesion, many urologists find it easiest to start on the periphery of the lesion and move across in a systematic fashion. For smaller lesions, the entire resection may be carried out using cold cup biopsy forceps rather than the resecting loop. Once the entire visible lesion has been resected, the coagulation current is used to achieve hemostasis. It is of paramount importance to avoid the ureteral orifices when using the coagulation current to avoid potential scarring and resultant obstruction.

In some instances when the diagnosis of a benign lesion has been previously established through biopsy, the lesion may be ablated rather than resected. This may be performed either by electrovaporization or via laser ablation. Electrovaporization simultaneously vaporizes the leading edge of tissue while desiccating the trailing edge at high power settings. A smooth roller ball is used with a cutting current at 240 W and is applied with the standard resectoscope. Hemostasis is then achieved with a setting of 40 W of coagulation current [55]. Since the tumor is vaporized, no specimen is available for pathological evaluation.

Another means is the use of laser ablation. Typically, the use of laser coagulation is limited to lesions 2.5 cm or smaller. The neodymium:yttrium-aluminum-garnet (Nd:YAG) laser is considered to be the optimal laser for bladder tumor ablation [56]. Holmium:YAG and KTP lasers are also effective for tissue ablation but lack deep coagulation [57]. The laser energy is transmitted via an end-fire laser fiber that is noncontact with a 5° to 15° angle of divergence. This allows a variable penetration depth of up to 5 mm [57]. After the entire resection or ablation has been completed, the bladder should be thoroughly inspected for signs of active bleeding or perforation.

Complications

Bladder perforation is among the most common complications of transurethral resection of bladder lesions and usually results from inadvertent full-thickness resection, trauma secondary to obturator reflex, or resecting a distended bladder. It may also occur in patients with large tumors in difficult locations or when resecting in a bladder diverticulum. Signs of perforation include visible fat at the resection site, less-than-expected return of irrigant, abdominal distention, and tachycardia. If perforation is suspected, a cystogram should be performed. A Foley catheter is inserted and contrast dye is allowed to fill the bladder by gravity. Extraperitoneal perforation is commonly demonstrated as a "flame-like" appearance from the extravasated contrast. Fortunately, most extraperitoneal bladder perforations can usually be managed conservatively with catheter drainage and antibiotics for 1–2 weeks postoperatively. In contrast, intraperitoneal perforation is a more troubling complication and is typically seen when perforation occurs at the bladder dome. Cystogram findings will often show contrast outlining loops of bowel. The vast majority will require open closure of the intraperitoneal perforation, though some clinicians will manage small intraperitoneal perforations conservatively with catheter drainage. Bleeding is another complication commonly seen after resection, though less so after ablative techniques. Meticulous hemostasis following resection is the best way to avoid this complication. If bleeding persists after the surgery is completed, a 3-way catheter (22-24Fr) may be inserted and continuous bladder irrigation (CBI) started. However, bladder perforation must be ruled out prior to starting CBI to avoid extravasation.

Conclusion

As described in this chapter, there are a number of lesions that can mimic neoplastic processes in the bladder. However, it is critical to differentiate these lesions from truly malignant lesions of the bladder to avoid overtreatment. A familiarity with the cystoscopic appearance of these lesions and the clinical presentation may provide some initial clues to a benign etiology. Ultimately, however, the diagnosis mostly relies upon an accurate pathologic diagnosis based on the histologic features of the lesion. A good working knowledge of the entities in this chapter is crucial for the surgical pathologist who examines pathologic specimens from bladder resections in order to provide the proper direction to the urologist. Finally, a dialogue between the pathologist and the urologist is essential and may help provide a definitive diagnosis for those cases in which either the clinical presentation and cystoscopic findings or the histologic features alone are insufficient to make an accurate diagnosis.

References

1. Young RH. Tumor-like lesions of the urinary bladder. Mod Pathol. 2009;22 Suppl 2:S37–52.
2. Volmar KE, Chan TY, De Marzo AM, Epstein JI. Florid von Brunn nests mimicking urothelial carcinoma: a morphologic and immunohistochemical comparison to the nested variant of urothelial carcinoma. Am J Surg Pathol. 2003;27(9):1243–52.
3. Smith AK, Hansel DE, Jones JS. Role of cystitis cystica et glandularis and intestinal metaplasia in development of bladder carcinoma. Urology. 2008;71(5):915–8.
4. Montironi R, Lopez-Beltran A, Scarpelli M, Mazzucchelli R, Cheng L. Morphological classification and definition of benign, preneoplastic and non-invasive neoplastic lesions of the urinary bladder. Histopathology. 2008;53(6):621–33.
5. Wiener DP, Koss LG, Sablay B, Freed SZ. The prevalence and significance of Brunn's nests, cystitis cystica and squamous metaplasia in normal bladders. J Urol. 1979;122(3):317–21.
6. Pantuck AJ, Bancila E, Das KM, Amenta PS, Cummings KB, Marks M, et al. Adenocarcinoma of the urachus and bladder expresses a unique colonic epithelial epitope: an immunohistochemical study. J Urol. 1997;158(5):1722–7.
7. Sung MT, Lopez-Beltran A, Eble JN, MacLennan GT, Tan PH, Montironi R, et al. Divergent pathway of intestinal metaplasia and cystitis glandularis of the urinary bladder. Mod Pathol. 2006;19(11):1395–401.
8. Yalla SV, Ivker M, Burros HM, Dorey F. Cystitis glandularis with perivesical lipomatosis. Frequent association of two unusual proliferative conditions. Urology. 1975;5(3):383–6.
9. Thrasher JB, Rajan RR, Perez LM, Humphrey PA, Anderson EE. Cystitis glandularis. Transition to adenocarcinoma of the urinary bladder. N C Med J. 1994;55(11):562–4.
10. Paulhac P, Maisonnette F, Bourg S, Dumas JP, Colombeau P. Adenocarcinoma in the exstrophic bladder. Urology. 1999;54(4):744.
11. Bryan RT, Nicholls JH, Harrison RF, Jankowski JA, Wallace DM. The role of beta-catenin signaling in the malignant potential of cystitis glandularis. J Urol. 2003;170(5):1892–6.
12. Corica FA, Husmann DA, Churchill BM, Young RH, Pacelli A, Lopez-Beltran A, et al. Intestinal metaplasia is not a strong risk factor for bladder cancer: study of 53 cases with long-term follow-up. Urology. 1997;50(3):427–31.
13. Jost SP, Dixon JS, Gosling JA. Ultrastructural observations on cystitis cystica in human bladder urothelium. Br J Urol. 1993;71(1):28–33.
14. Kaya C, Akpinar IN, Aker F, Turkeri LN. Large Cystitis glandularis: a very rare cause of severe obstructive urinary symptoms in an adult. Int Urol Nephrol. 2007;39(2):441–4.
15. Navarro JE, Huggins TJ. Cystitis glandularis: an unusual cause of ureteral obstruction. Urol Radiol. 1984;6(1):27–9.
16. Melicow MM, Hollowell JW. Intra-urothelial cancer: carcinoma in situ, Bowen's disease of the urinary system: discussion of thirty cases. J Urol. 1952;68(4):763–72.
17. Dhall D, Al-Ahmadie H, Olgac S. Nested variant of urothelial carcinoma. Arch Pathol Lab Med. 2007;131(11):1725–7.
18. Wasco MJ, Daignault S, Bradley D, Shah RB. Nested variant of urothelial carcinoma: a clinicopathologic and immunohistochemical study of 30 pure and mixed cases. Hum Pathol. 2010;41(2):163–71.
19. Murphy WM, Deana DG. The nested variant of transitional cell carcinoma: a neoplasm resembling proliferation of Brunn's nests. Mod Pathol. 1992;5(3):240–3.
20. Lin O, Cardillo M, Dalbagni G, Linkov I, Hutchinson B, Reuter VE. Nested variant of urothelial carcinoma: a clinicopathologic and immunohistochemical study of 12 cases. Mod Pathol. 2003;16(12):1289–98.
21. Oberg TN, Kipp BR, Campion MB, Voss JS, Jimenez RE, Sebo TJ, et al. Utilization of FISH to distinguish urothelial carcinoma with nested variant growth pattern from von Brunn's nests [Abstract]. Mod Pathol. 2010;23 Suppl 1:934.
22. Jimenez RE, Keane TE, Hardy HT, Amin MB. pT1 urothelial carcinoma of the bladder: criteria for diagnosis, pitfalls, and clinical implications. Adv Anat Pathol. 2000;7(1):13–25.
23. Mukhopadhyay S, Taylor W. Pathologic quiz case: bladder tumor in a 41-year-old man. Cystitis glandularis of intestinal type with mucin extravasation. Arch Pathol Lab Med. 2004;128(7):e89–90.
24. Davis TA. Hamartoma of the urinary bladder. Northwest Med. 1949;48(3):182–5.
25. Friedman NB, Kuhlenbeck H. Adenomatoid tumors of the bladder reproducing renal structures (nephrogenic adenomas). J Urol. 1950;64(5):657–70.
26. Kontothanassis D, Christophis J, Tamvakis N, Becopoulos T. Bladder washing flow cytometry assessment of nephrogenic adenoma of the bladder. Int Urol Nephrol. 1996;28(4):495–7.
27. Tse V, Khadra M, Eisinger D, Mitterdorfer A, Boulas J, Rogers J. Nephrogenic adenoma of the bladder in renal transplant and non-renal transplant patients: a review of 22 cases. Urology. 1997;50(5):690–6.
28. Mazal PR, Schaufler R, Altenhuber-Muller R, Haitel A, Watschinger B, Kratzik C, et al. Derivation of nephrogenic adenomas from renal tubular cells in

kidney-transplant recipients. N Engl J Med. 2002; 347(9):653–9.
29. Ingelfinger JR. Nephrogenic adenomas as renal tubular outposts. N Engl J Med. 2002;347(9):684–6.
30. Strand WR, Alfert HJ. Nephrogenic adenoma occurring in an ileal conduit. J Urol. 1987;137(3):491–2.
31. Fournier G, Menut P, Moal MC, Hardy E, Volant A, Mangin P. Nephrogenic adenoma of the bladder in renal transplant recipients: a report of 9 cases with assessment of deoxyribonucleic acid ploidy and long-term followup. J Urol. 1996;156(1):41–4.
32. Tong GX, Melamed J, Mansukhani M, Memeo L, Hernandez O, Deng FM, et al. PAX2: a reliable marker for nephrogenic adenoma. Mod Pathol. 2006;19(3): 356–63.
33. Porcaro AB, D'Amico A, Ficarra V, Balzarro M, Righetti R, Martignoni G, et al. Nephrogenic adenoma of the urinary bladder: our experience and review of the literature. Urol Int. 2001;66(3):152–5.
34. Weiss MA. Bladder lesion in a young man. Contemp Urol. 2001;13(3):15–9.
35. McIntire TL, Soloway MS, Murphy WM. Nephrogenic adenoma. Urology. 1987;29(3):237–41.
36. Oliva E, Young RH. Nephrogenic adenoma of the urinary tract: a review of the microscopic appearance of 80 cases with emphasis on unusual features. Mod Pathol. 1995;8(7):722–30.
37. Young RH, Scully RE. Nephrogenic adenoma. A report of 15 cases, review of the literature, and comparison with clear cell adenocarcinoma of the urinary tract. Am J Surg Pathol. 1986;10(4):268–75.
38. Rahemtullah A, Oliva E. Nephrogenic adenoma: an update on an innocuous but troublesome entity. Adv Anat Pathol. 2006;13(5):247–55.
39. Skinnider BF, Oliva E, Young RH, Amin MB. Expression of alpha-methylacyl-CoA racemase (P504S) in nephrogenic adenoma: a significant immunohistochemical pitfall compounding the differential diagnosis with prostatic adenocarcinoma. Am J Surg Pathol. 2004;28(6):701–5.
40. Xiao GQ, Burstein DE, Miller LK, Unger PD. Nephrogenic adenoma: immunohistochemical evaluation for its etiology and differentiation from prostatic adenocarcinoma. Arch Pathol Lab Med. 2006;130(6): 805–10.
41. Tong GX, Weeden EM, Hamele-Bena D, Huan Y, Unger P, Memeo L, et al. Expression of PAX8 in nephrogenic adenoma and clear cell adenocarcinoma of the lower urinary tract: evidence of related histogenesis? Am J Surg Pathol. 2008;32(9):1380–7.
42. Lane Z, Epstein JI. Polypoid/papillary cystitis: a series of 41 cases misdiagnosed as papillary urothelial neoplasia. Am J Surg Pathol. 2008;32(5):758–64.
43. Melchior S, Cudovic D, Jones J, Thomas C, Gillitzer R, Thuroff J. Diagnosis and surgical management of colovesical fistulas due to sigmoid diverticulitis. J Urol. 2009;182(3):978–82.
44. Najjar SF, Jamal MK, Savas JF, Miller TA. The spectrum of colovesical fistula and diagnostic paradigm. Am J Surg. 2004;188(5):617–21.
45. McKenney JK, Desai S, Cohen C, Amin MB. Discriminatory immunohistochemical staining of urothelial carcinoma in situ and non-neoplastic urothelium: an analysis of cytokeratin 20, p53, and CD44 antigens. Am J Surg Pathol. 2001;25(8): 1074–8.
46. Tsuzuki T, Epstein JI. Fibroepithelial polyp of the lower urinary tract in adults. Am J Surg Pathol. 2005;29(4):460–6.
47. Remick Jr DG, Kumar NB. Benign polyps with prostatic-type epithelium of the urethra and the urinary bladder. A suggestion of histogenesis based on histologic and immunohistochemical studies. Am J Surg Pathol. 1984;8(11):833–9.
48. Anjum MI, Ahmed M, Shrotri N, Azzopardi A, Mufti GR. Benign polyps with prostatic-type epithelium of the urethra and the urinary bladder. Int Urol Nephrol. 1997;29(3):313–7.
49. Young RH, Clement PB. Mullerianosis of the urinary bladder. Mod Pathol. 1996;9(7):731–7.
50. Denes FT, Pompeo AC, Montelatto NI, Lopes RN. Ureteral endometriosis. Int Urol Nephrol. 1980;12(3): 205–9.
51. Westney OL, Amundsen CL, McGuire EJ. Bladder endometriosis: conservative management. J Urol. 2000;163(6):1814–7.
52. Batler RA, Kim SC, Nadler RB. Bladder endometriosis: pertinent clinical images. Urology. 2001;57(4): 798–9.
53. Fedele L, Bianchi S, Raffaelli R, Portuese A. Preoperative assessment of bladder endometriosis. Hum Reprod. 1997;12(11):2519–22.
54. Young RH. Pseudoneoplastic lesions of the urinary bladder and urethra: a selective review with emphasis on recent information. Semin Diagn Pathol. 1997; 14(2):133–46.
55. Traxer O, Pasqui F, Gattegno B, Pearle MS. Technique and complications of transurethral surgery for bladder tumours. BJU Int. 2004;94(4):492–6.
56. Holzbeierlein JM, Smith JA, Jr. Surgical management of noninvasive bladder cancer (stages Ta/T1/CIS). Urol Clin North Am. 2000;27(1):15–24, vii-viii.
57. Smith Jr JA, Landau S. Neodymium: YAG laser specifications for safe intravesical therapy. J Urol. 1989;141(5):1238–9.

Diverticular Disease

3

W. Stuart Reynolds, Omar Hameed, and Harriette M. Scarpero

Urinary tract diverticula are common findings in patients presenting with symptoms of lower urinary tract (i.e., bladder and urethra) dysfunction. Diverticula in this setting can be the cause of primary symptoms or a concomitant result of an underlying abnormality. Diverticula are also incidental findings in patients undergoing routine, unrelated evaluations, and are typically not associated with serious clinical sequelae.

The most common structures affected by diverticula in the urinary tract are the bladder and urethra. While diverticula can be found in both structures, the mechanisms by which they develop and the underlying pathology are very different and largely unrelated. Additionally, the symptoms and signs by which diverticula in either structure affect patients are also very unique; thus, separate patient populations are typically afflicted based on the location of the diverticulum. Bladder and urethra diverticula are presented as separate discussions in this chapter.

W.S. Reynolds (✉)
Department of Urologic Surgery, Vanderbilt University Medical Center, A1302 Medical Center North, Nashville, TN 37232, USA
e-mail: William.Stuart.Reynolds@vanderbilt.edu

O. Hameed
Departments of Pathology and Surgery, The Comprehensive Cancer Center, University of Alabama at Birmingham, NP 3550, 1802 6th Avenue South, 619 19th Avenue South, Birmingham, AL 35249, USA
e-mail: ohameed@uab.edu

H.M. Scarpero
Associated Urologists of Nashville, 4230 Harding Road, Suite 521, Nashville, TN 37205, USA
e-mail: hscarpero@comcast.net

Bladder Diverticula

A bladder diverticulum is a protrusion or herniation of the bladder mucosa through the detrusor muscle fiber bundles of the bladder wall (i.e., the muscularis propria). This protrusion of the underlying mucosal lining and supporting lamina propria results in a thin-walled, saccular outpouching on the outer surface of the bladder; this structure can be of variable size and is lined by urothelium and typically filled with urine. The diverticulum maintains continuity with the bladder lumen via a neck or ostium that opens upon the lining of the bladder mucosa. Because of the virtual absence of any backing detrusor muscle fibers, a diverticulum does not contract as the bladder itself contracts during micturition. This results in poor emptying and stasis of urine in the diverticulum, which is the hallmark of diverticular pathophysiology.

Bladder diverticula can be broadly classified into two categories: congenital and acquired. Congenital diverticula can be further divided into primary and secondary types: Primary diverticula result from inherent weaknesses or abnormalities of the detrusor muscle layer, but are independent of voiding abnormalities or bladder outlet obstruction (BOO). These idiopathic diverticula are termed primary (nonobstructing) congenital

D.E. Hansel et al. (eds.), *The Urinary Tract: A Comprehensive Guide to Patient Diagnosis and Management*, DOI 10.1007/978-1-4614-5320-8_3, © Springer Science+Business Media New York 2012

bladder diverticula (PCBD) [1]. Secondary diverticula may also be antenatal and thus congenital, but cannot be PCBD by definition if associated with a primary bladder abnormality, such as BOO in the setting of posterior urethral valves. While occasionally seen in the pediatric population, acquired diverticula are still most commonly found in adults (usually men) and are strongly associated with BOO caused by obstruction of the prostate secondary to benign prostatic hyperplasia (BPH) or the urethra as a consequence of urethral stricture disease (USD) for example.

In the pediatric population congenital diverticula have a peak incidence in children younger than 10 years old [2]. They are typically solitary and located lateral and posterior to the ureteral orifices [3]. Boys are much more commonly affected than girls, with an overall incidence of approximately 1.7% [4]. PCBD are also associated with collagen and connective tissue disorders, and are found in patients with Williams–Beuren syndrome [5, 6], Ehlers–Danlos syndrome [7–9], prune belly [4], and Menkes [10, 11]. In these syndromic patients, the diverticula tend to be more numerous, but smaller than the solitary PCBD. Solitary PCBD in turn tend to be larger than those associated with neurogenic dysfunction or BOO [12], and generally are found in smooth-walled bladders without significant trabeculation [3]. Secondary congenital diverticula are most commonly associated with neurogenic bladder dysfunction and posterior urethral valves. Up to 60% of bladder diverticula in children are related to neurogenic bladder [4]. Ipsilateral vesicoureteral reflux (VUR) is also a common finding with congenital diverticula [13].

Acquired diverticula are much more common. They usually develop in older adults, presenting in the sixth decade, which corresponds to the development of BOO secondary to prostatic obstruction [14]. As such, more than 90% of diverticula are found in men as opposed to women [15]. In addition to prostatic obstruction (e.g., BPH, prostate cancer), other causes of BOO include USD and bladder neck contracture (BNC), which are also manifested in adulthood and contribute to diverticula formation. Characteristic changes of the bladder in the setting of BOO include detrusor hypertrophy, trabeculation, and diverticula [16]. In these cases, diverticula are often multiple and can be quite large [17]. Diverticula are estimated to develop in 4–13% of patients with BOO, most commonly associated with BPH or BNC [18] and up to 6% of men with "prostatism." [19] In one series, the etiology of diverticula was determined to be BPH in 70% of patients, BNC in 12%, and USD in 12% [20].

Clinical Presentation

Bladder diverticula do not necessarily result in symptoms themselves. Most commonly, they are discovered incidentally during evaluation for other lower urinary tract conditions—e.g., during the evaluation of hematuria or recurrent urinary tract infections (UTI)—often on endoscopic examination of the bladder or on radiographic imaging of the genitourinary tract. If signs or symptoms are present, they typically result from the pathologic sequelae related to incomplete emptying of urine from the diverticula and urinary stasis. A diverticulum may serve as a nidus for bacterial growth, causing persistent and recurrent UTIs. Urine stasis also contributes to urolithiasis formation within the diverticulum as well as neoplastic changes and tumor growth. If large enough, a diverticulum may promote symptoms related to mass effect in the pelvis and lower abdomen or related to urine volume, including incomplete bladder emptying, bladder fullness, and double voiding [14]. Determining if vague lower urinary tract symptoms are a result of a diverticulum or other lower tract pathology is difficult, given the high prevalence of BPH and associated symptoms. Several reports have been published describing bladder diverticula presenting in inguinal hernias [21, 22]. In children, the most common presentation may be recurrent UTI [1, 23].

When clinical signs and symptoms were reported in a review of acquired bladder diverticula in adults, the most common clinical finding was hematuria (49%), followed by urinary retention (22%), UTI (13%), urinary incontinence (11%), and dysuria (4%) [24].

Pathogenesis

Primary congenital and acquired (both secondary congenital and adult-onset) diverticula appear to have different mechanisms of formation and are thought to be pathologically distinct. PCBD develop at areas of weakness in the bladder wall where there is muscle failure (either embryologically or functionally) [25]. In this sense, PCBD are not so much herniations but rather aneurysmal dilatations. Given their predilections for developing posteriolaterally at the level of the trigone, it has been suggested that this is a location where muscle fusion is incomplete, as the joint between the trigone and the detrusor body represents the boundary of two distinct embryologic precursors [26].

PCBD can be categorized into three subtypes based on location and associated findings: posterolateral, paraureteral, and multiple (i.e., multidiverticular bladders) [1]. Posterolateral PCBD are located just as described, in a posterior-lateral position but are not related to the ureteral orifices and not associated with vesicoureteral reflux. They represent approximately 10% of the PCBD. Paraureteral diverticula are directly related to the ureteral hiatus through the detrusor and develop because of weakened muscle wall backing along the posterior aspect of the intramural ureter. The ureter and ureteral orifice may be adjacent to the diverticulum or may open into the diverticulum itself. In either case, VUR is virtually always present. These represent approximately 90% of PCBD and are widely known as Hutch diverticula, named eponymously after the first description [3]. Multidiverticular bladders are rare (<1%) and are associated with congenital conditions such as prune belly, Ehlers–Danlos, Menkes, and Williams–Beuren syndromes. The defects here are generally a direct or secondary dysfunction of connective tissue (or in the case of Ehlers–Danlos, collagen formation), leading to weakness of the viscoelastic properties of the bladder and diverticula formation [9].

Secondary congenital bladder diverticula are similar in pathogenesis to adult or acquired diverticula and develop as a result of a primary bladder or voiding dysfunction. In children, they are most commonly seen in the setting of posterior urethral valves and neurogenic bladders, both situations associated with elevated voiding and resting bladder pressures. Acquired bladder diverticula are traditionally described as mucosal protrusions through the detrusor muscle and are genuine mucosal hernias [27]. In the setting of abnormal voiding or high-pressure voiding against an obstructed bladder outlet, typical pathologic changes to the bladder result, including detrusor hypertrophy and trabeculation. Diverticula are thought to develop progressively under the effects of high pressure in the bladder lumen, first as cellules interdigitating between hypertrophied detrusor bundles, then as saccules and finally as diverticula [14]. As the detrusor hypertrophy continues, detrusor muscle bundles form a ring of muscle tissue around the diverticular ostium; during bladder contraction, this ostium is further constricted and traps urine inside the diverticulum. As acquired diverticula lack muscularis propria backing, they are not subjected to the pressures exerted by detrusor hypertrophy and they function as low-pressure reservoirs relative to the bladder lumen. Because of the low-pressure gradient between the diverticulum and bladder, reciprocal filling of the diverticulum with urine during voiding can occur [28]. As the BOO progresses, the cycle of increased bladder pressures and progressive detrusor hypertrophy continues, with expansion of existing diverticula and development of additional ones [14].

The pathologic result of urinary stasis within the diverticula is similar to the effects of stasis in the bladder at large. Recurrent or persistently infected urine initiates inflammatory reactions within the mucosa, submucosa, and lamina propria. Stasis and hyperconcentration of urine solutes promote sediment crystallization and stone formation. Presumably secondary to prolonged mucosal contact to urine substances and carcinogens, neoplastic changes occur and tumor growth ensues.

Clinical Examination and Cystoscopic Findings

Bladder diverticula may not be readily demonstrable on physical examination, given their rather insidious presentation. If markedly enlarged, they may be palpable through the lower abdominal wall as a fluctuant or cystic mass, and most often could be mistaken for a markedly distended bladder. A posteriorly or laterally located diverticulum may be palpable on digital rectal exam as a fluctuant mass or may cause prostate deviation [29].

Bladder diverticula are well visualized on radiographic studies and are often diagnosed incidentally at the time of imaging during evaluation of other lower urinary tract processes [30]. Both static and dynamic cystograms, as in the setting of video urodynamic bladder testing, can demonstrate diverticula as contrast filled structures immediately adjacent to the bladder. Cross-sectional imaging with contrast enhancement (e.g., computerized tomography (CT) or magnetic resonance imaging (MRI)) can also readily demonstrate diverticula as well as relations to surrounding anatomic structures. Finally, pelvic and abdominal sonography can also delineate bladder diverticula, as is typically used in children.

Cystoscopy is an essential component of the evaluation of bladder diverticula and diverticula often are diagnosed first during endoscopic inspection of the bladder. Typically a bladder diverticulum can be seen from within the bladder; however, inspection is limited by the diameter of the ostium leading into the diverticulum. In the case of acquired diverticula, the bladder is typically marked by associated trabeculation and if the ostium is small, identification may be difficult. The location and size of any diverticula should be noted as well as the relation to the ureteral orifices. Cystoscopic examination of bladder diverticula may reveal the presence of a stone within the diverticula or more rarely a tumor. Because of the association with neoplastic changes, complete and careful inspection of the entire diverticulum is warranted. A flexible cystoscope and possible dilation of the diverticular neck may be necessary to complete the inspection.

Similar to any bladder abnormality, any area of suspicious mucosa should be biopsied and submitted for pathological analysis. Several techniques for mucosal biopsy are available, including brush, cold-cup or forceps biopsy, and transurethral resection (TUR); however, as for any staging of carcinoma, adequate sampling must be assured. In the case of neoplasia in a diverticulum, the inherent difficulty in tissue biopsy arises from the paucity of submucosal tissue and detrusor muscle backing: too conservative a sampling of tissue may yield unsatisfactory results, while overaggressive sampling may risk diverticulum perforation. Therefore extreme care must be taken during biopsy of a tumor within a diverticulum to prevent perforation.

Although perforation is a known risk of TUR of bladder tumor (TURBT) within a diverticulum, it is not clear how frequently it occurs. The incidence of bladder perforation during TUR of a normal bladder is estimated to be 1.3–5% [31, 32], although the rate of asymptomatic or unrecognized perforation as measured with immediate post-TUR cystogram is reported to be 50–58% of cases [33, 34]. While immediate complications of hemorrhage or visceral injury are obvious results of perforation, the oncologic consequences of perforation are not clear as extravesical recurrence from tumor seeding is reportedly rare [35, 36].

Pathology

Primary congenital bladder diverticula are distinct pathologically from acquired or secondary diverticula because they represent different entities. PCBD are not true herniations of submucosa through the detrusor muscles, but instead may be more like dilatations or aneurysms. On histologic examination of PCBD, fine, attenuated muscle fibers can be found lining the diverticula, which is thought to represent rudimentary muscularis propria [1]. This finding may be supported by the hypothesis that PCBD are located at boundaries

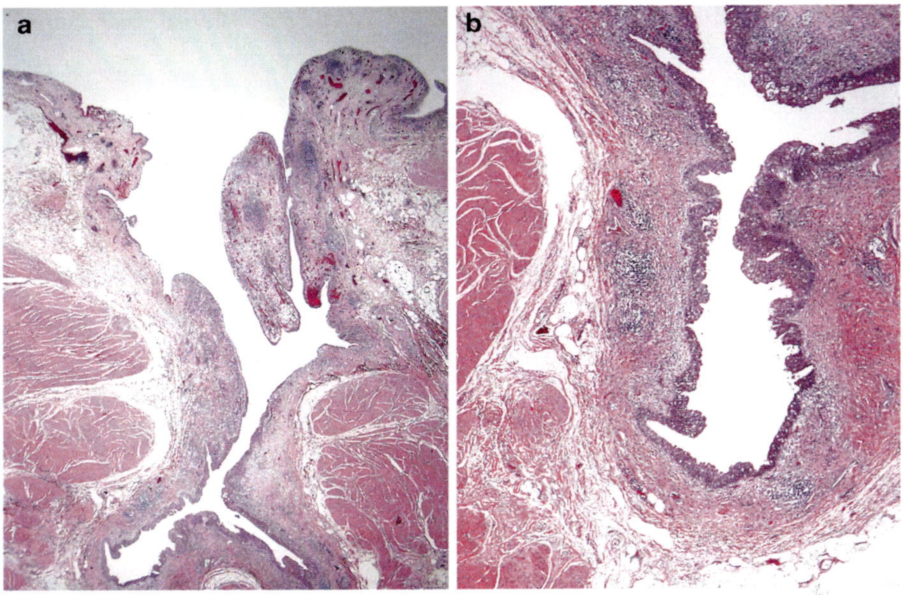

Fig. 3.1 Low power magnification (**a**) of bladder diverticulum showing deep extension between the thick eosinophilic bundles of the muscularis propria. On higher magnification (**b**) one can see that the diverticulum is lined by variably thick urothelium with an underlying inflamed and fibrotic lamina propria. Note that although there is muscularis propria on the side of the diverticulum, the deep portion is in direct continuity with the perivesical adipose tissue

where distinct embryological tissues meet and muscle fusion is incomplete. Diverticula develop primarily in this setting because of primitive muscularis propria failure [25, 26].

In acquired diverticula, the findings are more consistent with the concept of a true mucosal/submucosal herniation through the muscularis propria. On histological examination, the diverticulum wall is generally composed of mucosa and subepithelial connective tissue or lamina propria [27] with a markedly attenuated or absent muscularis propria (Fig. 3.1a, b). This lack of a true muscularis propria layer (detrusor muscle) in acquired bladder diverticula can lead to problems in staging invasive carcinomas arising in them [37], especially in distinguishing tumors limited to the lamina propria (T1) from those that have extended into the perivesical fat (T3; Fig. 3.2), with obvious therapeutic and prognostic implications. Given the unique challenge of accurate pathological staging of urothelial tumors arising within bladder diverticula, along with the inherent difficulty in staging bladder tumors in biopsy and TUR material, it is not surprising to find a significant rate of pathologic upstaging on more extensive resection [24].

Tamas et al. reviewed histopathologic samplings of 71 bladder diverticula treated between 1981 and 2006 at a tertiary referral center in order to address this issue of tumor staging [24]. In almost all cases, the boundary between the lamina propria and perivesical fat was readily defined by a variably thick band of dense fibrous tissue. The authors submitted that this band could be used to differentiate between the perivesical fat, which consisted almost entirely of fibroadipose tissue, and the lamina propria, which contained fibrovascular tissue and more abundant stromal tissue, and thus perhaps serves as a pathologic landmark to better identify the depth of tumor invasion. In their analysis of invasive tumors, the authors noted that diverticula with tumors limited to the lamina propria frequently demonstrated this connective tissue band to be intact, whereas in the case of tumors invasive into perivesical fat,

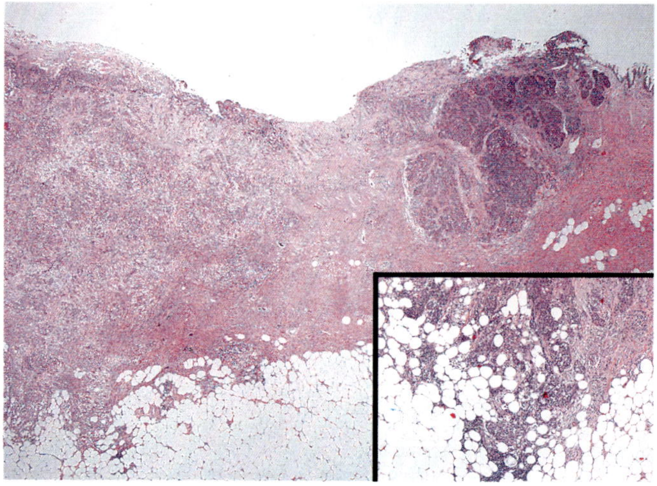

Fig. 3.2 Invasive urothelial carcinoma arising within a bladder diverticulum. Note that although the tumor on the right portion of the photomicrograph appears to be limited by thick fibroconnective tissue that otherwise would suggest growth limited to the lamina propria (T1), there is unequivocal extension into the perivesical adipose tissue (T3) in the *left portion* of the field, more evident on higher magnification (*inset*)

the tumor cells were readily demonstrated to extend beyond this landmark.

As might be inferred from above, neoplastic changes in bladder diverticula are not uncommon. In fact, it has been reported that up to 10% of all bladder diverticula will harbor neoplastic changes and that carcinomas arising in diverticula account for 1.5% of all bladder carcinomas [14, 37]. The most common histologic type of carcinoma reported in diverticula is urothelial carcinoma, while less common types include squamous cell carcinoma, adenocarcinoma, small cell carcinoma, and sarcomatoid carcinoma [14, 38]. There has been some suggestion that a higher proportion of unusual tumor types are seen within diverticula and may be related to the distinct microenvironment that influences the urothelium within the diverticulum specifically [24]. As for pathologic stage, extension beyond the bladder is common, with reports of 33–56% of malignant diverticular tumors invading the perivesical adipose tissue (T3) [24, 38].

Management

Basic Evaluation and Workup

The basic evaluation of a known or suspected bladder diverticulum overlaps with the workups of several lower urinary disorders and, as previously discussed, diverticula are most commonly detected incidentally during work-up for other urinary tract complaints. Therefore, the workup for diverticula must involve not only characterization of the diverticula, but also of any associated voiding dysfunction or abnormality, such as BOO, which may be a contributing etiologic agent. Aspects of patient history should focus on delineating lower urinary tract symptoms consistent with voiding dysfunction suggestive of BOO, assessing for any associated sequelae or symptoms specifically related to diverticulum and identifying any other medical or neurological condition that may contribute to urinary tract dysfunction. The essential elements of evaluation include cystoscopy to visually inspect the diverticula for any neoplastic epithelial changes or for stones, urinary cytology as an adjunct to visualization and/or mucosal biopsy of any suspicious lesions, voiding cystourethrography to assess diverticulum anatomy and drainage and to detect vesicoureteral reflux, and upper urinary tract imaging to evaluate for hydroureteronephrosis. A culture of urine sampled directly from the diverticulum can also be useful if recurrent UTI are a manifestation of diverticular disease. If malignancy is identified and confirmed with tissue biopsy, then appropriate staging studies and metastatic evaluations should be obtained. If significant voiding dysfunction or BOO is detected, further evaluations including multichannel urodynamics preferentially with fluoroscopy should be performed.

Indications for Treatment

For most patients, the presence of a small bladder diverticulum is incidental and causes no symptoms or sequelae. Treatment in such individuals is not warranted. In the case of acquired diverticula, treatment of the underlying condition predisposing to BOO and diverticulum formation should be considered primarily. This is usually sufficient to alleviate symptoms attributed to the diverticulum and no further treatment of the diverticulum specifically is needed if satisfactory emptying of the diverticulum is demonstrated and no complicating factors are present (e.g., stones, malignancy, infections, or reflux). There has been debate over the role of prophylactic excision of asymptomatic diverticula, primarily given the concern for malignant transformation [30]. Generally accepted indications for bladder diverticulectomy include: malignant disease, recurrent or persistent infections, stones, urinary obstruction or retention including a poorly draining diverticulum, bothersome urinary symptoms, or other complicating factors, such as ipsilateral vesicoureteral reflux or hydroureteronephrosis [14, 30]. If diverticulectomy is warranted and BOO exists, a procedure to relieve bladder obstruction is performed either before diverticulectomy or concurrently.

Conservative Management/ Observation

Observation of uncomplicated bladder diverticula is the preferred option for most patients. It is recommended that these patients be followed periodically with cystoscopy and urine cytology to monitor for malignant transformation [14]. However, there is no consensus on frequency of evaluations or duration of follow-up. There are few reports documenting subsequent tumor formation in diverticula under observation, although some authors have recommended prophylactic diverticulectomy because of the risk for tumor development years later and the relative poor prognosis of these patients [39]. Others have not advocated for prophylactic diverticulectomy, arguing that the risk of de novo malignancy is not increased [30, 40]. Aside from concerns for malignancy, patients should be regularly evaluated for progression of voiding dysfunction and bladder decompensation, particularly if the underlying BOO has not been definitively treated. As BOO progresses, bladder diverticula may progressively enlarge and become problematic and additional diverticula may develop. This can be monitored with symptom assessment as well as periodic uroflowmetry and postvoid residual measurements [30].

Treatment of Diverticula Without Malignancy

Endoscopic Management

Various endoscopic approaches to treatment of bladder diverticula have been reported. Transurethral incision or resection of the diverticular neck is one such approach [41]. Using a cold-cutting Collins knife or electrocautery resectoscope loop, the neck of the diverticulum is incised at the level of the ostium through the mucosa and submucosal tissue to the level of the bladder muscle fibers. This maneuver enlarges the neck of the diverticulum, allowing greater drainage of urine by releasing the obstructing sphincter-like mechanism of the bladder wall. Urinary retention has been reported after this technique secondary to a reversal of urine flow into the diverticulum through the enlarged hiatus during micturition [42].

Mucosal fulguration of the lining of the diverticulum can also result in shrinkage and ablation [43]; however, this technique is more effective when combined with incision of the diverticular neck. A four-point incision of the diverticular neck combined with mucosal fulguration using a roller ball electrode has been described [44–46].

Not only can this serve to ablate the diverticulum, but it also allows concomitant endoscopic management of stones within the diverticulum via endoscopic litholopaxy as well as TUR of a diverticular tumor that may be poorly accessible.

Open Surgical Excision

Traditionally, open surgical diverticulum excision has been performed most commonly through a transvesical approach, but extravesical and combined techniques have also been described [47]. Open surgical diverticulectomy proceeds via either a lower abdominal midline incision or through a Pfannenstial or Gibson incision, alternatively, with median separation of the rectus muscles and abdominal fascial layers to allow entry into the retropubic space. The anterior bladder wall is identified and a transverse cystotomy is performed after reflecting the peritoneum off the bladder dome. A self-retaining retractor can be placed to provide adequate exposure to the entire bladder. The entire bladder should be inspected and the locations of diverticula noted. If a diverticulum is large or in close proximity to a ureteral orifice, a ureteral catheter or stent should be placed to help identify the ureter and avoid inadvertent injury.

Once identified, small (<2.5 cm diameter) diverticulum can be pulled into the bladder lumen by grasping the apical component with a clamp inserted through the neck and gently everting the diverticulum (Fig. 3.3). The diverticular neck is then divided with cautery and bladder wall defect closed in two layers with separate muscular and mucosal sutures. If fibrosis or peridiverticular adhesions are present prohibiting simple diverticula eversion, then the bladder mucosa around the diverticular ostium is sharply incised and the diverticular neck is dissected free of the surrounding bladder musculature. The neck can be grasped with clamps and traction applied on the diverticulum; the underlying peridiverticular adhesions can be freed from the diverticular sac with a moist gauze as the diverticulum is pulled into the bladder. The bladder wall is then closed in two layers with absorbable suture.

Large diverticula can be approached via a combined intra- and extravesical technique in which the diverticular neck is first incised and dissected extravesically with careful attention to the location of the ipsilateral ureter and ureteral opening. Filling the diverticulum with moist gauze can better delineate the margins of the sac, especially if there is significant peridiverticular fibrosis and adhesions. Once the diverticulum is removed, the bladder wall defect is closed with a standard two-layer technique.

Minimally Invasive Surgical Excision: Laparoscopic and/or Robotic Diverticulectomy

Increasingly, bladder diverticulectomy has been performed with a minimally invasive approach by the use of standard laparoscopic instruments as well as robotic assistance. Both transperitoneal [48] and extraperitoneal [49] laparoscopic approaches have been described; robotic-assisted laparoscopic diverticulectomy via a transperitoneal approach has also recently been reported [50, 51]. Both standard and robotic-assisted laparoscopic techniques essentially emulate the standard principles of open surgical repair, with the notable difficulty of identifying the diverticulum intraoperatively. Several techniques have been described to facilitate visualization of diverticula during laparoscopic surgery, including cystoscopic transillumination [52], transurethral angiocatheter [51] and Foley catheter balloon insertion [49], and separate diverticulum and bladder catheterization.

Bladder Diverticulum Associated with Malignancy

Bladder diverticula harboring malignancy warrant treatment consistent with oncologic principles. Prognosis is poorly understood and a wide range of 2- and 5-year survival rates of patients with tumors in diverticula have been published. Two-year survival rates of 16–90% and 5-year rates of 72% have been published, albeit from relatively small, heterogeneous cohorts [38, 39, 53–56]. Clinical stage is the most important

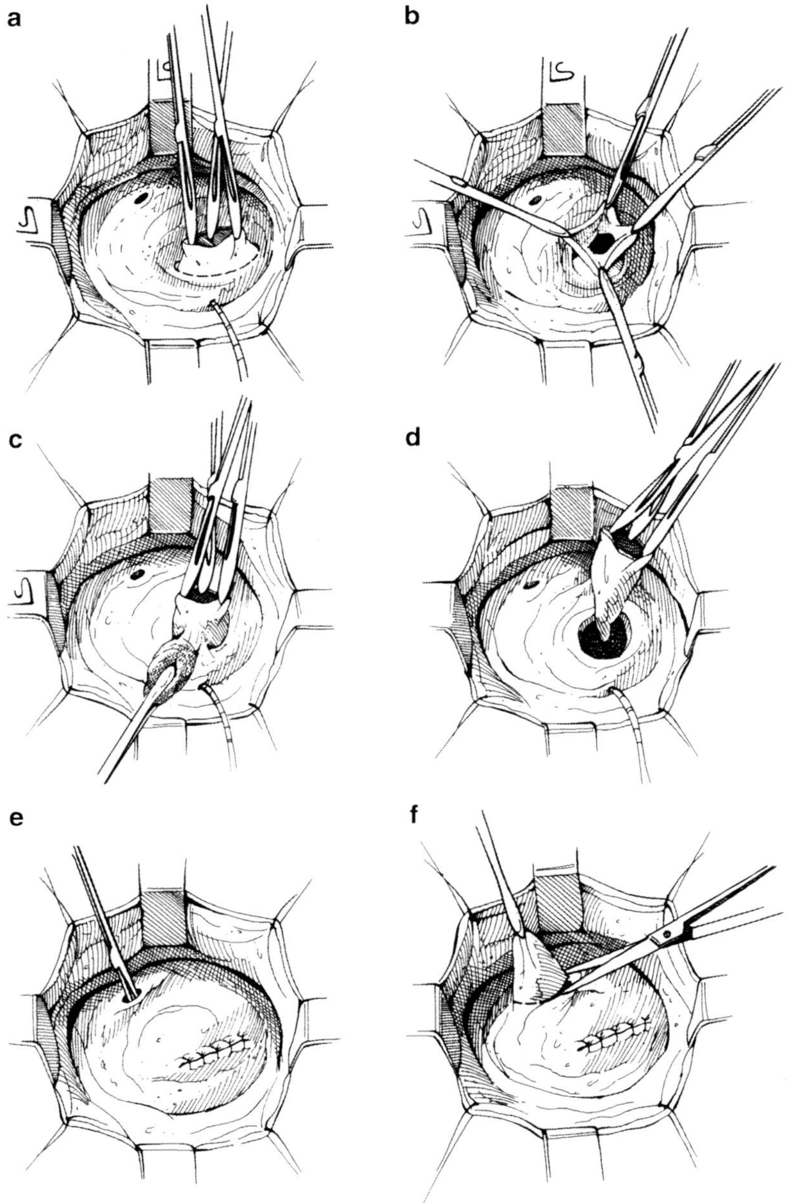

Fig. 3.3 Transvesical bladder diverticulectomy. Resection of medium-sized diverticula and those with significant peridiverticular adhesions is performed by incising around the neck of the diverticulum (**a**) and pulling the edges up into the bladder (**b**), while sweeping off the extravesical adhesions until freed (**c** and **d**). Small diverticula can be inverted into the lumen of the bladder and the neck transected before closing the bladder in two layers (**e** and **f**). Reproduced with permission from Cookson et al. [47]

prognostic indicator, as patients with noninvasive disease fare significantly better than those with invasion at 5 years (83% vs. 45% survival) [38]. TUR with intravesical therapy has been described; however, partial cystectomy or diverticulectomy with or without adjuvant intravesical chemotherapy as well as radical cystectomy are all preferred treatment modalities.

Urethral Diverticula

Urethral diverticula have traditionally been an enigmatic and elusive entity for the treating physician. Although relatively common in today's referral practice, urethral diverticula were not well described until the middle of the twentieth century, perhaps coinciding with improvement in radiographic techniques more sensitive to diverticula detection [14]. Indeed, urethral diverticula have been described as being "found in direct proportion to the avidity with which it is sought". [57] Urethral diverticula can be found in both men and women, although more commonly in women. In fact, differences in diverticula in men and women represent significantly divergent pathologic and etiologic entities, as diverticula occurring in men are almost exclusively related to postoperative consequences [58].

Female urethral diverticula are also primarily acquired and are estimated to occur in 1–6% of women [59]; however, the prevalence is higher (10%) when women with lower urinary tract symptoms are screened with dedicated pelvic MRI [60], suggesting that a significant number of diverticula are either asymptomatic or undiagnosed. Diverticula usually present in the third to fifth decades, but occur in women of all ages [61]. Racial differences have been described, with black women being affected more commonly than white women [62]; however, these differences have not been borne out in other series [63].

Clinical Presentation

The classical presentation of urethral diverticula is described as the "3 Ds": Dysuria, Dyspareunia, and Dribbling (postvoid). However, this symptom complex is neither specific nor sensitive for detecting urethral diverticula, and only a minority of patients will present with this trilogy of symptoms alone. Most patients present with nonspecific lower urinary tract complaints, including irritative voiding symptoms, dysuria, and recurrent UTI [14]. A majority will describe symptoms of frequency (40–100%) and dysuria (30–70%) [61], while up to 24% will report dyspareunia and up to 30% postvoid dribbling [62]. Recurrent UTI will present in up to a third of patients [62]. Additional presenting symptoms include hematuria, tender vaginal mass, retention, stones, urethral discharge, and urinary incontinence. Urinary incontinence may be present in up to 60% of patients and may be either genuine stress incontinence or paradoxical incontinence (loss of urine associated with intermittent drainage of the diverticulum) [64]. Symptoms can often be episodic with long periods (months to years) between flares [65]. Up to 20% of patients may be asymptomatic and may be diagnosed incidentally on imaging or physical examination [14].

Because of the nonspecific symptoms with which urethral diverticula present, a broad range of differential diagnoses may be considered, including vaginal wall cyst, cystocele, urethrocele, Skene's gland abscess, periurethral fibrosis, urethral carcinoma, urinary incontinence, interstitial cystitis, urgency-frequency syndrome, as well as idiopathic pelvic pain [66]. Furthermore, distinguishing between different etiologies of vaginal masses can also be subtle and misleading [67, 68]. Misdiagnosis is common and it is routine for patients to suffer a significant delay before the appropriate diagnosis is made. When specifically studied, mean intervals from symptom onset to diagnosis of 9.5 months to 5.2 years have been reported [65, 69], with an average of nine different physicians consulted before diagnosis made in one published series [65].

Pathogenesis

Urethral Anatomy

The female urethra is a 3- to 4-cm membranous tube connecting the bladder neck to the external urethral meatus and comprised of an epithelial lining invested in a thick envelope of smooth and skeletal muscle and fibroelastic tissue [14].

The urethra is lined proximally by urothelial or transitional epithelium and distally by nonkeratinized stratified squamous epithelium. Closely associated with the urethra and emptying posterolaterally into the distal third of the lumen are a series of 6–30 mucus-secreting tubuloalveolar glands homologous to the prostate gland in males, the periurethral glands [70]. The most distal ducts of these glands actually empty lateral the urethral meatus in the vulva and are known as Skene's ducts. Anatomic support for the urethra is provided by the urethropelvic ligament, a bilaminar sheet of connective tissue spanning the urogenital diaphragm, attached to both pelvic sidewalls at the tendinous arc of the obturator muscle. It is between these two laminae of the urethropelvic ligament that the urethra courses and the periurethral glands are located.

Pathogenesis

The true etiology of urethral diverticula is still unknown, but diverticula are generally thought to be acquired lesions related to pathology of the periurethral glands. Common hypothesis of formation suggests that repeated infection and obstruction of periurethral glands result in the formation of periurethral abscesses and cysts. These areas of focal purulent collection subsequently rupture and drain into the urethral lumen. With connections to the lumen, these areas become urethral outpouchings and can undergo epithelialization to become urethral diverticulum. Repeated inflammation/infection and urine trapping then lead to progression and enlargement. Alternatively, there have been a few reports of acquired diverticula after midurethral sling placement that suggest urethral diverticula develop from protrusion of urethral tissue through iatrogenic defects in the urethropelvic fascia under influence of proximal, elevated urethral pressures [71]. Congenital urethral abnormalities and birth trauma have also been hypothesized as etiologies, although urethral diverticula are rare in children [64] and 15–20% of nulliparous women present with diverticula [72].

Cystoscopic/Clinical Examination Findings

Physical examination of the anterior urethral wall with careful palpation may demonstrate a mass with or without tenderness. Urethral diverticula are typically located ventrally over the middle and proximal urethra, approximately 2–3 cm inside the introitus. The position and relation of a vaginal mass to the urethral meatus should be noted, as this can help differentiate a urethral diverticula from a Skenes gland abscess, which may present more distally and drain lateral to the meatus [68]. Classically, a urethral diverticulum may be demonstrated by "milking" a tender cystic mass or "stripping" the urethra with expression of pus or cloudy urine via the meatus; however, this classical sign is only present in a minority of patients [65]. A firm mass or nodule may suggest the presence of stone within the urethra or even carcinoma and a high index of suspicion should be aroused.

Endoscopic evaluation of the urethra and bladder should be performed, although urethral diverticula may be very difficult to visualize within the urethra, particularly if associated with a small ostium or the diverticulum is collapsed [73]. Diverticulum compression during urethroscopy may aid in the identification of the ostium by demonstrating the location of expressed diverticular contents into the urethra [74]. The use of a blunt-tip female cystourethroscope with a zero-degree lens may also help with visualization of the urethra.

Radiologic Imaging

A variety of radiographic techniques have been employed for identifying urethral diverticula. Historically, voiding cystourethrography (VCUG) was considered the best study to demonstrate urethral diverticula and has an overall reported accuracy of 85% [75] but a sensitivity of only 65% [72]. However, the study quality can be limited by patient factors, including discomfort and difficulty urinating, while locating the orifice can be very difficult and complex diverticular configurations may not be well visualized. Presently, VCUG is not considered a particularly useful study in the workup of suspected urethral diverticula.

Double-balloon or positive pressure urethrography as modification of retrograde urethrography was developed in 1959 [76] and has been demonstrated to be superior to VCUG in direct comparisons [77]. An overall accuracy of 90% has been reported [78]. Double-balloon urethrography (DBU) involves the use of a specialized urethral catheter with two balloons to "isolate" the urethra by obstructing the bladder neck and urethral meatus simultaneously. Iodinated contrast is injected into the isolated urethra under pressure, thereby filling any urethral communications or diverticula. The procedure can be cumbersome to perform and is associated with significant patient discomfort. Given these limitations and the advent of less invasive cross-sectional imaging and ultrasound, DBU is not used commonly today.

Ultrasonography (US) can be used for evaluation of urethral diverticula via transabdominal, transperineal, or transluminal techniques. Transabdominal and to some extent transperineal US techniques are limited for the detection of urethral diverticula as they are relatively insensitive to detecting smaller diverticula and thus suboptimal. Transluminal US, whether performed transvaginally, transurethrally, or transrectally, has greater sensitivity and provides better anatomic delineation. Transvaginal US can image the entire urethra from bladder neck to meatus and can provide such information as the size, number, location, structure, content, and wall thickness of diverticula [79]. Transvaginal US may be limited by compression of the urethral lumen causing distortion, which may be avoided alternatively by employing transrectal US [80]. Transurethral or endourethral US has been employed in select cases [81] and has demonstrated excellent sensitivity and specificity (100%) when used intraoperatively to delineate diverticular structure and location [82].

Conventional computed tomography (CT) has limited utility in the diagnosis and characterization of urethral diverticula, which may be demonstrated as a cystic mass adjacent to the urethra. However, more sophisticated CT image acquisition and processing techniques, including three-dimensional (3-D) reconstruction, have led to the development of new techniques of urethral evaluation, including CT voiding urethrography and virtual urethroscopy [83]. In this technique, CT scan images are rapidly acquired during voiding of bladder-instilled iodinated contrast material and then are used to generate two-dimensional (2-D) or 3-D images, including CT virtual urethroscopic images. Reconstructed 2-D images can demonstrate excellent cross-sectional anatomy of the urethra and associated structures in all imaging planes (axial, sagittal, and coronal), while 3-D surface rendering can be used to simulate a fiberoptic urethroscopic examination (CT virtual endoscopy), depicting, for example, the diverticular ostium within the lumen of the urethra. While experience with CT urethrography is limited, there are reports that correlate it well with MRI studies and findings at the time of surgery [70].

MRI is currently considered the mainstay of urethral diverticula imaging. Urethral MRI may be performed with a pelvic or torso phased-array coil or with an endoluminal coil (endorectal, endovaginal, or endourethral), which improves high-resolution imaging. Endoluminal MR imaging (i.e., with endovaginal coil) is the most accurate method for identifying and characterizing female urethral diverticula, being more sensitive than urethrography or endoscopy for the diagnosis of diverticula [70]. T2-weighted images best delineate the female urethra and urethral diverticulum, which appears as a hyperintense, fluid-filled structure (see Fig. 3.4). Gadolinium-enhanced images can improve soft tissue contrast and may be useful for detecting inflammation and malignancy within a diverticulum. Excellent cross-sectional imaging of axial anatomy of the urethra and adjacent structures can be achieved with MR imaging while avoiding ionizing radiation exposure or invasiveness associated with other forms of diverticular imaging.

Pathology

Pathologically, a urethral diverticulum is defined as a sac-like protrusion or pocket that is continuous with the lumen of the urethra [84]. A "true"

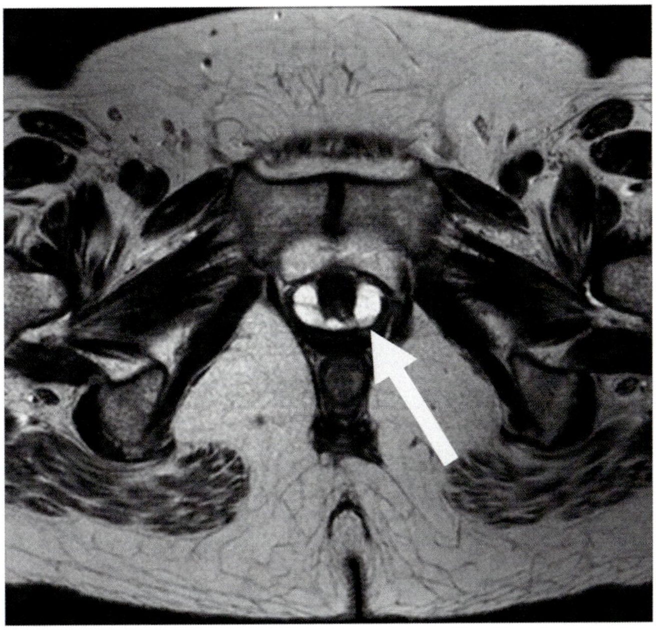

Fig. 3.4 On T2-weighted MRI, a urethral diverticulum appears as a hyperintense, fluid-filled structure in close proximity to the urethral lumen (*arrow*)

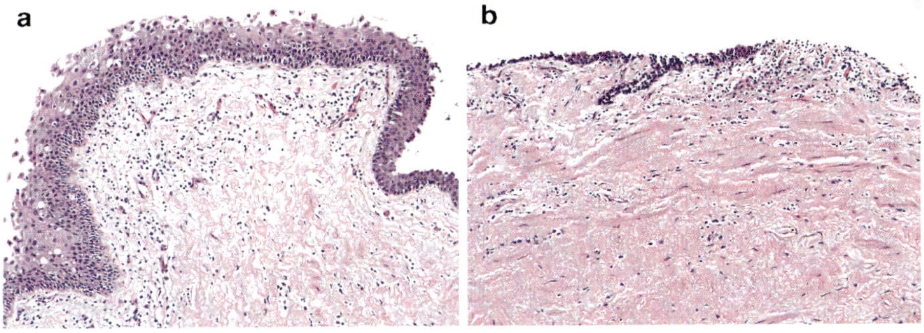

Fig. 3.5 Urethral diverticula can be lined by different types of epithelia including urothelial, squamous (**a**), and cuboidal/columnar (**b**) cells

diverticulum pathologically includes all urethral layers, including muscle tissue, while a "false" or pseudodiverticulum suggests a deficiency of urethral layers is present. Implicit in either definition is that the diverticular surface lining is in continuity with the urethra epithelium and thus would be similar in character to that of the urethra proper. The urethral lining proximally is characterized by urothelium, while the distal urethra is lined by stratified squamous epithelium. Both of these epithelial cell types are found lining diverticula, as well as columnar and cuboidal cell types (Fig. 3.5a, b) [85].

Typically, a narrow neck connects the urethral diverticulum to the urethral lumen, while the diverticulum protrudes into and through the periurethral smooth muscle to lie within the wall of the urethra in a ventral location. In the vast majority of cases, the ostium of the diverticulum is located posterolaterally in the mid or distal urethra, corresponding to the location of periurethral cyst ducts. Diverticula may be of variable sizes, ranging from a few millimeters to several centimeters. Several urethral connections may exist, and complex diverticula

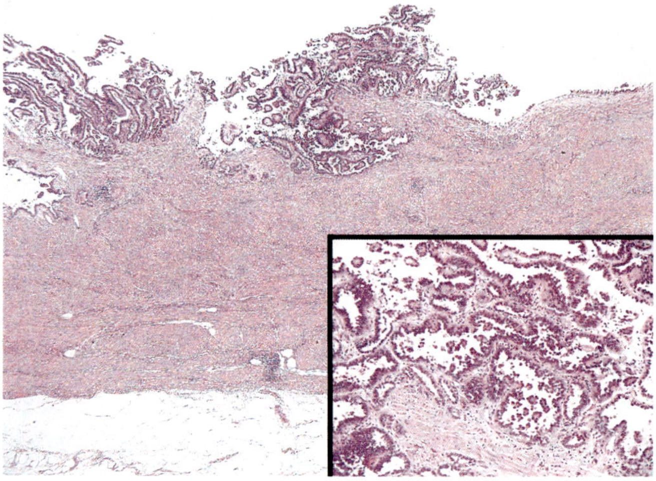

Fig. 3.6 A urethral diverticulum complicated by the development of adenocarcinoma, better depicted on higher magnification (*inset*)

structures can be seen with septations and extension around part ("saddlebag" or "horseshoe") or all of the urethra ("circumferential"). Noncommunicating diverticula have also been demonstrated with MRI [86].

A recent report of 22 histologically examined diverticula described a predominance of squamous (42%) and columnar (32%) epithelial types as well as combined squamous and columnar (18%) and cuboidal (14%); however, no diverticula demonstrated urothelial cell type lining [84]. Furthermore, no muscle tissue was detected within the wall of all diverticula, which was composed mainly of fibrous collagen tissue. The authors associated these histopathologic features with analogous pathological descriptions of paraurethral cysts and suggested both urethral diverticula and paraurethral cysts should be considered as common entities.

Epithelial metaplasia is a common finding in urethral diverticula, with progression to dysplasia and neoplasia well described. In a series of 90 urethral diverticula, only 16 (18%) demonstrated "normal" urothelial tissue and 18 (20%) demonstrated squamous metaplasia, while 10 (11%) had nephrogenic adenomas and 5 (6%) had intestinal metaplasia [87]. Nine (10%) diverticula were found to harbor neoplastic changes, including with 5 (6%) invasive adenocarcinoma (Fig. 3.6), 3 with high-grade dysplasia, and 1 with low-grade dysplasia. Generally, squamous cell carcinoma is the most common urethral carcinoma in women; however, this increased prevalence of adenocarcinomas in urethral diverticula has been reported by others as well [88–90]. Approximately 60% of neoplasias arising in urethral diverticula are adenocarcinomas, while 30% are urothelial and only 10% are squamous cell carcinomas [72]. The disproportionate number of adenocarcinomas arising in diverticula is consistent with the etiologic concept of diverticula developing from periurethral glandular structures, although mechanisms of metaplasia and epithelial degeneration are also likely contributory.

Some attempts have been made to standardize descriptions of urethral diverticula and classify them based on anatomic, pathologic, or etiologic factors. Leach et al. proposed a staging system, the *L/N/S/C3* classification system, which factors in diverticular *L*ocation, *N*umber, *S*ize, anatomic *C*onfiguration, site of *C*ommunication to the urethral lumen, and *C*ontinence status [91]. Although designed to be simple to use, the LNSC3 system has not been used widely in contemporary practice. Leng and McGuire proposed a dichotomous classification system to distinguish true diverticula (representing de novo diverticula, adherent to the classic periurethral cyst/infection etiology) from pseudodiverticula, which result from traumatic injury to urethral support tissues (specifically postsurgical defects in periurethral fascia) and protrusion of mucosa through this defect under the force of repeated hydrostatic/voiding pressure [71].

Management

Nonoperative Management

The natural history of urethral diverticula is unknown. For asymptomatic or mildly symptomatic diverticula, particularly if small, conservative management with observation may be warranted [61]. Antibiotics and even anticholinergic therapy can provide some relief in patients with mild symptoms [92]. Any associated finding, such as the presence of stones or diverticular mass, warrants further investigation and possibly surgical treatment.

Transurethral Procedures

Several transurethral procedures have been described for the treatment of urethral diverticula, although they are not widely accepted. Transurethral unroofing of the diverticulum with fulguration of the lining of the sac has been described and results in decompression as well as contraction and scarring of the sac [62, 93]. Additionally, transurethral enlargement of the diverticular ostium by a linear or longitudinal incision with a knife electrode [94] or cold-knife [95] urethrotome also decompresses the diverticulum to promote drainage and results in rapid symptomatic improvement. Long-term outcomes are lacking, however, and there are concerns regarding diverticular recurrence.

For distal diverticula, marsupialization via a posterior urethral meatotomy with incision of the urethrovaginal septum allows for drainage and closure by secondary intention [96]. Once the ostium is identified in the urethra, the urethral meatus and distal urethral lumen are incised sharply along the ventral aspect through the entire thickness of the urethrovaginal septum, incorporating the ostium proximally. A distal urethrovaginal fistula is essentially created, allowing free drainage of the diverticulum. This technique is only appropriate for distally located diverticular ostia; marsupialization too proximal or adjacent to the urinary sphincter mechanism may result in urinary incontinence.

Transvaginal Surgical Excision

Definitive surgical treatment for urethral diverticula involves complete excision of the diverticular sac and ostium and reconstruction of the urethral defect with watertight suture lines and interposition tissue layers [74]. This is approached via a transvaginal technique with the patient in the lithotomy position. The essential steps in urethral diverticulectomy are illustrated in Fig. 3.7. Care must be taken to dissect and preserve the periurethral fascia for closure purposes, while meticulous dissection and excision of the entire diverticular wall or sac are critical, so as to identify and excise the neck or ostium of the diverticulum. A watertight, tension-free urethral closure with multilayered tissue interposition layers is necessary, including the use of a labial fat pad (Martius flap) interposition if tissue quality is poor.

Concomitant SUI Procedures

Up to 50% of patients presenting with urethral diverticula will demonstrate urodynamically confirmed stress urinary incontinence (SUI) [64] and there is considerable debate as to the merits of performing concomitant SUI procedures at the time of diverticulectomy. Some authors have advocated for the routine use of autologous pubovaginal suburethral sling placement routinely in patients undergoing diverticular excision [97, 98], while others prefer a staged approach to treating the incontinence [61, 66]. It is generally agreed that the use of synthetic sling material should be avoided at the time of diverticulectomy because of concerns of infection and erosion [99].

Management of Diverticulum Associated with Malignancy

There is little consensus on managing urethral carcinomas arising within a urethral diverticulum [100]. Most diverticular carcinomas tend to

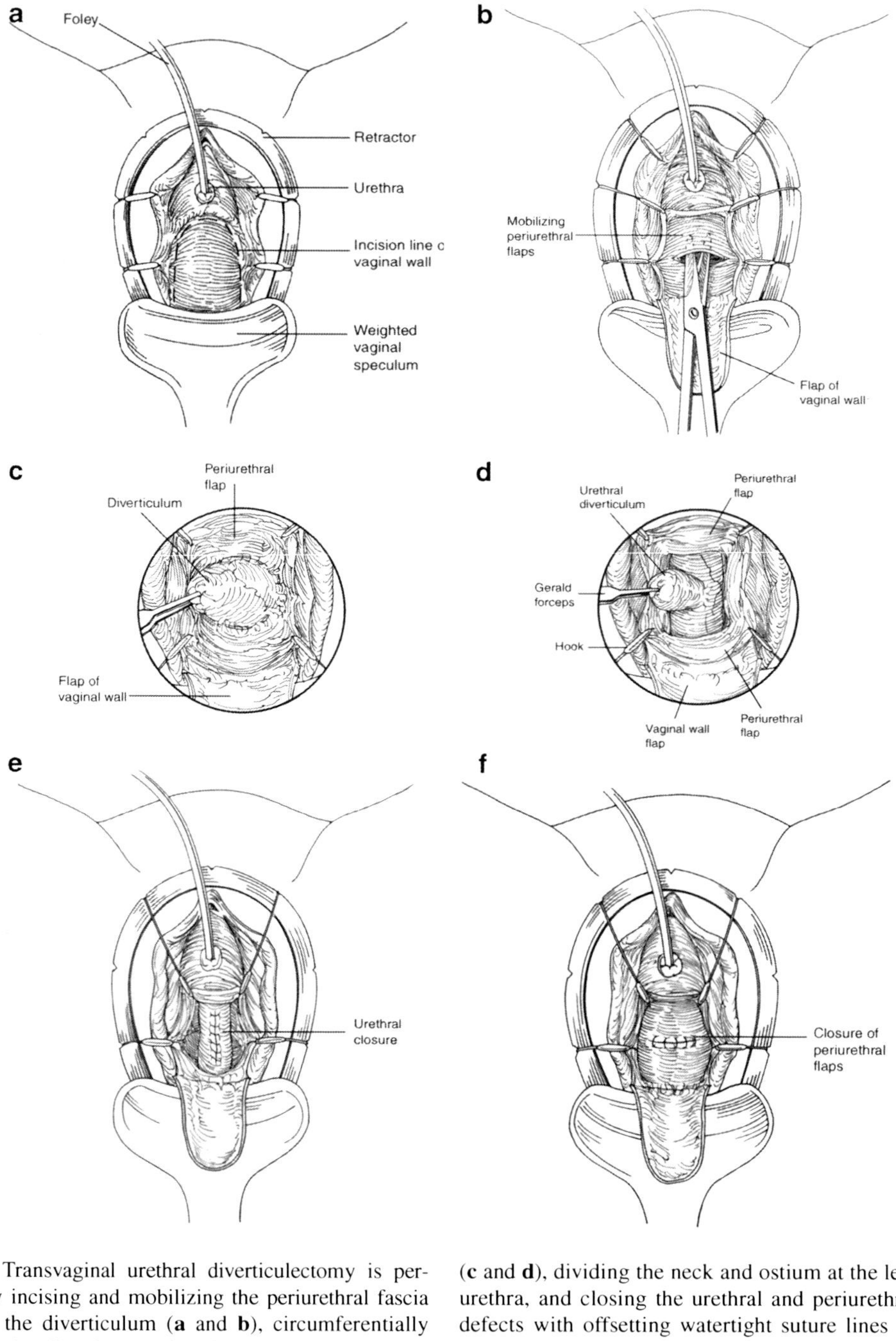

Fig. 3.7 Transvaginal urethral diverticulectomy is performed by incising and mobilizing the periurethral fascia overlying the diverticulum (**a** and **b**), circumferentially dissecting the diverticulum free from surrounding tissue (**c** and **d**), dividing the neck and ostium at the level of the urethra, and closing the urethral and periurethral fascial defects with offsetting watertight suture lines (**e** and **f**). Reproduced with permission from Scarpero et al. [74]

present with local invasion on tumor staging, with a higher predominance of stage T2 or higher lesions. For this reason, it is generally accepted that aggressive surgical excision, including pelvic exenteration, is warranted; however, the efficacy of diverticulectomy alone and the role of adjuvant chemotherapy or radiotherapy have not been studied.

References

1. Garat JM, Angerri O, Caffaratti J, Moscatiello P, Villavicencio H. Primary congenital bladder diverticula in children. Urology. 2007;70(5):984–8.
2. Boechat MI, Lebowitz RL. Diverticula of the bladder in children. Pediatr Radiol. 1978;7(1):22–8.
3. Hutch JA. Saccule formation at the ureterovesical junction in smooth walled bladders. J Urol. 1961; 86:390–9.
4. Blane CE, Zerin JM, Bloom DA. Bladder diverticula in children. Radiology. 1994;190(3):695–7.
5. Babbitt DP, Dobbs J, Boedecker RA. Multiple bladder diverticula in Williams "Elfin-Facies" syndrome. Pediatr Radiol. 1979;8(1):29–31.
6. Schulman SL, Zderic S, Kaplan P. Increased prevalence of urinary symptoms and voiding dysfunction in Williams syndrome. J Pediatr. 1996;129(3):466–9.
7. Burrows NP, Monk BE, Harrison JB, Pope FM. Giant bladder diverticulum in Ehlers-Danlos syndrome type I causing outflow obstruction. Clin Exp Dermatol. 1998;23(3):109–12.
8. Schippers E, Dittler HJ. Multiple hollow organ dysplasia in Ehlers-Danlos syndrome. J Pediatr Surg. 1989;24(11):1181–3.
9. Levard G, Aigrain Y, Ferkadji L, Elghoneimi A, Pichon J, Boureau M. Urinary bladder diverticula and the Ehlers-Danlos syndrome in children. J Pediatr Surg. 1989;24(11):1184–6.
10. Harcke Jr HT, Capitanio MA, Grover WD, Valdes-Dapena M. Bladder diverticula and Menkes' syndrome. Radiology. 1977;124(2):459–61.
11. Daly WJ, Rabinovitch HH. Urologic abnormalities in Menkes' syndrome. J Urol. 1981;126(2):262–4.
12. Frimberger D, Kropp BP. Bladder anomalies in children. In: Wein A, Kavoussi L, Novick A, Partin A, Peters C, editors. Campbell Walsh urology. 9th ed. Philadelphia, PA: Saunders Elsevier; 2007. p. 3573–82.
13. Amar AD. Vesicoureteral reflux associated with congenital bladder diverticulum in boys and young men. J Urol. 1972;107(6):966–8.
14. Rovner ES. Bladder and urethral diverticula. In: Wein AJ, Kavoussi LR, Novick AC, Partin AW, Peters CA, editors. Campbell-Walsh urology. 9th ed. Philadelphia: Saunders Elsevier; 2007. p. 2361–90.
15. Senger FL, Bottone JJ, Rothfeld SH. Bladder diverticulum in the female. J Urol. 1952;68(4): 699–702.
16. Roehrborn CG, McConnell JD. Benign prostatic hyperplasia: etiology, pathophysiology, epidemiology, and natural history. In: Wein AJ, Kavoussi LR, Novick AC, Partin AW, Peters CA, editors. Campbell-Walsh urology. 9th ed. Philadelphia: Saunders Elsevier; 2007. p. 2727–65.
17. Doehn C, Baumgärtel M, Fornara P, Jocham D. The largest bladder diverticulum ever? J Urol. 1999;162(3 Pt 1):793–4.
18. Hartung W, Flocks RH. Diverticulum of the bladder: a method of roentgen examination and roentgen and clinical findings in 200 cases. Radiology. 1943; 41:363.
19. Burns E. Diverticula of the urinary bladder. Ann Surg. 1944;119(5):656–64.
20. Gerridzen RG, Futter NG. Ten-year review of vesical diverticula. Urology. 1982;20(1):33–5.
21. Schewe J, Brands EH, Pannek J. The inguinal bladder diverticulum: a rare differential diagnosis of hernias. Int Urol Nephrol. 2000;32(2):255–6.
22. Buchholz NP, Biyabani R, Talati J. Bladder diverticulum as an unusual content of a femoral hernia. Br J Urol. 1998;82(3):457–8.
23. Pieretti RV, Pieretti-Vanmarcke RV. Congenital bladder diverticula in children. J Pediatr Surg. 1999;34(3):468–73.
24. Tamas EF, Stephenson AJ, Campbell SC, Montague DK, Trusty DC, Hansel DE. Histopathologic features and clinical outcomes in 71 cases of bladder diverticula. Arch Pathol Lab Med. 2009;133(5): 791–6.
25. Stephens FD. The vesicoureteral hiatus and paraureteral diverticula. J Urol. 1979;121(6):786–91.
26. Linke C, Mongiat-Artus P. [Management of vesical diverticula]. Ann Urol (Paris). 2004;38(3):103–11.
27. Peterson LJ, Paulson DF, Glenn JF. The histopathology of vesical diverticula. J Urol. 1973;110(1):62–4.
28. Wesselhoeft Jr CW, Perlmutter AD, Berg S, Unger L, Gherardi GJ, Harrison JH, et al. Pathogenesis and surgical treatment of diverticulum of the urinary bladder. Surg Gynecol Obstet. 1963;116:719–25.
29. Hsu HL, Huang KH, Chang CC, Liu KL. Which one is true bladder?—a giant urinary bladder diverticulum. QJM. 2011;104(2):169–70.
30. Powell CR, Kreder KJ. Treatment of bladder diverticula, impaired detrusor contractility, and low bladder compliance. Urol Clin North Am. 2009;36(4):511–25, vii.
31. Nieder AM, Meinbach DS, Kim SS, Soloway MS. Transurethral bladder tumor resection: intraoperative and postoperative complications in a residency setting. J Urol. 2005;174(6):2307–9.
32. Collado A, Chechile GE, Salvador J, Vicente J. Early complications of endoscopic treatment for superficial bladder tumors. J Urol. 2000;164(5):1529–32.
33. Balbay MD, Cimentepe E, Unsal A, Bayrak O, Koc A, Akbulut Z. The actual incidence of bladder perforation following transurethral bladder surgery. J Urol. 2005;174(6):2260–2, discussion 2–3.
34. El Hayek OR, Coelho RF, Dall'oglio MF, Murta CB, Ribeiro Filho LA, Nunes RLV, et al. Evaluation of the incidence of bladder perforation after transurethral bladder tumor resection in a residency setting. J Endourol. 2009;23(7):1183–6.
35. Mydlo JH, Weinstein R, Shah S, Solliday M, Macchia RJ. Long-term consequences from bladder perforation and/or violation in the presence of transitional cell carcinoma: results of a small series and a

review of the literature. J Urol. 1999;161(4): 1128–32.
36. Skolarikos A, Chrisofos M, Ferakis N, Papatsoris A, Dellis A, Deliveliotis C. Does the management of bladder perforation during transurethral resection of superficial bladder tumors predispose to extravesical tumor recurrence? J Urol. 2005;173(6):1908–11.
37. Messing EM. Urothelial tumors of the bladder. In: Wein AJ, Kavoussi LR, Novick AC, Partin AW, Peters CA, editors. Campbell-Walsh urology. 9th ed. Philadelphia, PA: Saunders Elsevier; 2007. p. 2407–46.
38. Golijanin D, Yossepowitch O, Beck SD, Sogani P, Dalbagni G. Carcinoma in a bladder diverticulum: presentation and treatment outcome. J Urol. 2003;170(5):1761–4.
39. Kelalis PP, McLean P. The treatment of diverticulum of the bladder. J Urol. 1967;98(3):349–52.
40. Fellows FJ. The association between vesical carcinoma and diverticulum of the bladder. Eur Urol. 1978;4(3):185–6.
41. Vitale PJ, Woodside JR. Management of bladder diverticula by transurethral resection: re-evaluation of an old technique. J Urol. 1979;122(6):744–5.
42. Schulze S, Hald T. Voiding inability after transurethral resection of a bladder diverticulum. Scand J Urol Nephrol. 1983;17(3):377–8.
43. Orandi A. Transurethral fulguration of bladder diverticulum: new procedure. Urology. 1977;10(1):30–2.
44. Clayman RV, Shahin S, Reddy P, Fraley EE. Transurethral treatment of bladder diverticula. Alternative to open diverticulectomy. Urology. 1984;23(6):573–7.
45. Adachi M, Nakada T, Yamaguchi T, Suzuki H, Hirano J, Hirano K, et al. Transurethral treatment of bladder diverticula. Eur Urol. 1991;19(2):104–8.
46. Yamaguchi K, Kotake T, Nishikawa Y, Yanagi S, Namiki T, Ito H. Transurethral treatment of bladder diverticulum. Urol Int. 1992;48(2):210–2.
47. Cookson MS, Change SS. Bladder diverticulectomy. In: Graham J, Sam D, editors. Glenn's urologic surgery. 6th ed. Philadelphia: Lippincott Williams & Wilkins; 2004. p. 178–83.
48. Parra RO, Jones JP, Andrus CH, Hagood PG. Laparoscopic diverticulectomy: preliminary report of a new approach for the treatment of bladder diverticulum. J Urol. 1992;148(3):869–71.
49. Nadler RB, Pearle MS, McDougall EM, Clayman RV. Laparoscopic extraperitoneal bladder diverticulectomy: initial experience. Urology. 1995;45(3): 524–7.
50. Myer EG, Wagner JR. Robotic assisted laparoscopic bladder diverticulectomy. J Urol. 2007;178(6):2406–10; discussion 10.
51. Tareen BU, Mufarrij PW, Godoy G, Stifelman MD. Robot-assisted laparoscopic partial cystectomy and diverticulectomy: initial experience of four cases. J Endourol. 2008;22(7):1497–500.
52. Jarrett TW, Pardalidis NP, Sweetser P, Badlani GH, Smith AD. Laparoscopic transperitoneal bladder diverticulectomy: surgical technique. J Laparoendosc Surg. 1995;5(2):105–11.
53. Faysal MH, Freiha FS. Primary neoplasm in vesical diverticula. A report of 12 cases. Br J Urol. 1981; 53(2):141–3.
54. Melekos MD, Asbach HW, Barbalias GA. Vesical diverticula: etiology, diagnosis, tumorigenesis, and treatment. Analysis of 74 cases. Urology. 1987; 30(5):453–7.
55. Baniel J, Vishna T. Primary transitional cell carcinoma in vesical diverticula. Urology. 1997;50(5): 697–9.
56. Montague DK, Boltuch RL. Primary neoplasms in vesical diverticula: report of 10 cases. J Urol. 1976;116(1):41–2.
57. Moore TD. Diverticulum of female urethra; an improved technique of surgical excision. J Urol. 1952;68(3):611–6.
58. Alphs HH, Meeks JJ, Casey JT, Gonzalez CM. Surgical reconstruction of the male urethral diverticulum. Urology. 2010;76(2):471–5.
59. Burrows LJ, Howden NLS, Meyn L, Weber AM. Surgical procedures for urethral diverticula in women in the United States, 1979-1997. Int Urogynecol J Pelvic Floor Dysfunct. 2005;16(2):158–61.
60. Lorenzo AJ, Zimmern P, Lemack GE, Nurenberg P. Endorectal coil magnetic resonance imaging for diagnosis of urethral and periurethral pathologic findings in women. Urology. 2003;61(6):1129–33; discussion 33–4.
61. Handel LN, Leach GE. Current evaluation and management of female urethral diverticula. Curr Urol Rep. 2008;9(5):383–8.
62. Davis BL, Robinson DG. Diverticula of the female urethra: assay of 120 cases. J Urol. 1970;104(6): 850–3.
63. Leach GE, Bavendam TG. Female urethral diverticula. Urology. 1987;30(5):407–15.
64. Ganabathi K, Leach GE, Zimmern PE, Dmochowski R. Experience with the management of urethral diverticulum in 63 women. J Urol. 1994;152(5 Pt 1): 1445–52.
65. Romanzi LJ, Groutz A, Blaivas JG. Urethral diverticulum in women: diverse presentations resulting in diagnostic delay and mismanagement. J Urol. 2000;164(2):428–33.
66. Patel AK, Chapple CR. Female urethral diverticula. Curr Opin Urol. 2006;16(4):248–54.
67. Dmochowski RR, Ganabathi K, Zimmern PE, Leach GE. Benign female periurethral masses. J Urol. 1994;152(6 Pt 1):1943–51.
68. Fletcher SG, Lemack GE. Benign masses of the female periurethral tissues and anterior vaginal wall. Curr Urol Rep. 2008;9(5):389–96.
69. Rufford J, Cardozo L. Urethral diverticula: a diagnostic dilemma. BJU Int. 2004;94(7):1044–7.
70. Chou C-P, Levenson RB, Elsayes KM, Lin Y-H, Fu T-Y, Chiu Y-S, et al. Imaging of female urethral diverticulum: an update. Radiographics. 2008;28(7): 1917–30.

71. Leng WW, McGuire EJ. Management of female urethral diverticula: a new classification. J Urol. 1998; 160(4):1297–300.
72. Lee JWS, Fynes MM. Female urethral diverticula. Best Pract Res Clin Obstet Gynaecol. 2005;19(6):875–93.
73. Saito S. Usefulness of diagnosis by the urethroscopy under anesthesia and effect of transurethral electrocoagulation in symptomatic female urethral diverticula. J Endourol. 2000;14(5):455–7.
74. Scarpero H, Dmochowski R, Leu P. Female urethral diverticula. Atlas Urol Clin. 2004;12(2):205–12.
75. Blander DS, Rovner ES, Schnall MD, Ramchandani P, Banner MP, Broderick GA, et al. Endoluminal magnetic resonance imaging in the evaluation of urethral diverticula in women. Urology. 2001;57(4): 660–5.
76. Lang EK, Davis HJ. Positive pressure urethrography: a roentgenographic diagnostic method for urethral diverticula in the female. Radiology. 1959; 72(3):401–5.
77. Jacoby K, Rowbotham RK. Double balloon positive pressure urethrography is a more sensitive test than voiding cystourethrography for diagnosing urethral diverticulum in women. J Urol. 1999;162(6):2066–9.
78. Drutz HP. Urethral diverticula. Obstet Gynecol Clin North Am. 1989;16(4):923–9.
79. Fontana D, Porpiglia F, Morra I, Destefanis P. Transvaginal ultrasonography in the assessment of organic diseases of female urethra. J Ultrasound Med. 1999;18(3):237–41.
80. Vargas-Serrano B, Cortina-Moreno B, Rodriguez-Romero R, Ferreiro-Arguelles I. Transrectal ultrasonography in the diagnosis of urethral diverticula in women. J Clin Ultrasound. 1997;25(1):21–8.
81. Siegel CL, Middleton WD, Teefey SA, Wainstein MA, McDougall EM, Klutke CG. Sonography of the female urethra. AJR Am J Roentgenol. 1998; 170(5):1269–74.
82. Chancellor MB, Liu JB, Rivas DA, Karasick S, Bagley DH, Goldberg BB. Intraoperative endo-luminal ultrasound evaluation of urethral diverticula. J Urol. 1995;153(1):72–5.
83. Chou CP, Huang JS, Wu MT, Pan HB, Huang FD, Yu CC, et al. CT voiding urethrography and virtual urethroscopy: preliminary study with 16-MDCT. AJR Am J Roentgenol. 2005;184(6):1882–8.
84. Tsivian M, Tsivian A, Shreiber L, Sidi AA, Koren R. Female urethral diverticulum: a pathological insight. Int Urogynecol J. 2009;20(8):957–60.
85. Rovner ES. Urethral diverticula: a review and an update. Neurourol Urodyn. 2007;26(7):972–7.
86. Daneshgari F, Zimmern PE, Jacomides L. Magnetic resonance imaging detection of symptomatic noncommunicating intraurethral wall diverticula in women. J Urol. 1999;161(4):1259–61; discussion 61–2.
87. Thomas AA, Rackley RR, Lee U, Goldman HB, Vasavada SP, Hansel DE. Urethral diverticula in 90 female patients: a study with emphasis on neoplastic alterations. J Urol. 2008;180(6):2463–7.
88. Clayton M, Siami P, Guinan P. Urethral diverticular carcinoma. Cancer. 1992;70(3):665–70.
89. Aspera AM, Rackley RR, Vasavada SP. Contemporary evaluation and management of the female urethral diverticulum. Urol Clin North Am. 2002;29(3): 617–24.
90. Seballos RM, Rich RR. Clear cell adenocarcinoma arising from a urethral diverticulum. J Urol. 1995;153(6):1914–5.
91. Leach GE, Sirls LT, Ganabathi K, Zimmern PE. L N S C3: a proposed classification system for female urethral diverticula. Neurourol Urodyn. 1993;12(6):523–31.
92. Fortunato P, Schettini M, Gallucci M. Diagnosis and therapy of the female urethral diverticula. Int Urogynecol J Pelvic Floor Dysfunct. 2001;12(1): 51–7.
93. Spencer WF, Streem SB. Diverticulum of the female urethral roof managed endoscopically. J Urol. 1987;138(1):147–8.
94. Lapides J. Transurethral treatment of urethral diverticula in women. J Urol. 1979;121(6):736–8.
95. Vergunst H, Blom JH, De Spiegeleer AH, Miranda SI. Management of female urethral diverticula by transurethral incision. Br J Urol. 1996;77(5): 745–6.
96. Spence HM, Duckett Jr JW. Diverticulum of the female urethra: clinical aspects and presentation of a simple operative technique for cure. J Urol. 1970;104(3):432–7.
97. Migliari R, Pistolesi D, D'urso L, Muto G. Recurrent pseudodiverticula of female urethra: five-year experience. Urology. 2010;73(6):1218–22.
98. Faerber GJ. Urethral diverticulectomy and pubovaginal sling for simultaneous treatment of urethral diverticulum and intrinsic sphincter deficiency. Tech Urol. 1998;4(4):192–7.
99. Dmochowski RR, Blaivas JM, Gormley EA, Juma S, Karram MM, Lightner DJ, et al. Update of AUA guideline on the surgical management of female stress urinary incontinence. J Urol. 2010;183(5): 1906–14.
100. Ahmed K, Dasgupta R, Vats A, Nagpal K, Ashrafian H, Kaj B, et al. Urethral diverticular carcinoma: an overview of current trends in diagnosis and management. Int Urol Nephrol. 2010;42(2):331–41.

Infection and Inflammatory Disorders

4

Charles C. Guo and Courteney K. Moore

Introduction

Cystitis is the broad term encompassing the inflammatory response of the urinary bladder to various harmful stimuli. In the acute phase, cystitis is characterized by enhanced blood flow to the urinary bladder that results in leakage and accumulation of leukocytes and plasma in the bladder wall. In the chronic phase, cystitis is generally a healing process characterized by simultaneous tissue destruction and repair. Although cystitis rarely results in the death of a patient, it often leads to significant morbidity. Patients may develop general symptoms, such as fever, chill, malaise, and lethargy, as well as urinary symptoms, such as dysuria, frequency, urgency, and suprapubic pain. Patients may also have marked changes in urine, including hematuria, bacteriuria, and/or pyuria.

A variety of "injuries" can cause cystitis. The most common injury is infection from various microorganisms. Bacteria, most commonly *Escherichia coli*, account for the majority of pathogens. Bacteria infect the bladder most commonly by ascending the urethra. In females, adherence of pathogens to the introital and urothelial mucosa plays a significant role in ascending infections. Occasionally, bacteria may infect the bladder via a hematogenous or lymphatic route. Fungal and viral infections usually occur in immunocompromised patients. Protozoa, such as schistosomiasis, are rarely seen in the United States, but are prevalent in some areas of Africa and the Middle East. Noninfectious injuries—such as physical trauma (e.g., instrumentation, catheterization, and bladder stones), radiation, and chemotherapeutic agents—can also evoke a cystitis-type response. In some cases, such as interstitial cystitis, malakoplakia, and eosinophilic cystitis, the exact etiology is unclear despite distinctive manifestations and histologic features.

In this chapter, cystitis is divided into two broad categories, infectious cystitis and inflammatory cystitis, based on the presence or absence of infectious pathogens. Under each category, a variety of specific entities with distinct pathological and clinical features will be discussed.

Infectious Cystitis

Bacterial Cystitis

Infectious cystitis, or urinary tract infection (UTI), is the second most common infectious disease in humans, second only to respiratory tract

C.C. Guo (✉)
Department of Pathology, University of Texas MD Anderson Cancer Center, 1515 Holcombe Boulevard, Unit 085, Houston, TX 77030, USA
e-mail: ccguo@mdanderson.org

C.K. Moore
Department of Surgery, Cleveland Clinic Lerner College of Medicine of Case Western Reserve University, 9500 Euclid Avenue, Q-10, Cleveland, OH 44195, USA
e-mail: moorec6@ccf.org

D.E. Hansel et al. (eds.), *The Urinary Tract: A Comprehensive Guide to Patient Diagnosis and Management*, DOI 10.1007/978-1-4614-5320-8_4, © Springer Science+Business Media New York 2012

infections. UTI is the most common urological disease in the United States and leads to 8 million visits to physicians' offices, 1.5 million visits to emergency rooms, and 300,000 hospital admissions every year [1, 2]. UTIs account for 1.2% of all office visits by women and 0.6% of all office visits by men [3]. The annual cost to treat UTIs is about $3.5 billion US dollars [1]. Women are more frequently affected than men partly due to female pelvic and urethral anatomy. In women, the urethra is relatively short and in close proximity to the anus, making the urinary bladder easily accessible to bacteria.

Bacterial cystitis, the most common bacterial infection in humans, accounts for the overwhelming majority of UTIs. More than 80% of bacterial cystitis is caused by *E. coli*, a normal flora in the lower gastrointestinal tract [4]. Other bacterial species, such as *Staphylococcus saprophyticus*, *Klebsiella pneumoniae*, *Streptococcus faecalis*, *Proteus vulgaris*, *Neisseria gonorrhoeae*, *Salmonella typhi*, and *diphtheroids*, have also been implicated in bacterial cystitis. Risk factors include urinary obstruction, catheterization, cystoscopy, pregnancy, and diabetes. Frequent sexual activity also significantly increases the risk of bacterial cystitis [5].

Normal urine is generally sterile in the urinary bladder. When bacteria colonize the urine, patients may develop bacterial cystitis. Bacteriuria is defined as the presence of bacteria in the urine. Bacteria may be identified by microscopic examination of the urine or indirectly detected by a dipstick test for nitrite. Bacterial culture, the gold standard, not only confirms the diagnosis, but also provides valuable information regarding the sensitivity of bacteria to antibiotics. The microbiologic diagnosis of acute cystitis requires greater than or equal to 10^5 colony forming units (CFU) per mL. Because the urine is prone to contamination during the specimen collection and transfer, midstream clean-catch voided urine or catheterized urine may reduce the likelihood of contamination. Pyuria is defined as the presence of four or more neutrophils per high power field of unspun, voided midstream urine. Although it is most commonly associated with bacterial cystitis, pyuria can also be seen in other conditions, such as stones, Kawasaki disease, tuberculosis, and reaction to acetaminophen [6].

Bladder biopsy specimens generally show similar histologic features regardless of the type of bacteria involved in cystitis. In the acute phase, the urothelial mucosa may be ulcerated and covered by fibrinous exudate that contains abundant neutrophils sometimes mixed with bacterial colonies. The lamina propria is edematous and hyperemic with an intense neutrophilic infiltrate. In severe cases, suppuration and abscess may develop in the bladder wall. In the chronic phase, the neutrophils are gradually replaced with lymphocytes, eosinophils, macrophages, and plasma cells. Granulation tissue and fibrosis may be seen in the lamina propria. In general, bladder biopsy has limited value in establishing the diagnosis, which can be better accomplished by clinical presentation, urine examination, and urine culture.

Acute uncomplicated UTIs or acute uncomplicated cystitis is characterized by dysuria, frequency, urgency, suprapubic pressure, or pain, hematuria and occasionally nausea and vomiting. In the elderly and spinal cord injury patients, the symptoms may be subtle, consisting of abdominal discomfort, worsening incontinence, or they may be completely asymptomatic. Although urine culture is the gold standard of diagnosis, new onset frequency, dysuria, and urgency have a positive predictive value of 90% for acute cystitis [7]. As many as 10–20% of symptomatic patients may have negative urine cultures due to lower than 10^5 CFU [7].

In uncomplicated UTIs, *E. coli* is the most common pathogen, isolated in more than 80% of community acquired UTIs [8]. *Staphyloccoccus saprophyticus* accounts for 5–15%, especially in sexually active younger females, with the remaining 5–10% caused by aerobic gram-negative rods, such as *Klebsiella*, *Proteus*, and *enterococci* [8].

The North American Urinary Tract Infection Collaborative Alliance study from 2003 to 2004 determined the resistance rate of *E. coli* to ampicillin was 38%, trimethoprim-sulfamethoxazole (TMP/SMX) 21%, nitrofurantoin 1%, and ciprofloxacin 6% [8]. Several more recent studies have shown that aminopenicillins and fluoroquinolones have lost effectiveness against

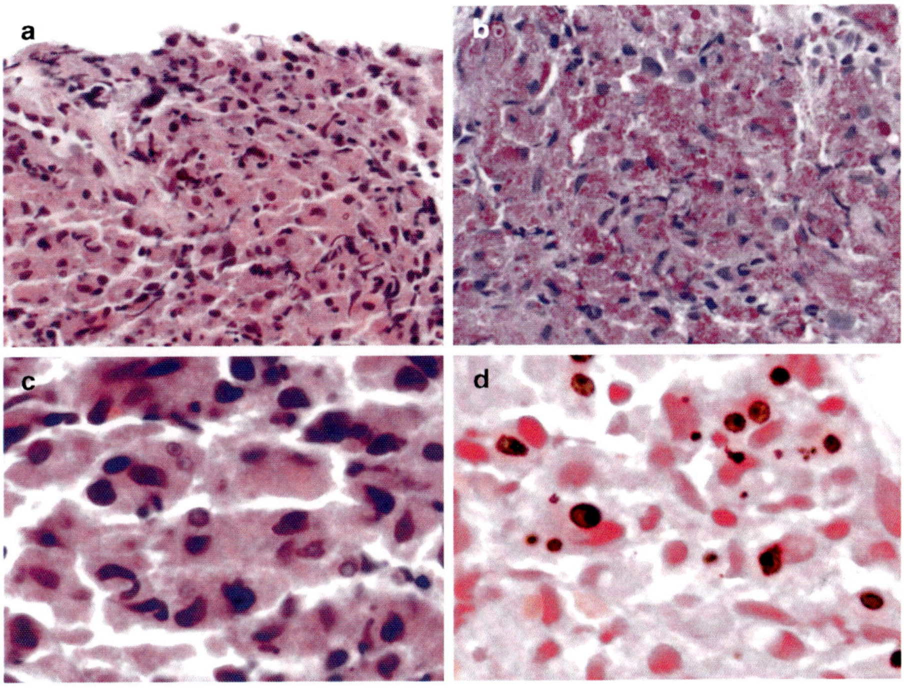

Fig. 4.1 (**a**) Malakoplakia shows abundant histiocytes with granular eosinophilic cytoplasm infiltrating the lamina propria. (**b**) Granular eosinophilic cytoplasm in histiocytes is highlighted on periodic acid-Schiff stain. (**c**) Target-like Michaelis-Guttman bodies are present in some histiocytes. (**d**) Michaelis-Gutman bodies are highlighted on von Kossa stain

typical acute cystitis pathogens due to increasing resistance [9]. Therefore, drugs with low resistance rates, such as TMP/SMX, fosfomycin, and nitrofurantoin, should be considered first-line in the treatment of uncomplicated UTIs. The Infectious Diseases Society of America Guidelines recommend TMP/SMX for 3 days as first-line treatment for acute uncomplicated cystitis [10]. In areas where the prevalence of *E. coli* resistance to TMP/SMZ is >20%, treatment with nitrofurantoin for 7 days or fluoroquinolone for 3 days is recommended.

Malakoplakia

Malakoplakia is a descriptive term used for soft plaque lesions in the urothelial mucosa. The word *malakoplakia* was derived from the Greek roots of *malakos* (soft) and *plakos* (plaque) [11]. Since it was first described in the urinary bladder by Michaelis and Gutmann, malakoplakia has also been reported in the skin, lymph nodes, bones, lungs, brain, and gastrointestinal tract [12, 13]. While malakoplakia may occur in children, it is most commonly seen in adults, with a peak incidence in the fifth decade. Most patients are women with a female: male ratio of 4:1. Patients may also have various degrees of suppressed immune status.

On cystoscopy, the lesions are characteristic of multiple, yellow-white, soft plaques on the urothelial mucosa. The plaques are often raised with an indentation at the center and a rim of congestion in the periphery. They are usually less than 2 cm and are more common at the bladder base. Microscopically, the plaque lesion is characterized by abundant histiocytes in the lamina propria (Fig. 4.1a). The histiocytes, or the so-called von Hansemann cells, contain granular eosinophilic cytoplasm that can be highlighted on the periodic acid-Schiff (PAS) stain (Fig. 4.1b). The histologic hallmark is the presence of intracytoplasmic inclusions, known as Michaelis-Gutmann bodies, in the histiocytes (Fig. 4.1c). Michaelis-Gutmann bodies, ranging from 2 to 10 μm in diameter, have a target-like appearance with a dense dot at the center and a lucent space in the periphery. They often contain calcium and sometimes iron that can be highlighted on von Kossa (calcium) (Fig. 4.1d) and Prussian blue (iron) stains, respectively. Mineralization occurs later in the disease process, so early lesions of malakoplakia may only stain with PAS. On electromicroscopy, Michaelis-Gutmann bodies consist of a dense crystalline core surrounded by a homogeneous zone of myelin figures. In later stages of malakoplakia, the diagnosis may be complicated by extensive fibrosis and granulation tissue response. An associated acute or chronic inflammatory infiltrate may also obscure the histiocytes at any phase. The most critical differential diagnostic consideration for the histologic diagnosis of malakoplakia is urothelial carcinoma with a sheet-like pattern of growth. The more striking nuclear pleomorphism and the cytokeratin immunoreactivity in the neoplastic cells of carcinomas should allow distinction in the majority of cases.

The etiology of malakoplakia is unclear. It was initially thought to be a response to bladder cancer or an infectious disease of fungi, tubercles bacilli, or virus. Recent studies have suggested that malakoplakia is likely to represent an impaired granulomatous reaction in which histiocytes cannot sufficiently eliminate phagocytosed bacteria [14]. *E. coli* is the most frequently cultured from the urine of patients with malakoplakia, and other bacteria, including *P. vulgaris*, *Aerobacter Aerogenes*, *K. pneumoniae*, and *Alpha-hemolytic streptococci*, have also been isolated [15]. Furthermore, ultrastructural studies reveal the presence of fragments of the *E. coli* wall in the histiocytes, supporting the premise that the histiocytes have a decreased ability to kill the bacteria in malakoplakia [16].

The typical presentation is bladder irritability and hematuria in a debilitated or immunosuppressed patient with chronic *E. coli* infections. Cystoscopy reveals yellow mucosal plaques or nodules within the bladder. As the disease progresses these nodules can grow and create radiographic filling defects of the bladder and eventually compression of the distal ureter leading to renal obstruction or ultimately renal failure.

Management should be aimed at eradicating the UTIs that perpetuate the disease process. Treatment with sulfonamides, rifampin, doxycycline, and TMP are very effective given their intracellular bactericidal activity [17]. Fluoroquinolones, because of macrophage ingestion, have also proven effective in the management of malakoplakia [18]. Several studies have demonstrated the beneficial effects of combination therapy, ascorbic acid or bethanechol and antimicrobial therapy, in treating malakoplakia [14, 19, 20]. Both agents are believed to increase intracellular cyclic guanosine monophosphate levels, the biologic defect causing macrophage dysfunction [21].

Tuberculous Cystitis

Tuberculous infection is rare in the USA, but its incidence has increased recently. The risk factors include human immunodeficiency virus (HIV) infection, organ transplantation, and immigration from developing countries [22]. The majority of tuberculous infection occurs in the lungs. In 10% of cases, tuberculous bacteria may also infect extrapulmonary sites. The genitourinary tract is the most common extrapulmonary site of tuberculous infection [23]. Most tuberculous infections of the urinary tract occur in the kidney, and tuberculous cystitis is usually secondary to renal tuberculosis due to a downstream effect. *Mycobacterium tuberculosis* is identified in most cases while *Mycobacterium bovis* is reported in only 3% of cases [24].

Microscopically, the characteristic lesions are composed of tuberculous granulomas, in which central caseous necrosis is surrounded by multinucleated giant cells, plasma cells, and lymphocytes. Acid-fast or auramine-rhodamine-stained sections will usually disclose mycobacteria, but the organisms may be very few in number and

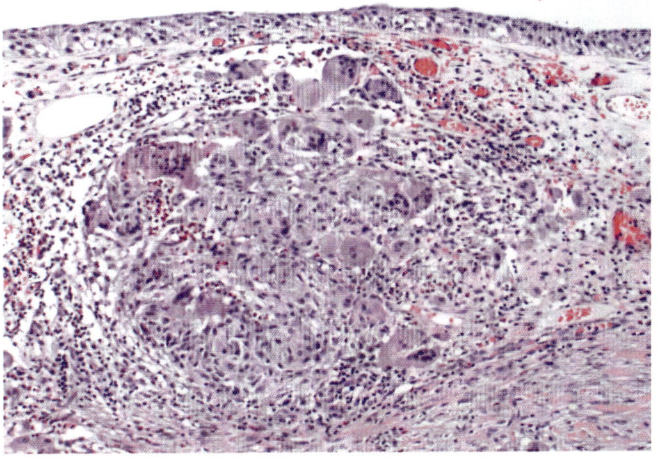

Fig. 4.2 BCG granuloma is composed of epithelioid histiocytes, multinucleated giant cells, and other inflammation cells

very careful and prolonged evaluation at high power magnification is often necessary for identification of the organisms. The absence of acid-fast bacilli by special stains and microscopy does not entirely exclude the diagnosis. In highly suspicious cases where organisms are not identified, additional tissue or urine cultures or molecular testing for *Mycobacterium* by polymerase chain reaction (PCR) methodology on the paraffin-embedded tissue may be utilized for diagnosis if needed.

Bacillus Calmette-Guérin (BCG) is an attenuated mycobacteria that is used to treat urothelial carcinoma in situ and superficially invasive urothelial carcinoma [25]. In the bladder, the live BCG organisms bind to the urothelium through the interaction of a fibronectin attachment protein on the bacteria surface with fibronectin in the urothelium. Although controversial, it has been proposed that BCG organisms are then internalized by the urothelial cells, leaving the mycobacterial surface glycoproteins, which serve as antigens to initiate a local immune response [26]. On bladder biopsy, the urothelium is often ulcerated. The characteristic finding is the presence of marked chronic granulomatous inflammation (Fig. 4.2). The granulomas are composed of epithelioid histiocytes, lymphocytes, and multinucleated giant cells. Occasionally, eosinophils are numerous. The granulomas typically have relatively round contours with no central necrosis; acid-fast stains may identify organisms, but special stains are not typically utilized in this setting. Nephrogenic adenoma has also been reported in patients who receive intravesical BCG therapy [27].

The presenting symptoms of tubercular cystitis are similar to those of any UTI: frequency, urgency, hematuria, and dysuria. Patients may also have systemic symptoms of tuberculosis, such as fever, night sweats, and weight loss.

If tuberculosis infection is suspected, at least 3, but preferably 5, consecutive early morning urines should be collected. The urine is classically characterized by a sterile pyuria; however, up to 20% of patients will not have leukocytes in the urine. Overt hematuria is present in only 10% of patients, but microscopic hematuria is present in up to 50% [21].

Cystoscopy is rarely indicated in the diagnosis of genitourinary TB and bladder biopsies are only indicated to rule out malignancy. Tuberculous cystitis often affects the ureteral orifices and trigone regions. In the acute phase, the urothelial mucosa may be congested and edematous. There are often tiny elevated yellow or white spots in the urothelial mucosa that may become ulcerated. In the chronic phase, the bladder wall becomes fibrotic and contracted, leading to a low capacity bladder; the ureteral orifices may be obstructed, causing hydronephrosis and hydroureter; in severe cases, fistula may develop and penetrate the bladder wall, resulting in peritonitis.

The current recommendation of the US Centers for Disease Control (CDC) is to treat compliant patients with drug-sensitive genitourinary TB for 6–9 months with rifampin, INH, pyrazinamide, and ethambutol [21]. Patients should have three consecutive early morning specimens of urine done at 3, 6, and 12 months. In the last decade, multidrug-resistant tuberculosis (MDR TB) emerged as a major public health problem. In this population, treatment regimens should be tailored to the organism's sensitivity and continued for 18–24 months or 12–18 months after cultures become negative [21].

Fungal Cystitis

Fungal cystitis is more commonly seen in immunocompromised patients. Other predisposing factors include indwelling catheters, antimicrobial therapy, diabetes mellitus, and hospitalization. Most patients with fungal cystitis are asymptomatic. Only 4% of patients are symptomatic and present with urgency, frequency, and hematuria [28]. The majority of fungal cystitis is caused by *Candida* species, particularly *C. albicans* [29]. Rarely fungal cystitis may be caused by *Aspergillus* species. Fungal cystitis can be due to either hematogenous spread or ascending infection via the urethra.

Cystoscopy may reveal sharply demarcated white plaques in the urothelial mucosa. The plaques are usually irregular in shape and are most commonly seen in the trigone. Occasionally, a fungus ball may be present in the bladder or in the upper tracts.

Microscopically, the urothelial mucosa may be ulcerated, and there is usually marked acute and chronic inflammation in the lamina propria. Fungal hyphae and budding yeast forms may be seen in routine sections, which can be highlighted on PAS or Gomori's methenamine silver stains.

Fungal infection is a difficult problem to diagnose. Blood and urine culture may detect fungi; however, fungemia and funguria are often transient. Bacterial cystitis is far more common and should be excluded before reaching the diagnosis of fungal cystitis. Recently, the detection of fungi using PCR methodology promises to be a valuable diagnostic tool with high sensitivity and specificity [30].

Treatment of funguria is recommended in symptomatic or immunocompromised patients. Removal of indwelling Foley catheters (and other foreign bodies such as ureteral stents) and cessation of antibiotics should be first-line therapy and may eradicate colonization or infection. In a prospective multicenter study of patients with nosocomial funguria, Kauffman et al. reported that in 116 patients who had catheter removal as the only treatment, the funguria resolved in 41 (35.3%) [28]. If candiduria does not resolve after removal of the indwelling urinary catheter or cessation of antibiotic therapy, then antifungal therapy should be initiated. This could include bladder irrigation, oral, and/or parenteral administration of antifungal agents. In a study by Lee et al., bladder irrigation with amphotericin B was faster at eradicating candiduria than oral or intravenous therapy. However, successful eradication rates 1–4 weeks after treatment were similar for all three regimens [31].

Viral Cystitis

Viral cystitis is rare in immunocompetent hosts, but it has been increasingly seen in immunocompromised patients. The common risk factors for immunosuppression include stem cell and solid organ transplantation, cancer chemotherapy, and HIV infection. Viral infections by BK virus, adenovirus, and cytomegalovirus have been associated with hemorrhagic cystitis [32]. Bladder biopsy evaluation, even with the use of specific immunohistochemical antibodies directed against viral antigens, is generally ineffective in diagnosing a specific viral infection. In some cases, the specific viral inclusions may be identified. Culture-based tests may be useful, but usually

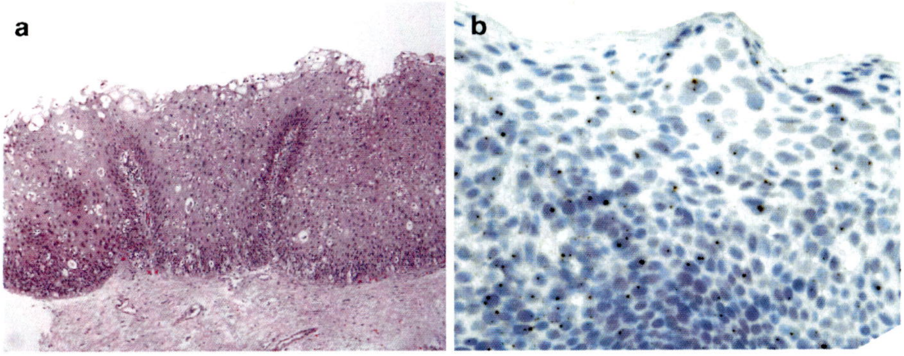

Fig. 4.3 (**a**) Condyloma acuminatum of the bladder shows papillary squamous hyperplasia with koilocytosis and wrinkled nuclei. (**b**) HPV in situ hybridization demonstrates punctuate nuclear stain of HPV DNA

take days or weeks. Furthermore, the sensitivity of viral culture is influenced by several factors, such as specimen transfer, blood transfusion, and therapy. Molecular technology, particularly real-time PCR, has become the diagnostic method of choice [33]. PCR is a rapid and sensitive test that can not only detect the specific viral pathogen but also quantify the viral load.

Studies have found that human papillomavirus (HPV) may cause condyloma acuminatum in the bladder [34, 35]. Most patients have concurrent condyloma of the external genitalia, urethra, and perineum, but some patients may have condylomata only in the bladder. Cystoscopy often reveals papillary lesions in the bladder trigone that may closely mimic papillary urothelial carcinoma. Microscopically, the lesions are characterized by papillary squamous hyperplasia with koilocytosis, clear cytoplasm, and wrinkled nuclei (Fig. 4.3a). HPV in situ hybridization often demonstrates punctate staining of HPV DNA in the nuclei (Fig. 4.3b). Condyloma of the urinary bladder may be associated with or progress to carcinoma and patients should be closely followed [34].

The clinical presentation of viral cystitis varies depending upon the immune status of the patient. In immunocompetent patients, symptoms are similar to bacterial cystitis: dysuria, urgency, frequency, hematuria, and suprapubic pressure. In immunocompromised hosts, fever, malaise, and significant gross hematuria are often present.

The diagnosis of viral cystitis is made primarily by ruling out a positive bacterial culture. In immunocompromised patients, cytology, enzyme-linked immunosorbent assay (ELISA), and PCR are often employed.

Like clinical manifestations, treatments vary depending on the status of the patient, with immunocompetent patients treated conservatively. In immunocompromised patients, the treatment depends on the virus and the degree of gross hematuria. Cidofovir is the drug of choice for human polyomavirus, adenovirus, and cytomegalovirus [32].

Schistosomal Cystitis

Schistosomiasis is one of the most common parasitic diseases in the world. There are more than 200 million people infected with Schistosoma worldwide, with most patients found in Africa and the Middle East [36]. Schistosomal infection is rare in the United States and other developed countries. Schistosomal cystitis, also known as bilharziasis, is a chronic infection of the urinary bladder by Schistosoma. Although four schistosomal species can infect humans, most schistosomal cystitis is caused by the species *S. haematobium*. Schistosoma infects humans when they come into contact with contaminated water [37]. The parasites, in the form of cercariae, penetrate the skin and enter the blood vessels.

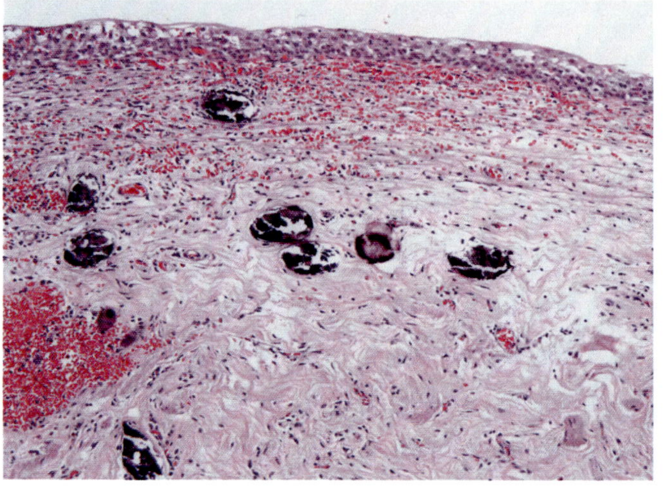

Fig. 4.4 Schistosoma shows calcified parasitic eggs in the bladder wall

The cercariae reach the liver via the bloodstream and mature into adult flukes. Then the flukes migrate to the venous plexuses around the bladder where the female fluke lays thousands of eggs every day. The eggs transverse the bladder wall and enter into the urinary bladder lumen. After the eggs are released from the host into the water supply, the eggs hatch and form miracardiae, which infect freshwater snails, the intermediate hosts. Inside snails, miracardiae evolve into cercariae and release into water. The free-swimming cercariae become infective to humans.

Schistosomal cystitis can be divided into active and chronic phases. In the acute phase, schistosomal eggs deposit in the muscularis propria and lamina propria of the bladder wall, eliciting an inflammatory reaction. The urothelial mucosa may become ulcerated, leading to hematuria and clot retention. There are usually abundant neutrophils, eosinophils, and lymphocytes in the bladder wall, which will be followed by chronic granulomatous inflammation with giant cell reaction. Large inflammatory polyps may form in the trigone and ureteral orifices, which may obstruct the ureters or the bladder outlet. In the chronic phase, eggs become calcified in the bladder wall (Fig. 4.4) and inflammatory polyps become fibrotic. Urothelial ulcers may still persist. Metaplastic changes, such as squamous and intestinal metaplasia, are common.

The diagnosis of schistosomal cystitis is usually made by examination of the urine for eggs in the acute phase. The presence of terminally spined eggs in urinary sediment is pathognomonic of active *S. haematobium* infection. In the chronic phase, eggs may be difficult to find and serological and immunological tests may be helpful. Schistosomiasis should also be suspected in patients with chronic or recurrent UTIs caused by *Salmonella* species. *Salmonella* organisms reside in the apical invaginations of the schistosome tegument, where they are protected from host defenses and antibiotics.

Acutely, 3–6 weeks after infection, patients develop Katayama fever, characterized by lymphadenopathy, splenomegaly, eosinophilia, and urticaria. During the early chronic phase of the disease, 2–3 months after infection, eggs are excreted in the urine, accounting for the classic hematuria with terminal dysuria presentation. Hematuria can be very pronounced resulting in anemia or clot retention. Patients may also develop polypoid lesions of the bladder leading to urethral or ureteral obstruction.

The late chronic active stage, 4–7 months after infection, is characterized by schistosomal "contracted bladder" syndrome: constant, deep lower abdominal and pelvic pain, urgency, frequency, and incontinence [38]. During this phase the trigone appears normal or minimally hyperemic and

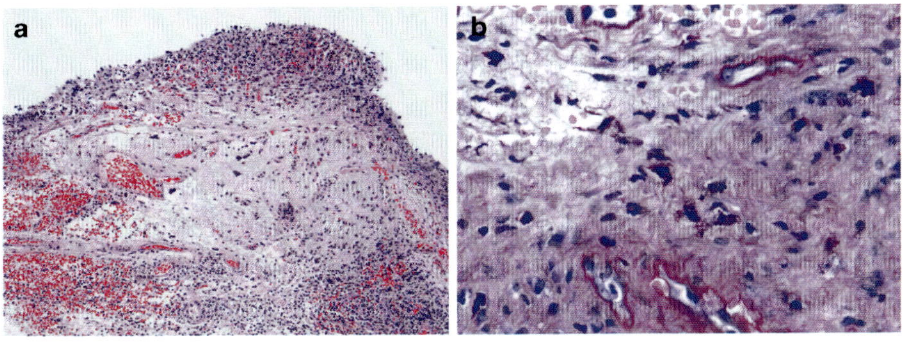

Fig. 4.5 (**a**) Interstitial cystitis shows inflammatory cells infiltrating the urothelial mucosa and lamina propria associated with hemorrhage. (**b**) Giemsa stain highlights mast cells infiltrating the muscularis propria in interstitial cystitis (courtesy of Dr. Steven Shen)

edematous, however, the entire bladder wall thickens, reducing the lumen and hence the bladder capacity to as little as 50 mL. Several years after active infection, patients enter the chronic inactive phase, in which viable eggs are no longer detected in urine or tissues. Signs and symptoms at this stage are caused by sequelae and complications rather than by the schistosomal infection.

All patients with schistosomiasis should be treated regardless of the intensity or apparent activity of their infection. Praziquantel is the drug of choice for all *Schistosoma* species with cure rates ranging from 83 to 100% [39]. It is well known that patients with schistosomal cystitis have an increased risk for the development of squamous cell carcinoma of the bladder and these patients should be followed with cystoscopy [40].

Bladder Inflammation Diseases

Interstitial Cystitis

Interstitial cystitis is a chronic inflammatory disease characterized by a triad of bladder pain, urinary frequency, and urgency. It was first described by Hunner, and, therefore, has also been referred to as Hunner's ulcer [41]. Interstitial cystitis varies in symptoms and severity. For the patients who suffer from chronic bladder pain but do not meet the strict criteria for interstitial cystitis, the term painful bladder syndrome (PBS) has been used [42, 43]. Recently the European Society for the Study of Interstitial Cystitis has adopted the term "bladder pain syndrome/interstitial cystitis" to include all cases of chronic bladder pain that cannot be attributed to other specific causes [44]. According to this broad definition, the prevalence of the disease is estimated to be 300 in women and 30 in men per 100,000 [45]. Interstitial cystitis poses a diagnostic challenge for both urologists and pathologists, and the diagnosis can only be made after other specific causes have been ruled out and repeated urine cultures for microorganisms are negative.

Cystoscopy may reveal punctate hemorrhage and fissure in the urothelial mucosa after bladder distention. Radiating scars may be seen in the late phase of disease. Interstitial cystitis often affects the dome, posterior and lateral walls, but is rarely present in the trigone.

Bladder biopsy specimens have a variety of appearances. There is usually an infiltrate of lymphocytes and plasma cells in the lamina propria (Fig. 4.5a). Hemorrhage and edema may also be seen in the lamina propria. When present, Hunner ulcers in the urothelial mucosa are wedge-shaped and covered by fibrin and necrotic material. An increased number of mast cells are often seen in the specimen, particularly in the muscularis propria. Mast cells may become numerous when an ulcer is present. However, there is lack of consensus in the literature regarding what is the "normal" concentration of mast cells in the bladder wall, partly due to the difficulty of counting mast cells on routine hematoxylin and eosin stained sections and their increased numbers in other unrelated inflammatory conditions. Special chemical stains, such as Toluidine blue and Giemsa (Fig. 4.5b) or immunostains for CD117 (c-kit), may be helpful in the counting. Overall, however, the diagnosis of interstitial cystitis is based on clinical features, and the pathologic features are not specific. The major role of bladder biopsy is not to specifically diagnose interstitial cystitis, but rather to rule out other conditions, particularly urothelial carcinoma in situ, which may clinically mimic interstitial cystitis.

Interstitial cystitis or PBS, the terminology preferred by the International Continence Society (ICS), is defined as "the complaint of suprapubic pain related to bladder filling, accompanied by other symptoms such as increased daytime and nighttime frequency, in the absence of proven urinary infection or other obvious pathology." [46] However, the ICS does reserve the diagnosis of IC for patients with "typical cystoscopic and histological features."

The diagnosis of IC/PBS is a diagnosis of exclusion, requiring a complete history, physical examination, appropriate cultures, and local cystoscopy to rule out infectious, malignant, and muscular etiologies of frequency, urgency, and pelvic pain.

Urodynamic evaluation typically demonstrates decreased bladder capacity and hypersensitivity. The characteristic findings on cystoscopy are glomerulations and Hunner ulcers. However, glomerulations can be seen in other disease processes such as radiation cystitis and carcinoma. Conversely, in a study by Messing et al., 8.7% of patients undergoing cystoscopy with hydrodistention for IC/PBS had no cystoscopic evidence of glomerations [47].

First-line treatment of IC/PBS involves dietary manipulation (avoidance of spicy and acidic food and beverages), nonprescription analgesics, and pelvic floor physical therapy. When these modalities fail, oral medications (amitriptyline, Elmiron, anti-muscarinics), intravesical treatment, or hydrodistention are prescribed or performed. There are numerous agents used in intravesical treatment, depending on the institution, with varying levels of evidence, which is beyond the scope of this book. Those patients refractory to oral and intravesical therapy are candidates for more invasive and aggressive modalities such as neuromodulation, pain clinic consultation, and narcotic analgesia. Should patients not respond to third-line therapy, surgical intervention such as augmentation cystoplasty or urinary diversion with or without cystectomy may be necessary.

Eosinophilic Cystitis

Eosinophilic cystitis (EC) is a rare variant of cystitis characterized by a prominent eosinophilic infiltrate in the bladder wall. It has been reported at all ages (5 days to 87 years), with 20% of cases occurring in children [48]. It is equally distributed between males and females. The common presenting symptoms are urinary frequency, dysuria, and hematuria. Based on the etiology, EC may be divided into two groups: one group is associated with allergic diseases (asthma, eosinophilic gastroenteritis, and eosinophilia in the peripheral blood) and the other group is associated with bladder injury (transurethral resection, urothelial carcinoma, and benign prostatic hyperplasia) [49]. While most patients in the first group are women and children, the majority of patients in the second group are elderly men. Rarely, EC is associated with parasitic infection. EC might be considered a pattern of inflammation that is not a specific entity as some patients with EC do not have a specific identifiable risk factor.

Cystoscopy usually finds erythematous changes in the urothelial mucosa. Sometimes there may be polypoid lesions resembling polypoid cystitis. Bladder biopsy is mandatory to establish the diagnosis of eosinophilic cystitis. In the acute phase, there is a prominent infiltrate of eosinophils in the bladder wall with edema and congestion (Fig. 4.6). Muscle necrosis may be present and is often associated with even more eosinophils. Popescu et al. have suggested a criterion of at least one eosinophil per high power

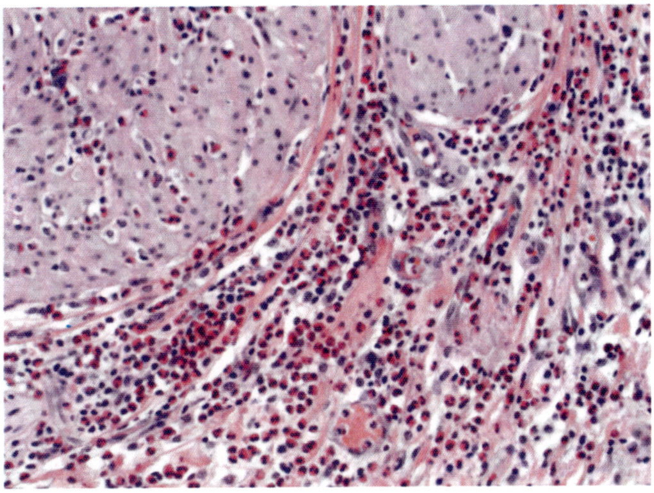

Fig. 4.6 Eosinophilic cystitis shows abundant eosinophils infiltrating the muscularis propria

field (40× magnification) [50]. In the chronic phase, the eosinophilic infiltrate may not be prominent and often mixed with lymphocyte, plasma cells, and mast cells.

The clinical manifestations of EC vary from mild irritative symptoms, urgency, and frequency dysuria to urinary retention and flank pain caused by an infiltrative mass causing upper tract obstruction [51, 52].

While physical exam is typically unremarkable, there are several case reports of patients presenting with lower abdominal masses [52]. Urinalysis is characterized by hematuria and pyuria, with a negative urine culture. Urine eosinophilia can occur, but is rare as eosinophils are rapidly degraded and urothelial shedding is minimal [52]. As with interstitial cystitis, other disease processes, such as carcinoma in situ, must be ruled out.

Radiographic findings may also vary from normal to bladder and ureteral filling defects resulting in hydronephrosis [51–53]. Cystoscopy reveals erythematous and polypoid lesions that mimic several urothelial neoplasms, making biopsies mandatory for the diagnosis.

Treatment of EC is primarily conservative. In patients with allergic EC, removal of the inciting agent and treatment with mitomycin-C and tranilast have yielded cure rates. In idiopathic cases of EC, antihistamines and nonsteroidals provide first-line treatment. In patients that do not respond to first-line modalities, corticosteroids, intravesical dimethylsulfoxide, and cyclosporine-A have been used [52]. In obstructing lesions, transurethral resection of the lesion is required. Those with significant symptoms, such as gross hematuria, clot retention, and/or pain, who do not respond to medical or transurethral resection may require more radical surgery, even cystectomy and urinary diversion [52].

Follicular Cystitis

Follicular cystitis is a histologic pattern of inflammation that is characterized by the presence of lymphoid follicles with germinal centers in the lamina propria of bladder (Fig. 4.7). It is usually discovered incidentally in bladder biopsy specimens. Cystoscopy may find small white or pink nodules on an erythematous urothelial mucosa. These lesions are more commonly seen in the trigone. The etiology of follicular cystitis is uncertain. Although it is often seen in patients with UTIs, follicular cystitis is also highly prevalent in bladder biopsy specimens from patients who do not have any evidence of UTIs. While Marsh et al. reported follicular cystitis in 35% of patients with UTIs, Sarma reported that up to 40% of patients with bladder cancer had

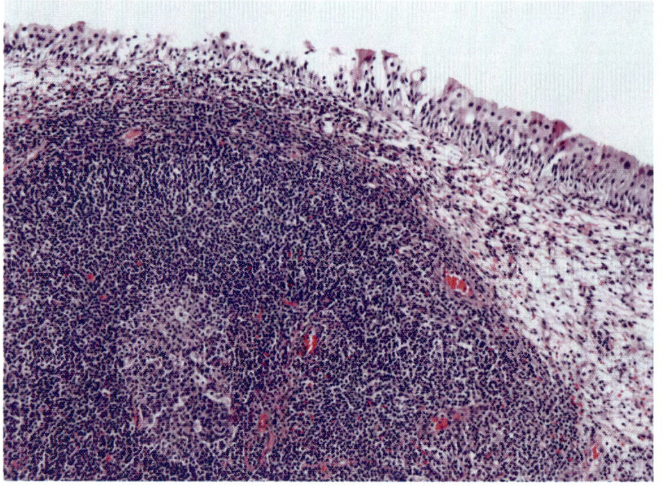

Fig. 4.7 Follicular cystitis shows a hyperplastic lymphoid follicle with a germinal center in the lamina propria (courtesy of Dr. Steven Shen)

follicular cystitis and half of these patients had sterile urine [54, 55]. The diagnosis of follicular cystitis is solely based on histologic examination, and occasionally follicular lymphoma may be considered in the differential diagnosis. In difficult cases, immunophenotypic studies may be utilized to distinguish reactive follicles from a lymphoma.

Clinically, patients present with irritative urinary symptoms consistent with acute cystitis and a negative urine culture. Treatment regimens vary with one case report citing successful remission with ciprofloxacin, vitamin A, and prednisone [56].

Hemorrhagic Cystitis

Hemorrhagic cystitis manifests as variable degrees of hematuria, ranging from microscopic hematuria to massive gross hematuria with clot retention. Blood clots irritate the bladder, leading to urinary frequency, urgency, and dysuria. The etiology of hemorrhagic cystitis is varied. Hemorrhagic cystitis most commonly occurs in cancer patients who have undergone chemotherapy or radiation therapy, but may be associated with UTIs. Cyclophosphamide is the drug most frequently responsible for hemorrhagic cystitis. It was reported that approximately 8% of patients who were treated with cyclophosphamide developed hemorrhagic cystitis [57]. Occasionally, the hematuria may be massive and intractable, requiring cystectomy. Radiation-induced hemorrhagic cystitis mostly commonly results from pelvic radiation. Hemorrhagic cystitis may develop acutely or months to years after therapy. Frequent hematuria has been reported in 0.5% of prostate cancer patients who undergo pelvic radiation [58].

Bladder biopsy specimens show nondescript hemorrhage and edema in the lamina propria (Fig. 4.8). The urothelium may be ulcerated and covered with fibropurulent exudate. Intravesical irrigation with mitomycin C and thiotepa may induce marked cytologic atypia that may be mistaken as urothelial carcinoma in situ; however, the cytologic atypia is usually limited to the superficial urothelium and lacks significant mitotic activity [59].

Hemorrhagic cystitis can range from mild to life-threatening hematuria. First-line treatment is bladder irrigation to prevent clot retention and the formation of organized clots. Several oral agents, sodium pentosan polysulfate, aminocaproic acid, and estrogen, as well as intravesical agents including alum, silver nitrate, prostaglandins, and formalin, have been used with varying degrees of success and possible side effects. If conservative options fail, life-saving measures may be required, including urinary diversion, cystectomy, or selective embolization of the hypogastric arteries.

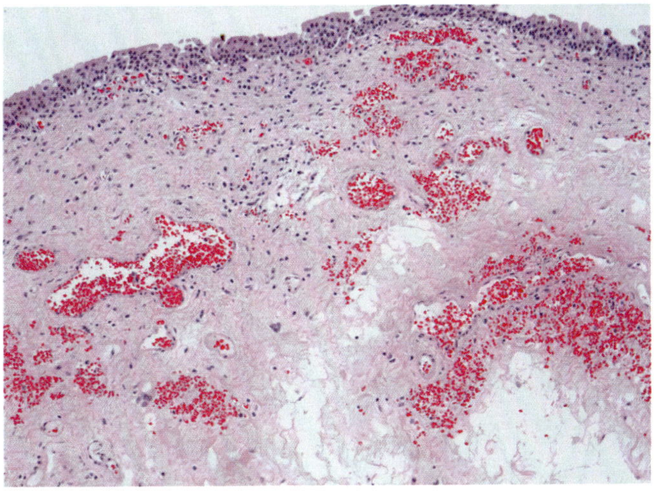

Fig. 4.8 Hemorrhagic cystitis shows diffuse hemorrhage and edema in the lamina propria. (courtesy of Dr. Steven Shen)

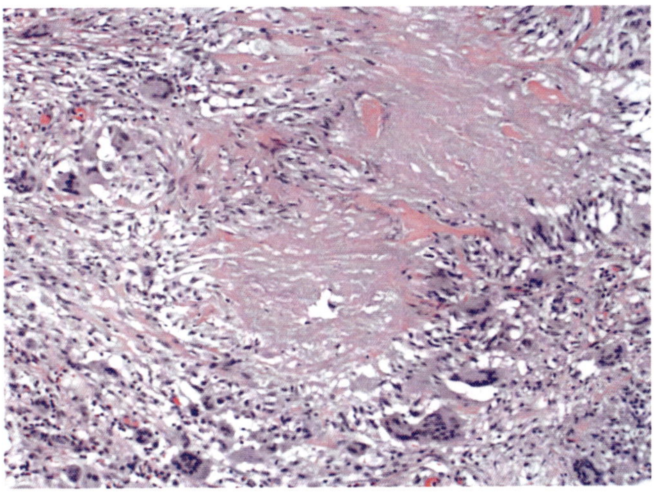

Fig. 4.9 Postsurgical granuloma (necrobiotic type) shows acellular eosinophilic fibrinoid material associated with histiocytes and multinuclear giant cells

Hyperbaric oxygen therapy—which induces capillary angiogenesis; increases fibroblast concentration; induces healing of tissue damage; and decreases edema, necrosis, and leukocyte infiltration—has shown some success in patients failing conservative therapies.

Postsurgical Granulomas

Granulomas may develop in surgical sites of the bladder after transurethral surgery using diathermic cautery. The occurrence of postsurgical granuloma is increased with the number of surgical procedures. Spagnolo and Waring reported that granulomas were present in 3% of patients who had bladder biopsy or resection, and the frequency increased to 13.6% in patients who had at least two surgical procedures [60]. Postsurgical granulomas may be either necrobiotic type or foreign body type [60, 61]. The necrobiotic granulomas are typically long and narrow with acellular eosinophilic fibrinoid material in the center and a band of palisading histiocytes in the periphery (Fig. 4.9). The foreign body type granulomas have abundant epithelioid histiocytes and foreign body giant cells. Both types of granulomas are often present in the same specimen. Eventually,

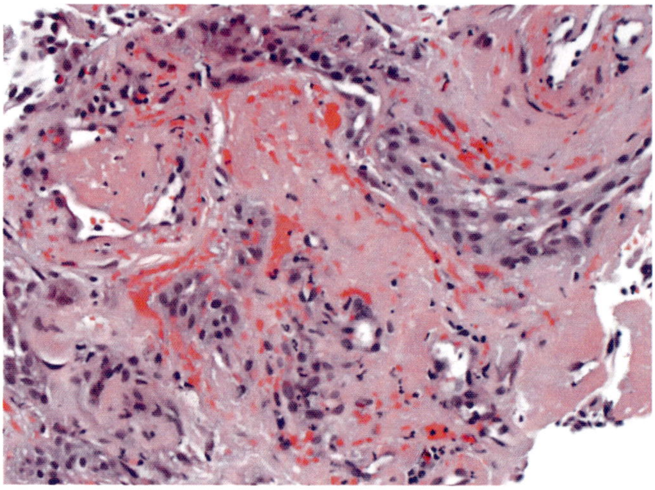

Fig. 4.10 Radiation cystitis shows nests of urothelial cells admixed with fibrin deposition wrapping around the blood vessels

the granulomas result in fibrous scars, sometimes with dystrophic calcification.

Postsurgical granulomas occur as a local reaction to tissue necrosis caused by surgical procedures. Although they resemble the granulomatous reaction induced by mycobacteria, postsurgical granulomas should not be subject to extensive evaluation of infectious etiology nor to antimicrobial therapy.

Radiation Cystitis

In men, about one-third of all cancers arise from the pelvic organs, including the prostate, rectum, and urinary bladder; in women, about one-fifth of all cancers are from this region, including the uterus, ovary, urinary bladder, and rectum [62]. Patients with cancers of the pelvic region often receive brachytherapy or external radiation therapy. Although radiation therapy aims to deliver a high dose of energy to a target pelvic organ carrying cancer, it often damages the urinary bladder due its close proximity to the other pelvic organs.

The urinary bladder shows various histologic responses to radiation therapy. In the early phase, the urothelial mucosa often develops acute inflammation with focal denudation of the urothelium. The remaining urothelium may show epithelial proliferations with mild-to-moderate nuclear atypia. Intracytoplasmic vacuolization in the urothelial cells and nucleomegaly with smudgy degenerative chromatin are common. There may be hemorrhage and edema in the lamina propria. Atypical reactive fibroblasts are often present in the lamina propria. Blood vessels may develop hyalinization and thrombosis. In the late phase, ulcers and fibrosis may be prominent in the bladder wall.

Sometimes radiation cystitis may show areas of epithelial proliferation mimicking an invasive cancer within the lamina propria [63]. A characteristic feature is the presence of pseudo-invasive urothelial nests wrapping around the blood vessels associated with fibrin deposition (Fig. 4.10). This feature is often associated with other reactive changes, such as acute inflammation, edema, hemorrhage, fibrin deposition, and fibrin thrombi, which can be helpful in distinguishing it from an invasive cancer.

Radiation cystitis can occur anywhere from 6 month to >10 years post-pelvic irradiation and is characterized by gross hematuria [64]. Studies show that 6.5% of women who received radiation for stage 1b cervical cancer and 3–5% of men receiving radiation for prostate cancer developed radiation-induced hemorrhagic cystitis [64]. Other urinary symptoms include dysuria, frequency, painful voiding, and urgency.

The first-line treatment for radiation hemorrhagic cystitis is bladder irrigation to prevent clot retention and the formation of organized clot. The other treatments would be the ones used for the treatment of hemorrhagic cystitis [64, 65]. The treatment for voiding symptoms includes anticholinergic medications.

Chemotherapy Cystitis

Chemotherapeutic drugs affect the urinary bladder through secretion of active metabolites in the urine. Although most histologic changes induced by chemotherapy consist of mild-to-moderate urothelial atypia, chemotherapy may occasionally induce pseudocarcinomatous changes. It has been described previously that cyclophosphamide may cause transient or persistent hemorrhagic cystitis. Cyclophosphamide, an alkylating agent, has been used to treat lymphoma, leukemia, and myeloma, and also employed to treat non-neoplastic diseases, such as rheumatoid arthritis, systemic lupus erythematosus, and nephrotic syndrome. The toxicity of cyclophosphamide is caused by acrolein, a liver metabolite [66]. The hemorrhage may be aggravated by thrombocytopenia, which is often associated with chemotherapy. Hemorrhagic cystitis may occur at any time after the administration and is related to the dose of drug.

Intravesical topical chemotherapy has been used to treat urothelial carcinoma in situ and superficially invasive urothelial carcinoma. Chemical agents, such as triethylenethiophosphoramide (thiotepa), doxorubicin, and mitomycin C, can induce denudation of the urothelial mucosa and inflammation. The remaining urothelium may show urothelial hyperplasia and atypia. Sometimes the atypia is so prominent that it may mimic residual urothelial carcinoma in situ [67, 68]. Intracytoplasmic vacuolization and prominent cytoplasmic eosinophilia are common post-therapy changes. However, the atypia is typically limited to the superficial urothelial cells and it also lacks robust mitotic activity, which is often seen in urothelial carcinoma in situ. In bladder biopsies taken within the first few months of therapy, the degree of morphologic overlap between therapy-induced atypia and carcinoma in situ may preclude a definitive diagnosis. Diagnostic caution should be used in this setting and clinical follow-up is warranted before rendering a definitive diagnosis of carcinoma in situ in the acute post-therapy period.

Chemotherapic hemorrhagic cystitis can present in as many as 70% of patients who receive cyclophosphamide without intravesicular 2-sodium mercaptoethane sulfonate, which binds acrolein [69]. Hemorrhagic cystitis can occur after as few as one dose of cyclophosphamide [69]. Treatments include oral agents (sodium pentosan polysulfate, aminocaproic acid, and estrogen), intravesical agents (alum, silver nitrate, prostaglandins, and formalin), intravesical clot evacuation, urinary diversion, cystectomy, and selective embolization of the hypogastric arteries.

Conclusion

Cystitis is the broad term encompassing the inflammatory response of the urinary bladder to various harmful stimuli. In this chapter cystitis was divided into two broad categories, infectious cystitis and inflammatory cystitis, based on the presence or absence of infectious pathogens. While each type of cystitis is different in its histological features, all forms adversely affect patients. The key to successful treatment is based on the correct clinical and histological diagnosis.

References

1. Litwin MS, Saigal CS, Yano EM, et al. Urologic diseases in America Project: analytical methods and principal findings. J Urol. 2005;173:933.
2. Foxman B, Brown P. Epidemiology of urinary tract infections: transmission and risk factors, incidence, and costs. Infect Dis Clin North Am. 2003;17:227.
3. Schappert SM. Ambulatory care visits of physician offices, hospital outpatient departments, and emergency departments: United States, 1995. Vital Health Stat 13. 1997;129:1.
4. Ronald A. The etiology of urinary tract infection: traditional and emerging pathogens. Dis Mon. 2003;49:71.
5. Brown PD, Foxman B. Pathogenesis of urinary tract infection: the role of sexual behavior and sexual transmission. Curr Infect Dis Rep. 2000;2:513.

6. Dieter RS. Sterile pyuria: a differential diagnosis. Compr Ther. 2000;26:150.
7. Nicolle LE. Uncomplicated urinary tract infection in adults including uncomplicated pyelonephritis. Urol Clin North Am. 2008;35:1.
8. Wagenlehner FM, Weidner W, Naber KG. Antibiotics in urology: new essentials. Urol Clin North Am. 2008;35:69.
9. Killgore KM, March KL, Guglielmo BJ. Risk factors for community-acquired ciprofloxacin-resistant Escherichia coli urinary tract infection. Ann Pharmacother. 2004;38:1148.
10. Warren JW, Abrutyn E, Hebel JR, et al. Guidelines for antimicrobial treatment of uncomplicated acute bacterial cystitis and acute pyelonephritis in women. Infectious Diseases Society of America (IDSA). Clin Infect Dis. 1999;29:745.
11. McClure J. Malakoplakia. J Pathol. 1983;140:275.
12. Michaelis L, Gutman C. Ueber Einschliisse in Blasentumoren. Z Klin Med. 1902;47:208.
13. Yousef GM, Naghibi B, Hamodat MM. Malakoplakia outside the urinary tract. Arch Pathol Lab Med. 2007;131:297.
14. Abdou NI, NaPombejara C, Sagawa A, et al. Malakoplakia: evidence for monocyte lysosomal abnormality correctable by cholinergic agonist in vitro and in vivo. N Engl J Med. 1977;297:1413.
15. McClurg FV, D'Agostino AN, Martin JH, et al. Ultrastructural demonstration of intracellular bacteria in three cases of malakoplakia of the bladder. Am J Clin Pathol. 1973;60:780.
16. Qualman SJ, Gupta PK, Mendelsohn G. Intracellular Escherichia coli in urinary malakoplakia: a reservoir of infection and its therapeutic implications. Am J Clin Pathol. 1984;81:35.
17. Maderazo EG, Berlin BB, Morhardt C. Treatment of malakoplakia with trimethoprim-sulfamethoxazole. Urology. 1979;13:70.
18. Vallorosi CJ, Putzi MJ, Wolf Jr JS. Renal malacoplakia. Tech Urol. 1999;5:43.
19. Zornow DH, Landes RR, Morganstern SL, et al. Malacoplakia of the bladder: efficacy of bethanechol chloride therapy. J Urol. 1979;122:703.
20. Stanton MJ, Lynch JH, Maxted WC, et al. Malacoplakia of the bladder: a case report of resolution with bethanechol, trimethoprim-sulfamethoxazole and ascorbic acid. J Urol. 1983;130:1174.
21. Wein A, Kavoussi L, Novick AC, et al. Campbells-Walsh urology. Philadelphia: Saunders; 2007.
22. Wise GJ, Marella VK. Genitourinary manifestations of tuberculosis. Urol Clin North Am. 2003;30:111.
23. Figueiredo AA, Lucon AM. Urogenital tuberculosis: update and review of 8961 cases from the world literature. Rev Urol. 2008;10:207.
24. Christensen WI. Genitourinary tuberculosis: review of 102 cases. Medicine (Baltimore). 1974;53:377.
25. Gontero P, Bohle A, Malmstrom PU, et al. The role of bacillus Calmette-Guerin in the treatment of non-muscle-invasive bladder cancer. Eur Urol. 2010; 57:410.
26. Bevers RF, Kurth KH, Schamhart DH. Role of urothelial cells in BCG immunotherapy for superficial bladder cancer. Br J Cancer. 2004;91:607.
27. Oyama N, Tanase K, Akino H, et al. Nephrogenic adenoma in a patient with transitional cell carcinoma of the bladder receiving intravesical bacillus Calmette-Guerin. Int J Urol. 1998;5:185.
28. Sobel JD, Kauffman CA, McKinsey D, et al. Candiduria: a randomized, double-blind study of treatment with fluconazole and placebo. The National Institute of Allergy and Infectious Diseases (NIAID) Mycoses Study Group. Clin Infect Dis. 2000;30:19.
29. Roy JB, Geyer JR, Mohr JA. Urinary tract candidiasis: an update. Urology. 1984;23:533.
30. Schabereiter-Gurtner C, Selitsch B, Rotter ML, et al. Development of novel real-time PCR assays for detection and differentiation of eleven medically important Aspergillus and Candida species in clinical specimens. J Clin Microbiol. 2007;45:906.
31. Leu HS, Huang CT. Clearance of funguria with short-course antifungal regimens: a prospective, randomized, controlled study. Clin Infect Dis. 1995;20:1152.
32. Paduch DA. Viral lower urinary tract infections. Curr Urol Rep. 2007;8:324.
33. Smith TF, Espy MJ, Mandrekar J, et al. Quantitative real-time polymerase chain reaction for evaluating DNAemia due to cytomegalovirus, Epstein-Barr virus, and BK virus in solid-organ transplant recipients. Clin Infect Dis. 2007;45:1056.
34. Guo CC, Fine SW, Epstein JI. Noninvasive squamous lesions in the urinary bladder: a clinicopathologic analysis of 29 cases. Am J Surg Pathol. 2006;30:883.
35. Cheng L, Leibovich BC, Cheville JC, et al. Squamous papilloma of the urinary tract is unrelated to condyloma acuminata. Cancer. 2000;88:1679.
36. Chitsulo L, Engels D, Montresor A, et al. The global status of schistosomiasis and its control. Acta Trop. 2000;77:41.
37. Gryseels B, Polman K, Clerinx J, et al. Human schistosomiasis. Lancet. 2006;368:1106.
38. Duvie SO. Cup-patch ileocystoplasty in the treatment of bilharzial contracted bladder. J R Coll Surg Edinb. 1986;31:56.
39. Mott KE, Dixon H, Osei-Tutu E, et al. Effect of praziquantel on hematuria and proteinuria in urinary schistosomiasis. Am J Trop Med Hyg. 1985;34:1119.
40. Badawi AF, Mostafa MH, Probert A, et al. Role of schistosomiasis in human bladder cancer: evidence of association, aetiological factors, and basic mechanisms of carcinogenesis. Eur J Cancer Prev. 1995;4:45.
41. Hunner GL. A rare type of bladder ulcer in women report of cases. Tans South Surgical Gynecology. 1914;27:247.
42. Gillenwater JY, Wein AJ. Summary of the National Institute of Arthritis, Diabetes, Digestive and Kidney Diseases Workshop on Interstitial Cystitis, National Institutes of Health, Bethesda, Maryland, August 28-29, 1987. J Urol. 1988;140:203.
43. Abrams P, Cardozo L, Fall M, et al. The standardisation of terminology of lower urinary tract function:

report from the Standardisation Sub-committee of the International Continence Society. Am J Obstet Gynecol. 2002;187:116.
44. van de Merwe JP, Nordling J, Bouchelouche P, et al. Diagnostic criteria, classification, and nomenclature for painful bladder syndrome/interstitial cystitis: an ESSIC proposal. Eur Urol. 2008;53:60.
45. Hanno P, Lin A, Nordling J, et al. Bladder Pain Syndrome Committee of the International Consultation on Incontinence. Neurourol Urodyn. 2010;29:191.
46. Abrams P, Cardozo L, Fall M, et al. The standardisation of terminology in lower urinary tract function: report from the standardisation sub-committee of the International Continence Society. Urology. 2003;61:37.
47. Messing E, Pauk D, Schaeffer A, et al. Associations among cystoscopic findings and symptoms and physical examination findings in women enrolled in the Interstitial Cystitis Data Base (ICDB) Study. Urology. 1997;49:81.
48. van den Ouden D. Diagnosis and management of eosinophilic cystitis: a pooled analysis of 135 cases. Eur Urol. 2000;37:386.
49. Hellstrom HR, Davis BK, Shonnard JW. Eosinophilic cystitis. A study of 16 cases. Am J Clin Pathol. 1979;72:777.
50. Popescu OE, Landas SK, Haas GP. The spectrum of eosinophilic cystitis in males: case series and literature review. Arch Pathol Lab Med. 2009;133:289.
51. Salman M, Al-Ansari AA, Talib RA, et al. Eosinophilic cystitis simulating invasive bladder cancer: a real diagnostic challenge. Int Urol Nephrol. 2006;38:545.
52. Teegavarapu PS, Sahai A, Chandra A, et al. Eosinophilic cystitis and its management. Int J Clin Pract. 2005;59:356.
53. Popert RJ, Ramsay JW, Owen RA, et al. Eosinophilic cystitis mimicking invasive bladder tumour: discussion paper. J R Soc Med. 1990;83:776.
54. Marsh FP, Banerjee R, Panchamia P. The relationship between urinary infection, cystoscopic appearance, and pathology of the bladder in man. J Clin Pathol. 1974;27:297.
55. Sarma KP. On the nature of cystitis follicularis. J Urol. 1970;104:709.
56. Mateos BJ, Lavalle MF, Ramirez ZA, et al. Follicular cystitis. Case report and bibliographic review. Arch Esp Urol. 2007;60:77.
57. Lawrence HJ, Simone J, Aur RJ. Cyclophosphamide-induced hemorrhagic cystitis in children with leukemia. Cancer. 1975;36:1572.
58. Crook J, Esche B, Futter N. Effect of pelvic radiotherapy for prostate cancer on bowel, bladder, and sexual function: the patient's perspective. Urology. 1996;47:387.
59. Polat O, Gundogdu C, Demirel A, et al. The effects of thiotepa, mitomycin C, BCG and interferon instillation on urothelium. Int Urol Nephrol. 1996;28:43.
60. Spagnolo DV, Waring PM. Bladder granulomata after bladder surgery. Am J Clin Pathol. 1986;86:430.
61. Eble JN, Banks ER. Post-surgical necrobiotic granulomas of urinary bladder. Urology. 1990;35:454.
62. Jemal A, Siegel R, Ward E, et al. Cancer statistics, 2009. CA Cancer J Clin. 2009;59:225.
63. Chan TY, Epstein JI. Radiation or chemotherapy cystitis with "pseudocarcinomatous" features. Am J Surg Pathol. 2004;28:909.
64. Corman JM, McClure D, Pritchett R, et al. Treatment of radiation induced hemorrhagic cystitis with hyperbaric oxygen. J Urol. 2003;169:2200.
65. Yoshida T, Kawashima A, Ujike T, et al. Hyperbaric oxygen therapy for radiation-induced hemorrhagic cystitis. Int J Urol. 2008;15:639.
66. Cox PJ. Cyclophosphamide cystitis–identification of acrolein as the causative agent. Biochem Pharmacol. 1979;28:2045.
67. Murphy WM, Soloway MS, Lin CJ. Morphologic effects of thio-TEPA on mammalian urothelium. Changes in abnormal cells. Acta Cytol. 1978;22:550.
68. Murphy WM, Soloway MS, Finebaum PJ. Pathological changes associated with topical chemotherapy for superficial bladder cancer. J Urol. 1981;126:461.
69. Kaplan JR, Wolf Jr JS. Efficacy and survival associated with cystoscopy and clot evacuation for radiation or cyclophosphamide induced hemorrhagic cystitis. J Urol. 2009;181:641.

Part III

Bladder Neoplasia

5 Bladder Cancer Overview and Staging

Todd M. Morgan, Michael S. Cookson, George J. Netto, and Jonathan I. Epstein

Epidemiology and Demographics

In 2011, approximately 69,250 new cases of bladder cancer and 14,990 deaths from bladder cancer were predicted in the USA [1]. While population-adjusted incidence rates have remained stable for the past 35 years, bladder cancer remains the fifth-leading new cancer diagnosis in the USA and is the fourth most common cancer among men. When considering the fact that most newly diagnosed bladder cancer is noninvasive, coupled with a high rate of recurrence, it is estimated that in the USA alone there are more than 500,000 patients who have been or are currently undergoing treatment from bladder cancer. Currently, one in 42 people born in the USA is predicted to be diagnosed with bladder cancer during his or her lifetime including one in 26 men. Additionally, in worldwide incidence, bladder cancer ranks seventh among men and is seventeenth in women.

T.M. Morgan (✉)
Department of Urology, University of Michigan, 3875 Taubman Center, Ann Arbor, MI 48109, USA
e-mail: tomorgan@med.umich.edu

M.S. Cookson
Department of Urologic Surgery, Vanderbilt University Medical Center, A1302 Medical Center North, Nashville, TN 37232, USA

G.J. Netto
Department of Pathology, Johns Hopkins University, 401 N Broadway/Weinberg 2242, Baltimore, MD 21231, USA

J.I. Epstein
Department of Pathology, Urology, Oncology, The Johns Hopkins Medical Institutions, 401 N. Broadway Street, Room 2242, Baltimore, MD 21231, USA

Gender and Race

The difference in bladder cancer incidence between men and women has been longstanding and persistent; [1] however, the prognosis is significantly worse for women than it is for men. In an analysis of the Surveillance, Epidemiology, and End Results (SEER) registry, Scosyrev et al. [2] found that women have a significant increased risk of death compared to men, even while controlling for key prognostic variables such as age, stage, grade, and histologic subtype. Additionally, women tended to be older and have higher stage tumors at the time of presentation.

Although a number of studies have reported significant differences in presentation and survival between men and women [3–5], the explanation for these findings is not clear. One possible cause is a delay in diagnosing and treating women with bladder cancer, and Johnson et al. have shown women to be 40% less likely than men to be referred to a urologist for hematuria [6]. Additionally, women are more likely to be older and have more advanced tumors at diagnosis, supporting the presence of a delay [2, 5]. However, in the study by Scosyrev and colleagues, differences in key prognostic factors explained no

D.E. Hansel et al. (eds.), *The Urinary Tract: A Comprehensive Guide to Patient Diagnosis and Management*, DOI 10.1007/978-1-4614-5320-8_5, © Springer Science+Business Media New York 2012

more than 30% of the increased mortality seen in women. This excess mortality among women despite multivariate adjustment suggests that there may be other explanations for the gender disparity. While differences in quality of care or even treatment choice may exist, there may also be intrinsic host factors responsible for the observed differences. For example, it has been proposed that androgens promote oncogenesis in bladder tissue while estrogens may have an inhibitory effect.

Bladder cancer incidence also varies by race. White men are approximately two times as likely as black men to develop bladder cancer, and bladder cancer occurs approximately 50% more frequently in white compared to black women [7–9]. In Hispanic Americans, the incidence is less than half that of white individuals [10]. Black patients with bladder cancer are significantly more likely than white patients to present with aggressive tumors: studies consistently demonstrate differences in both grade and stage at diagnosis [2, 11–13]. In a SEER review spanning nearly three decades, Lee et al. [11] demonstrated that black Americans presented with tumors of higher stage and grade than whites, and this trend persisted throughout the entire period of the study. Black patients presented with nonlocalized bladder cancer 11% more frequently than white patients, and this phenomenon was most pronounced in women where the rate of regional or distant disease was far higher among black individuals (39% vs. 22%).

Bladder-cancer-specific survival is significantly worse in black compared to white patients, even controlling for relevant clinical and pathological variables. Lee et al. [11] controlled for age, grade, treatment, and stage, and found that black patients still had a 35% greater risk of disease-specific mortality than whites. The 10-year disease-specific survival was 4.6–10.5% lower in grade-matched black versus white patients. Scosyrev et al. [2] also demonstrated significant mortality differences between black and white patients. While controlling for relevant clinicopathologic factors mitigated some of the disparity, the increased bladder cancer mortality in black patients still persisted.

Potential causes for these findings may include differences in access to care, differences in exposures, and/or differences in tumor biology. Lee and associates found that the likelihood of undergoing treatment with curative intent was significantly lower in black vs. white patients [11]. Hollenbeck et al. [14] evaluated treatment differences by race in a more recent subset of the SEER database. While some minor differences in treatment were detected, aggressive therapies were utilized equally in black and white patients, and no clear disparities in the quality of care were identified. Another population-based assessment of quality of care found a 66% greater likelihood of perioperative mortality in black patients and prolonged hospitalizations in 38% of black patients compared with 25% of white patients [15]. These findings may be primarily a function of hospital setting, with black individuals undergoing surgery at lower volume centers [16, 17]. Some have also speculated that genetic differences may explain some of the observed disparities [18].

Age

Bladder cancer is primarily a disease of patients more than 50 years old. The median age of diagnosis is 69 years in men and 71 years in women, and the risk of developing bladder cancer increases sharply with increasing age [12]. In men, the risk of developing bladder cancer between 40 and 59 years of age is only 0.41%; it increases to 0.96% between ages 60 and 69 and to 3.57% for diagnosis at age 70 or later. In women, there is a 0.26% probability of bladder cancer diagnosis between 60 and 69, compared to a 1.01% likelihood at 70 years or older [1]. An analysis of the California Cancer Registry demonstrated a peak incidence of bladder cancer in individuals 85 or older [19]. With the expected significant population growth and overall aging, bladder cancer is likely to become an increasingly prevalent disease [20].

There are many forces driving the association between aging and bladder cancer. Increasing age can allow for greater exposure to potential carcinogens such as cigarettes. There is also a long delay between the carcinogenic exposure and its clinical effect, increasing the number of years before the potential development of bladder cancer. Additionally, age itself can lead to the accumulation of sufficient genetic and cellular events to result in a neoplastic process. Finally, voiding dysfunction in the elderly may lead to increased urothelial contact with urinary toxins.

Bladder cancer prognosis is significantly worse with advanced age. In patients with superficial bladder cancer, increasing age has been associated with a greater likelihood of having a high-grade tumor [21]. Older patients are also more likely to suffer tumor recurrence. In patients who have undergone radical cystectomy, greater patient age is associated with higher stage disease and a marked decrease in cancer-specific survival [22, 23]. The greater mortality in the elderly may be due to a number of factors, including characteristics of the cancer itself (e.g., stage and grade), decreased use of neoadjuvant or adjuvant chemotherapy, and delays in management stemming from reluctance to pursue aggressive surgical management. While cystectomy can offer a significant survival benefit in the elderly [14], it is infrequently employed. In an analysis of the SEER database, only 14% of those older than 75 with muscle-invasive cancer underwent radical cystectomy, compared with 45% of those younger than 75 [24].

Risk Factors

Smoking

Cigarette smoking is the primary risk factor for bladder cancer. Up to 50% of bladder cancer in men and 35% of bladder cancer in women is attributable to cigarette smoking [25]. These large differences reflect the historic disparity in smoking rates between men and women as these estimates come from a large meta-analysis in which the average prevalence of smoking was 43% in men and 28% in women. In the same meta-analysis, current male smokers were found to have an adjusted odds ratio of 3.18 for developing bladder cancer, suggesting they have more than three times the risk of developing bladder cancer than nonsmokers. The findings were similar in women (OR 2.90) [25]. In a prospective study of more than 120,000 men and women in the Netherlands, current smokers had a 3.3-fold increased risk of bladder cancer compared to those who have never smoked [26]. The relative risk was 1.03 (CI 1.02–1.04) per one-year increment of smoking duration. Furthermore, a large population-based study found a significant increase in smoking-related bladder cancer risk over time [27]. The odds ratio for current smokers compared to nonsmokers increased from 2.9 to 4.2 to 5.5 over the years 1994–1998, 1998–2001, and 2001–2004.

Smoking cessation significantly reduces the risk of bladder cancer; however, the risk does not appear to return to the level of never smokers. Individuals who stop smoking experience a decrease in the risk of bladder cancer of approximately 35% after one to four years and of over 60% after 25 years [28]. In the Netherlands study, while the relative risk of bladder cancer was 3.3 in current smokers, former smokers had a relative risk of 2.1 compared to never smokers [26]. Zeegers et al. [25] found a relative risk in former smokers of 1.7, while it was 2.6 in a combined analysis of current male and female smokers. Importantly, patients with non-muscle-invasive bladder cancer (NMIBC) who stop smoking may experience a decrease in their risk of recurrence. Fleshner et al. [29] demonstrated a 40% increased risk of recurrence for current smokers over ex-smokers (those quitting prior to their diagnosis), and the risk of recurrence was nearly 30% lower for those stopping at the time of diagnosis compared to continued smokers [30]. In another study of 265 patients with NMIBC, continued smokers had a 2.2-fold greater risk of recurrence than nonsmokers after controlling for relevant clinicopathologic variables. These data underscore the need for smoking cessation counseling by those caring for patients with bladder cancer [31–33].

The biologic mechanism responsible for the association between cigarette smoking and urothelial cancer has not been clearly delineated. A number of candidate carcinogenic compounds are present in cigarette smoke. Most of these are aromatic amines, including 2-naphthylamine, 4-aminobiphenyl, benzidine, and 4-chloro-ortho-toluidine [34–36]. Host interactions may play an important role, with some studies demonstrating that individuals with specific genetic polymorphisms are more susceptible to bladder cancer when exposed to cigarette smoke [37–39]. One enzyme of particular interest is N-acetyltransferase 2 (NAT2), an acetylating enzyme important in the detoxification of aromatic amines. In comparison to the more common intermediate- or rapid-acetylation genotypes, patients with the NAT2 slow-acetylation genotype appear to have a significantly increased risk of bladder cancer in the setting of cigarette use [40].

Due to exposure to compounds similar to those found in cigarettes, certain occupations have been associated with an increased incidence of bladder cancer. Aniline dyes, used in the textile industry, were first identified as a bladder carcinogen well over 100 years ago [41]. The carcinogenic compounds in these dyes are aromatic amines that are also found around painters, hairdressers, and individuals working in the rubber industry [42]. Individuals working in aluminum production, roofing, and coal gasification are all at increased risk of bladder cancer, stemming from exposure to polycyclic aromatic hydrocarbons [43].

Other Risk Factors

There are a number of other important risk factors for bladder cancer. Phenacetin-containing analgesics confer an increased risk of urothelial cancer [44, 45], although no association has been found with other analgesics [46, 47]. The chemotherapeutic agent cyclophosphamide confers a significant risk of bladder cancer, exerting a dose-dependent effect that increases the risk of bladder cancer up to 14-fold [48, 49]. The carcinogenic chemical, acrolein, is a urinary metabolite of cyclophosphamide. Oral administration of 2-mercaptoethanesulfonic acid (mesna) inactivates acrolein in the genitourinary tract, providing a uroprotective effect. Coffee and tea have both long been proposed as potential bladder carcinogens; however, studies have been inconsistent and any potential increased risk may be limited to men drinking at least seven cups of coffee per day [50, 51].

Other risk factors include catheter- or stone-induced chronic cystitis and Schistosoma haematobium cystitis—classically associated with squamous cell carcinoma of the bladder [52, 53]. Patients who have received pelvic radiation for ovarian, cervical, or prostate cancer are all at an increased risk of developing bladder cancer [54–56]. Additionally, patients with a family history of bladder cancer have a significantly elevated risk of developing the disease. First-degree relatives of patients with bladder cancer have up to an 80% increased risk of bladder cancer [57–59].

Diagnosis

Cystoscopy

Hematuria is the most common presenting symptom in patients with bladder cancer, and it may be either intermittent or continuous. However, patients with asymptomatic microhematuria also require thorough evaluation when three or more red blood cells per high-power field are present in two of three urinalysis specimens [60, 61]. In addition to a careful history and physical exam, all patients with gross or microscopic hematuria require cystoscopic examination—the gold standard for the diagnosis of bladder cancer. Bladder cancer may also present with irritative voiding symptoms, such as urinary frequency and urgency; however, these are typically associated with microhematuria in the setting of a urothelial malignancy.

While white light cystoscopy is the current standard in the diagnosis of bladder cancer, a number of techniques have been studied to improve the ability to visualize these tumors. Fluorescence cystoscopy has greater sensitivity than white light cystoscopy, but this has not yet translated into decreased progression rates or improved survival [62, 63]. Newer technologies are under development that may improve the precision of identifying bladder tumors while also providing real-time pathologic information. Optical coherence tomography (OCT) allows cross-sectional imaging of bladder tissue using a small probe, potentially allowing identification of bladder tumors while also showing their depth of invasion [64]. When coupled to fluorescence cystoscopy, OCT demonstrated a sensitivity of 97.5% and a specificity of 97.9% for the identification of malignant bladder lesions [65]. Another technique, confocal laser endomicroscopy, utilizes a 2.6-mm probe to show some degree of cellular architecture and could potentially allow immediate differentiation between normal urothelium, low-grade tumors, and high-grade tumors [66]. However, further improvements in image quality will likely be necessary before this technology can be utilized in the management of patients with bladder cancer.

Imaging

The initial evaluation of a patient with hematuria also includes evaluation of the upper urinary tracts. Computed tomography (CT) with and without contrast has become the imaging modality of choice for detecting any abnormalities in the kidneys or ureters. Noncontrast CT will demonstrate most urinary tract stones, and CT urography allows detection of upper urinary tract lesions. These typically appear as filling defects and may be associated with hydronephrosis when present in the ureter [67]. In addition, CT allows assessment of any renal parenchymal lesions and provides cross-sectional imaging for potential nodal and distant metastases. Magnetic resonance (MR) urography has been studied as an alternative to CT urography. However, because MR urography requires gadolinium and is generally inferior to CT urography, its use is typically restricted to those with allergies to iodine-based contrast agents [67, 68]. In general, patients with renal insufficiency may be imaged by ultrasound and retrograde pyelography [69]. Retrograde pyelography should also be performed when the upper tracts are not adequately visualized on CT.

Cytology

Urinary cytology is another critical component of the bladder cancer evaluation, although it is not very sensitive for the detection of low-grade papillary urothelial neoplasms. Since the large majority of urothelial carcinomas are lowgrade, it drives down the overall sensitivity of the test. However, urinary cytology has good sensitivity for the detection of high-grade urothelial carcinoma, such that the test's main role is in the diagnosis and follow-up of high-grade urothelial carcinoma (carcinoma in situ or papillary) [70].

Voided urine samples should come from the second morning midstream urine specimen after hydration, which, if collected over three consecutive days, optimizes the detection of urothelial malignancies [71]. Urine obtained through catheterization of the bladder is more cellular and can induce a false-positive diagnosis, and urologists should therefore note on a cytology specimen if it is voided or instrumented.

Papillomas and papillary urothelial neoplasms of low malignant potential (PUNLMP) cannot be reliably diagnosed by cytology since these lesions are cytologically identical to normal urothelial cells [72]. Low-grade papillary urothelial carcinomas are heterogeneous in urine specimens with the presence of small and large clusters of urothelial cells with enlarged nuclei, slightly higher nuclear to cytoplasmic ratios and a small nucleolus [73–75]. The changes seen in low-grade papillary urothelial carcinoma can be hard to distinguish from those seen due to lithiasis, inflammation, or even instrumentation. High-grade papillary urothelial carcinoma cytology specimens contain clusters and single markedly atypical cells with pleomorphic nuclei, coarse chromatin, and, frequently, prominent nucleoli. Invasion cannot be reproducibly diagnosed [75, 76]. Urine cytology represents a major tool in the diagnosis of carcinoma in situ (CIS) since cystoscopy has a lower sensitivity due to several factors, including denudation of the urothelium. The voided specimens from cases with CIS contain a population of atypical cells of intermediate size that are present mostly as single cells, although clusters and large pleomorphic cells might be present. The nuclear to cytoplasmic ratio is high and the cytoplasm is dense (Fig. 5.1). Treatment effect in patients receiving intravesical *Bacillus Calmette-Guérin* (BCG) or chemotherapy can lead to a false-positive diagnosis. Urine cytology will be discussed in greater detail in Chap. 16.

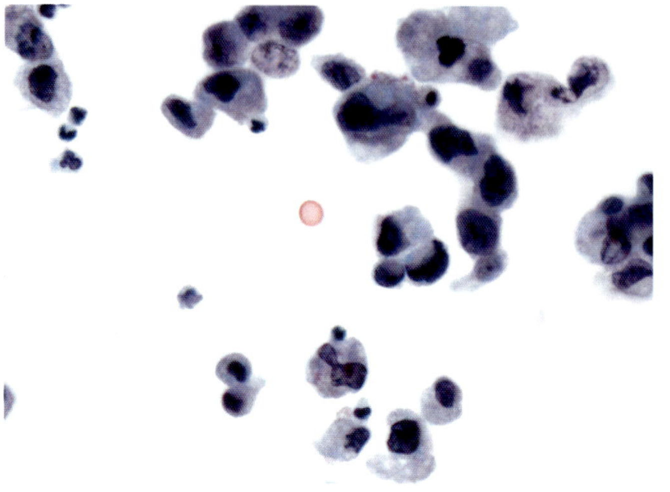

Fig. 5.1 CIS consisting of markedly atypical cells with hyperchromatic angulated nuclei, coarse chromatin pattern, irregular nuclear contours and occasional prominent nucleoli, and increased nuclear to cytoplasmic ratio

Transurethral Resection

The central component in the diagnosis of bladder carcinoma is transurethral resection (TUR). Ideally, TUR involves resection of all visible tumors in the bladder and/or urethra. This is critical from both a therapeutic and a diagnostic standpoint, as staging and grading accuracy are essential to determining the course of additional treatment. In order to facilitate accurate pathological evaluation, it is important to minimize the use of coagulation, include muscularis propria in the tumor specimen, and carefully handle the resected tissue. Following these basic principles will help eliminate artifacts within the specimen and significantly improve the ability to correctly identify the stage and grade of the tumor [77, 78].

In order to determine whether patients with pTa or pT1 bladder tumors have unrecognized CIS, random bladder biopsies from normal-appearing urothelium may be obtained. CIS can be found in approximately 15% of these patients [79], and, in a nonrandomized study, Thorstenson et al. [80] showed that patients who underwent random bladder biopsy were significantly more likely to receive intravesical BCG and to undergo radical cystectomy. Patients who did not undergo random biopsies were found to have a significantly greater risk of disease-specific mortality. However, some have suggested that urothelial injury from these biopsies may increase the likelihood of tumor implantation and therefore recurrence [81, 82]. The 2008 European Association of Urology (EAU) guidelines on NMIBC cancer note the low likelihood of detecting CIS in patients with low-risk tumors and suggest that the random biopsy result will not alter the choice of adjuvant treatment patients with higher risk tumors [83, 84]. These guidelines recommend that random biopsies be obtained only in the setting of an abnormal urinary cytology or a non-papillary exophytic tumor. Thus, while not routinely performed in all patients, the role of random bladder biopsies remains somewhat controversial but may be of benefit in those patients with high-risk features and/or those suspected of harboring carcinoma in situ.

Pathology

Currently, there is convincing evidence that noninvasive low-grade papillary tumors (PUNLMP and low-grade urothelial carcinoma) on the one hand and flat urothelial CIS and invasive high-grade urothelial carcinoma on the other hand follow two relatively distinct oncogenic pathways. These molecular differences are not totally surprising given the stark differences in the natural history and clinical behavior of the two groups of neoplasms. Noninvasive low-grade papillary urothelial tumors are characterized by the frequent presence of alterations in the receptor tyrosine kinase (RTK)-Ras pathways. Structural and functional alterations in tumor suppressor genes p53 and RB are implicated in the development and progression of CIS and high-grade invasive urothelial carcinoma.

The majority of urothelial tumors (60–70%) present as noninvasive (pTa) tumors at time of first diagnosis. Of these, 50% will recur as noninvasive tumors and only 5–10% will progress. Muscle-invasive high-grade urothelial carcinoma represents 20–30% of all bladder cancers. It is estimated that 15% of muscle-invasive urothelial carcinomas have a history of prior superficial urothelial carcinoma while the remaining 80–90% are "primary" muscle-invasive urothelial carcinoma.

The combined World Health Organization and International Society of Urologic Pathology (WHO/ISUP) grading system has gained wider use since its introduction in 1998 [85]. The system classifies noninvasive urothelial neoplasms into the following five categories:

- Urothelial papilloma: lowest risk of recurrence and no progression
- PUNLMP: 35% (25–47%) risk of recurrence, virtually no progression
- Noninvasive low-grade papillary urothelial carcinoma: 50% (30–76%) recurrence rate, 10% progress
- Noninvasive high-grade papillary urothelial carcinoma: most frequent recurrence rate (50–69%), 25–65% progress
- Urothelial carcinoma in situ (CIS): almost similar rates as high-grade papillary urothelial carcinoma in terms of recurrence rates and progression

Invasive carcinomas of the bladder are predominantly of urothelial histology (90%) with less frequent tumors being of pure epidermoid squamous (squamous cell carcinoma: 4%), pure glandular (adenocarcinoma: 2%), or small cell differentiation (small cell carcinoma: 1%). A histologic mixture of all previous types may exist in a given lesion.

Invasive urothelial carcinomas of the bladder should be considered for all practical purposes as high-grade tumors based on their cytologic morphology with the exception of a rare subtype (nested variant) that may display a low-grade cytology that betrays its aggressive behavior. Other rare subtypes of urothelial carcinoma include undifferentiated large cell, osteoclast cell like, lymphoepithelial cell like, and sarcomatoid (carcinosarcoma) (see Chap. 7 for further details). Regardless of histologic type, bladder tumors are staged in an identical fashion using the 2010 pTNM staging scheme.

Grading

In 1973, the WHO system proposed that tumors be categorized into benign urothelial papillomas and three grades of carcinoma (grades 1, 2, and 3) [86, 87]. A major limitation of the WHO (1973) grading system was its vague definition of the various grades and its lack of specific histologic criteria. In 1998, members of WHO and ISUP published the WHO/ISUP consensus classification of urothelial (transitional cell) neoplasms of the urinary bladder, which is the currently recommended system by WHO [85]. This new classification system arose out of the need to develop a more detailed classification system for bladder neoplasia and because many of the tumors classified as "transitional cell carcinoma, grade 1" had no potential for malignant behavior once completely excised.

A major misconception in the application of the WHO/ISUP classification is that there is a one-to-one translation between it and the WHO (1973) classification system (Fig. 5.2). Only at the extremes of grades in the WHO (1973) classification does this one-to-one correlation hold true. Lesions called papilloma in the WHO (1973) classification system are also called papilloma in the WHO/ISUP system and lesions

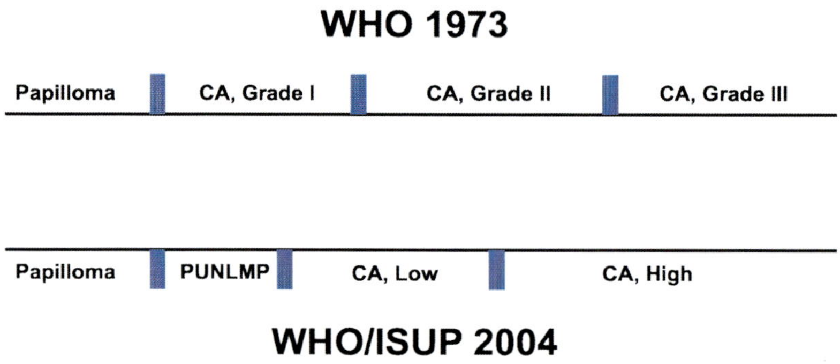

Fig. 5.2 Comparison of the WHO (1973) classification with the WHO/ISUP (2004) classification system for grading urothelial tumors

called WHO (1973) grade 3 are by definition high-grade carcinoma in the WHO/ISUP system. WHO (1973) grade 1 tumors may be either PUNLMP or low-grade urothelial carcinoma depending on their morphology. WHO (1973) system grade 2 tumors represent either WHO/ISUP papillary urothelial low-grade carcinoma or high-grade carcinoma. In the old WHO (1973) system, a large percentage of patients with non-invasive papillary urothelial carcinomas were called grade 2, an ambiguous group that the urologists did not know how to treat. In the WHO/ISUP grading system, these grade 2 tumors can be segregated roughly equally into low- and high-grade cancers with correspondingly low and high risks of progression [88–90]. When WHO (1973) grade 2 tumors are reclassified as high-grade tumors, they show molecular aberrations usually associated with cancers of higher grade and poor outcome, further supporting that WHO (1973) grade 2 tumors form a heterogeneous group that can be subdivided into low-and high-grade cancer [91].

There have been several studies comparing WHO (1973) and the current WHO/ISUP system. Most have demonstrated a superiority of WHO/ISUP in predicting recurrence and progression or interobserver reproducibility [88, 92–95]. Others have reported no difference in interobserver reproducibility of WHO/ISUP compared to WHO (1973), although in some of these works the WHO/ISUP grade was merely translated from the WHO (1973) grade, which as described earlier is inaccurate [96–98]. In another study comparing the two grading systems, there was no difference in survival; yet, one would not expect a difference in survival as the vast majority of papillary urothelial neoplasms do not result in the death of the patient. The more appropriate endpoints to evaluate are either progression (in grade or stage) or recurrence [99].

Papilloma

The WHO/ISUP system has very restrictive histologic features for the diagnosis of papilloma, requiring papillary fronds to be lined by normal-appearing urothelium (Table 5.1 and Fig. 5.3). Most papillomas present as single lesions that are relatively small; however, multifocal tumors and larger lesions may be seen.

Papillomas are rare and typically, but not exclusively, occur in younger patients. Papillomas may occur in association with a prior or concurrent history of other urothelial tumors. If a papilloma is the first manifestation of urothelial neoplasia, only about 7–8% recur, typically within 5 years of the initial diagnosis [98, 100–103]. Lesions typically recur as papilloma and, less commonly, as PUNLMP or noninvasive low-grade papillary urothelial carcinoma. Of the three largest series on papillomas totaling 112 patients, only one patient experienced stage progression;

Table 5.1 Histologic features of papillary urothelial lesions

	Papilloma	Papillary neoplasm of low malignant potential	Low-grade papillary carcinoma	High-grade papillary carcinoma
Architecture papillae	Delicate	Delicate; occasionally fused	Fused; branching; delicate	Fused; branching; delicate
Organization of cells	Identical to normal	Polarity identical to normal; any thickness; cohesive	Predominantly ordered, yet minimal crowding and minimal loss of polarity; any thickness; cohesive	Predominantly disordered with frequent loss of polarity; any thickness; often discohesive
Cytology nuclear size	Identical to normal	May be uniformly enlarged	Enlarged with variation in size	Enlarged with variation in size
Nuclear shape	Identical to normal	Elongated; round-oval; uniform	Round-oval; slight variation in shape and contour	Moderate-marked pleomorphism
Nuclear chromatin	Fine	Fine	Mild variation within and between cells	Moderate-marked variation within and between cells with hyperchromasia
Nucleoli	Absent	Absent to inconspicuous	Usually inconspicuous[a]	Multiple prominent nucleoli may be present
Mitoses	Absent	Rare; basal	Occasional, at any level	Usually frequent, at any level; may be atypical
Umbrella cells	Uniformly present	Present	Usually present	May be present

Reprinted with permission from Epstein JI, Amin MB, Reuter VE. Bladder biopsy interpretation (chapter 3). 2nd edn. Philadelphia: Lippincott Williams & Wilkins; 2010

[a]If present, small and regular and not accompanied by other features of high-grade carcinoma

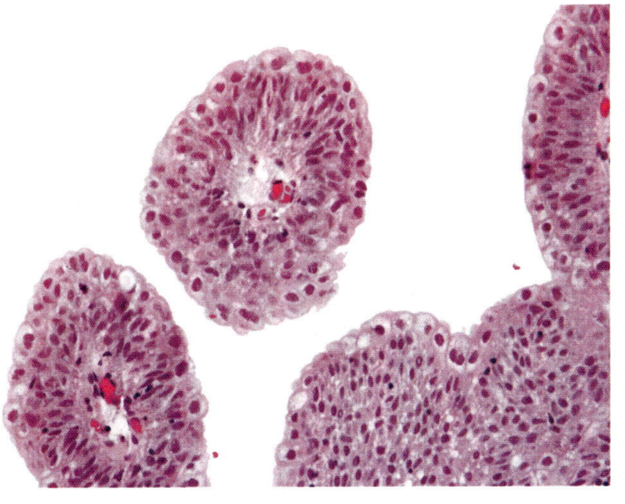

Fig. 5.3 Urothelial papilloma

invasive urothelial carcinoma was found extending out of the bladder 4 years after the diagnosis of papilloma [100, 101, 103]. A caveat to this exceptional case is that the patient was immunosuppressed following renal transplantation.

Papillary Urothelial Neoplasm of Low Malignant Potential

PUNLMPs at low power differ from papillomas by having thicker urothelium. At most, nuclei

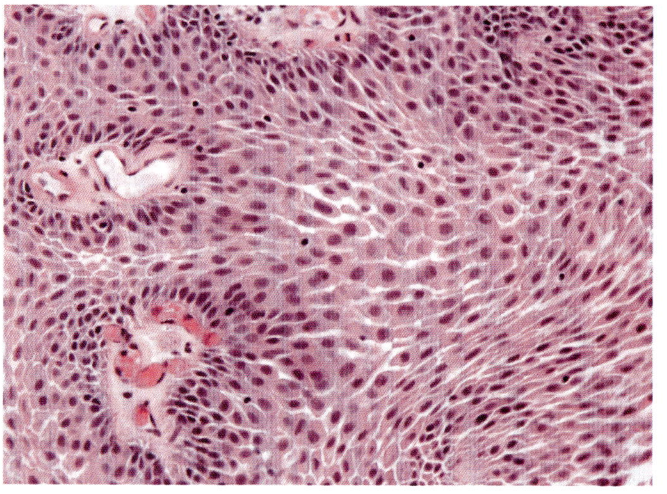

Fig. 5.4 Papillary urothelial neoplasm of low malignant potential

Table 5.2 Risk of recurrence according to grade of papillary neoplasm

Author	Papilloma (%)	PUNLMP (%)	Low-grade carcinoma (%)	High-grade carcinoma (%)
Magi-Galuzzi [16]	18			
McKenney [17]	14			
Cheng [19]	10			
Herr [18]	31	52	72	
Oosterhius [14]	14	32	34	43
Fujii [26]		60		
Campbell [22]		25	75	67
Desai [23]		33	64	56
Holmang [24]		35	71	73
Ramos [12]		62	65	
Pich [11]		47	78	
Alsheikh [21]		25	48	

Reprinted with permission from Epstein JI, Amin MB, Reuter VE. Bladder biopsy interpretation (chapter 3). 2nd edn. Philadelphia: Lippincott Williams & Wilkins; 2010

are slightly enlarged and more crowded relative to those in normal urothelial nuclei (Table 5.1 and Fig. 5.4). The chromatin is uniformly even without the scattered hyperchromatic nuclei seen in low-grade papillary carcinoma. Mitoses are exceedingly rare and usually limited to the basal layer.

A few studies have demonstrated a low level of agreement in the histological distinction between PUNLMP and low-grade carcinoma or have failed to show a difference in prognosis between the two entities [93, 96, 98, 104]. However, a much larger number of studies have demonstrated that PUNLMP have a lower risk of recurrence than low-grade urothelial carcinoma (Table 5.2) [89, 95, 102, 105–109]. In addition, whereas a small percentage of noninvasive low-grade papillary urothelial carcinomas progress either to invasive carcinoma or to high-grade noninvasive papillary carcinoma, the majority of studies have reported that PUNLMPs do not progress either in stage or grade (Table 5.3) [95, 102, 105, 107, 109, 110]. Having a category of PUNLMP avoids labeling a patient as having cancer, which has psychosocial

Table 5.3 Risk of progression[a] according to grade of papillary neoplasm

Author	(%)	PUNLMP (%)	Low-grade carcinoma (%)	High-grade carcinoma (%)
Magi-Galuzzi [16]	0			
McKenney [17]	0			
Cheng [19]	0			
Samaratunga [5]	0	7	10	35
Oosterhius [14]	0	3	4	8
Campbell [22]		0	4	22
Desai [23]		0	3	8
Holmang [24]		0	4	23
Fujii [26]		0		

Reprinted with permission from Epstein JI, Amin MB, Reuter VE. Bladder biopsy interpretation (chapter 3). 2nd edn. Philadelphia: Lippincott Williams & Wilkins; 2010

[a]Progression defined as recurrence with high-grade or invasive cancer

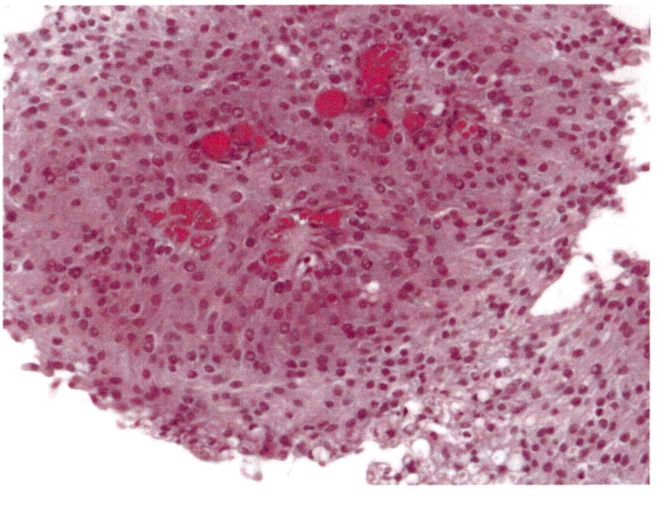

Fig. 5.5 Noninvasive low-grade papillary urothelial carcinoma

and financial (e.g., insurance) implications, but neither is a benign lesion (e.g., papilloma) diagnosed, so the patient will be adequately followed. PUNLMP is especially useful as a diagnosis for the younger patient with a newly diagnosed non-invasive papillary tumor that does not fulfill the criteria of papilloma but is still very low grade [111]. Some investigators have proposed that patients with PUNLMP may be submitted to fewer follow-up cystoscopies if there are few lesions and no recurrences are seen during the initial surveillance period.

Low-Grade Papillary Carcinoma

Low-grade papillary urothelial carcinoma exhibits an overall orderly appearance (i.e., maintains polarity) but has minimal variability in nuclear size, shape, and chromatin texture (Table 5.1 and Figure 5.5). Although mitoses may be seen at any level of the urothelium, they are usually limited to the lower half and are relatively infrequent. Scattered hyperchromatic nuclei and scattered "typical" mitotic figures best distinguish this lesion from PUNLMP.

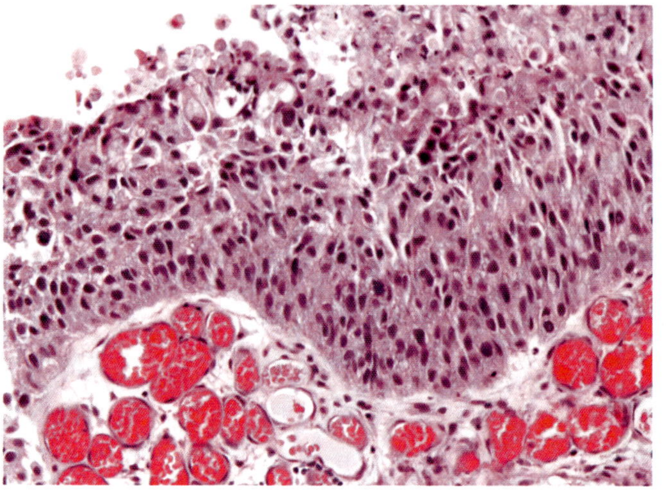

Fig. 5.6 Noninvasive high-grade papillary urothelial carcinoma

Occasionally one sees similar cytologic features in thickened urothelium adjacent to a papillary neoplasm.

High-Grade Papillary Carcinoma

High-grade papillary urothelial carcinomas are characterized by a disorderly appearance resulting from marked architectural and cytologic abnormalities, for the most part recognizable at low magnification (Fig. 5.6). Architecturally, high-grade papillary urothelial carcinomas are irregularly oriented and disorganized (Table 5.1). Cellular pleomorphism ranges from moderate to marked. The nuclear chromatin tends to be clumped and nucleoli may be prominent and irregular; occasionally, multiple nucleoli and nucleolar pleomorphism may be present. Mitotic figures, including atypical forms, may be frequently seen at all levels of the urothelium. As with CIS, high-grade papillary urothelial carcinomas are more likely than lower grade papillary neoplasms to have dyscohesive cells and some denudation.

A single papillary urothelial neoplasm may occasionally contain a mixture of both low- and high-grade morphology. These tumors should be graded according to the highest grade, although current practice is to note minor components (<5%) of high-grade tumor, but still grade the tumor as low grade [87]. In order to account for different grades within a given tumor, a combined grading system has been proposed adding the primary (most common) and secondary (second most common) grade of bladder cancer, regardless of extent, analogous to the Gleason grading for prostate cancer [88, 112, 113].

Although a combined grading system for papillary urothelial carcinoma appears to improve prediction of prognosis, further studies are needed before this system can be recommended for routine clinical practice. Given the inherent problems of interobserver reproducibility the authors doubt this approach will become standard of practice in the foreseeable future.

It is recognized that high-grade cancer has a spectrum of atypia with some cases showing marked anaplasia and that cases with marked anaplasia have a worse prognosis than other high grade cancers [88, 108]. The major argument against subdividing high-grade cancers is that high-grade noninvasive papillary cancers with marked anaplasia comprise only a small percentage of noninvasive papillary cancers. In Holmang's study of the 363 noninvasive papillary carcinomas, only 13 (3.6%) were classified as WHO (1973) grade 3, compared with 28% of the cases classified as high-grade carcinoma by the WHO/ISUP system [24]. These data are similar to those from Hopkins where only 4.5% of noninvasive papillary tumors were WHO (1973) grade 3 compared with 21.6% classified as WHO/ISUP high-grade [89]. There are so few WHO (1973) grade 3 noninvasive papillary carcinomas because most cases of WHO (1973) grade 3 are aggressive tumors in which there is already coexisting invasive cancer. Because patients with high-grade noninvasive papillary carcinoma are not treated with definitive therapy (e.g., cystectomy), the goal should not be to restrict the high-risk group to a small population but to expand it to be more inclusive of all patients at significant risk of progression so that they can be monitored closely and treated earlier in the course of the disease.

Conclusions

The WHO/ISUP system has the following benefits:

1. Establishment of uniform terminology and common definitions for papillary neoplasms.
2. Establishment of detailed criteria of various preneoplastic conditions and various grades of tumor.
3. Correlation with urine cytology terminology, facilitating cytohistologic correlation and making it easier for urologists to manage patients.
4. Creation of a category of tumor that identifies a tumor with a negligible risk of progression (PUNLMP), whereby patients avoid the label of having cancer, which has psychosocial and financial implications. Neither is a benign lesion diagnosed in these patients, so they may still be followed up closely.
5. Approximately half the cases occurring in young patients are now diagnosed as PUNLMP instead of TCC grade 1, obviating a carcinoma diagnosis in patients with biologically indolent tumors and in keeping with their stable molecular profile.
6. Identification of a distinct group of patients (high-grade papillary urothelial carcinoma) who would be ideal candidates for intravesical therapy.
7. Identification of a larger group of patients at high risk for progression for urologists to follow up more closely.
8. Removal of ambiguity in diagnostic categories in WHO 1973 system (e.g., TCC grade I-II, TCC grade II-III).
9. Stratification of bladder tumors into prognostically significant categories.

Bladder Staging

The main staging system in bladder cancer is the joint International Union Against Cancer (UICC) and the American Joint Committee on Cancer (AJCC) system. The 2010 UICC-AJCC staging system is given in Table 5.4, and has been modified from the prior 2002 staging system [114]. As before, noninvasive papillary tumors are classified as stage Ta, and tumors invading the lamina propria are classified as stage T1. T2 tumors are those invading into the muscularis propria, and T3 invade into the perivesical fat. Tumors invading the pelvic viscera such as the prostate continue to be classified as T4; however, this now includes only prostatic stromal invasion and not subepithelial invasion of the prostatic urethra. pT4 is gross macroscopic invasion extending from the bladder wall into the prostate. Invasion arising from CIS or a papillary CA in the urethra is not pT4.

The classification of regional lymph node disease in the 2010 system has been altered from the previous version and no longer relies on size of lymph node involvement. Patients with N1 disease are those with a single positive node in the primary drainage regions of the bladder—the hypogastric, obturator, internal iliac, external iliac, perivesical, sacral, and presacral lymph nodes. Patients with multiple positive nodes in the primary drainage regions are classified as having N2 disease. The common iliac lymph nodes are considered secondary drainage regions in the current staging system, and tumors involving these lymph nodes are classified as N3. Laterality is not a factor in lymph node staging. Patients with disease beyond the regional lymph nodes, such as lung, bone, and retroperitoneal lymph nodes, are classified as stage M1. Patients are considered Nx or Mx if the status of their lymph nodes or distant sites has not been determined.

Table 5.4 TNM staging system for bladder cancer

Definitions of TNM	
Primary tumor (T)	
TX	Primary tumor cannot be assessed
T0	No evidence of primary tumor
Ta	Noninvasive papillary carcinoma
Tis	Carcinoma in situ: "flat tumor"
T1	Tumor invades subepithelial connective tissue
T2	Tumor invades muscularis propria
pT2a	Tumor invades superficial muscularis propria (inner half)
pT2b	Tumor invades deep muscularis propria (outer half)
T3	Tumor invades perivesical tissue
pT3a	Microscopically
pT3b	Macroscopically (extravesical mass)
T4	Tumor invades any of the following: prostatic stroma, seminal vesicles, uterus, vagina, pelvic wall, abdominal wall
T4a	Tumor invades prostatic stroma, uterus, vagina
T4b	Tumor invades pelvic wall, abdominal wall
Regional lymph nodes (N)	
Regional lymph nodes include both primary and secondary drainage regions. All other nodes above the aortic bifurcation are considered distant lymph nodes.	
NX	Lymph nodes cannot be assessed
N0	No lymph node metastasis
N1	Single regional lymph node metastasis in the true pelvis (hypogastric, obturator, external iliac, or presacral lymph node)
N2	Multiple regional lymph node metastasis in the true pelvis (hypogastric, obturator, external iliac, or presacral lymph node metastasis)
N3	Lymph node metastasis to the common iliac lymph nodes
Distant metastasis (M)	
M0	No distant metastasis
M1	Distant metastasis

Used with the permission of the American Joint Committee on Cancer (AJCC), Chicago, Illinois. The original source for this material is the AJCC Cancer Staging Manual, Seventh Edition (2010) published by Springer-Verlag New York, http:\\www.springer.com

The initial assessment of tumor depth is made with TUR and bimanual exam under anesthesia. TUR should include resection of muscularis propria; [78] accurate discrimination between T1 and T2 tumors dictates initial management, and understaging of T1 lesions in the absence of muscularis propria may be as high as 62% [115]. Re-resection of T1 tumors is recommended by most guidelines when no muscle is present in the specimen. However, most experts recommend repeat resection for all patients with T1 tumors in whom bladder conservation is being considered [116]. This allows for improved detection of occult muscle invasive disease, and also ensures that all T1 disease has been resected prior to initiation of intravesical therapy.

Pathologic Staging

Pathologically, T1 disease is not a uniform entity. The region between the urothelium and the muscularis propria is divided by a thin layer of smooth muscle fibers (muscularis mucosae) [117]. Occasionally, muscularis mucosae bundles undergo hypertrophy, and in such situations the

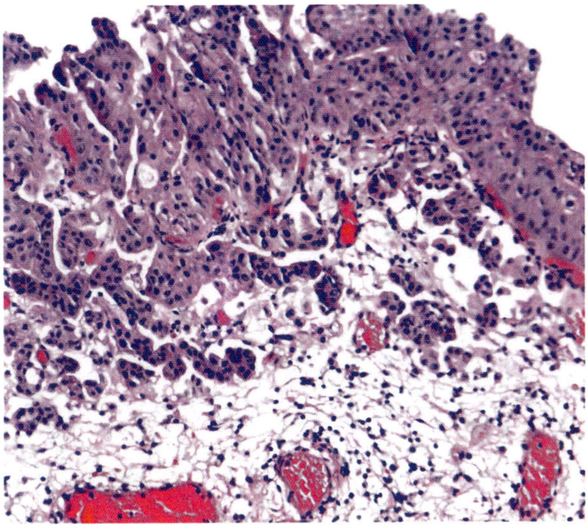

Fig. 5.7 Urothelial carcinoma with lamina propria invasion

distinction between muscularis mucosae and muscularis propria (detrusor muscle) may be difficult, especially in biopsy or TURBT specimens. There are several different types of lamina propria invasion: (1) CIS with invasion, (2) papillary urothelial carcinoma with invasion into stalk, and (3) invasion into underlying lamina propria at the base of a papillary neoplasm (Fig. 5.7). Diagnosis of lamina propria invasion in TURBT specimens is often difficult due to (1) tangential sectioning and poor orientation, (2) thermal injury, (3) obscuring inflammation, (4) CIS involving von Brunn nests, and (5) muscle invasion indeterminate for type of muscle. Due to the reasons described previously, it may be difficult to distinguish between hypertrophic muscularis mucosae or muscularis propria bundles, and the pathologist is unable to determine whether the muscle involved belongs to the muscularis mucosae or the muscularis propria. It is recommended that, when faced with this situation, pathologists should clearly state their uncertainty in establishing the depth of invasion. Smoothelin, a novel smooth muscle-specific contractile protein expressed only by fully differentiated smooth muscle cells and not by proliferative or noncontractile smooth muscle cells and myofibroblasts, has potential diagnostic utility in the distinction of muscularis mucosae from muscularis propria, yet in the hands of the authors there is too much overlap to be reliably used for diagnostic purposes [118].

Several studies have evaluated the issue of substaging T1 urothelial carcinomas using the muscularis mucosae as an anatomic landmark to assess the depth of invasion (tumors above or into muscularis mucosae are T1a; tumors invasive below are T1b) [119–121]. However, either muscularis mucosae or large vessels that are a substitute for muscularis mucosae are only present in about 50% of TUR specimens. Others have used the depth of invasion in millimeters from the basement membrane [122]. Although deep lamina propria invasion identifies a subset of patients with T1 disease with a more adverse prognosis, at this point substaging of T1 tumors is not standard practice because there is no consistently applicable and reproducible method. Nevertheless, in cases with T1 disease, pathologists should make some attempt to convey in their report the extent of lamina propria invasion even if it is with subjective terms such as "focal" versus "extensive." In cases of T1 disease, pathologists should always note whether muscularis propria is present. In the absence of muscularis propria, additional tissue sampling is recommended.

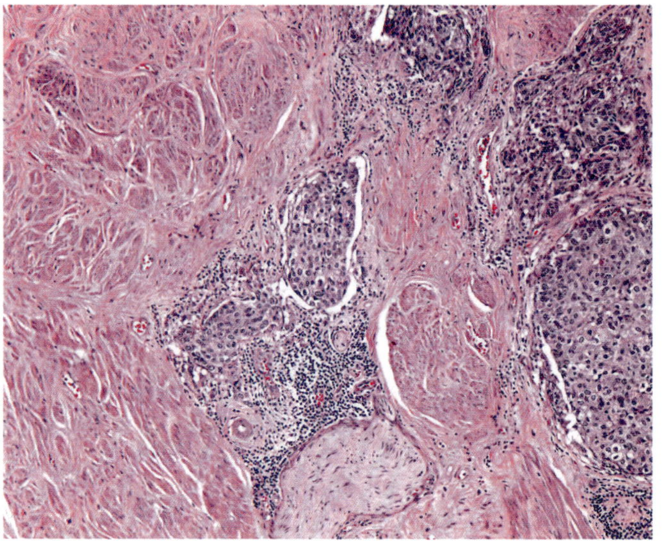

Fig. 5.8 Muscularis propria invasion by urothelial carcinoma

In patients with muscle invasion, clinical assessment of the depth of tumor invasion is challenging. Because TURBT specimens lack orientation with respect to bladder anatomy, pathological substaging of T2 disease should be performed in cystectomy specimens alone. Also, because there is often abundant adipose tissue between muscularis propria bundles, the presence of tumor in adipose tissue in a TURBT specimen does not necessarily equate to perivesical fat involvement [123]. Hence, pathologic staging in TURBT specimens is limited to whether the tumor is Ta, T1, or T2 (Fig. 5.8). The distinction between T2a, T2b, and pT3 cancer is, hence, performed in cystectomy specimens alone.

Imaging

Imaging of the bladder to help stage the primary tumor has limited value. Overall, the sensitivity of CT in detecting bladder cancer ranges from 79 to 89.7% with a specificity of 91–94.7% [124, 125]. However, the accuracy of CT in staging invasive bladder cancers is approximately 55%. Given that CT cannot accurately distinguish organ-confined from non-organ-confined disease, it is rarely utilized for this purpose [126, 127]. While techniques such as instillation of contrast into the bladder and air insufflation can be used to improve the staging accuracy of CT, these tests have limited clinical value [128, 129]. Although MRI is superior to CT in staging of the primary tumor, it cannot reliably distinguish the layers of the bladder wall and is rarely used for this purpose. The staging accuracy of contrast-enhanced dynamic MRI ranges from 62 to 85%; but when performed after TUR, perivesical inflammation from tumor resection can lead to overstaging tumors that are confined to the bladder [127, 130–132]. El-Assmy et al. compared diffusion-weighted MRI with T2-weighted MRI [133]. Diffusion-weighted imaging outperformed T2 MRI but was only 63.6% accurate in differentiating superficial from invasive tumors and 69.6% accurate in differentiating organ-confined from non-organ-confined tumors.

In contrast to their role in local staging of bladder tumors, CT and MRI are integral to the metastatic survey of patients with muscle-invasive or high-risk NMIBC. CT is the imaging modality most often used to evaluate for nodal and distant abdominal/pelvic metastases, though the sensitivity of CT for detecting nodal involvement is as low as 14–19% [126, 134]. Both MRI and CT are limited by the inability to recognize cancer in normal-sized lymph nodes, and a number of techniques for improving their performance have been evaluated. For example, using three-dimensional T1-weighted imaging, Jager et al. [135] demonstrated a sensitivity of 75% for detecting nodal metastases. Ferumoxtran-10, an ultra-small superparamagnetic iron oxide particle, has been used as an enhancing agent, with a reported sensitivity of 96%, specificity of 95%, and negative predictive value of 98% in the identification of individual lymph nodes harboring tumor [136]. In 12 normal-sized nodes with metastatic cancer, ten were correctly identified as harboring tumor. Thoeny et al. [137] have reported a novel approach combining ferumoxtran-10 with diffusion-weighted MRI. Evaluating only patients with normal-sized nodes, they reported negative predictive values of 86–93% and sensitivities of 60–80%, while significantly shortening MRI reading times from the previously employed pre- and post-contrast T2 technique (13 vs. 80 min).

Finally, ^{18}F-FDG positron emission tomography (PET) has been utilized in the evaluation of regional and distant sites of metastasis with sensitivity and specificity reported as 76.9% and 97.1%, respectively, for detecting metastatic disease [138]. The role of ^{18}F-FDG PET in pelvic imaging is limited due to urinary excretion of ^{18}F-FDG [139], and other agents such as ^{11}C-choline and ^{11}C-methionine are undergoing investigation as PET tracers for bladder cancer. While combined PET/CT holds promise in the evaluation of bladder cancer patients with suspected recurrent, nodal, or metastatic disease, its use is controversial and currently limited to investigational applications. To complete the metastatic evaluation in patients with muscle-invasive cancer, a chest radiograph should be performed, and a bone scan is required in the setting of an elevated alkaline phosphatase. A CT chest should be obtained in lieu of a chest radiograph in patients with clinical T3 or node-positive disease and those with high-risk histologic variants such as micropapillary carcinoma.

Secondary Tumors

Carcinomas of the prostate (see later), rectosigmoid, and uterine cervix are the most common primary neoplasms to involve the bladder by direct extension [140, 141]. Additionally, urachal carcinomas are a separate entity from primary bladder adenocarcinoma, and most urachal cancers invade the bladder.

Colorectal

Colorectal carcinoma most commonly involves the bladder by direct invasion, but also by discontinuous metastases. Histologically, it is impossible to distinguish a colon or urachal adenocarcinoma extending into the bladder from a bladder primary adenocarcinoma [142, 143]. Only if there is a mixed urothelial carcinoma with enteric differentiation can a bladder primary be established. A history of high-grade, high-stage colon cancer is important and, if present, an adenocarcinoma in the bladder with enteric histology should be considered as a metastasis. Immunohistochemical studies can in some cases suggest a colon primary (strong diffuse nuclear Beta-catenin expression; CK7 negative/CK20 positive) although other "intestinal" markers (CDX2, villin) may be expressed in both [143–148]. As immunohistochemical studies are not definitive, we report cases with this differential diagnosis as: "Although this tumor may be primary in the bladder, an intestinal adenocarcinoma with spread to the bladder should be excluded on clinical grounds."

Uterine Cervix

Routine pathology cannot distinguish squamous cell carcinoma primary in the uterine cervix from urothelial or squamous carcinoma of the bladder. In situ hybridization for HPV 16 and 18 may also be useful, as, with rare exception, urothelial and squamous carcinoma of the bladder are not related to HPV [149, 150]. Immunohistochemistry for p16 is not useful diagnostically because it is expressed in both bladder and uterine cervical cancer [151, 152].

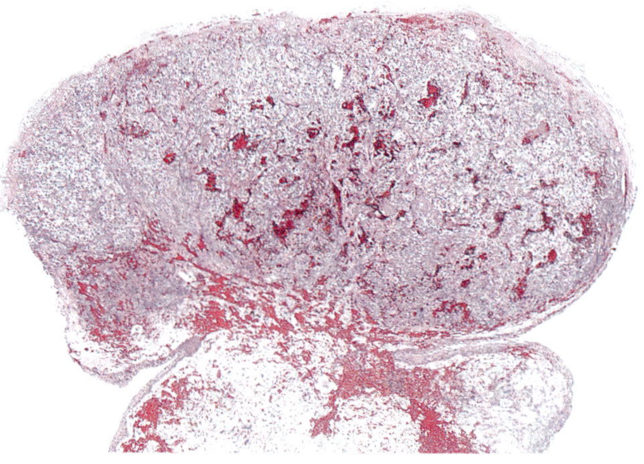

Fig. 5.9 Polypoid nodule of metastatic clear cell renal cell carcinoma to the bladder

Metastases to the Bladder

Melanoma is the most common tumor to metastasize to the bladder [140]. Other relatively common tumors include breast, stomach, lung, and kidney (Fig. 5.9) [140, 141, 153–158]. Rare examples of other primary sites with tumors metastatic to the bladder are pancreas, testis, gallbladder, liver, uterus, skin, appendix, and tongue [140, 141, 159–163]. Carcinomas with micropapillary morphology can occur in the bladder, breast, ovary, and lung and can be distinguished with an immunohistochemical panel [164, 165]. Metastatic small cell carcinoma to the bladder from the lung is histologically and immunohistochemically identical to primary small cell carcinoma arising in the bladder, with the exception that in some bladder small cell carcinomas, identification of CIS or invasive urothelial carcinoma can verify a bladder primary [166]. If at the time of diagnosis of small cell carcinoma involving the bladder, tumor appears localized to the bladder, it unlikely represents spread from an occult pulmonary primary.

Prostate Staging

Prostatic urothelial carcinoma has its own staging system independent of any concomitant bladder carcinoma. TNM stage is determined by depth of invasion, and the 2010 UICC-AJCC staging system is given in Table 5.5. CIS involving the prostate is distinguished by the suffix "is pd" for involvement of the prostatic ducts and "is pu" for involvement of the prostatic urethra. This staging system applies only to tumors originating from the prostatic urethra and involving prostatic ducts and acini with or without associated prostatic stromal invasion. In contrast, when invasive urothelial carcinoma from the bladder directly extends into the prostatic stroma, it is designated as pT4a disease.

The prostatic urethra is frequently involved with urothelial carcinoma in the setting of bladder carcinoma—prostatic urothelial carcinoma has been identified in up to 48% of cystoprostatectomy specimens [167, 168]. Stromal invasion of the prostate is present in 7–17% patients undergoing radical cystectomy [168–171], and the prostate is the primary source of urothelial carcinoma in 3% of patients [168]. Three patterns of bladder cancer invasion into the prostate have been characterized: extension along the urethra, extravesically into the prostate, and submucosally through the bladder neck [172]. Key risk factors for prostatic involvement include bladder CIS, multifocal disease, and bladder tumors located in the trigone or bladder neck [173–177]. Prostatic stromal invasion from prostatic urothelial carcinoma originating in the prostate carries an approximately 2.5-fold increased risk of mortality independent of other clinical and pathologic variables [178, 179].

Table 5.5 TNM staging system for urethral carcinoma of the prostate

Definitions of TNM	
Primary tumor (T) (male and female)	
TX	Primary tumor cannot be assessed
T0	No evidence of primary tumor
Ta	Noninvasive papillary, polypoid, or verrucous carcinoma
Tis	Carcinoma in situ
T1	Tumor invades subepithelial connective tissue
T2	Tumor invades any of the following: corpus spongiosum, prostate, periurethral muscle
T3	Tumor invades any of the following: corpus cavernosum, beyond prostatic capsule, anterior vagina, bladder neck
T4	Tumor invades other adjacent organs
Urothelial (transitional cell) carcinoma of the prostate (T)	
Tis pu	Carcinoma in situ, involvement of the prostatic urethra
Tis pd	Carcinoma in situ, involvement of the prostatic ducts
T1	Tumor invades urethral subepithelial connective tissue
T2	Tumor invades any of the following: prostatic stroma, corpus spongiosum, periurethral muscle
T3	Tumor invades any of the following: corpus cavernosum, beyond prostatic capsule, bladder neck (extraprostatic extension)
T4	Tumor invades other adjacent organs (invasion of the bladder)
Regional lymph nodes (N)	
NX	Regional lymph nodes cannot be assessed
N0	No regional lymph node metastasis
N1	Metastasis in a single lymph node 2 cm or less in greatest dimension
N2	Metastasis in a single node more than 2 cm in greatest dimension, or in multiple nodes
Distant metastasis (M)	
M0	No distant metastasis
M1	Distant metastasis

Adapted from Edge et al. [114]. Used with the permission of the American Joint Committee on Cancer (AJCC), Chicago, Illinois. The original source for this material is the AJCC Cancer Staging Manual, Seventh Edition (2010) published by Springer-Verlag New York, http:\\www.springer.com

Given the high incidence and prognostic significance of prostatic urothelial carcinoma in patients with bladder cancer, staging of bladder cancer should include independent evaluation of the prostatic urethra. Prostatic lesions should be biopsied to assess for stromal invasion, and patients with known prostatic urothelial carcinoma should have an intraoperative frozen section of the apical distal urethral margin at the time of cystectomy. Some have recommended TUR or mucosal biopsy of the prostatic urethra in all patients with high-grade cancer, with biopsies taken at the level of the verumontanum where there is the highest concentration of prostatic ducts [180–182]. However, TUR does not detect prostatic involvement with great accuracy [183]. Donat et al. [183] reported sensitivity and specificity of 53% and 77%, respectively, in patients who underwent TUR prior to cystectomy, and many have suggested that the decision to perform an orthotopic diversion may be based on the results of frozen section analysis of the apical margin at the time of cystectomy [167, 184]. While both prostatic stromal invasion and a positive apical margin significantly increase the risk of urethral recurrence; the latter may be the one absolute indication for urethrectomy in patients undergoing radical cystectomy [185–187]. It is important to note that the risk of urethral recurrence is significantly less with an orthotopic than a cutaneous diversion, even among patients with no prostatic urethral involvement [187].

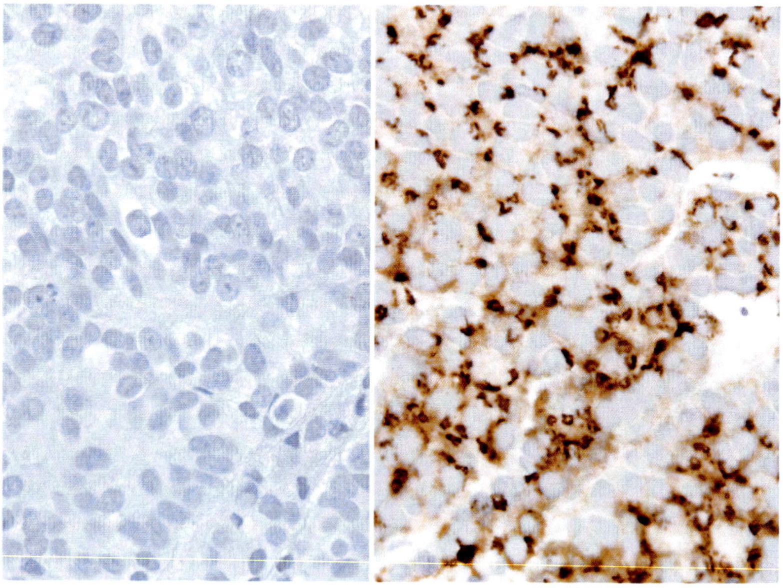

Fig. 5.10 Poorly differentiated prostate adenocarcinoma with negative stains for PSA (*left*), yet demonstrating characteristic granular immunoreactivity for P501s (*right*)

The mechanism for this disparity is not known, and may simply reflect selection bias. Staging biopsy showing prostatic ductal CIS may alter the management strategy for a patient who is otherwise deemed eligible for bladder preservation with TUR +/- BCG. CIS of the prostatic ducts is difficult to monitor and may not respond to BCG as CIS occurring at other sites. These patients may be at risk for silent progression in the prostatic ducts—thus, these patients may be considered for immediate cystoprostatectomy.

Pathologic Staging

A common diagnostic problem is in differentiating poorly differentiated urothelial carcinoma of the bladder from poorly differentiated prostatic adenocarcinoma on TURP [188]. In many cases, there are histological clues that can separate out these entities. However, there are rare cases of prostate adenocarcinoma with marked pleomorphism termed "pleomorphic giant cell adenocarcinoma of the prostate" that are microscopically identical to urothelial carcinoma [189]. Consequently, in a poorly differentiated tumor involving the bladder and prostate without any glandular differentiation typical of prostate adenocarcinoma, the case should be worked up immunohistochemically.

Approximately 90% of poorly differentiated prostatic adenocarcinomas show prostate-specific antigen (PSA) and prostate-specific acid phosphatase (PSAP) staining, although it may be focal [190–192]. With only a few exceptions, immunoperoxidase staining for "prostatic markers" is very specific for prostatic tissue [193–196]. Immunohistochemical stains used to label urothelial carcinoma, which are in general negative in prostate cancer, include high molecular weight cytokeratin, p63, thrombomodulin, and GATA3 [160, 197, 198]. The authors propose that a first-line panel for this differential should include PSA (expected positive for prostate cancer) and p63 and high molecular weight cytokeratin (expected negative in prostate cancer). In cases not fully resolved by this panel, a second line panel including NKX3.1 and P501S (expected positive in prostate) should help resolve most cases (Fig. 5.10).

Management

Non-Muscle-Invasive Bladder Cancer

Although up to 80% of bladder cancers are non-muscle-invasive (NMIBC) at the time of diagnosis, 15–25% will eventually progress to invasive disease. Most patients with NMIBC may be followed with close cystoscopic surveillance and re-resection when new tumors arise [199]. Additionally, there is level I evidence supporting the use of a single, prophylactic postoperative instillation of intravesical chemotherapy in patients with NMIBC [200]. This is based on a 39% decrease in the odds of tumor recurrence and is reflected in the published guidelines [83, 199]. However, the predicted effectiveness of a single instillation of perioperative chemotherapy has been estimated by the American Urological Association (AUA) Guidelines Panel to be a more modest 17% reduction in recurrence [199]. Additionally, the benefit is reduced in patients with multiple tumors as compared to solitary lesions.

Patients with NMIBC may also benefit from further induction and maintenance intravesical therapy regimens. BCG has been consistently shown to be superior to mitomycin C (MMC) in the treatment of NMIBC, but only with inclusion of a maintenance regimen [201]. The response to BCG is greatest in patients with CIS, and up to 68% experience a complete response [202]. Notably, patients may continue to respond to BCG up to 6 months after induction therapy due to the nature of the immune response [203]. In patients who suffer a recurrence after one induction course of BCG, another induction course of BCG may still be of benefit. In fact, in patients who fail a single 6-week course, up to one-third of patients may be salvaged with an additional course of BCG. Those with persistent disease despite two courses of BCG are unlikely to benefit from additional intravesical BCG and alternative strategies should be discussed [204].

A number of potential intravesical treatments exist for patients with BCG-refractory NMIBC; however, all offer only limited success rates. Administration of MMC via microwave hyperthermia [205] or electromotive drug administration [206] has shown benefit over MMC alone and may be effective in patients with BCG-refractory disease. A derivative of MMC, apaziquone, has also demonstrated potential as an intravesical agent [207]. In patients with BCG-refractory CIS, valrubicin is currently the only US Food and Drug Administration (FDA)-approved drug [208]. Other promising agents include mycobacterial cell wall–DNA complex, with response rates up to 46% in a mostly pretreated population [209], and DTA-H19, a DNA plasmid carrying the diptheria toxin A gene [210]. The available evidence suggests that intravesical salvage strategies for BCG-refractory NMIBC may decrease recurrence rates over the short term, but most patients will ultimately develop recurrent disease requiring cystectomy.

Patients with T1 bladder cancer present a particularly difficult group of patients to treat. While these patients may be appropriately managed endoscopically, they also carry a high risk of recurrence and progression, and there are not yet clear criteria delineating which patients should undergo aggressive surgical management. Early cystectomy in patients with T1 cancer does appear to offer a survival advantage. Hautmann et al. [211] reported a 10-year cancer-specific survival of 78.7% in a large nonrandomized cohort undergoing early cystectomy and 64.5% in those undergoing delayed cystectomy. This survival benefit is at the expense of "overtreating" a substantial proportion of patients, and, in order to help select patients for early cystectomy, a number of predictors have been identified. The presence of CIS and/or muscularis mucosa invasion is clearly associated with upstaging at cystectomy [212–215]. Other predictors of understaging and disease progression include lymphovascular invasion, small-cell or micropapillary components, and urethral involvement [215–217].

Muscle-Invasive Bladder Cancer

In patients with muscle-invasive tumors, the standard treatment is radical cystectomy. In those without lymph node involvement and using prior staging criteria, Stein et al. [218] reported 10-year recurrence-free survival rates of 87% in T2, 76% in T3, and 45% in T4 disease. Lymph node involvement varied with tumor stage, ranging from 18% of patients with T2a disease to 45% of patients with T3/T4 disease, and the 10-year recurrence-free survival rate in these patients was 34%. There is a clear relationship between survival after cystectomy and the number of lymph nodes removed at the time of surgery. Herr et al. [219] showed significant differences in survival among 68 node-positive patients depending on the number of lymph nodes obtained. Additionally, among 258 node-negative patients, the number of lymph nodes removed remained an important predictor of survival [219]. This association between increasing lymph node counts and improved overall survival after cystectomy has also been demonstrated in a population-based study [220].

Bladder-sparing therapies, which generally include endoscopic resection followed by chemotherapy and radiation, may obviate the need for radical cystectomy. No randomized trials have compared these regimens with immediate radical cystectomy; however, some series have demonstrated survival rates that are similar to cystectomy series. In these studies, selection of appropriate candidates is essential based on a variety of clinical and pathologic characteristics. Candidates for bladder-preserving protocols generally are recommended to have a solitary tumor <5 cm in size, clinical stage T2 or lower, no hydronephrosis, and no evidence of lymphatic or distant metastases. Of note, patients who recur with invasive disease after attempted bladder preservation should be strongly reconsidered to undergo cystectomy. Rodel et al. reported a 10-year disease-specific survival of 42% with over 80% of survivors preserving their bladder [221].

Chemotherapy

The administration of chemotherapy before or after radical cystectomy is an area of ongoing debate, with only neoadjuvant chemotherapy supported by level 1 evidence. Neoadjuvant chemotherapy offers a number of potential advantages, including early treatment of microscopic metastases, downstaging of the primary tumor, and improved patient tolerance relative to adjuvant chemotherapy. A potential disadvantage; however, is the delay in cystectomy, as longer waiting periods between TUR and cystectomy are associated with worse outcomes [222–224].

Use of neoadjuvant chemotherapy is supported by a number of studies. The Southwest Oncology Group's study 8710 (SWOG 8710) randomized 307 patients with locally advanced bladder cancer to cystectomy with or without neoadjuvant chemotherapy [225]. Patients randomized to the chemotherapy group received methotrexate, vinblastine, adriamycin, and cisplatin (MVAC) and had significantly improved overall and disease-specific survival. The greatest benefit was to patients with T3 or T4 disease, while there appeared to be little impact on patients with T2 cancer. A meta-analysis of 3,005 patients from 11 randomized trials found that neoadjuvant chemotherapy provided a 5% absolute overall survival benefit at 5 years ($p=0.003$) [226]. While adjuvant chemotherapy has the advantage of selecting patients at highest risk for failure, most adjuvant chemotherapy trials have failed to demonstrate a significant benefit [227]. However, most adjuvant chemotherapy studies following cystectomy suffer from methodological flaws including small sample size as compared to the neoadjuvant studies that limit definitive conclusions. In patients with persistent node-positive disease at cystectomy despite neoadjuvant treatment, Kassouf et al. found a significant improvement in recurrence-free survival with the administration of adjuvant chemotherapy (13 vs. 5 month, $p=0.02$) [228].

Conclusion

Significant differences in bladder cancer incidence and survival by race and gender exist, and ongoing research continues to advance our understanding of the factors behind these disparities. From a clinical standpoint, further development of cystoscopic and imaging technologies to assist with the detection and staging of bladder cancers holds significant promise. The appropriate management of bladder cancer patients relies heavily on accurate staging and grading at the time of TURBT. The pathological identification of T1 disease can be particularly challenging, but careful tissue handling, minimal use of electrocautery, and inclusion of muscularis during endoscopic resection can facilitate an accurate pathologic diagnosis. While there is continued debate over how best to manage patients with T1 cancer, it is important to counsel patients on the risks and benefits of early cystectomy versus bladder-sparing regimens. Additional progress continues to be made in the treatment of muscle-invasive bladder cancer, including the increasing use of neoadjuvant chemotherapy and minimally invasive approaches to radical cystectomy, however, the importance of an appropriate lymph node dissection remains paramount regardless of approach. Hopefully, continued advances in systemic chemotherapy will provide further improvements in survival and quality of life for these patients in the near future.

Disclosures Dr. Cookson: Endo, Allergan, GE Healthcare

References

1. Siegel R, Ward E, Brawley O, et al. Cancer statistics, 2011: the impact of eliminating socioeconomic and racial disparities on premature cancer deaths. CA Cancer J Clin. 2011;61:212.
2. Scosyrev E, Noyes K, Feng C, et al. Sex and racial differences in bladder cancer presentation and mortality in the US. Cancer. 2009;115:68.
3. Horstmann M, Witthuhn R, Falk M, et al. Gender-specific differences in bladder cancer: a retrospective analysis. Gend med. 2008;5:385.
4. Mungan NA, Aben KK, Schoenberg MP, et al. Gender differences in stage-adjusted bladder cancer survival. Urology. 2000;55:876.
5. Puente D, Malats N, Cecchini L, et al. Gender-related differences in clinical and pathological characteristics and therapy of bladder cancer. Eur Urol. 2003;43:53.
6. Johnson EK, Daignault S, Zhang Y, et al. Patterns of hematuria referral to urologists: does a gender disparity exist? Urology. 2008;72:498.
7. Glaser S, Satariano E, Leung R, et al. Cancer incidence by race/ethnicity in the San Francisco Bay Area: twenty years of cancer reporting, 1973-1992. Union City: Northern California Cancer Center; 1995.
8. Hankey B. Urinary bladder. In: Miller B, Ries LAG, Hankey B, et al., editors. Cancer statistics review 1973-1989. Bethesda: National Cancer Institute; 1992.
9. Smart CR. Bladder cancer survival statistics. J Occup Med. 1990;32:926.
10. Canto MT, Chu KC. Annual cancer incidence rates for Hispanics in the United States: surveillance, epidemiology, and end results, 1992-1996. Cancer. 2000;88:2642.
11. Lee CT, Dunn RL, Williams C, et al. Racial disparity in bladder cancer: trends in tumor presentation at diagnosis. J Urol. 2006;176:927.
12. Lynch CF, Cohen MB. Urinary system. Cancer. 1995;75:316.
13. Prout GR, Wesley MN, Greenberg RS, et al. Bladder cancer: race differences in extent of disease at diagnosis. Cancer. 2000;89:1349.
14. Hollenbeck BK, Dunn RL, Ye Z, et al. Racial differences in treatment and outcomes among patients with early stage bladder cancer. Cancer. 2010;116(1):50–6.
15. Taub DA, Hollenbeck BK, Cooper KL, et al. Racial disparities in resource utilization for cystectomy. Urology. 2006;67:288.
16. Lucas FL, Stukel TA, Morris AM, et al. Race and surgical mortality in the United States. Ann Surg. 2006;243:281.
17. Liu JH, Zingmond DS, McGory ML, et al. Disparities in the utilization of high-volume hospitals for complex surgery. JAMA. 2006;296:1973.
18. Yu MC, Ross RK, Chan KK, et al. Glutathione S-transferase M1 genotype affects aminobiphenyl-hemoglobin adduct levels in white, black and Asian smokers and nonsmokers. Cancer Epidemiol Biomarkers Prev. 1995;4:861.
19. Schultzel M, Saltzstein SL, Downs TM, et al. Late age (85 years or older) peak incidence of bladder cancer. J Urol. 2008;179:1302.
20. Edwards BK, Howe HL, Ries LAG, et al. Annual report to the nation on the status of cancer, 1973-1999, featuring implications of age and aging on U.S. cancer burden. Cancer. 2002;94:2766.
21. Shi B, Zhang K, Zhang J, et al. Relationship between patient age and superficial transitional cell carcinoma characteristics. Urology. 2008;71:1186.
22. Nielsen ME, Shariat SF, Karakiewicz PI, et al. Advanced age is associated with poorer bladder cancer-specific survival in patients treated with radical cystectomy. Eur Urol. 2007;51:699.
23. Resorlu B, Beduk Y, Baltaci S, et al. The prognostic significance of advanced age in patients with bladder cancer treated with radical cystectomy. BJU Int. 2009;103:480.

24. Prout GR, Wesley MN, Yancik R, et al. Age and comorbidity impact surgical therapy in older bladder carcinoma patients: a population-based study. Cancer. 2005;104:1638.
25. Zeegers MP, Tan FE, Dorant E, et al. The impact of characteristics of cigarette smoking on urinary tract cancer risk: a meta-analysis of epidemiologic studies. Cancer. 2000;89:630.
26. Zeegers MPA, Goldbohm RA, van den Brandt PA. A prospective study on active and environmental tobacco smoking and bladder cancer risk (The Netherlands). Cancer Causes Control. 2002;13:83.
27. Baris D, Karagas MR, Verrill C, et al. A case-control study of smoking and bladder cancer risk: emergent patterns over time. J Natl Cancer Inst. 2009; 101:1553.
28. Brennan P, Bogillot O, Cordier S, et al. Cigarette smoking and bladder cancer in men: a pooled analysis of 11 case-control studies. Int J Cancer. 2000;86:289.
29. Fleshner N, Garland J, Moadel A, et al. Influence of smoking status on the disease-related outcomes of patients with tobacco-associated superficial transitional cell carcinoma of the bladder. Cancer. 1999;86:2337.
30. Aveyard P, Adab P, Cheng K, et al. Does smoking status influence the prognosis of bladder cancer? A systematic review. BJU Int. 2002;90:228.
31. Strope SA, Montie JE. The causal role of cigarette smoking in bladder cancer initiation and progression, and the role of urologists in smoking cessation. J Urol. 2008;180:31.
32. Schroeder SA. What to do with a patient who smokes. JAMA. 2005;294:482.
33. Bao Y, Duan N, Fox SA. Is some provider advice on smoking cessation better than no advice? An instrumental variable analysis of the 2001 National Health Interview Survey. Health Serv Res. 2006;41:2114.
34. Hoffman D, Masuda Y, Wynder EL. Alpha-naphthylamine and beta-naphthylamine in cigarette smoke. Nature. 1969;221:255.
35. Johansson SL, Cohen SM. Epidemiology and etiology of bladder cancer. Semin Surg Oncol. 1997;13:291.
36. Ross RK, Jones PA, Yu MC. Bladder cancer epidemiology and pathogenesis. Semin Oncol. 1996;23:536.
37. Cao W, Cai L, Rao J-Y, et al. Tobacco smoking, GSTP1 polymorphism, and bladder carcinoma. Cancer. 2005;104:2400.
38. Lin J, Spitz MR, Dinney CP, et al. Bladder cancer risk as modified by family history and smoking. Cancer. 2006;107:705.
39. García-Closas M, Malats N, Real FX, et al. Genetic variation in the nucleotide excision repair pathway and bladder cancer risk. Cancer Epidemiol Biomarkers Prev. 2006;15:536.
40. García-Closas M, Malats N, Silverman D, et al. NAT2 slow acetylation, GSTM1 null genotype, and risk of bladder cancer: results from the Spanish Bladder Cancer Study and meta-analyses. Lancet. 2005;366:649.
41. Rehn L. Blasengeschwulste bei Fuchsin-Arbeitern. Arch Klin Chir. 1895;50:588.
42. Golka K, Hermes M, Selinski S, et al. Susceptibility to urinary bladder cancer: relevance of rs9642880[T], GSTM1 0/0 and occupational exposure. Pharmacogenet Genomics. 2009;19(11):903–6.
43. Boffetta P, Jourenkova N, Gustavsson P. Cancer risk from occupational and environmental exposure to polycyclic aromatic hydrocarbons. Cancer Causes Control. 1997;8:444.
44. Castelao JE, Yuan JM, Gago-Dominguez M, et al. Non-steroidal anti-inflammatory drugs and bladder cancer prevention. Br J Cancer. 2000;82:1364.
45. Piper JM, Tonascia J, Matanoski GM. Heavy phenacetin use and bladder cancer in women aged 20 to 49 years. N Engl J Med. 1985;313:292.
46. Derby LE, Jick H. Acetaminophen and renal and bladder cancer. Epidemiology. 1996;7:358.
47. Rosenberg L, Rao RS, Palmer JR, et al. Transitional cell cancer of the urinary tract and renal cell cancer in relation to acetaminophen use (United States). Cancer Causes Control. 1998;9:83.
48. Pedersen-Bjergaard J, Ersbøll J, Hansen VL, et al. Carcinoma of the urinary bladder after treatment with cyclophosphamide for non-Hodgkin's lymphoma. N Engl J Med. 1988;318:1028.
49. Travis LB, Curtis RE, Glimelius B, et al. Bladder and kidney cancer following cyclophosphamide therapy for non-Hodgkin's lymphoma. J Natl Cancer Inst. 1995;87:524.
50. Cohen SM, Johansson SL. Epidemiology and etiology of bladder cancer. Urol Clin North Am. 1992;19:421.
51. Zeegers MP, Dorant E, Goldbohm RA, et al. Are coffee, tea, and total fluid consumption associated with bladder cancer risk? Results from the Netherlands Cohort Study. Cancer Causes Control. 2001;12:231.
52. Gouda I, Mokhtar N, Bilal D, et al. Bilharziasis and bladder cancer: a time trend analysis of 9843 patients. J Egypt Natl Canc Inst. 2007;19:158.
53. Locke JR, Hill DE, Walzer Y. Incidence of squamous cell carcinoma in patients with long-term catheter drainage. J Urol. 1985;133:1034.
54. Boice JD, Engholm G, Kleinerman RA, et al. Radiation dose and second cancer risk in patients treated for cancer of the cervix. Radiat Res. 1988;116:3.
55. Bostrom PJ, Soloway MS. Secondary cancer after radiotherapy for prostate cancer: should we be more aware of the risk? Eur Urol. 2007;52:973.
56. Nieder AM, Porter MP, Soloway MS. Radiation therapy for prostate cancer increases subsequent risk of bladder and rectal cancer: a population based cohort study. J Urol. 2008;180:2005.
57. Aben KKH, Witjes JA, Schoenberg MP, et al. Familial aggregation of urothelial cell carcinoma. Int J Cancer. 2002;98:274.

58. Kantor AF, Hartge P, Hoover RN, et al. Familial and environmental interactions in bladder cancer risk. Int J Cancer. 1985;35:703.
59. Goldgar DE, Easton DF, Cannon-Albright LA, et al. Systematic population-based assessment of cancer risk in first-degree relatives of cancer probands. J Natl Cancer Inst. 1994;86:1600.
60. Grossfeld GD, Wolf JS, Litwan MS, et al. Asymptomatic microscopic hematuria in adults: summary of the AUA best practice policy recommendations. Am Fam Physician. 2001;63:1145.
61. Khan MA, Shaw G, Paris AMI. Is microscopic haematuria a urological emergency? BJU Int. 2002;90:355.
62. Denzinger S, Wieland WF, Otto W, et al. Does photodynamic transurethral resection of bladder tumour improve the outcome of initial T1 high-grade bladder cancer?A long-term follow-up of a randomized study. BJU Int. 2008;101:566.
63. Grossman HB, Gomella L, Fradet Y, et al. A phase III, multicenter comparison of hexaminolevulinate fluorescence cystoscopy and white light cystoscopy for the detection of superficial papillary lesions in patients with bladder cancer. J Urol. 2007;178:62.
64. Goh AC, Tresser NJ, Shen SS, et al. Optical coherence tomography as an adjunct to white light cystoscopy for intravesical real-time imaging and staging of bladder cancer. Urology. 2008;72:133.
65. Schmidbauer J, Remzi M, Klatte T, et al. Fluorescence cystoscopy with high-resolution optical coherence tomography imaging as an adjunct reduces false-positive findings in the diagnosis of urothelial carcinoma of the bladder. Eur Urol. 2009;56:914.
66. Sonn GA, Jones S-NE, Tarin TV, et al. Optical biopsy of human bladder neoplasia with in vivo confocal laser endomicroscopy. J Urol. 2009; 182:1299.
67. Browne RFJ, Meehan CP, Colville J, et al. Transitional cell carcinoma of the upper urinary tract: spectrum of imaging findings. Radiographics. 2005;25:1609.
68. Vikram R, Sandler CM, Ng CS. Imaging and staging of transitional cell carcinoma: part 2, upper urinary tract. AJR Am J Roentgenol. 2009;192:1488.
69. Grossfeld GD, Litwin MS, Wolf JS, et al. Evaluation of asymptomatic microscopic hematuria in adults: the American Urological Association best practice policy–part II: patient evaluation, cytology, voided markers, imaging, cystoscopy, nephrology evaluation, and follow-up. Urology. 2001;57:604.
70. Droller MJ. Bladder cancer: state-of-the-art care. CA Cancer J Clin. 1998;48:269.
71. Koss LG, Deitch D, Ramanathan R, et al. Diagnostic value of cytology of voided urine. Acta Cytol. 1985;29:810.
72. Wolinska WH, Melamed MR, Klein FA. Cytology of bladder papilloma. Acta Cytol. 1985;29:817.
73. Esposti PL, Zajicek J. Grading of transitional cell neoplasms of the urinary bladder from smears of bladder washings. A critical review of 326 tumors. Acta Cytol. 1972;16:529.
74. Kern WH. The cytology of transitional cell carcinoma of the urinary bladder. Acta Cytol. 1975;19:420.
75. Murphy WM, Soloway MS, Jukkola AF, et al. Urinary cytology and bladder cancer. The cellular features of transitional cell neoplasms. Cancer. 1984;53:1555.
76. Rife CC, Farrow GM, Utz DC. Urine cytology of transitional cell neoplasms. Urol Clin North Am. 1979;6:599.
77. Cauberg EC, de la Rosette JJ, de Reijke TM. How to improve the effectiveness of transurethral resection in nonmuscle invasive bladder cancer? Curr Opin Urol. 2009;19:504.
78. Maruniak NA, Takezawa K, Murphy WM. Accurate pathological staging of urothelial neoplasms requires better cystoscopic sampling. J Urol. 2002;167:2404.
79. Taguchi I, Gohji K, Hara I, et al. Clinical evaluation of random biopsy of urinary bladder in patients with superficial bladder cancer. Int J Urol. 1998;5:30.
80. Thorstenson A, Schumacher MC, Wiklund NP, et al. Diagnostic random bladder biopsies: reflections from a population-based cohort of 538 patients. Scand J Urol Nephrol. 2010;44(1):11–9.
81. Kiemeney LA, Witjes JA, Heijbroek RP, et al. Should random urothelial biopsies be taken from patients with primary superficial bladder cancer?A decision analysis. Members of the Dutch South-East Co-Operative Urological Group. Br J Urol. 1994;73:164.
82. Weldon TE, Soloway MS, Persky L. Urothelial susceptibility to neoplastic cellular implantation. Surg Forum. 1974;25:547.
83. Babjuk M, Oosterlinck W, Sylvester R, et al. EAU guidelines on non-muscle-invasive urothelial carcinoma of the bladder. Eur Urol. 2008;54:303.
84. van der Meijden A, Oosterlinck W, Brausi M, et al. Significance of bladder biopsies in Ta, T1 bladder tumors: a report from the EORTC Genito-Urinary Tract Cancer Cooperative Group. EORTC-GU Group Superficial Bladder Committee. Eur Urol. 1999;35:267.
85. Epstein JI, Amin MB, Reuter VR, et al. The World Health Organization/International Society of Urological Pathology consensus classification of urothelial (transitional cell) neoplasms of the urinary bladder. Bladder Consensus Conference Committee. Am J Surg Pathol. 1998;22:1435.
86. Mostofi F, Sobin L, Torloni H. Histological typing of urinary bladder tumors. In: Mostofi FK, editor. International classification of tumors, vol. 10. Geneva: World Health Organization; 1973.
87. Eble J, Sauter G, Epstein J, et al. Pathology and genetics: tumors of the urinary system and male genital organs. WHO classification of tumors. Lyon: IARC Press; 2004.
88. Bircan S, Candir O, Serel TA. Comparison of WHO 1973, WHO/ISUP 1998, WHO 1999 grade and

combined scoring systems in evaluation of bladder carcinoma. Urol Int. 2004;73:201.

89. Samaratunga H, Makarov DV, Epstein JI. Comparison of WHO/ISUP and WHO classification of noninvasive papillary urothelial neoplasms for risk of progression. Urology. 2002;60:315.
90. Genega EM, Kapali M, Torres-Quinones M, et al. Impact of the 1998 World Health Organization/International Society of Urological Pathology classification system for urothelial neoplasms of the kidney. Mod Pathol. 2005;18:11.
91. Brunner A, Schonhuber G, Waldner M, et al. Chromosomal aberrations in urothelial carcinoma of the bladder and the World Health Organization 2004 grading system. Anal Quant Cytol Histol. 2008;30:297.
92. Burger M, Denzinger S, Wieland WF, et al. Does the current World Health Organization classification predict the outcome better in patients with noninvasive bladder cancer of early or regular onset? BJU Int. 2008;102:194.
93. Gonul II, Poyraz A, Unsal C, et al. Comparison of 1998 WHO/ISUP and 1973 WHO classifications for interobserver variability in grading of papillary urothelial neoplasms of the bladder. Pathological evaluation of 258 cases. Urol Int. 2007;78:338.
94. Mamoon N, Iqbal MA, Jamal S, et al. Urothelial neoplasia of the urinary bladder–comparison of interobserver variability for WHO Classification 1972 with WHO/ISUP Consensus Classification 1998. J Ayub Med Coll Abbottabad. 2006;18:4.
95. Pich A, Chiusa L, Formiconi A, et al. Biologic differences between noninvasive papillary urothelial neoplasms of low malignant potential and low-grade (grade 1) papillary carcinomas of the bladder. Am J Surg Pathol. 2001;25:1528.
96. Ramos D, Navarro S, Villamon R, et al. Cytokeratin expression patterns in low-grade papillary urothelial neoplasms of the urinary bladder. Cancer. 2003;97:1876.
97. Yorukoglu K, Tuna B, Dikicioglu E, et al. Reproducibility of the 1998 World Health Organization/International Society of Urologic Pathology classification of papillary urothelial neoplasms of the urinary bladder. Virchows Arch. 2003;443:734.
98. Oosterhuis JW, Schapers RF, Janssen-Heijnen ML, et al. Histological grading of papillary urothelial carcinoma of the bladder: prognostic value of the 1998 WHO/ISUP classification system and comparison with conventional grading systems. J Clin Pathol. 2002;55:900.
99. Schned AR, Andrew AS, Marsit CJ, et al. Survival following the diagnosis of noninvasive bladder cancer: WHO/International Society of Urological Pathology versus WHO classification systems. J Urol. 2007;178:1196.
100. Magi-Galluzzi C, Epstein JI. Urothelial papilloma of the bladder: a review of 34 de novo cases. Am J Surg Pathol. 2004;28:1615.
101. McKenney JK, Amin MB, Young RH. Urothelial (transitional cell) papilloma of the urinary bladder: a clinicopathologic study of 26 cases. Mod Pathol. 2003;16:623.
102. Herr HW, Donat SM, Reuter VE. Management of low grade papillary bladder tumors. J Urol. 2007;178:1201.
103. Cheng L, Darson M, Cheville JC, et al. Urothelial papilloma of the bladder. Clinical and biologic implications. Cancer. 1999;86:2098.
104. Murphy WM, Takezawa K, Maruniak NA. Interobserver discrepancy using the 1998 World Health Organization/International Society of Urologic Pathology classification of urothelial neoplasms: practical choices for patient care. J Urol. 2002;168:968.
105. Alsheikh A, Mohamedali Z, Jones E, et al. Comparison of the WHO/ISUP classification and cytokeratin 20 expression in predicting the behavior of low-grade papillary urothelial tumors. World/Health Organization/International Society of Urologic Pathology. Mod Pathol. 2001;14:267.
106. Campbell PA, Conrad RJ, Campbell CM, et al. Papillary urothelial neoplasm of low malignant potential: reliability of diagnosis and outcome. BJU Int. 2004;93:1228.
107. Desai S, Lim SD, Jimenez RE, et al. Relationship of cytokeratin 20 and CD44 protein expression with WHO/ISUP grade in pTa and pT1 papillary urothelial neoplasia. Mod Pathol. 2000;13:1315.
108. Holmang S, Andius P, Hedelin H, et al. Stage progression in Ta papillary urothelial tumors: relationship to grade, immunohistochemical expression of tumor markers, mitotic frequency and DNA ploidy. J Urol. 2001;165:1124.
109. Holmang S, Hedelin H, Anderstrom C, et al. Recurrence and progression in low grade papillary urothelial tumors. J Urol. 1999;162:702.
110. Fujii Y, Kawakami S, Koga F, et al. Long-term outcome of bladder papillary urothelial neoplasms of low malignant potential. BJU Int. 2003;92:559.
111. Fine SW, Humphrey PA, Dehner LP, et al. Urothelial neoplasms in patients 20 years or younger: a clinicopathological analysis using the world health organization 2004 bladder consensus classification. J Urol. 2005;174:1976.
112. Billis A, Carvalho RB, Mattos AC, et al. Tumor grade heterogeneity in urothelial bladder carcinoma–proposal of a system using combined numbers. Scand J Urol Nephrol. 2001;35:275.
113. Cheng L, Neumann RM, Nehra A, et al. Cancer heterogeneity and its biologic implications in the grading of urothelial carcinoma. Cancer. 2000;88:1663.
114. Edge SB, Byrd DR, Compton CC, Fritz AG, Greene FL, Trotti A, editors. AJCC cancer staging manual. 7th ed. New York: Springer; 2010.
115. Dutta SC, Smith JA, Shappell SB, et al. Clinical under staging of high risk nonmuscle invasive urothelial carcinoma treated with radical cystectomy. J Urol. 2001;166:490.

116. Kulkarni G, Hakenberg O, Gschwend J, et al. An updated critical analysis of the treatment strategy for newly diagnosed high-grade T1 (previously T1G3) bladder cancer. Eur Urol. 2010;57(1):60–70.
117. Ro JY, Ayala AG, el-Naggar A. Muscularis mucosa of urinary bladder. Importance for staging and treatment. Am J Surg Pathol. 1987;11:668.
118. Paner GP, Shen SS, Lapetino S, et al. Diagnostic utility of antibody to smoothelin in the distinction of muscularis propria from muscularis mucosae of the urinary bladder: a potential ancillary tool in the pathologic staging of invasive urothelial carcinoma. Am J Surg Pathol. 2009;33:91.
119. Jimenez RE, Keane TE, Hardy HT, et al. pT1 urothelial carcinoma of the bladder: criteria for diagnosis, pitfalls, and clinical implications. Adv Anat Pathol. 2000;7:13.
120. Holmang S, Hedelin H, Anderstrom C, et al. The importance of the depth of invasion in stage T1 bladder carcinoma: a prospective cohort study. J Urol. 1997;157:800.
121. Younes M, Sussman J, True LD. The usefulness of the level of the muscularis mucosae in the staging of invasive transitional cell carcinoma of the urinary bladder. Cancer. 1990;66:543.
122. Cheng L, Weaver AL, Neumann RM, et al. Substaging of T1 bladder carcinoma based on the depth of invasion as measured by micrometer: a new proposal. Cancer. 1999;86:1035.
123. Philip AT, Amin MB, Tamboli P, et al. Intravesical adipose tissue: a quantitative study of its presence and location with implications for therapy and prognosis. Am J Surg Pathol. 2000;24:1286.
124. Knox MK, Cowan NC, Rivers-Bowerman MD, et al. Evaluation of multidetector computed tomography urography and ultrasonography for diagnosing bladder cancer. Clin Radiol. 2008;63:1317.
125. Sadow CA, Silverman SG, O'Leary MP, et al. Bladder cancer detection with CT urography in an Academic Medical Center. Radiology. 2008;249:195.
126. Paik ML, Scolieri MJ, Brown SL, et al. Limitations of computerized tomography in staging invasive bladder cancer before radical cystectomy. J Urol. 2000;163:1693.
127. Tanimoto A, Yuasa Y, Imai Y, et al. Bladder tumor staging: comparison of conventional and gadolinium-enhanced dynamic MR imaging and CT. Radiology. 1992;185:741.
128. Caterino M, Giunta S, Finocchi V, et al. Primary cancer of the urinary bladder: CT evaluation of the T parameter with different techniques. Abdom Imaging. 2001;26:433.
129. Kim JK, Park S-Y, Ahn HJ, et al. Bladder cancer: analysis of multi-detector row helical CT enhancement pattern and accuracy in tumor detection and perivesical staging. Radiology. 2004;231:725.
130. Beyersdorff D, Taupitz M, Giessing M, et al. The staging of bladder tumors in MRT: the value of the intravesical application of an iron oxide-containing contrast medium in combination with high-resolution T2-weighted imaging. Rofo. 2000;172:504.
131. Tachibana M, Baba S, Deguchi N, et al. Efficacy of gadolinium-diethylenetriaminepentaacetic acid-enhanced magnetic resonance imaging for differentiation between superficial and muscle-invasive tumor of the bladder: a comparative study with computerized tomography and transurethral ultrasonography. J Urol. 1991;145:1169.
132. Tekes A, Kamel I, Imam K, et al. Dynamic MRI of bladder cancer: evaluation of staging accuracy. AJR Am J Roentgenol. 2005;184:121.
133. El-Assmy A, Abou-El-Ghar ME, Mosbah A, et al. Bladder tumour staging: comparison of diffusion- and T2-weighted MR imaging. Eur Radiol. 2009;19:1575.
134. deVere White R, Gold RP, et al. Sensitivity of computed tomography in evaluation of pelvic lymph node metastases from carcinoma of bladder and prostate. Urology. 1983;21:81.
135. Jager GJ, Barentsz JO, Oosterhof GO, et al. Pelvic adenopathy in prostatic and urinary bladder carcinoma: MR imaging with a three-dimensional TI-weighted magnetization-prepared-rapid gradient-echo sequence. AJR Am J Roentgenol. 1996;167:1503.
136. Deserno WM, Harisinghani MG, Taupitz M, et al. Urinary bladder cancer: preoperative nodal staging with ferumoxtran-10-enhanced MR imaging. Radiology. 2004;233:449.
137. Thoeny HC, Triantafyllou M, Birkhaeuser FD, et al. Combined ultrasmall superparamagnetic particles of iron oxide-enhanced and diffusion-weighted magnetic resonance imaging reliably detect pelvic lymph node metastases in normal-sized nodes of bladder and prostate cancer patients. Eur Urol. 2009;55:761.
138. Liu IJ, Lai Y-H, Espiritu JI, et al. Evaluation of fluorodeoxyglucose positron emission tomography imaging in metastatic transitional cell carcinoma with and without prior chemotherapy. Urol Int. 2006;77:69.
139. Jana S, Blaufox MD. Nuclear medicine studies of the prostate, testes, and bladder. Semin Nucl Med. 2006;36:51.
140. Velcheti V, Govindan R. Metastatic cancer involving bladder: a review. Can J Urol. 2007;14:3443.
141. Klinger ME. Secondary tumors of the genito-urinary tract. J Urol. 1951;65:144.
142. Silver SA, Epstein JI. Adenocarcinoma of the colon simulating primary urinary bladder neoplasia. A report of nine cases. Am J Surg Pathol. 1993;17:171.
143. Tamboli P, Mohsin SK, Hailemariam S, et al. Colonic adenocarcinoma metastatic to the urinary tract versus primary tumors of the urinary tract with glandular differentiation: a report of 7 cases and investigation using a limited immunohistochemical panel. Arch Pathol Lab Med. 2002;126:1057.

144. Thomas AA, Stephenson AJ, Campbell SC, et al. Clinicopathologic features and utility of immunohistochemical markers in signet-ring cell adenocarcinoma of the bladder. Hum Pathol. 2009;40:108.
145. Raspollini MR, Nesi G, Baroni G, et al. Immunohistochemistry in the differential diagnosis between primary and secondary intestinal adenocarcinoma of the urinary bladder. Appl Immunohistochem Mol Morphol. 2005;13:358.
146. Suh N, Yang XJ, Tretiakova MS, et al. Value of CDX2, villin, and alpha-methylacyl coenzyme A racemase immunostains in the distinction between primary adenocarcinoma of the bladder and secondary colorectal adenocarcinoma. Mod Pathol. 2005; 18:1217.
147. Werling RW, Yaziji H, Bacchi CE, et al. CDX2, a highly sensitive and specific marker of adenocarcinomas of intestinal origin: an immunohistochemical survey of 476 primary and metastatic carcinomas. Am J Surg Pathol. 2003;27:303.
148. Wang HL, Lu DW, Yerian LM, et al. Immunohistochemical distinction between primary adenocarcinoma of the bladder and secondary colorectal adenocarcinoma. Am J Surg Pathol. 2001; 25:1380.
149. Westenend PJ, Stoop JA, Hendriks JG. Human papillomaviruses 6/11, 16/18 and 31/33/51 are not associated with squamous cell carcinoma of the urinary bladder. BJU Int. 2001;88:198.
150. Maloney KE, Wiener JS, Walther PJ. Oncogenic human papillomaviruses are rarely associated with squamous cell carcinoma of the bladder: evaluation by differential polymerase chain reaction. J Urol. 1994;151:360.
151. Abdulamir AS, Hafidh RR, Kadhim HS, et al. Tumor markers of bladder cancer: the schistosomal bladder tumors versus non-schistosomal bladder tumors. J Exp Clin Cancer Res. 2009;28:27.
152. Yang CC, Chu KC, Chen HY, et al. Expression of p16 and cyclin D1 in bladder cancer and correlation in cancer progression. Urol Int. 2002;69:190.
153. Shiraishi K, Mohri J, Inoue R, et al. Metastatic renal cell carcinoma to the bladder 12 years after radical nephrectomy. Int J Urol. 2003;10:453.
154. Sim SJ, Ro JY, Ordonez NG, et al. Metastatic renal cell carcinoma to the bladder: a clinicopathologic and immunohistochemical study. Mod Pathol. 1999;12:351.
155. Silverstein LI, Plaine L, Davis JE, et al. Breast carcinoma metastatic to bladder. Urology. 1987;29:544.
156. Matsuo M, Koga S, Nishikido M, et al. Renal cell carcinoma with solitary metachronous metastasis to the urinary bladder. Urology. 2002;60:911.
157. van Driel MF, Ypma AF, van Gelder B. Gastric carcinoma metastatic to the bladder. Br J Urol. 1987;59:193.
158. Coltart RS, Stewart S, Brown CH. Small cell carcinoma of the bronchus: a rare cause of haematuria from a metastasis in the urinary bladder. J R Soc Med. 1985;78:1053.
159. Strasser H, Amann K, Schrott KM, et al. Solitary metastasis of a Merkel cell tumor to the urinary bladder. Anticancer Res. 2008;28:1361.
160. Chung SD, Ho CH, Hung SF, et al. Metastatic hepatocellular carcinoma in the urinary bladder with radiation-induced hemorrhagic cystitis. J Formos Med Assoc. 2007;106:861.
161. Chalbaud RA, Johnson DE. Adenocarcinoma of tongue metastatic to bladder. Urology. 1974;4:454.
162. Young RH, Johnston WH. Serous adenocarcinoma of the uterus metastatic to the urinary bladder mimicking primary bladder neoplasia. A report of a case. Am J Surg Pathol. 1990;14:877.
163. Henry R, Bracken RB, Ayala A. Appendiceal carcinoma mimicking primary bladder cancer. J Urol. 1980;123:590.
164. Ramalingam P, Middleton LP, Tamboli P, et al. Invasive micropapillary carcinoma of the breast metastatic to the urinary bladder and endometrium: diagnostic pitfalls and review of the literature of tumors with micropapillary features. Ann Diagn Pathol. 2003;7:112.
165. Lotan T, Ye H, Shih I, et al. Immunohistochemical panel to distinguish micropapillary urothelial carcinoma from breast, lung and ovarian micropapillary carcinomas. Am J Surg Pathol. 2009;33(7): 1037–41.
166. Jones TD, Kernek KM, Yang XJ, et al. Thyroid transcription factor 1 expression in small cell carcinoma of the urinary bladder: an immunohistochemical profile of 44 cases. Hum Pathol. 2005;36:718.
167. Revelo MP, Cookson MS, Chang SS, et al. Incidence and location of prostate and urothelial carcinoma in prostates from cystoprostatectomies: implications for possible apical sparing surgery. J Urol. 2004;171:646.
168. Wood DP, Montie JE, Pontes JE, et al. Transitional cell carcinoma of the prostate in cystoprostatectomy specimens removed for bladder cancer. J Urol. 1989;141:346.
169. Njinou Ngninkeu B, Lorge F, Moulin P, et al. Transitional cell carcinoma involving the prostate: a clinicopathological retrospective study of 76 cases. J Urol. 2003;169:149.
170. Pagano F, Bassi P, Ferrante G, et al. Is stage pT4a (D1) reliable in assessing transitional cell carcinoma involvement of the prostate in patients with a concurrent bladder cancer?A necessary distinction for contiguous or noncontiguous involvement. J Urol. 1996;155:244.
171. Reese JH, Freiha FS, Gelb AB, et al. Transitional cell carcinoma of the prostate in patients undergoing radical cystoprostatectomy. J Urol. 1992;147:92.
172. Donat SM, Genega EM, Herr HW, et al. Mechanisms of prostatic stromal invasion in patients with bladder cancer: clinical significance. J Urol. 2001;165: 1117.
173. Grabstald H. Prostatic biopsy in selected patients with carcinoma in situ of the bladder: preliminary report. J Urol. 1984;132:1117.

174. Patel SG, Cookson MS, Barocas DA, et al. Risk factors for urothelial carcinoma of the prostate in patients undergoing radical cystoprostatectomy for bladder cancer. BJU Int. 2009;104(7):934–7.
175. Hardeman SW, Soloway MS. Urethral recurrence following radical cystectomy. J Urol. 1990;144:666.
176. Mazzucchelli R, Barbisan F, Santinelli A, et al. Prediction of prostatic involvement by urothelial carcinoma in radical cystoprostatectomy for bladder cancer. Urology. 2009;74:385.
177. Tongaonkar HB, Dalal AV, Kulkarni JN, et al. Urethral recurrences following radical cystectomy for invasive transitional cell carcinoma of the bladder. Br J Urol. 1993;72:910.
178. Ayyathurai R, Gomez P, Luongo T, et al. Prostatic involvement by urothelial carcinoma of the bladder: clinicopathological features and outcome after radical cystectomy. BJU Int. 2007;100:1021.
179. Barocas DA, Patel SG, Chang SS, et al. Outcomes of patients undergoing radical cystoprostatectomy for bladder cancer with prostatic involvement on final pathology. BJU Int. 2009;104:1091.
180. Lerner SP, Shen S. Pathologic assessment and clinical significance of prostatic involvement by transitional cell carcinoma and prostate cancer. Urol Oncol. 2008;26:481.
181. Rikken CH, van Helsdingen PJ, Kazzaz BA. Are biopsies from the prostatic urethra useful in patients with superficial bladder carcinoma? Br J Urol. 1987;59:145.
182. Sakamoto N, Tsuneyoshi M, Naito S, et al. An adequate sampling of the prostate to identify prostatic involvement by urothelial carcinoma in bladder cancer patients. J Urol. 1993;149:318.
183. Donat S, Wei D, McGuire M, et al. The efficacy of transurethral biopsy for predicting the long-term clinical impact of prostatic invasive bladder cancer. J Urol. 2001;165:1580.
184. Lebret T, Hervé JM, Barré P, et al. Urethral recurrence of transitional cell carcinoma of the bladder. Predictive value of preoperative latero-montanal biopsies and urethral frozen sections during prostatocystectomy. Eur Urol. 1998;33:170.
185. Cho KS, Seo JW, Park SJ, et al. The risk factor for urethral recurrence after radical cystectomy in patients with transitional cell carcinoma of the bladder. Urol Int. 2009;82:306.
186. Freeman JA, Tarter TA, Esrig D, et al. Urethral recurrence in patients with orthotopic ileal neobladders. J Urol. 1996;156:1615.
187. Stein JP, Clark P, Miranda G, et al. Urethral tumor recurrence following cystectomy and urinary diversion: clinical and pathological characteristics in 768 male patients. J Urol. 2005;173:1163.
188. Epstein JI, Netto GJ. Biopsy interpretation of the prostate. 4th ed. Philadelphia, PA: Lippincott Williams Wilkins; 2008.
189. Parwani AV, Herawi M, Epstein JI. Pleomorphic giant cell adenocarcinoma of the prostate: report of 6 cases. Am J Surg Pathol. 2006;30:1254.
190. Ellis DW, Leffers S, Davies JS, et al. Multiple immunoperoxidase markers in benign hyperplasia and adenocarcinoma of the prostate. Am J Clin Pathol. 1984;81:279.
191. Ford TF, Butcher DN, Masters JR, et al. Immunocytochemical localisation of prostate-specific antigen: specificity and application to clinical practice. Br J Urol. 1985;57:50.
192. Svanholm H. Evaluation of commercial immunoperoxidase kits for prostatic specific antigen and prostatic specific acid phosphatase. Acta Pathol Microbiol Immunol Scand A. 1986;94:7.
193. Lane Z, Hansel DE, Epstein JI. Immunohistochemical expression of prostatic antigens in adenocarcinoma and villous adenoma of the urinary bladder. Am J Surg Pathol. 2008;32:1322.
194. Heyderman E, Brown BM, Richardson TC. Epithelial markers in prostatic, bladder, and colorectal cancer: an immunoperoxidase study of epithelial membrane antigen, carcinoembryonic antigen, and prostatic acid phosphatase. J Clin Pathol. 1984;37:1363.
195. Epstein JI, Kuhajda FP, Lieberman PH. Prostate-specific acid phosphatase immunoreactivity in adenocarcinomas of the urinary bladder. Hum Pathol. 1986;17:939.
196. Nadji M, Tabei SZ, Castro A, et al. Prostatic-specific antigen: an immunohistologic marker for prostatic neoplasms. Cancer. 1981;48:1229.
197. Varma M, Morgan M, Amin MB, et al. High molecular weight cytokeratin antibody (clone 34betaE12): a sensitive marker for differentiation of high-grade invasive urothelial carcinoma from prostate cancer. Histopathology. 2003;42:167.
198. Chuang AY, DeMarzo AM, Veltri RW, et al. Immunohistochemical differentiation of high-grade prostate carcinoma from urothelial carcinoma. Am J Surg Pathol. 2007;31:1246.
199. Hall MC, Chang SS, Dalbagni G, et al. Guideline for the management of nonmuscle invasive bladder cancer (stages Ta, T1, and Tis): 2007 update. J Urol. 2007;178:2314.
200. Sylvester RJ, Oosterlinck W, van der Meijden APM. A single immediate postoperative instillation of chemotherapy decreases the risk of recurrence in patients with stage Ta T1 bladder cancer: a meta-analysis of published results of randomized clinical trials. J Urol. 2004;171:2186.
201. Malmström P-U, Sylvester RJ, Crawford DE, et al. An individual patient data meta-analysis of the long-term outcome of randomised studies comparing intravesical mitomycin C versus bacillus Calmette-Guérin for non-muscle-invasive bladder cancer. Eur Urol. 2009;56:247.
202. Lamm DL, Blumenstein BA, Crissman JD, et al. Maintenance bacillus Calmette-Guerin immunotherapy for recurrent TA, T1 and carcinoma in situ transitional cell carcinoma of the bladder: a randomized Southwest Oncology Group Study. J Urol. 2000; 163:1124.

203. Herr HW, Dalbagni G. Defining bacillus Calmette-Guerin refractory superficial bladder tumors. J Urol. 2003;169:1706.
204. Montie JE, Clark PE, Eisenberger MA, et al. Bladder cancer. J Natl Compr Canc Netw. 2009;7:8.
205. Witjes AJ, Hendricksen K, Gofrit O, et al. Intravesical hyperthermia and mitomycin-C for carcinoma in situ of the urinary bladder: experience of the European Synergo working party. World J Urol. 2009;27:319.
206. Di Stasi SM, Riedl C. Updates in intravesical electromotive drug administration of mitomycin-C for non-muscle invasive bladder cancer. World J Urol. 2009;27:325.
207. Jain A, Phillips RM, Scally AJ, et al. Response of multiple recurrent TaT1 bladder cancer to intravesical apaziquone (EO9): comparative analysis of tumor recurrence rates. Urology. 2009;73:1083.
208. Steinberg G, Bahnson R, Brosman S, et al. Efficacy and safety of valrubicin for the treatment of Bacillus Calmette-Guerin refractory carcinoma in situ of the bladder. The Valrubicin Study Group. Urol J. 2000;163:761.
209. Morales A, Phadke K, Steinhoff G. Intravesical mycobacterial cell wall-DNA complex in the treatment of carcinoma in situ of the bladder after standard intravesical therapy has failed. J Urol. 2009;181:1040.
210. Sidi AA, Ohana P, Benjamin S, et al. Phase I/II marker lesion study of intravesical BC-819 DNA plasmid in H19 over expressing superficial bladder cancer refractory to bacillus Calmette-Guerin. J Urol. 2008;180:2379.
211. Hautmann RE, Volkmer BG, Gust K. Quantification of the survival benefit of early versus deferred cystectomy in high-risk non-muscle invasive bladder cancer (T1 G3). World J Urol. 2009;27:347.
212. Holmäng S, Hedelin H, Anderström C, et al. The importance of the depth of invasion in stage T1 bladder carcinoma: a prospective cohort study. J Urol. 1997;157:800.
213. Masood S, Sriprasad S, Palmer JH, et al. T1G3 bladder cancer–indications for early cystectomy. Int Urol Nephrol. 2004;36:41.
214. Orsola A, Trias I, Raventós CX, et al. Initial high-grade T1 urothelial cell carcinoma: feasibility and prognostic significance of lamina propria invasion microstaging (T1a/b/c) in BCG-treated and BCG-non-treated patients. Eur Urol. 2005;48:231.
215. Weizer AZ, Wasco MJ, Wang R, et al. Multiple adverse histological features increase the odds of under staging T1 bladder cancer. J Urol. 2009;182:59.
216. Andius P, Johansson SL, Holmäng S. Prognostic factors in stage T1 bladder cancer: tumor pattern (solid or papillary) and vascular invasion more important than depth of invasion. Urology. 2007;70:758.
217. Cho K, Seo H, Joung J, et al. Lymphovascular invasion in transurethral resection specimens as predictor of progression and metastasis in patients with newly diagnosed T1 bladder urothelial cancer. J Urol. 2009;182:2625.
218. Stein JP, Lieskovsky G, Cote R, et al. Radical cystectomy in the treatment of invasive bladder cancer: long-term results in 1,054 patients. J Clin Oncol. 2001;19:666.
219. Herr HW. Superiority of ratio based lymph node staging for bladder cancer. J Urol. 2003;169:943.
220. Wright JL, Lin DW, Porter MP. The association between extent of lymphadenectomy and survival among patients with lymph node metastases undergoing radical cystectomy. Cancer. 2008;112:2401.
221. Rodel C, Grabenbauer GG, Kuhn R, et al. Combined-modality treatment and selective organ preservation in invasive bladder cancer: long-term results. J Clin Oncol. 2002;20:3061.
222. Chang SS, Hassan JM, Cookson MS, et al. Delaying radical cystectomy for muscle invasive bladder cancer results in worse pathological stage. Urol J. 2003;170:1085.
223. Gore JL, Lai J, Setodji CM, et al. Mortality increases when radical cystectomy is delayed more than 12 weeks: results from a Surveillance, Epidemiology, and End Results-Medicare analysis. Cancer. 2009;115:988.
224. Kulkarni GS, Urbach DR, Austin PC, et al. Longer wait times increase overall mortality in patients with bladder cancer. J Urol. 2009;182:1318.
225. Grossman HB, Natale RB, Tangen CM, et al. Neoadjuvant chemotherapy plus cystectomy compared with cystectomy alone for locally advanced bladder cancer. N Engl J Med. 2003;349:859.
226. Advanced Bladder Cancer (ABC) Meta-analysis Collaboration. Neoadjuvant chemotherapy in invasive bladder cancer: update of a systematic review and meta-analysis of individual patient data advanced bladder cancer (ABC) meta-analysis collaboration. Eur Urol. 2005;48:202.
227. Calabrò F, Sternberg CN. Neoadjuvant and adjuvant chemotherapy in muscle-invasive bladder cancer. Eur Urol. 2009;55:348.
228. Kassouf W, Agarwal PK, Grossman HB, et al. Outcome of patients with bladder cancer with pN+disease after preoperative chemotherapy and radical cystectomy. Urology. 2009;73:147.

6 Non-Muscle-Invasive Low- and High-Grade Neoplasia

Robert Jackson, Hikmat Al-Ahmadie, Victor E. Reuter, and Cheryl T. Lee

Introduction

Bladder cancer imposes a considerable burden on patients and health care systems around the world. Estimates predict more than 70,000 new cases of bladder cancer and more than 14,000 deaths in 2010 in the USA [1]. Bladder cancer is three times more common in men than in women and roughly twice as common in Caucasians as African-Americans. For unknown reasons, relative mortality rates are lower for men and for Caucasians [2, 3]. The risk of bladder cancer increases with age, peaking between the sixth and eighth decades of life, creating unique challenges in treatment related to existing comorbidities [4, 5]. At the time of diagnosis, 75% of patients present with non-muscle-invasive bladder cancers (NMIBC); 70–80% are limited to the mucosa (Ta, Tis) and the remaining 20–30% invade the lamina propria (T1) [6].

Bladder cancer's propensity for recurrence and progression requires long-term surveillance, making bladder cancer the most expensive solid neoplasm to treat from diagnosis to death, ranging from $96,000 to $187,000 per patient in 2001 dollars [7]. This disease remains an important health condition that poses many clinical, pathologic, and social challenges. The complexities of the disease have even created controversies in the pathologic description of the disease (urothelial vs. transitional), grading of tumors, and in disease classification (superficial vs. NMIBC) [8]. Changes in disease descriptors have improved our ability to examine the many different diseases that make up bladder cancer. In this chapter, we will evaluate several "categories" of NMIBC that present varying levels of patient risk necessitating a spectrum of management intensity. A multidisciplinary approach to this disease is essential. In managing NMIBC, a close relationship with pathology can greatly clarify the threat of the tumor.

Clinical Presentation

Hematuria is the most common presentation of bladder cancer, seen in up to 80% of patients [9]. Rates of bladder cancer are higher in those presenting with gross hematuria (13–35%) than microscopic hematuria (0.5–11%) [10]. Irritative

R. Jackson
Department of Urology, University of Michigan, 3875 TC/SPC 5330 1500 E Medical Center Drive 48109 Ann Arbor, MI, USA
e-mail: robejack@med.umich.edu

H. Al-Ahmadie • V.E. Reuter
Department of Pathology, Memorial Sloan-Kettering Cancer Center, 1275 York Avenue, New York, NY 10065, USA
e-mail: alahmadh@mskcc.org; reuterv@mskcc.org

C.T. Lee (✉)
Department of Urology, University of Michigan, 1500 East Medical Center Drive 7303 CCGC SPC 5946, Ann Arbor, MI 48109-5946, USA
e-mail: ctlee@umich.edu

D.E. Hansel et al. (eds.), *The Urinary Tract: A Comprehensive Guide to Patient Diagnosis and Management*, DOI 10.1007/978-1-4614-5320-8_6, © Springer Science+Business Media New York 2012

voiding symptoms, (urinary urgency and frequency) are also common signs at presentation, and, in the absence of an obvious cause, these symptoms warrant further investigation as they may be associated with urothelial carcinoma, particularly carcinoma in situ (CIS) [4]. Less often, patients present with signs and symptoms resulting from urinary tract obstruction such as recurrent urinary tract infection, hydronephrosis, flank or abdominal pain, pyelonephritis, and renal insufficiency. Hydronephrosis has traditionally been associated with invasive and extravesical disease; this association is stronger for patients with bilateral hydronephrosis. More than 90% of patients with bilateral hydronephrosis will have advanced disease (i.e., > p3b, or N^+) at the time of presentation; approximately 67% of those with unilateral hydronephrosis have advanced disease at the time of presentation [5, 11].

Pathogenesis and Natural History

The pathogenesis of bladder cancer is multifactorial, with both exogenous and endogenous factors playing important roles. The strongest risk factor for development of urothelial carcinoma is smoking. The link between bladder cancer and smoking is well established. Smokers have a two to fourfold higher chance of developing bladder cancer, and as many as 50% of bladder cancer cases may be attributable to smoking [3, 12, 13]. Smoking risk increases with the number of cigarettes smoked and the duration of smoking. Smoking cessation has been shown to reduce the risk of bladder cancer [14].

Well-established environmental exposures also increase the risk of bladder cancer. These include aromatic amines, acrolein, aniline dyes, coal, arsenic, nitrates, and nitrites [9, 15]. Consequently, professions linked to increased rates of bladder cancer include painters, truck drivers, machine operators, auto workers, metal workers, leather workers, dry cleaners, paper manufacturers, barbers, beauticians, physicians, and plumbers [3, 16, 17]. The latency time for chemical exposure and the increasing incidence in industrialized countries lend credence to the theory that prolonged carcinogenic exposures in the urine play a critical role in the formation of urothelial tumors [2, 14].

Endogenous molecular and genetic factors also contribute to the development of urothelial carcinoma; however, evidence does not exist for a purely heritable cause [14]. Derangements of established molecular mechanisms that promote urothelial carcinogenesis include altered metabolism/detoxification pathways, inactivation of tumor-suppressor genes, activation of oncogenes, and overexpression of normal genes. Pathways involved in metabolism of exogenous carcinogens include cytochrome P450, glutathione *S*-transferase, and *N*-acetyltransferase. Each of these pathways has been implicated in bladder cancer [18–20].

Abnormalities in tumor-suppressor genes also result in cell cycle dysregulation and tumor development. Tumor-suppressor genes implicated in the development of urothelial carcinoma include p21, p16, p53, and Rb [2, 21–23]. Genetic alterations can also lead to induction of oncogenes, leading normal genes to encode for a malignant phenotype. Oncogenes associated with urothelial carcinoma include those of the *myc* and *ras* families [24–26]. Overexpression of normal genes encoding for growth factors and growth factor receptors, such as epidermal growth factor (EGF) and its receptors (ERBB1 and ERBB2), has also been implicated in urothelial carcinogenesis [27–29].

The molecular alterations observed in bladder cancer may cooperate with chemical exposures resulting in the recurrent nature of the disease. Much of the morbidity and mortality associated with NMIBC results from disease recurrence and progression. Even after a complete endoscopic resection, 50–70% of tumors will recur and 10–30% will subsequently progress to muscle-invasive disease [6, 30, 31]. The majority of recurrences happen within the first 5 years after treatment [32]. The risks of recurrence and progression vary according to tumor grade and stage. High-grade (HG) tumors with invasion into the lamina propria (T1) have been estimated to progress in more than half of patients over 15 years [30]. Similarly, 39% of patients with carcinoma in situ (CIS), another high-grade lesion, will suffer progression within 3 years of

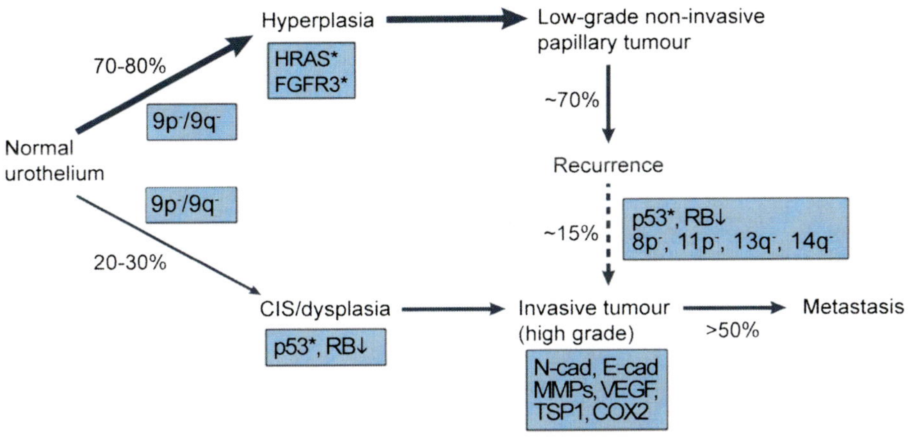

Fig. 6.1 Important genetic and epigenetic defects that characterize the divergent pathways of urothelial tumorigenesis. Clinical data and experimental evidence indicate that urothelial tumors arise and progress along two distinct pathways. The first of these (*top pathway*), which accounts for 70–80% of urothelial tumors, is often preceded by simple and papillary hyperplasia and exhibits a tumor morphology that is low grade, superficial, and papillary. About 70% of these tumors will recur, but only ~15% will proceed to infiltrate the musculature (*dashed line*). These tumors harbor frequent mutations in the HRAS gene (30–40%) and fibroblast growth factor receptor 3 (FGFR3) gene (~70%), indicating that RTK-Ras activation has an early and crucial role in this tumorigenesis pathway. Deletions in the short arms of chromosomes 8 and 11 (8p- and 11p-) and long arms of chromosomes 13 and 14 (13q- and 14q-) are often associated with tumor progression to the invasive stages. The second tumor pathway (*bottom pathway*) (accounting for 20–30% of the urothelial tumors) is characterized by high-grade muscle-invasive tumors, which either originate from flat carcinoma in situ (CIS)/severe dysplasia or arise de novo. Over half of these tumors contain structural and functional defects in the tumor suppressors p53 and/or the retinoblastoma protein (RB) and over 50% of these tumors progress to local and distant metastases despite radical cystectomy and chemotherapy. Invasion and metastases are promoted by several factors that alter the tumor microenvironment, including the aberrant expression of N- and E-cadherins (N-cad and E-cad), matrix metalloproteinases (MMPs), angiogenic factors such as vascular endothelial growth factor (VEGF), and antiangiogenic factors such as thrombospondin 1 (TSP1) and cyclooxygenase 2 (COX2). Deletion of both arms of chromosome 9 (9p-/9q-) occurs early during urothelial tumorigenesis, but they do not seem to be markers that differentiate the two tumor pathways. Elucidating the genetic and epigenetic causes of the two distinct pathways of urothelial tumorigenesis should have a tremendous impact on the rational management of different urothelial carcinomas. *Asterisk* indicates mutated proteins. Reprinted with permission from Wu [38]

treatment [33]. In contrast, 15-year progression-free survival rates for high-grade Ta urothelial carcinoma are 61% and for low-grade (LG) Ta are 95% [34]. Tumor grade, then, will greatly influence a patient's risk of recurrence and progression. This distinction in clinical behavior is a clear reflection of the variation in tumor biology seen in low- and high-grade lesions (Fig. 6.1). Low-grade tumors typically have relatively few chromosomal abnormalities (most often loss of all or part of chromosome 9), while higher grade lesions display more numerous and varied abnormalities including alterations in chromosomes 7, 9, and 17 [10, 35–38].

Clinical Evaluation

A thorough history is important in the evaluation of bladder cancer patients. Often, patients have had a variety of recurrences and have been treated with intravesical and endoscopic therapies. The course of the disease is important as it outlines the capabilities of the tumor and the consequent patient risk. The social history is particularly relevant, as it can inform the provider about cancer etiology and ongoing hazardous exposures. A complete physical examination is essential with particular attempts to identify: (1) cervical, supraclavicular, and inguinal adenopathy; (2) flank pain or a palpable abdominal mass; (3) lower extremity edema; (4) bone pain; and (5) mass effect on rectal examination in men or pelvic examination in women. The clinical stage of the tumor along with complications of the disease may be readily apparent. In patients with disease confined to the bladder, the physical assessment is often unremarkable.

Urine cytology is also an essential part of patient evaluation both initially and when monitoring for recurrence. A cytopathologic assessment of urothelial cells shed into the urine is accomplished from a voided or instrumented urine sample. The strength of cytology as a diagnostic test is its specificity, which can be high as 94% [5, 39]. In certain cases, positive cytology may actually precede the development of visible tumors [40]. The sensitivity of the test, however, is somewhat low, primarily due to its very poor performance in detecting low-grade tumors [41]. Consequently, its role as a urinary marker is much greater in the detection of high-grade lesions, likely resulting from the discohesive nature of these tumors, which contributes to the shedding of cells into the urine. The sensitivity of cytology may be improved when cells are collected from a bladder wash, rather than a voided sample, as the irrigation leads to a specimen with higher cellularity. Ultimately, the most significant limitation of urine cytology may be the variation in interpreter evaluation [42]. One must truly know their local cytopathologist to gauge the level of suspicion of an "atypical" or "dysplastic" cytology result. A multitude of urinary assays have been developed to improve the sensitivity of cytology yet maintain its specificity (Table 6.1). These tests have often provided point-of-care-based alternatives to cytology. Because many of these tests are new, their clinical utility is still uncertain.

Imaging

Radiographic imaging is an essential part of clinical staging. The computerized tomography urogram (CTU) has replaced the intravenous pyelogram (IVP) as the radiographic test of choice. In addition to an evaluation of the upper urinary tract, it provides important anatomic detail within the abdomen and pelvis permitting assessment of lymph nodes, viscera, perivesical tissue, and detailed changes in the appearance of the renal pelvis, calyces, and ureter. In the case of renal insufficiency, ultrasound and magnetic resonance imaging (MRI) are typically used as alternatives to CTU in the upper-tract evaluation, although concerns regarding nephrogenic systemic fibrosis have limited the use of MRI in those patients with severe renal impairment [5].

While CTU is an improvement over IVP, there are still a substantial number of patients that are clinically understaged. This is in part due to the inability of CT to detect micrometastases, especially in lymph nodes, where 40–70% of metastases can go undetected [43, 44]. Consequently alternative imaging techniques and modalities are being investigated. These include dynamic MRI, virtual cystoscopy using either CT or MRI, and positron emission tomography (PET) alone or in combination with CT [44–47]. Although the more expensive modalities such as MRI and PET may have a potential role in staging muscle-invasive tumors, their role in staging NMIBC is less well defined and may not provide sufficient additional information to justify routine use.

Cystoscopy

White-light cystoscopy has long been the standard of care for bladder cancer detection since it allows direct visualization of bladder pathology. Flexible cystoscopy is a quick and relatively well-tolerated office procedure for the majority of patients. Direct visualization of the urothelium allows assessment of the number of tumors, their location and relation to other important structures such as the ureteral orifices, bladder neck, and prostatic urethra. Urothelial carcinoma can have a papillary, sessile, or nodular appearance. Carcinoma in situ typically appears as a velvety, erythematous patch of mucosa alongside the otherwise smooth and pale urothelium. Studies have shown that cystoscopy can accurately discriminate between benign and malignant lesions, with

Table 6.1 Review of current bladder tumor markers

Marker	Point of service	Target	FDA approved	Comments
Urine cytology	No	Urothelial cells	Yes	Poor sensitivity for low-grade disease; dependence on expertise of pathologist
UroVysion™ fluorescence in situ hybridization (FISH)	No	chromosomes 3, 7, 17, and 9p21	Yes	Lack of standardization of criteria for positive test; expensive; specially trained personnel
NMP-22	Yes	Nuclear mitotic protein involved in distribution of chromatin during replication	Yes	Results can be influenced by benign urologic conditions
BTA stat	Yes	Complement factor H-related protein	Yes	Specificity is low among patients with benign urologic conditions
BTA-TRAK	No	Complement factor H-related protein	Yes	Same as BTA stat
uCyt	No	Sulfated mucin glycoproteins and glycosylated carcinoembryonic antigen	No	Need significant experience for interpreting and time to examine slides
BLCA-4	No	Nuclear mitotic protein	No	Found in both tumor and normal regions of bladder
BLCA-1	No	Nuclear mitotic protein	No	Expressed only in tumor areas of bladder
Aurora kinase A (AURKA)	No	Gene that encodes a key regulator of mitosis	No	Overexpression of AURKA can cause aneuploidy in urothelial cells
CXCL1	No	Secreted protein that is part of CXC chemokine family	No	CXCL1 may be associated with tumorigenesis; may have increased levels in invasive bladder cancer
Matrix metalloproteinase (MMP) complexes	No	Zinc-dependent endopeptidases	No	MMPs are key regulators of tumor growth and angiogenesis
FGFR3	No	Glycoprotein that is part of tyrosine kinase receptor family	No	FGFR3 mutations are associated with non-muscle-invasive bladder cancers
Methylation markers	No	Methylation of a gene locus	No	Hypermethylation of promoter sequence DNA is a mechanism for silencing tumor-suppressor genes

Adapted with permission from Jacobs et al. [5]

sensitivity, specificity, and positive predictive values of up to 100% in some series [48]. Prediction of pathologic stage based on endoscopic appearance, however, is somewhat less accurate, although sessile tumors and those with visible areas of necrosis are more likely to be invasive high-grade lesions [10, 48, 49].

Newer technologies are currently being studied that address the shortcomings of cystoscopy including difficulties in the detection of flat neoplastic lesions, and the lack of immediate grade and stage information. Fluorescence cystoscopy (FC) is a technology that uses intravesical instillation of 5-aminolevulinic acid. This compound is a precursor in the heme biosynthesis pathway and induces an accumulation of fluorescent endogenous porphyrins in tissues of epithelial origin. It is preferentially taken up by cells with an elevated metabolism and can therefore highlight neoplastic cells that display fluorescence when viewed with a blue light and an observation filter on the cystoscope [50]. Studies suggest that FC improves detection of superficial tumors compared to white-light cystoscopy [51, 52].

Denzinger and colleagues reported the 8-year results of a randomized, prospective trial in which patients underwent either conventional cystoscopy and transurethral resection of bladder tumor (TURBT) or fluorescence cystoscopy and TURBT. All patients then underwent TURBT to identify residual tumor. Patients evaluated with FC had a lower incidence of residual tumors and a significantly higher 8-year recurrence-free survival [53]. In a phase III multicenter trial by Grossman and colleagues, FC detected at least one more Ta or T1 tumor than conventional cystoscopy in roughly a third of patients [50]. This technique, available in Europe for several years, is now available in the USA.

Narrow band imaging cystoscopy (NBI) is another new technology being evaluated as a possible adjunct to conventional, white-light cystoscopy. In NBI, white light is filtered into two narrow bands (415 and 540 nm) absorbed by hemoglobin, improving visualization of surface capillaries and blood vessels in the submucosa. This enhances the contrast between normal bladder mucosa and urothelial carcinomas (which are more vascular). Herr and colleagues evaluated 427 patients for recurrence of NMIBC using conventional cystoscopy followed by NBI. In the 24% of patients with a recurrence, 87% were visible by conventional methods, while 100% were visualized with NBI. The mean number of tumors visualized by NBI was higher, and NBI revealed additional papillary tumors or more extensive CIS in 56% of patients with recurrences [54].

Optical coherence tomography (OCT) employs near-infrared light and analysis of unique tissue backscatter patterns to provide real-time cross-sectional imaging of biologic tissues. This allows in vivo assessment of the microarchitectural features of bladder lesions. In a study of 32 patients undergoing either bladder biopsy or TURBT, Lerner and colleagues obtained OCT images of suspicious lesions and correlated them with biopsy results. Lesions confined to the mucosa were correctly identified by OCT with 90% sensitivity and 89% specificity. For muscle-invasive lesions, sensitivity was 100% and specificity was 90% [55].

In vivo confocal laser endomicroscopy (ICLE) employs laser light and fluorescent dyes to provide real-time, cellular-resolution histologic data, giving the user an "optical biopsy" of the tissue being examined (Fig. 6.2). Sonn and colleagues reported the first use of ICLE in the urinary tract in 2009. In this preliminary study, 27 patients scheduled to undergo TURBT were evaluated by conventional cystoscopy and ICLE; 19 patients were found to have urothelial carcinoma. Using ICLE, marked differences were appreciated in the appearance of normal urothelium and urothelial carcinomas. The authors concluded that further investigation of the technology might lead to a useful adjunct to conventional cystoscopy [56].

All of the technologies previously discussed illustrate the exciting potential for improved detection and diagnosis of NMIBC. The exact role of these new technologies awaits further study, and, for patients in the USA, Food and Drug Administration (FDA) approval.

Pathology

Urothelial Neoplasia

The vast majority (approximately 98%) of malignant tumors arising in the urinary bladder are of epithelial origin, and of these, 90% are "typical" urothelial carcinomas (previously called transitional cell carcinoma (TCC)) [57]. Most urothelial carcinomas at initial diagnosis are papillary and superficial, and as many as 70% follow a prolonged clinical course characterized by multiple recurrences following local resection without tumor progression [58]. There is, however, a smaller but significant percentage of patients whose tumors present with an aggressive clinical course over a short period of time. A number of pathologic features have been identified that are accurate predictors of the clinical course of bladder cancer, the most important of which are depth of invasion, if any, at presentation, tumor multifocality, a history of prior urothelial tumors, tumor size, and grade [58]. As a rule, only high-grade tumors develop regional lymph node metastasis.

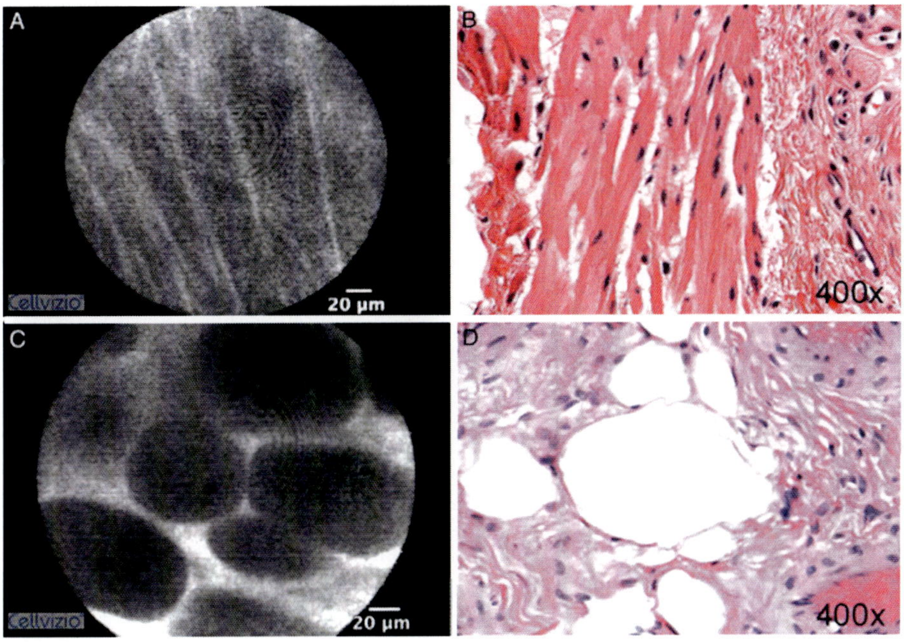

Fig. 6.2 (**a**) Endomicroscopic image of tumor resection bed after TURBT showing fibers of muscularis propria. (**b**) H and E stain of biopsy from this site demonstrating fibers of muscularis propria. (**c**) Endomicroscopic image of resection bed revealing distinctive appearance of fat lobules. (**d**) H and E stain of biopsy from this site confirming presence of fat in specimen [56]

Cytologically, benign papillary tumors may and do recur, but do not invade. Tumors are as likely to recur at a different site in the bladder, indicating multifocal occurrence rather than recurrence of the original tumor.

Classification/Grading of Urothelial Tumors

Classification of urothelial tumors has undergone many revisions in the past, but in this chapter we will follow the latest classification of World Health Organization (WHO) of 2003 (Table 6.2). This classification was adopted after the WHO guided and sponsored consensus meeting of urologic pathologists in 2002 in Lyon, France. During that meeting, the 1998 classification of WHO and the International Society of Urological Pathologists (ISUP) [8] was accepted with few changes and few dissenting votes, and now has become the 2003 WHO classification of urothelial tumors [59].

Table 6.2 The World Health Organization/International Society of Urological Pathology consensus classification of urothelial (transitional cell) neoplasms of the urinary bladder

Normal
Flat lesions
Flat hyperplasia
Flat lesions with atypia
Reactive (inflammatory) atypia
Atypia of unknown significance
Dysplasia (low-grade intraurothelial neoplasia)
Carcinoma in situ (high-grade intraurothelial neoplasia)
Papillary lesions
Papillary hyperplasia
Papillary neoplasms
Papilloma
Papillary urothelial neoplasm of low malignant potential
Papillary carcinoma, low grade
Papillary carcinoma, high grade

Adapted from Epstein et al. [8]

Hyperplasia

Urothelial hyperplasia can be flat or papillary. Flat hyperplasia consists of a markedly thickened mucosa without cytological atypia. Although this lesion may be seen adjacent to low-grade papillary urothelial lesions, it is still debatable whether it represents a premalignant process. Papillary hyperplasia is characterized by undulating urothelium or papillary growth lined by urothelium of varying thickness and lacking atypia and generally lacking a well-developed fibrovascular core or branching of the papillary structures. This lesion is usually asymptomatic and generally found on routine follow-up cystoscopy for papillary urothelial neoplasms.

Flat Urothelial Lesions

Reactive Atypia

Reactive (inflammatory) atypia consists of nuclear abnormalities of the urothelium occurring in the setting of acutely or chronically inflamed urothelium. The nuclei are enlarged but often contain a single prominent nucleolus and evenly distributed vesicular chromatin. Generally, there is no nuclear pleomorphism and the cells maintain their polarity and order. Mitoses may be observed but are usually located in the basal or middle urothelium and without atypical forms. An acute or chronic inflammatory infiltrate is commonly seen in the urothelial mucosa and a history of reactive conditions is usually present such as calculi, trauma, instrumentation, or infection [60].

Atypia of Unknown Significance

This term is reserved for situations when it is difficult to differentiate between reactive and neoplastic atypia. There may be a greater degree of pleomorphism and/or hyperchromatism out of proportion to the extent of the inflammation such that dysplasia or urothelial CIS cannot be confidently excluded. This designation allows patients to be followed more closely for reevaluation.

Dysplasia (Low-Grade Intraurothelial Neoplasia)

The term urothelial dysplasia has been used when the urothelium exhibits appreciable cytologic and architectural abnormalities felt to be preneoplastic, yet falling short of the diagnostic threshold for CIS. The dysplastic urothelium is usually of normal thickness and shows loss of polarity as well as nuclear atypia and irregular chromatin distribution. This term has inherent problems with interobserver reproducibility and lack of a uniform definition, which complicates interpretation of reports in the literature. Some genitourinary pathologists diagnose such lesions as atypia of unknown significance given these diagnostic problems, especially in the absence of any other concomitant urothelial neoplasm.

Carcinoma in Situ (High-Grade Intraurothelial Neoplasia)

Urothelial CIS is a flat lesion of the urothelium with unequivocal severe cytologic atypia that is a documented precursor of invasive cancer in many cases. It is characterized by the presence of cells with large, irregular, hyperchromatic nuclei that may be present either throughout the entire thickness of the epithelium or only part of it (Fig. 6.3). Mitoses are commonly seen in the mid to upper urothelium. Carcinoma in situ may have a pagetoid spread or may be present as isolated cells in a partially denuded surface. It is an exclusively high-grade lesion often found in association with papillary or invasive carcinoma, where it has been reported in as many as 90% of cases [61–65], or in patients with a history of prior tumors. A substantial proportion of patients with CIS alone are asymptomatic. Symptoms, when they appear, suggest cystitis: dysuria, frequency, and nocturia [63, 64, 66–71]. Most patients with CIS have microscopic hematuria, but gross hematuria is not uncommon. The epithelium in areas of CIS is only loosely cohesive and the cells readily desquamate, resulting in extensive exfoliation from even limited areas of CIS, which when biopsied will show a predominantly denuded bladder wall (the so-called erosive cystitis). This makes urine cytology a very important and sensitive means to establish the correct diagnosis. Although some patients may have only a limited focus of CIS, the majority will have multifocal or diffuse involvement. If left untreated, most cases of CIS will progress to

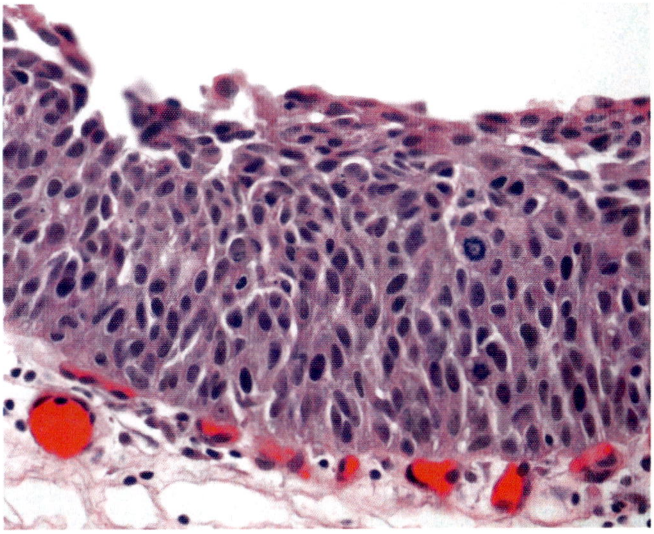

Fig. 6.3 Urothelial carcinoma in situ. Markedly hyperchromatic and pleomorphic cells lacking polarity in relation to the basement membrane. Mitotic figures are readily identified

invasive carcinoma, and in patients who underwent cystectomy for CIS, invasion was detected in approximately one-third of them [71–73]. Nevertheless, not all patients with CIS develop subsequent invasive disease [74].

Papillary Urothelial Lesions

Grading of Papillary Urothelial Lesions

Although tumor stage is the most important prognostic factor of urothelial carcinoma, outcome of patients with noninvasive papillary tumors is largely dependent on the pathological grade. The issue of grading papillary urothelial tumors has been vigorously debated among urologic pathologists. The classification system outlined in Table 6.2 relies on changes in the architectural and cytologic features within the urothelium. The architectural features primarily include the overall organization of the cells in the papillary structures and the cytologic features include nuclear size and shape, chromatin distribution, presence of nucleoli, and mitoses. Before the current classification was adopted, numerous other classification systems for grading papillary urothelial neoplasms have been proposed in attempts to more precisely predict the prognosis. These systems, however, had poor interobserver reproducibility among pathologists. Of all these classification systems, the most commonly used was the one proposed by the WHO in 1973, in which papillary tumors were categorized into benign urothelial papilloma and three grades of carcinoma (grades 1, 2, and 3) [75]. Although this system had been most commonly used, its definition of the various grades was vague, without regard to specific histological criteria, which resulted in most cases falling into the intermediate category often as the default diagnosis [76, 77]. In December 1998 the WHO/ISUP consensus classification system was developed in an effort to achieve a universally acceptable system for bladder tumors. This system became the basis for the 2003 WHO/ISUP system for classifying urothelial tumors [8, 59]. The WHO/ISUP (2003) system classifies papillary urothelial neoplasms into four types: papilloma, papillary urothelial neoplasm of low malignant potential (PUNLMP), low-grade carcinoma, and high-grade carcinoma, with detailed description of the specific architectural and cytological criteria.

Although in both the WHO (1973) system and in the WHO/ISUP (2003) system papillary urothelial tumors were divided into four categories, a one-to-one translation between the two systems is not intended, except for tumors at the

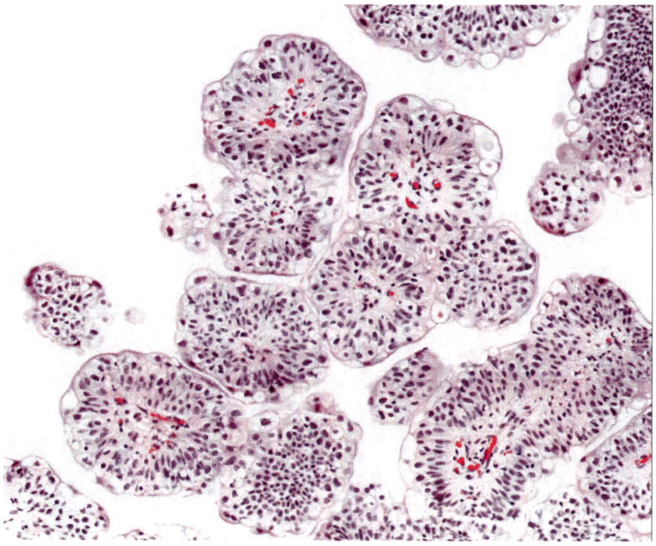

Fig. 6.4 Urothelial papilloma. Discrete exophytic papillary growth. The lining urothelium is of normal thickness and cytology

extremes of the grading spectrum. Lesions called papilloma in the WHO (1973) system are also called papilloma in the WHO/ISUP (2003) system. At the other end of the grading extreme, the grade 3 in the WHO (1973) system is assigned to the high-grade carcinoma category in the WHO/ISUP (2003) system. By contrast, for grades 1 and 2 of the WHO (1973) system, there is no direct correlation with the WHO/ISUP (2003) classification. These lesions must be graded using the criteria of the newer system without regard to how they were diagnosed in the old system. Some lesions that were called grade 1 carcinoma according to WHO (1973) would be classified as PUNLMP in the WHO/ISUP (2003) system, if they show no cytological atypia and merely thickened urothelium with, at most, nuclear enlargement. Other WHO (1973) grade 1 tumors with definite yet slight cytological atypia would be diagnosed as low-grade carcinoma in WHO/ISUP (2003) system. Grade 2 tumors in WHO (1973) comprise a rather broad category. It includes tumors that are relatively bland and would have been diagnosed as grade 1–2 according to the WHO (1973) system but would fall into the low-grade carcinoma category in the WHO/ISUP (2003) system. In other cases that are classified as high grade according to the WHO/ISUP (2003) system, they would have been called grade 2–3 in the WHO (1973) system.

In the 1973 WHO system, a large percentage of noninvasive papillary urothelial carcinomas were called grade 2, which, as we now know, represents an ambiguous and heterogeneous group. In the 2003 WHO/ISUP system, however, these grade 2 tumors can be segregated approximately equally into low- and high-grade carcinomas with correspondingly low and high risks of progression. In addition, several studies have compared the 1973 WHO and newer WHO/ISUP systems. Most have demonstrated a superiority of the WHO/ISUP system in predicting recurrence and progression as well as interobserver reproducibility [78–83]. On the other hand, some other studies have reported no difference in interobserver reproducibility between the two grading systems [84, 85].

Urothelial Papilloma

This is a rare benign condition typically occurring as a small, isolated growth seen primarily, but not exclusively, in younger patients. Morphologically it is a discrete, exophytic papillary growth with a central fibrovascular core lined by urothelium of normal thickness and cytology

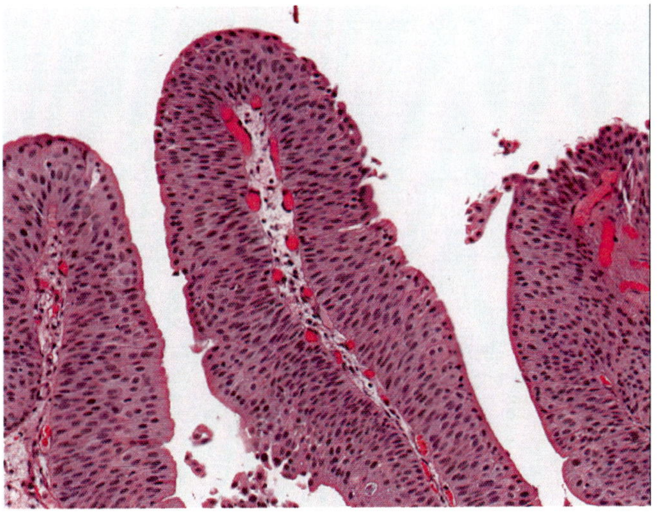

Fig. 6.5 Papillary urothelial neoplasm of low malignant potential (PUNLMP). Papillary fronds urothelial lining surrounding fibrovascular cores. The cells maintain an orderly arrangement and lack cytologic atypia or pleomorphism. The chromatin pattern is homogeneous

(Fig. 6.4). In some papillomas, complex anastomosing and branching may be seen and stromal edema within the papillae may be prominent. Additionally, umbrella cells may exhibit variable degrees of atypia, which is acceptable as long as it is not present beyond the umbrella cells. Recurrences of papilloma are rare and progression to carcinoma is exceedingly rare [86, 87].

Inverted Urothelial Papilloma

This lesion is, by definition, an endophytic mass that shares several features with exophytic urothelial papilloma. Histologically, these tumors usually exhibit a trabecular arrangement of tumor cells into the lamina propria, accompanied by a smooth urothelial surface. The trabeculae are orderly with uniform width but also show marked branching and anastomosis. Squamous metaplasia without keratinization may be seen. Inverted papillomas have a low risk of recurrence when completely excised. Rarely, hybrid cases exist with portions of the lesion being endophytic and others exophytic. They may be seen in patients with a history of urothelial carcinoma, and rarely, urothelial carcinoma may arise within inverted urothelial papilloma.

Papillary Urothelial Neoplasm of Low Malignant Potential (PUNLMP)

This term describes a papillary urothelial neoplasm with an orderly arrangement of cells within papillae with minimal architectural abnormalities and minimal nuclear atypia (Fig. 6.5). In comparison with papillomas, PUNLMPs typically have thicker urothelium at low magnification without architectural abnormalities. The cells composing PUNLMPs are uniform and identical to each other, maintaining an orderly arrangement. They may be enlarged and more crowded compared to adjacent normal urothelium. There is no (or minimal) nuclear atypia with fine chromatin and absent to inconspicuous nucleoli. Nuclear grooves may be seen and mitoses are infrequent and usually limited to the basal layer. PUNLMPs may occasionally exhibit inverted growth pattern. When strictly defined, PUNLMP is not associated with invasion or metastasis. Nevertheless, these patients are at risk of developing new bladder tumors, usually of similar histology [88–90]. Subsequent lesions may manifest as urothelial carcinoma in 7–10% of cases, so follow-up of the patient is warranted. The PUNLMP category avoids overdiagnosis of cancer but also avoids a completely benign diagnosis

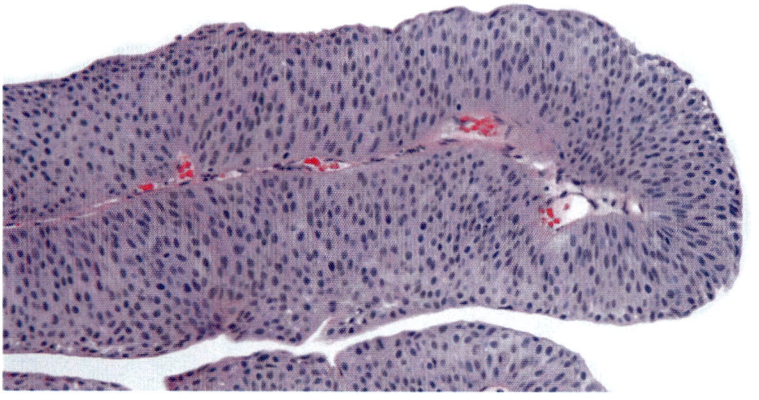

Fig. 6.6 Noninvasive papillary urothelial carcinoma, low grade. A papillary neoplasm with minimal architectural disorder and mild cellular atypia and pleomorphism

such as papilloma. The introduction of this entity to the current WHO/ISUP classification, however, has been criticized [91]. Some have argued that all papillary tumors should be dichotomized into low-grade neoplasms vs. high-grade carcinoma [89]. These arguments were supported by a few studies that demonstrated a low level of agreement in the histological distinction between PUNLMP and low-grade carcinoma or no significant difference in prognosis between these two categories [82, 84, 92]. On the other hand, more and larger studies have shown that PUNLMP has a distinct risk of recurrence intermediate between papillomas and low-grade papillary carcinomas, and a lower risk of progression than low-grade carcinomas [89].

Low-Grade Noninvasive Papillary Urothelial Carcinoma

Low-grade carcinomas maintain an overall orderly appearance but exhibit architectural or cytologic atypia that is easily recognizable at scanning magnification (Fig. 6.6). Papillae are slender and frequently branched and may show fusion with adjacent papillae. Variability in polarity, nuclear size, shape, and chromatin texture are minimal but comprise the hallmarks of the cytologic atypia seen in low-grade papillary urothelial carcinoma. Mitotic figures are infrequent. Although mitoses may be seen at any level of the urothelium, they are not atypical and usually are limited to the lower half. Fusion of papillae and examination of tangentially sectioned tumor may lead to erroneous overgrading of these lesions as high-grade carcinoma. These tumors frequently recur and have a low (<5%) risk of progression.

High-Grade Noninvasive Papillary Urothelial Carcinoma

High-grade carcinomas are characterized by a disorderly appearance and exhibit marked architectural and cytologic abnormalities easily recognizable at low magnification (Fig. 6.7). Cellular pleomorphism ranges from moderate to marked, and mitotic figures, including atypical forms, are frequently seen at all levels of the urothelium. The thickness of the urothelium varies considerably and tumor cells may be discohesive resulting in denudation of the mucosa. They are commonly associated with invasive carcinoma at the time of initial presentation and the adjacent mucosa may show evidence of carcinoma in situ. The Progression rate varies from 15 to 40%, much higher than low-grade lesions.

In a papillary urothelial neoplasm with variable histology, the tumor should be graded

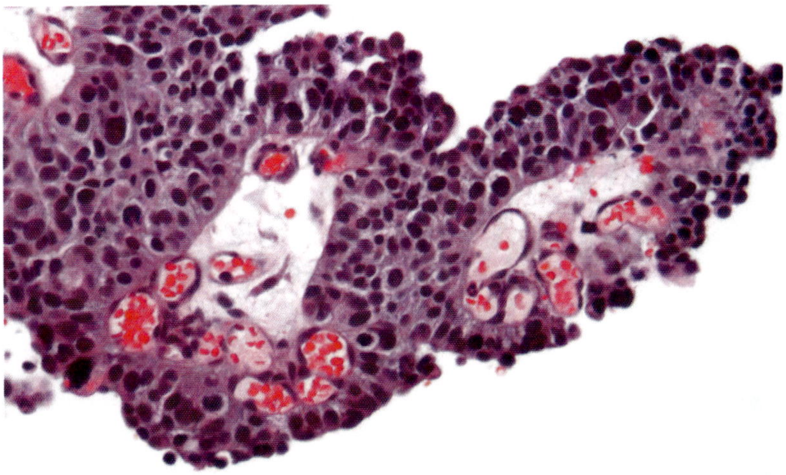

Fig. 6.7 Noninvasive papillary urothelial carcinoma, high grade. Neoplastic cells with marked pleomorphism, hyperchromasia, and disorder

according to the highest grade, although it is not uncommon for minuscule areas of higher grade morphology to be ignored in a tumor with an overwhelming low-grade component. It is yet to be determined how significant a minor component must be in order to have an impact on the prognosis of low-grade tumors.

Urothelial Carcinoma with Lamina Propria Invasion

The assessment of the depth of invasion of urothelial carcinoma is of paramount importance as it has prognostic considerations and greatly impacts treatment. The histology of invasive urothelial carcinoma has no specific features and shows cohesive nests of cells with moderate to abundant cytoplasm and large hyperchromatic nuclei. Nuclear pleomorphism is common with irregular nuclear contours, occasionally prominent nucleoli, and readily identifiable mitotic figures.

Descriptors of T1 bladder cancer may be confusing. In an effort to distinguish T1 disease from noninvasive or "superficial" tumors, the term non-muscle-invasive bladder cancer (NMIBC) has been popularized. However, this newer terminology may cause confusion for pathologists since the term "muscle invasion," when used without further qualification, does not distinguish between invasion of the muscularis mucosae and the muscularis propria. Most agree that the term "superficial bladder cancer" should not be used as it groups three biologically different lesions: CIS, noninvasive papillary neoplasia, and carcinoma with lamina propria invasion. Currently, NMIBC is used widely in clinical circles, referring to early stage tumors that have not invaded the muscularis propria.

Table 6.3 Morphologic criteria to determine invasion into lamina propria

Histologic grade
Invasion more common in high-grade lesion
Characteristics of the invading epithelium
Irregular nests or single infiltrating cells
Irregular or absent basement membrane
Irregular invasive nests with more cytoplasm than the overlying noninvasive component (paradoxic differentiation)
Characteristics of stromal-host reaction
Presence of retraction artifact
Presence of stromal desmoplasia or myxoid stroma
Inflammatory reaction

There are several morphologic criteria useful in the determination of lamina propria invasion (Table 6.3). The presence of urothelial nests,

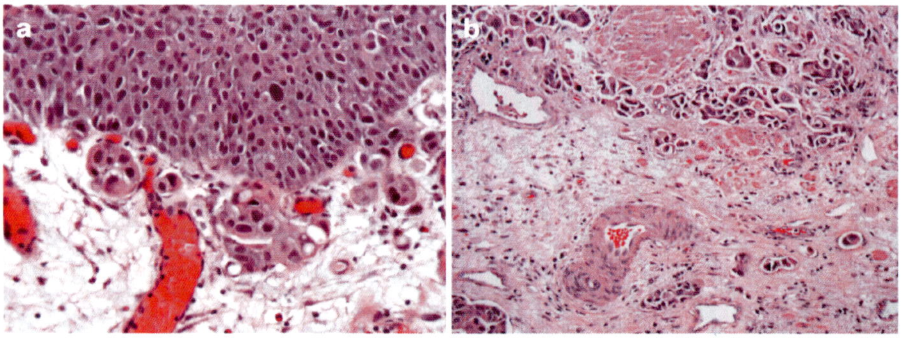

Fig. 6.8 Invasive urothelial carcinoma. (**a**) Invasion into superficial lamina propria. Irregular clusters of tumor cells with abundant eosinophilic cytoplasm are seen. (**b**) Invasion into deep lamina propria. Irregular tumor clusters and nests surrounding muscularis mucosae and large vessels of the deep lamina propria

clusters, or single cells within the lamina propria, sometimes with prominent retraction artifact, is characteristic. The invasive tumor cells may show abundant eosinophilic cytoplasm at the advancing edge of the infiltrating nests (Fig. 6.8a, b). Another feature of invasive tumor is the presence of associated desmoplastic or inflammatory stromal response. Invasive tumors are invariably high grade and only a small minority is of low-grade morphology, but the outcome of these tumors is determined by their stage not grade.

Assessing lamina propria invasion may be difficult and problematic with lack of reproducibility among pathologists [77, 93–95]. Some of the factors that contribute to pitfalls in the diagnosis of lamina propria invasion include tangential sectioning and poor orientation of tumor specimen, thermal or cautery artifact that may produce severe distortion of the specimen, and intense inflammation that may obscure isolated tumor cells or nests of invasive tumor. Urothelial carcinoma in situ involving von Brunn nests may appear as if invading the lamina propria [96, 97]. Additionally, when limited to the lamina propria, urothelial carcinoma with deceptively bland morphology (such as microcystic carcinoma nested variant of urothelial carcinoma) may make the identification of lamina propria invasion very difficult, which may be overlooked instead for a benign entity such as von Brunn nests and proliferative cystitis [98–100]. Special attention should be paid to the general features of the tumor to assess invasion such as cytologic atypia, infiltrative architecture, desmoplasia, and architectural complexity, especially since these changes may be subtle in superficial biopsies [97].

Overdiagnosis of vascular invasion may complicate the assessment of invasion in urothelial carcinoma since invasion into lamina propria is usually associated with retraction artifact of the stroma, which can be easily misinterpreted as lymphatic or vascular invasion. Because of this, data on the impact of vascular invasion in urothelial carcinoma are conflicting and may be difficult to interpret [97].

Attempts to subclassify T1 tumors based on their depth of invasion may be difficult because of the variability in tumor specimen. It may be feasible in cases with well-delineated anatomic landmarks used for subclassification, including muscularis mucosae or distinctive large vessels in the deep lamina propria. These landmarks, however, are not always easily identified in transurethral resection or biopsy specimens and such assessment may become difficult [97, 101, 102]. Nonetheless, when possible, some assessment of the extent of invasion should be provided in the pathology report. But before substaging of pT1 tumors becomes required in routine practice, more work is necessary to arrive at criteria that can be universally adopted and applied to all transurethral resection and biopsy specimens [8].

Carcinomas with Divergent (Aberrant) Differentiation

Urothelial carcinomas, particularly high-grade tumors, may show divergent differentiation. This feature is seen primarily in invasive and advanced tumors but may occasionally be present in noninvasive tumors as well. Different morphologic variants have been reported including glandular, villoglandular papillary (adeno), micropapillary, small cell, and plasmacytoid [103–105]. A number of noninvasive squamous lesions have been reported in the bladder including keratinizing squamous metaplasia, verrucous squamous hyperplasia, squamous papilloma, condyloma acuminatum, and squamous cell carcinoma in situ [106, 107]. Most of these lesions, however, were associated with subsequent or concurrent in situ or invasive squamous carcinoma or carcinoma with squamous differentiation, underscoring the importance of following these lesions closely. In a series of 300 consecutive cystectomies performed at Memorial Sloan-Kettering Cancer Center, 27% of cancer-bearing specimens contained some form of divergent differentiation. This incidence, however, was lower in transurethral resection specimens at approximately 7%. When divergent differentiation is seen together with usual urothelial carcinoma, the pathologist should use the terminology *urothelial carcinoma with ____ differentiation,* inserting the type of differentiation observed.

Disease Management

Endoscopic Management

Patients with any combination of abnormal findings on physical examination, cytology, imaging, or cystoscopy require further assessment. In most cases, this entails endoscopic tumor resection and bimanual examination under anesthesia under anesthesia, with or without upper tract with or without upper-tract evaluation as dictated by intraoperative findings and the patient's previous workup. At the time of endoscopic assessment, a bimanual pelvic bladder examination should be performed in all patients, particularly those with large and/or suspected invasive tumors. Palpable masses are associated with a high probability of extravesical tumor extension, and bladder fixation usually indicates inoperability and need for systemic therapy.

Transurethral resection of a bladder tumor is the initial step in therapy for any visible lesion found on cystoscopy. The TURBT is both diagnostic and therapeutic in that it provides tissue for pathologic diagnosis and also removes any visible tumor. In most cases, complete eradication of the tumor through a combination of resection and fulguration is the goal. For large tumors, or tumors in poorly accessible locations, such as the anterior wall, staged resection may be required. For patients with high-volume, high-grade lesions who will clearly need a cystectomy, total eradication of disease may be impossible and/or unnecessary. Still, the tumor must be adequately sampled to provide pathologic parameters that will influence therapeutic decision-making, including grade, depth of invasion (if any), histology, and presence of lymphovascular invasion. For patients who are not candidates for cystectomy, a complete resection of large tumors should be attempted if the patient is to receive subsequent chemoradiation as this may improve the response to therapy. Other settings in which complete resection may not be accomplished include medical instability and substantial risk of bladder perforation.

At the time of TURBT, directed biopsies may also be appropriate. Areas suspicious for CIS can be biopsied with cold-cup biopsy forceps. In patients with positive cytology without visible disease, or with multifocal CIS, the prostatic urethra should be sampled with a resectoscope [108]. Random bladder biopsies may be helpful in the setting of multiple tumors, or positive cytology; however, they are not recommended for low-risk patients—i.e., those with single papillary tumors and negative cytology [109, 110].

Many patients will derive additional benefit from a restaging TURBT. This is most often performed within 4–6 weeks of the initial resection. Restaging TURBT may detect residual disease in

26–83% of cases [111]. For high-risk tumors, a second resection shows worse prognostic findings in roughly 20% of cases, and changes treatment decisions in ~30% of cases [112, 113]. Many experts recommend restaging TUR for all patients with T1 and HG Ta disease [4, 10]. Given the prognostic implications of upstaging from Ta to T1, re-resection is also recommended when pathology results are equivocal or when lamina propria invasion is uncertain.

Restaging TURBT for T1 lesions becomes even more important if there is no muscularis propria identified in the initial resection. Dutta and colleagues found that there is a 64% risk of understaging for T1 lesions when no muscle is present in the specimen compared with a 30% risk when muscle is present [114]. Because the presence of muscularis propria in the specimen is so important for accurate staging, a sample of the tumor base should be procured as a distinct specimen after the bulk of the tumor has been resected. This technique may facilitate identification of muscularis propria and can be especially helpful with large, high-grade appearing lesions.

The findings on restaging TURBT may be predictive of future recurrence. Patients with T1 tumor on restaging evaluation have a ~80% risk of progression within 5 years. These patients are ideal candidates for early cystectomy [115]. As a result, the authors restage all T1 tumors with the exception of those in patients opting for immediate cystectomy. Another benefit to restaging is that it improves the initial response to *Bacillus Calmette-Guérin* (BCG) therapy. A 2005 study by Herr compared response to BCG after a single TUR to response following a restaging TUR. Patients in the latter group had a lower incidence of residual or recurrent tumor at first cystoscopy and a lower incidence of disease progression with 3 years of follow-up [116].

Knowing the advantages of restaging TURBT for T1 tumors, one may consider the role of re-resection for Ta tumors. The data are less clear in this situation, but these tumors can be understaged in up to 40% of high-risk patients [117]. Those tumors that may be good candidates include bulky lesions, particularly HG tumors. Muscularis propria should be adequately sampled in this setting. For low-volume Ta tumors, the choice to re-resect remains a matter of clinical judgment. In the setting of recurrent LG disease, gross resection without evidence of lamina propria invasion is often sufficient without the presence of muscularis propria, in part due to the low risk of tumor progression. In this setting, the resectionist must weigh the costs and risks of a second surgery with the potential benefit, which is diminished for low-volume LG Ta disease.

Other important findings in a TURBT specimen or biopsy include the presence of divergent or mixed or aberrant histologies. The presence of mixed histology is associated with a higher incidence of muscle invasion at TURBT and extravesical extension at cystectomy [118]. Although this is seen uncommonly in noninvasive tumors, one must consider the implication in T1 disease. Complete resection is essential, if feasible, as the response of these histologic variants to intravesical agents is uncertain. Reports of mixed histologies should therefore prompt re-resection, and potentially aggressive treatment. The authors consider early cystectomy in T1 patients with micropapillary, squamous, sarcomatoid, or glandular tumors and also in those with aggressive (nested or inverted) growth patterns in view of the aggressive nature of the clinical course [119–123]. The rare patient with small cell carcinoma in a T1 lesion should be considered for systemic chemotherapy [124, 125].

Intravesical Therapy

Following definitive TURBT, further therapeutic planning is based on tumor characteristics. Cystectomy with or without neoadjuvant chemotherapy is the standard treatment for those with muscle-invasive disease. However, for the majority of patients with NMIBC, the next step is adjuvant intravesical therapy aimed at decreasing the risk of tumor recurrence, and possibly progression. The type and duration of therapy depends on the characteristics of the patient and the tumor. Most intravesical therapy can be classified into two broad categories, immunotherapy and chemotherapy. Table 6.4 summarizes the mecha-

Table 6.4 Summary of intravesical therapies

Intravesical therapies	Mechanism of action	Primary efficacy[a] (absolute % reduction in recurrence vs. TURBT alone)	Cystitis [128] (%)	Other side effects [128] (%)
Chemotherapeutic agents				
Mitomycin C	Antibiotic; inhibits DNA synthesis	3–18 [2, 127]	30–40	Rash (8–19), contracted bladder (5)
Thiotepa	DNA alkylating agent; crosslinks nucleic acids	12 [127]	10–30	Myelosuppression (8–19)
Gemcitabine	Deoxycytidine analog; inhibits DNA synthesis	2 [126]	Mild	Occasional nausea
Doxorubicin	Intercalating agent; inhibits DNA synthesis	15 [127]	20–40	Fever, allergy (~5)
Epirubicin	Intercalating agent; inhibits DNA synthesis	12 [127]	10–30	Contracted bladder rare
Immunomodulatory agents				
BCG	Inflammatory host response, cytokine release	24–42 [2, 127]	60–80	Serious infection (5)
Interferon	Lymphocyte activation, cytokine release, also antiproliferative and antiangiogenic actions	8 [129]	<5	Flu-like symptoms (20)

[a]Defined as the total percent of patients free from recurrence following TURBT + intravesical therapy minus the percent of patients free from recurrence after TURBT alone. Length of follow-up, patient, and tumor characteristics vary between studies making statistical comparisons between studies not appropriate, with the exception of those reported by the original authors [128]

nisms of action, side effects, and primary efficacy of common agents [2, 126–129].

Intravesical chemotherapy exposes the tumor to high drug concentrations, while avoiding systemic effects. A number of chemotherapeutic agents have been used intravesically including: doxorubicin, epirubicin, thiotepa, gemcitabine, and mitomycin C (MMC). For most clinicians, mitomycin is the agent of choice for primary intravesical chemotherapy due to its low cost and its high molecular weight, which results in minimal systemic absorption and a low side-effect profile.

Intravesical chemotherapy has an added benefit when used in the perioperative setting. In a meta-analysis of seven randomized controlled trials with a median follow-up time of 3.4 years, Sylvester and colleagues demonstrated a 37–48% reduction in the risk of recurrence when a single postoperative dose of intravesical thiotepa, epirubicin, pirarubicin, or MMC was instilled within 24 hours of TURBT. Efficacy was similar among the chemotherapeutics studied, and unfortunately, there was no indication that any of the drugs decreased the risk of progression [130]. A recent study evaluating a single dose of postoperative gemcitabine found that it was not superior to placebo in terms of recurrence-free survival [126]. Perioperative therapy is contraindicated in cases of suspected bladder perforation or extensive tumor resection because of the risks of chemical cystitis, systemic absorption, and extravesical extravasation.

Intravesical immunotherapy is another effective means of reducing recurrence of NMIBC. *Bacillus Calmette-Guérin* is the most widely used intravesical immunotherapeutic agent. This is an attenuated mycobacterium, initially developed as a tuberculosis vaccine. Multiple strains of BCG exist and are used for treatment of NMIBC. These include Connaught, Tice, Armand, Frappier, Pasteur, Tokyo, and RIVM

[10]. Administration of BCG results in an exaggerated local immune response. The antineoplastic mechanism of action is not entirely understood, but is thought to be related to activation of cell-mediated cytotoxic mechanisms [131].

Rarely, BCG can be used to treat residual tumor after incomplete resection of papillary tumors in patients that will not tolerate another endoscopic procedure. Success rates for treatment of local tumor are roughly 60% [132]. Much more frequently, BCG is used either to treat CIS, since the nature of this lesion prevents endoscopic resection, or as prophylaxis in patients that have undergone complete TUR. In the treatment of CIS, a complete response rate of 70% can be expected, although only 64% of those complete responders will have a durable response at 5 years [133]. By 10 years, however, only 30% will remain disease free [134], indicating the importance of continued surveillance.

Maintenance BCG administration can delay recurrence following complete resection of Ta or T1 lesions. The best results are seen when patients undergo an initial induction course of BCG followed by maintenance therapy. The efficacy of regimens containing induction and maintenance therapy was recently demonstrated in a meta-analysis of 25 studies including a total of 4,767 patients [135]. The ideal dosing schedule for induction and maintenance courses has not yet been determined. Some of the best results to date have been reported by the Southwest Oncology Group (SWOG), using a induction course of 1 instillation per week for 6 weeks followed by three weekly instillations at 3, 6, 12, 18, 24, and 36 months from the initial induction. Median recurrence-free survival was 76.8 months for those receiving induction and maintenance therapy compared with 35.7 months for those receiving induction therapy alone [136].

The effects of BCG on progression have been less clear-cut, with some studies showing a decrease in progression and some studies showing no effect. However, two recent meta-analyses have found reductions in the risk of progression of more than 20% when patients receive both induction and maintenance BCG [32, 137]. Neither study was able to demonstrate a survival advantage.

Interferon-alpha is another form of intravesical immunotherapy. As a primary treatment, it is both less effective and more expensive than BCG [138]. However, there is evidence showing that the combination of the two drugs may be superior to either drug alone, and that using the two drugs together could allow for BCG dose reductions, thereby decreasing side effects while preserving efficacy [139]. Further studies are necessary to confirm these observations.

BCG can be poorly tolerated. As high as 70–90% of patients treated with BCG will experience some level of toxicity [2, 108, 140]. The majority of this toxicity is associated with the immunostimulatory effects of BCG. This most often results in lower urinary tract symptoms such as dysuria, urgency, and frequency, and can also manifest as mild systemic symptoms such as fatigue, malaise, and low-grade fever [2, 140]. Severe local complications such as bladder contracture and severe systemic complications such as BCG sepsis can also occur. Fortunately, these complications are rare, and the vast majority of adverse reactions to BCG are manageable Grade I and II toxicities [108, 131, 141, 142].

Because BCG is given over a prolonged time period, with many patients receiving multiple maintenance courses, studies have also looked at the timing of BCG toxicity. A 2003 meta-analysis by Bohle et al. showed no difference in toxicities between those receiving BCG induction and maintenance and those receiving an induction course only [131]. The European Organization for Research and Treatment of Cancer (EORTC) phase III study of maintenance BCG showed that patients experienced the majority of side effects during induction and the first 6 months of maintenance therapy, and that there was no increase in side effects with further therapy [143]. While the majority of BCG complications are manageable, they are still irritating enough to patients to cause a considerable number to discontinue therapy. In the phase III EORTC trial previously cited, 20.3% of patients treated with BCG stopped therapy because of side effects [143]. In a Southwest Oncology Group study only 16% of patients were able to tolerate the full maintenance regimen of eight courses over a 3-year period [136].

To minimize the symptoms associated with BCG maintenance, clinicians must be prepared to reduce the dosage relatively quickly after symptoms begin. A 2002 study by the Spanish Oncology Group (CUETO) evaluating standard dose BCG (81 mg) and 1/3 standard dose (27 mg) showed no significant differences in recurrence (28% vs. 31%) or progression rates (11.5% vs. 13.3%) between the two groups, except in the case of multifocal tumors, where the standard dose was superior. There was also a suggestion of lower recurrence rates for other types of high-risk tumors with the standard dose, although this did not reach statistical significance. The reduced-dose was better tolerated, with fewer patients in that group requiring a treatment delay or withdrawing, and with a larger percentage of reduced-dose patients reporting no toxicity. However, severe systemic toxicity was not significantly different between the two groups. The authors concluded that patients with high-risk tumors should still receive full-dose treatment, but that reduced dose treatment would be acceptable for low- to intermediate-risk tumors and for maintenance regimens [144]. CUETO also evaluated further dose reduction to 1/6 the standard dose. However, this was less effective than 1/3 dose BCG against intermediate-risk bladder cancer [145]. Other groups have reported decreased toxicity and equivalent efficacy with a regimen employing longer intervals between doses of BCG during the induction therapy [146]. As the studies previously discussed were conducted in Europe where BCG vaccination against tuberculosis is common, there is some question as to how well these studies translate to the BCG-naive North American population [10].

Numerous studies have compared the efficacy and side effects of MMC and BCG in preventing recurrence of Ta or T1 urothelial carcinoma. A 1995 SWOG study randomized 377 patients with Ta or T1 bladder cancer to receive adjuvant BCG or MMC after TURBT. Patients in the BCG arm had a significantly higher recurrence-free survival than those treated with MMC. Patients in the BCG group also experienced more side effects, although no grade 4 (life-threatening) toxicity was seen in either arm [142]. Similar findings have been observed in other randomized trials and in large meta-analyses. A meta-analysis by Bohle et al. evaluated 11 trials including 2,749 patients comparing BCG to MMC for treatment of NMIBC. A significantly lower rate of recurrence in the BCG group (38.6%) compared to the MMC group (46.4%) was observed at 26 months of follow-up. However, patients in the BCG group (53.8%) were more likely to experience cystitis than patients in the MMC group (39.2%). An independent meta-analysis by Shelley et al. demonstrated a 31% decrease in the risk of recurrence for those patients receiving BCG compared to those receiving MMC for high-risk NMIBC. The incidence of local and systemic toxicity was, again, higher in the BCG group [147].

A follow-up meta-analysis reviewed nine randomized trials encompassing 2,410 patients to assess tumor progression in the setting of adjuvant BCG or MMC after TURBT [137]. At a median follow-up of 26 months, there was no statistically significant difference in progression rates. However, subset analysis was performed in five studies that utilized maintenance therapy. Within the subgroup receiving maintenance therapy, the relative risk of progression was significantly lower in patients treated with BCG than for those receiving MMC [137].

Studies have also demonstrated that BCG is superior to chemotherapy for the treatment of CIS. A meta-analysis by Sylvester et al. showed a complete response in 68.1% of CIS patients treated with BCG and a 51.5% response in those treated with chemotherapy (including MMC), corresponding to a 47% decrease in the odds of treatment failure for BCG patients compared to those on chemotherapy [148]. At a median follow-up of 3.6 years, a greater recurrence-free survival was observed in the BCG cohort (46.7%), compared with patients receiving chemotherapy (26.2%). Subgroup analysis demonstrated even greater efficacy for BCG when a maintenance strategy was utilized [5, 148].

Decisions regarding the type and duration of intravesical therapy must consider patient characteristics and the risk of tumor recurrence and progression. In an effort to better quantify these issues, the EORTC developed a system of risk stratification derived from data from seven different EORTC trials that included 2,596 patients with NMIBC [149]. A scoring system was developed to incorporate several clinical and pathologic factors: number of tumors, tumor size, prior recurrence rate, T-stage category, presence of CIS, and tumor grade. Using these criteria, patients are stratified by risk, and probabilities of recurrence and progression at 1 and 5 years are calculated. These tables can be a useful tool for educating patients, informing treatment decisions, and devising surveillance strategies [149].

Despite the large body of evidence showing the benefits of intravesical therapy in appropriate patients, studies show that intravesical therapy is underutilized. Data from the Surveillance, Epidemiology and End Results (SEER) Program 2003 Bladder Cancer Patterns of Care project showed that only 42% of high-risk bladder cancer patients in the studied population received intravesical therapy [150]. In an effort to help guide the use of intravesical therapy for NMIBC, both the American Urological Association (AUA) and the European Association of Urology (EAU) have released guidelines evaluating the existing evidence and providing treatment recommendations. There is agreement between the two organizations about the major principles of therapy including: (1) the use of a single perioperative dose of chemotherapy for low-risk patients; (2) intravesical chemotherapy or immunotherapy for intermediate-risk patients; (3) induction and maintenance BCG for high-risk patients; and (4) consideration of cystectomy for those at highest risk, including BCG failures. Presentation of these treatment options differs, with the AUA presenting recommendations in terms of a set of "index patients," and the EAU presenting its guidelines in terms of risks groups based on the aforementioned EORTC risk calculator. Tables 6.5 and 6.6 summarize recommendations from these organizations for specific clinical scenarios [2, 151].

Table 6.5 Summary of AUA recommendations for treatment of non-muscle-invasive urothelial carcinoma [2]

Tumor type	Recommended treatment options
Small volume, LG Ta	Single perioperative dose of intravesical chemotherapy
Large volume, multifocal LGTa or recurrent LGTa	Induction BCG (or MMC)
HG Ta or T1 +/– CIS	Repeat resection Induction and maintenance BCG
Recurrent T1, CIS; or high-risk T1	Consider radical cystectomy

Table 6.6 Summary of EAU recommendations for treatment of non-muscle-invasive urothelial carcinoma [151]

Risk group	Recommended treatment options
Low-risk tumors	Single perioperative dose of intravesical chemotherapy
Intermediate-risk tumors	Repeat resection Induction intravesical chemo- or immunotherapy
High-risk tumors	Repeat resection Induction and maintenance BCG (≥1 year)
Highest risk tumors, or BCG failure	Consider radical cystectomy

Management of Recurrent or Refractory Disease

Up to 70% of NMIBC will recur. The majority of recurrences develop within 2 years after the initial treatment; however, late recurrences and tumor progression occur frequently, thus, careful long-term surveillance is necessary [152]. The presence or absence of recurrence at the first follow-up cystoscopy (3 months after resection) may have prognostic implications. A negative cystoscopic assessment at this time period has been associated with a decreased risk of recurrence and progression 5 years after treatment [153]. Although patients with early recurrence tend to have a more aggressive course, patients with late recurrences, more than 2 years after initial treatment, are still likely to suffer future recurrences and thus require definitive therapy [154].

The treatment paradigm for management of a recurrent tumor mirrors the management of primary tumors—i.e., endoscopic resection and appropriate imaging with subsequent treatment based on histology, tumor staging, and patient risk. Recurrence of papillary, low-grade appearing lesions in patients with an established history of low-grade Ta poses minimal risk of progression. This constitutes the one situation in which urologists may consider tumor ablation rather than resection. In this setting, management of small recurrences with in-office fulguration has equivalent disease-specific survival compared to TUR, and spares the patient the risk and expense of an anesthetic. Some clinicians even advocate observation for these types of recurrence [155, 156].

For patients with high-risk disease, even those receiving BCG have a recurrence rate of 20–40%. Historically, BCG failure was defined broadly, referring to any tumor recurrence after treatment. More recently, there has been an effort to selectively define a patient's response to therapy. Patients that progress or fail to improve despite BCG therapy are considered "BCG-refractory." Those with recurrent or persistent tumor of a lesser grade or stage after initial BCG therapy are termed "BCG-resistant." With retreatment, these tumors ultimately resolve within 6 months of initial therapy. Patients that recur after an initial disease-free interval are classified as "BCG-relapsing." Those that recur after an inadequate course of therapy, typically due to toxicity, are termed "BCG-intolerant" [108, 157].

For those failing BCG with refractory or recurrent high-grade disease, treatment options include a second course of BCG, a salvage intravesical agent, or cystectomy. Up to 35% of BCG-relapsing patients will have a durable response to a second course of BCG induction [158]. The efficacy of standard chemotherapeutics in BCG-refractory patients is somewhat less, ranging from 10 to 20%. Malmstrom and colleagues reported a 19% 3-year disease-free survival rate in patients receiving MMC after BCG failure [159]. Studies with valrubicin, an anthracycline similar to doxorubicin, showed only a 21% complete response rate at 6 months, and 8% at 24 months in patients with recurrent CIS after BCG treatment [160]. These studies suggest that the efficacy of standard intravesical chemotherapy in BCG-refractory disease is limited [161]. Newer chemotherapeutics are being evaluated as alternative salvage therapies. A recent phase II trial of intravesical gemcitabine for BCG-refractory disease showed a 21% complete response rate [162].

Ultimately, continued use of intravesical therapies after two failed courses of BCG should be avoided, since the patient will suffer continued relapse up to 80% of the time. Patients in this situation should be urged to consider cystectomy [10]. In the setting of recurrent high-risk disease, there are several benefits of "early" cystectomy: (1) there is a high likelihood that rapidly recurring, high-risk disease will eventually progress to muscle invasion [163, 164], (2) a 5–10% chance of metastases is associated with every recurrent T1 tumor [165], (3) high-risk NMIBC is understaged in 25–45% of cases [166], and (4) disease-free survival in patients who progress to muscle invasion is no better (and may even be worse) than those who present with muscle invasion [165, 166].

In some cases, the management of recurrent NMIBC is not straightforward. Patients with an initial high-grade Ta or T1 tumor may present with low-grade Ta disease. In these cases, a less aggressive treatment path may be considered as compared to the patient with recurrent T1 tumor. Consideration must be given to patient characteristics, the pattern of recurrence, and tumor characteristics, including tumor volume, tumor location, ease of resection, and histologic characteristics. If the completeness of the resection is uncertain, restaging TURBT should be performed. If the clinical scenario is favorable with a less risky recurrence, TURBT and intravesical therapy may be a reasonable treatment approach [161]. For low-grade tumors that recur after prior use of BCG for high-grade disease, the authors often utilize MMC as an adjuvant strategy. Aggressive, regular surveillance should be continued in these patients, with further treatment decisions based on the pathology of subsequent recurrences.

A more ominous situation is the patient with low- or intermediate-risk disease that suffers grade and/or stage progression. Again, patient and tumor factors must be weighed, along with the timing of recurrence. The development of grade progression in those with noninvasive disease should prompt the use of intravesical BCG after resection. The development of stage progression to T1 disease is worrisome and should prompt a discussion about more aggressive therapies, including cystectomy and its benefits when delivered "early." Progression to muscle invasion certainly requires radical treatment with cystectomy in the surgical candidate, along with a discussion about neoadjuvant systemic chemotherapy. Chemoradiation may be another option for the motivated patient desiring bladder preservation and also for the surgically unfit.

Surveillance

Due to the high risk of recurrence and progression of NMIBC, patients with this disease are surveyed vigorously. Since the risk of progression and recurrence continues over the long term, most patients are followed for years, or even for life [167, 168]. Surveillance typically entails regular cystoscopy, periodic imaging, and urine cytology or other markers. Surveillance schedules have not been based in evidence, and thus there is variability.

The NCCN recommends an initial 3-month cystoscopy and cytology for patients with papilloma or LG Ta followed by regular cystoscopy at increasing intervals; no follow-up imaging is required [4]. For HG Ta, T1, CIS, and recurrent disease, it recommends cystoscopy every 3 months for 2 years, every 6 months for 2 years, and then annually for life, with upper-tract imaging every 1–2 years. The EAU schedule is more relaxed. In consideration of recent data on the prognostic implications of a negative initial surveillance cystoscopy, the EAU suggests an initial 3-month cystoscopy, and if negative, repeat cystoscopy at 9 months, and then yearly for 5 years in patients with low-grade Ta tumors [151, 153]. Regardless of the schedule followed, surveillance should be tailored to the individual patient and tumor characteristics, with the goal being the minimum amount of surveillance necessary to facilitate early detection of recurrence and minimize the risk of progression.

A tailored surveillance schedule is particularly important for patients diagnosed with PUNLMP or papilloma. Multiple studies have shown that both recurrence and progression can occur with PUNLMP, but at far lower rates than with low-grade Ta tumors [89, 169]. Rarely is the progression to a high-grade tumor. Thus, patients with PUNLMP should be followed, but on a less frequent schedule than those with low- or high-grade Ta lesions. When papillomas occur in isolation, they have a very low rate of recurrence and an essentially negligible risk of progression, thus regular surveillance is not required, particularly in the patient with a small, single papilloma [86, 89]. However, papillomas may uncommonly occur in patients with a previous or concomitant diagnosis of urothelial carcinoma [89]. In such cases, surveillance should be dictated by the requirements of the bladder carcinoma. Moreover, the decision to survey a patient with papilloma may be reasonable in the case of large or multifocal disease.

Molecular Alterations and Targeted Therapy

As previously mentioned, multiple chromosomal alterations have been identified that are associated with UC, including alterations and subsequent inactivation of tumor-suppressor genes such as p53 and RB1, activation of oncogenes such as those from the *myc* and *ras* families, and overexpression of normal genes encoding for growth factors and growth factor receptors such as ERBB1 and ERBB2. As illustrated in Fig. 6.1, UC is thought to arise from at least two separate mechanisms [170]. These mechanisms result in a heterogeneous group of diseases that consist of two main phenotypes, low-grade papillary tumor and invasive tumor [38]. These entities have drastically different biological behaviors and prognoses, as has been described previously. Low-grade noninvasive tumors are characterized by mutations in the

HRAS and fibroblast growth factor receptor 3 (FGFR3) genes, while high-grade invasive tumors frequently have defects in the p53 and pRb tumor-suppressor pathways [38]. Tumor invasion and progression in bladder cancer appear to be a multifactorial process, promoted by microenvironmental changes (Fig. 6.1) [38].

Therapies targeted at these genes and their products are being investigated and may play a role in treatment of NMIBC in the future. Examples of targeted therapies currently being investigated include trastuzumab, an anti-ERBB2-related monoclonal antibody being evaluated for treatment of patients with muscle-invasive, urothelial carcinoma whose tumors overexpress ERBB-2; and multiple studies investigating the role of the tyrosine-kinase inhibitors, sorafenib and sunitinib [9, 171].

Conclusion

Despite advances in diagnosis and treatment, NMIBC remains a common disorder. Its tendency to recur and progress necessitates long-term follow-up and makes treatment expensive and often challenging. Understanding the pathology of NMIBC, its presentation, and its treatment will enable healthcare providers to give care that is consistent with current guidelines, yet integrate treatment advances in a timely and cost-effective manner. The economic impact of the management of NMIBC must be appreciated. Common clinical practices have been perpetuated over time, but are often not based in evidence. Careful scrutiny of disease management is necessary to optimally utilize effective strategies and to reduce surveillance or treatments that do not improve patient outcomes.

References

1. Jemal A, Siegel R, Xu J, Ward E, Cancer statistics. CA Cancer J Clin. 2010;60(5):277–300.
2. Hall MC, Chang SS, Dalbagni G, Pruthi RS, Seigne JD, Skinner EC, et al. Guideline for the management of non-muscle invasive bladder cancer (stages Ta, T1, and Tis): 2007 update. J Urol. 2007;178(6):2314–30.
3. Messing EM. Urothelial tumors of the bladder. In: Wein AJ, Kavoussi LR, Novick AC, Partin AW, Peters CA, editors. Campbell-Walsh urology. 9th ed. Philadelphia: Saunders-Elsevier; 2007.
4. Montie JE, Clark PE, Eisenberger MA, El-Galley R, Greenberg RE, Herr HW, et al. Bladder cancer. J Natl Compr Canc Netw. 2009;7(1):8–39.
5. Jacobs BL, Lee CT, Montie JE. Bladder cancer in 2010: how far have we come? CA Cancer J Clin. 2010:caac.20077.
6. Soloway MS, Sofer M, Vaidya A. Contemporary management of stage T1 transitional cell carcinoma of the bladder. J Urol. 2002;167(4):1573–83.
7. Botteman MF, Pashos CL, Redaelli A, Laskin B, Hauser R. The health economics of bladder cancer: a comprehensive review of the published literature. Pharmacoeconomics. 2003;21(18):1315–30.
8. Epstein JI, Amin MB, Reuter VR, Mostofi FK. The World Health Organization/International Society of Urological Pathology consensus classification of urothelial (transitional cell) neoplasms of the urinary bladder. Bladder Consensus Conference Committee. Am J Surg Pathol. 1998;22(12):1435–48.
9. Kaufman DS, Shipley WU, Feldman AS. Bladder cancer. Lancet. 2009;374(9685):239–49.
10. Jones SMD, Campbell SMDPD. Non-muscle-invasive bladder cancer (Ta, T1, and CIS). In: Wein AJ, Kavoussi LR, Novick AC, Partin AW, Peters CA, editors. Campbell-Walsh urology. 9th ed. Philadelphia: Saunders Elsevier; 2007.
11. Haleblian GE, Skinner EC, Dickinson MG, Lieskovsky G, Boyd SD, Skinner DG. Hydronephrosis as a prognostic indicator in bladder cancer patients. J Urol. 1998;160(6 Pt 1):2011–4.
12. Strope SA, Montie JE. The causal role of cigarette smoking in bladder cancer initiation and progression, and the role of urologists in smoking cessation. J Urol. 2008;180(1):31–7; discussion 7.
13. Wynder EL, Goldsmith R. The epidemiology of bladder cancer: a second look. Cancer. 1977;40(3):1246–68.
14. Golijanin DJ, Kakiashvili D, Madeb RR, Messing EM, Lerner SP. Chemoprevention of bladder cancer. World J Urol. 2006;24(5):445–72.
15. Lamm SH, Engel A, Penn CA, Chen R, Feinleib M. Arsenic cancer risk confounder in southwest Taiwan data set. Environ Health Perspect. 2006;114(7):1077–82.
16. Silverman DT, Levin LI, Hoover RN. Occupational risks of bladder cancer in the United States: II Nonwhite men. J Natl Cancer Inst. 1989;81(19):1480–3.
17. Silverman DT, Levin LI, Hoover RN, Hartge P. Occupational risks of bladder cancer in the United States: I. White men. J Natl Cancer Inst. 1989;81(19):1472–80.
18. Choi JY, Lee KM, Cho SH, Kim SW, Choi HY, Lee SY, et al. CYP2E1 and NQO1 genotypes, smoking and bladder cancer. Pharmacogenetics. 2003;13(6):349–55.

19. Engel LS, Taioli E, Pfeiffer R, Garcia-Closas M, Marcus PM, Lan Q, et al. Pooled analysis and meta-analysis of glutathione S-transferase M1 and bladder cancer: a HuGE review. Am J Epidemiol. 2002; 156(2):95–109.
20. Marcus PM, Vineis P, Rothman N. NAT2 slow acetylation and bladder cancer risk: a meta-analysis of 22 case–control studies conducted in the general population. Pharmacogenetics. 2000;10(2):115–22.
21. Cordon-Cardo C, Zhang ZF, Dalbagni G, Drobnjak M, Charytonowicz E, Hu SX, et al. Cooperative effects of p53 and pRB alterations in primary superficial bladder tumors. Cancer Res. 1997;57(7): 1217–21.
22. Esrig D, Elmajian D, Groshen S, Freeman JA, Stein JP, Chen SC, et al. Accumulation of nuclear p53 and tumor progression in bladder cancer. N Engl J Med. 1994;331(19):1259–64.
23. Grossman HB, Liebert M, Antelo M, Dinney CP, Hu SX, Palmer JL, et al. p53 and RB expression predict progression in T1 bladder cancer. Clin Cancer Res. 1998;4(4):829–34.
24. Shinohara N, Koyanagi T. Ras signal transduction in carcinogenesis and progression of bladder cancer: molecular target for treatment? Urol Res. 2002;30(5):273–81.
25. Theodorescu D. Molecular pathogenesis of proliferative and progressive (invasive) urothelial cancer. In: Droller MJ, Goldsmith K, Goldsmith C, editors. Urothelial tumors. Hamilton, British Colombia: Decker; 2004. p. 28–43.
26. Hazra AG, Gu J, Wu X. Genetic susceptibility to bladder cancer. In: Lerner SP, Schoenberg MP, Sternberg CN, editors. Textbook of bladder cancer. Oxford: Taylor and Francis; 2006. p. 2–36.
27. Mellon K, Wright C, Kelly P, Horne CH, Neal DE. Long-term outcome related to epidermal growth factor receptor status in bladder cancer. J Urol. 1995;153(3 Pt 2):919–25.
28. Messing EM. Clinical implications of the expression of epidermal growth factor receptors in human transitional cell carcinoma. Cancer Res. 1990;50(8): 2530–7.
29. Neal DE, Sharples L, Smith K, Fennelly J, Hall RR, Harris AL. The epidermal growth factor receptor and the prognosis of bladder cancer. Cancer. 1990;65(7):1619–25.
30. Herr HW. Tumour progression and survival in patients with T1G3 bladder tumours: 15-year outcome. Br J Urol. 1997;80(5):762–5.
31. Saad A, Hanbury DC, McNicholas TA, Boustead GB, Morgan S, Woodman AC. A study comparing various noninvasive methods of detecting bladder cancer in urine. BJU Int. 2002;89(4):369–73.
32. Sylvester RJ, van der Meijden AP, Lamm DL. Intravesical bacillus Calmette-Guerin reduces the risk of progression in patients with superficial bladder cancer: a meta-analysis of the published results of randomized clinical trials. J Urol. 2002; 168(5):1964–70.
33. Smits G, Schaafsma E, Kiemeney L, Caris C, Debruyne F, Witjes JA. Microstaging of pT1 transitional cell carcinoma of the bladder: identification of subgroups with distinct risks of progression. Urology. 1998;52(6):1009–13; discussion 13–4.
34. Herr HW. Tumor progression and survival of patients with high grade, noninvasive papillary (TaG3) bladder tumors: 15-year outcome. J Urol. 2000;163(1):60–1; discussion 1–2.
35. Droller MJ. Biological considerations in the assessment of urothelial cancer: a retrospective. Urology. 2005;66(5 Suppl):66–75.
36. Richter J, Jiang F, Gorog JP, Sartorius G, Egenter C, Gasser TC, et al. Marked genetic differences between stage pTa and stage pT1 papillary bladder cancer detected by comparative genomic hybridization. Cancer Res. 1997;57(14):2860–4.
37. Degtyar P, Neulander E, Zirkin H, Yusim I, Douvdevani A, Mermershtain W, et al. Fluorescence in situ hybridization performed on exfoliated urothelial cells in patients with transitional cell carcinoma of the bladder. Urology. 2004;63(2):398–401.
38. Wu XR. Urothelial tumorigenesis: a tale of divergent pathways. Nat Rev Cancer. 2005;5(9):713–25.
39. Glas AS, Roos D, Deutekom M, Zwinderman AH, Bossuyt PM, Kurth KH. Tumor markers in the diagnosis of primary bladder cancer. A systematic review. J Urol. 2003;169(6):1975–82.
40. Nabi G, Greene D, O'Donnell MO. Suspicious urinary cytology with negative evaluation for malignancy in the diagnostic investigation of haematuria: how to follow up? J Clin Pathol. 2004;57(4): 365–8.
41. Halling KC, King W, Sokolova IA, Meyer RG, Burkhardt HM, Halling AC, et al. A comparison of cytology and fluorescence in situ hybridization for the detection of urothelial carcinoma. J Urol. 2000;164(5):1768–75.
42. Lokeshwar VB, Habuchi T, Grossman HB, Murphy WM, Hautmann SH, Hemstreet 3rd GP, et al. Bladder tumor markers beyond cytology: International Consensus Panel on bladder tumor markers. Urology. 2005;66(6 Suppl 1):35–63.
43. Paik ML, Scolieri MJ, Brown SL, Spirnak JP, Resnick MI. Limitations of computerized tomography in staging invasive bladder cancer before radical cystectomy. J Urol. 2000;163(6):1693–6.
44. Saksena MA, Dahl DM, Harisinghani MG. New imaging modalities in bladder cancer. World J Urol. 2006;24(5):473–80.
45. Arslan H, Ceylan K, Harman M, Yilmaz Y, Temizoz O, Can S. Virtual computed tomography cystoscopy in bladder pathologies. Int Braz J Urol. 2006;32(2):147–54; discussion 54.
46. Kibel AS, Dehdashti F, Katz MD, Klim AP, Grubb RL, Humphrey PA, et al. Prospective study of [18F]fluorodeoxyglucose positron emission tomography/computed tomography for staging of muscle-invasive bladder carcinoma. J Clin Oncol. 2009; 27(26):4314–20.

47. Tekes A, Kamel I, Imam K, Szarf G, Schoenberg M, Nasir K, et al. Dynamic MRI of bladder cancer: evaluation of staging accuracy. AJR Am J Roentgenol. 2005;184(1):121–7.
48. Cina SJ, Epstein JI, Endrizzi JM, Harmon WJ, Seay TM, Schoenberg MP. Correlation of cystoscopic impression with histologic diagnosis of biopsy specimens of the bladder. Hum Pathol. 2001;32(6):630–7.
49. Mitropoulos D, Kiroudi-Voulgari A, Nikolopoulos P, Manousakas T, Zervas A. Accuracy of cystoscopy in predicting histologic features of bladder lesions. J Endourol. 2005;19(7):861–4.
50. Grossman HB, Gomella L, Fradet Y, Morales A, Presti J, Ritenour C, et al. A phase III, multicenter comparison of hexaminolevulinate fluorescence cystoscopy and white light cystoscopy for the detection of superficial papillary lesions in patients with bladder cancer. J Urol. 2007;178(1):62–7.
51. Babjuk M, Soukup V, Petrik R, Jirsa M, Dvoracek J. 5-aminolaevulinic acid-induced fluorescence cystoscopy during transurethral resection reduces the risk of recurrence in stage Ta/T1 bladder cancer. BJU Int. 2005;96(6):798–802.
52. Riedl CR, Daniltchenko D, Koenig F, Simak R, Loening SA, Pflueger H. Fluorescence endoscopy with 5-aminolevulinic acid reduces early recurrence rate in superficial bladder cancer. J Urol. 2001; 165(4):1121–3.
53. Denzinger S, Burger M, Walter B, Knuechel R, Roessler W, Wieland WF, et al. Clinically relevant reduction in risk of recurrence of superficial bladder cancer using 5-aminolevulinic acid-induced fluorescence diagnosis: 8-year results of prospective randomized study. Urology. 2007;69(4):675–9.
54. Herr HW, Donat SM. A comparison of white-light cystoscopy and narrow-band imaging cystoscopy to detect bladder tumour recurrences. BJU Int. 2008;102(9):1111–4.
55. Goh AC, Tresser NJ, Shen SS, Lerner SP. Optical coherence tomography as an adjunct to white light cystoscopy for intravesical real-time imaging and staging of bladder cancer. Urology. 2008;72(1):133–7.
56. Sonn GA, Jones SN, Tarin TV, Du CB, Mach KE, Jensen KC, et al. Optical biopsy of human bladder neoplasia with in vivo confocal laser endomicroscopy. J Urol. 2009;182(4):1299–305.
57. Oyasu R. World Health Organization and International Society of Urological Pathology classification and two-number grading system of bladder tumors. Cancer. 2000;88(7):1509–12.
58. Loening S, Narayana A, Yoder L, Slymen D, Penick G, Culp D. Analysis of bladder tumor recurrence in 178 patients. Urology. 1980;16(2):137–41.
59. Eble JN, Sauter G, Epstein J, Sesterhenn I, editors. Pathology and genetics of tumours of the urinary system and male genital organs. Lyon: IARC press; 2004.
60. McKenney JK, Desai S, Cohen C, Amin MB. Discriminatory immunohistochemical staining of urothelial carcinoma in situ and non-neoplastic urothelium: an analysis of cytokeratin 20, p53, and CD44 antigens. Am J Surg Pathol. 2001;25(8): 1074–8.
61. Murphy WM, Beckwith JB, Farrow GM. Tumors of the kidney, bladder and related urinary structures. In: Rosai J, editor. Atlas of tumor pathology. Washington, D.C.: Armed Forces Institute of Pathology; 1994.
62. Murphy WM. Current topics in the pathology of bladder cancer. Pathol Annu. 1983;18(Pt 1):1–25.
63. Murphy WM, Irving CC. The cellular features of developing carcinoma in murine urinary bladder. Cancer. 1981;47(3):514–22.
64. Murphy WM, Soloway MS. Developing carcinoma (dysplasia) of the urinary bladder. Pathol Annu. 1982;17(Pt 1):197–217.
65. Nagy GK, Frable WJ, Murphy WM. Classification of premalignant urothelial abnormalities. A Delphi study of the National Bladder Cancer Collaborative Group A. Pathol Annu. 1982;17(Pt 1):219–33.
66. Koss LG, Nakanishi I, Freed SZ. Nonpapillary carcinoma in situ and atypical hyperplasia in cancerous bladders: further studies of surgically removed bladders by mapping. Urology. 1977;9(4):442–55.
67. Murphy WM, Nagy GK, Rao MK, Soloway MS, Parija GC, Cox 2nd CE, et al. "Normal" urothelium in patients with bladder cancer: a preliminary report from the National Bladder Cancer Collaborative Group A. Cancer. 1979;44(3):1050–8.
68. Prout Jr GR, Griffin PP, Daly JJ, Heney NM. Carcinoma in situ of the urinary bladder with and without associated vesical neoplasms. Cancer. 1983;52(3):524–32.
69. Kakizoe T, Matumoto K, Nishio Y, Ohtani M, Kishi K. Significance of carcinoma in situ and dysplasia in association with bladder cancer. J Urol. 1985;133(3):395–8.
70. Utz DC, Farrow GM, Rife CC, Segura JW, Zincke H. Carcinoma in situ of the bladder. Cancer. 1980;45(7 Suppl):1842–8.
71. Zincke H, Utz DC. Review of Mayo Clinic experience with carcinoma in situ. Urology. 1986; 27(3):288.
72. Melamed MR, Voutsa NG, Grabstald H. Natural history and clinical behavior of in situ carcinoma of the human urinary bladder. 1964. CA Cancer J Clin. 1993;43(6):348–70.
73. Farrow GM, Utz DC, Rife CC, Greene LF. Clinical observations on sixty-nine cases of in situ carcinoma of the urinary bladder. Cancer Res. 1977;37(8 Pt 2): 2794–8.
74. Weinstein RS, Miller 3rd AW, Pauli BU. Carcinoma in situ: comments on the pathobiology of a paradox. Urol Clin North Am. 1980;7(3):523–31.
75. Mostofi FK, Sobin LH, Torloni H. Histological typing of urinary bladder tumors: international classification of tumors. 10th ed. Geneva: WHO, editor; 1973.
76. Epstein JI. The new World Health Organization/ International Society of Urological Pathology (WHO/ISUP) classification for TA, T1 bladder

tumors: is it an improvement? Crit Rev Oncol Hematol. 2003;47(2):83–9.
77. Abel PD, Henderson D, Bennett MK, Hall RR, Williams G. Differing interpretations by pathologists of the pT category and grade of transitional cell cancer of the bladder. Br J Urol. 1988;62(4):339–42.
78. Pich A, Chiusa L, Formiconi A, Galliano D, Bortolin P, Navone R. Biologic differences between noninvasive papillary urothelial neoplasms of low malignant potential and low-grade (grade 1) papillary carcinomas of the bladder. Am J Surg Pathol. 2001; 25(12):1528–33.
79. Samaratunga H, Makarov DV, Epstein JI. Comparison of WHO/ISUP and WHO classification of noninvasive papillary urothelial neoplasms for risk of progression. Urology. 2002;60(2):315–9.
80. Bircan S, Candir O, Serel TA. Comparison of WHO 1973, WHO/ISUP 1998, WHO 1999 grade and combined scoring systems in evaluation of bladder carcinoma. Urol Int. 2004;73(3):201–8.
81. Genega EM, Kapali M, Torres-Quinones M, Huang WC, Knauss JS, Wang L-P, et al. Impact of the 1998 World Health Organization//International Society of Urological Pathology classification system for urothelial neoplasms of the kidney. Mod Pathol. 2004;18(1):11–8.
82. Gonul II, Poyraz A, Unsal C, Acar C, Alkibay T. Comparison of 1998 WHO/ISUP and 1973 WHO classifications for interobserver variability in grading of papillary urothelial neoplasms of the bladder. Pathological evaluation of 258 cases. Urol Int. 2007;78(4):338–44.
83. Burger M, Denzinger S, Wieland W-F, Stief CG, Hartmann A, Zaak D. Does the current World Health Organization classification predict the outcome better in patients with noninvasive bladder cancer of early or regular onset? BJU Int. 2008;102(2):194–7.
84. Oosterhuis JWA, Schapers RFM, Janssen-Heijnen MLG, Pauwels RPE, Newling DW, ten Kate F. Histological grading of papillary urothelial carcinoma of the bladder: prognostic value of the 1998 WHO/ISUP classification system and comparison with conventional grading systems. J Clin Pathol. 2002;55(12):900–5.
85. Yorukoglu K, Tuna B, Dikicioglu E, Duzcan E, Isisag A, Sen S, et al. Reproducibility of the 1998 World Health Organization/International Society of Urologic Pathology classification of papillary urothelial neoplasms of the urinary bladder. Virchows Arch. 2003;443(6):734–40.
86. Cheng L, Darson M, Cheville JC, Neumann RM, Zincke H, Nehra A, et al. Urothelial papilloma of the bladder. Clinical and biologic implications. Cancer. 1999;86(10):2098–101.
87. McKenney JK, Amin MB, Young RH. Urothelial (transitional cell) papilloma of the urinary bladder: a clinicopathologic study of 26 cases. Mod Pathol. 2003;16(7):623–9.
88. Holmang S, Andius P, Hedelin H, Wester K, Busch C, Johansson SL. Stage progression in Ta papillary urothelial tumors: relationship to grade, immunohistochemical expression of tumor markers, mitotic frequency and DNA ploidy. J Urol. 2001;165(4):1124–8; discussion 8–30.
89. Miyamoto H, Miller JS, Fajardo DA, Lee TK, Netto GJ, Epstein JI. Non-invasive papillary urothelial neoplasms: the 2004 WHO/ISUP classification system. Pathol Int. 2010;60(1):1–8.
90. Desai S, Lim SD, Jimenez RE, Chun T, Keane TE, McKenney JK, et al. Relationship of cytokeratin 20 and CD44 protein expression with WHO/ISUP grade in pTa and pT1 papillary urothelial neoplasia. Mod Pathol. 2000;13(12):1315–23.
91. MacLennan GT, Kirkali Z, Cheng L. Histologic grading of noninvasive papillary urothelial neoplasms. Eur Urol. 2007;51(4):889–97; discussion 97–8.
92. Murphy WM, Takezawa K, Maruniak NA. Interobserver discrepancy using the 1998 World Health Organization/International Society of Urologic Pathology classification of urothelial neoplasms: practical choices for patient care. J Urol. 2002;168(3):968–72.
93. Lamina propria microinvasion of bladder tumors, incidence on stage allocation (pTa vs pT1): recommended approach. Pathologists of the French Association of Urology Cancer Committee. World J Urol. 1993;11(3):161–4.
94. Bol MG, Baak JP, Buhr-Wildhagen S, Kruse AJ, Kjellevold KH, Janssen EA, et al. Reproducibility and prognostic variability of grade and lamina propria invasion in stages Ta, T1 urothelial carcinoma of the bladder. J Urol. 2003;169(4):1291–4.
95. Tosoni I, Wagner U, Sauter G, Egloff M, Knonagel H, Alund G, et al. Clinical significance of interobserver differences in the staging and grading of superficial bladder cancer. BJU Int. 2000;85(1):48–53.
96. Lopez-Beltran A, Cheng L. Stage pT1 bladder carcinoma: diagnostic criteria, pitfalls and prognostic significance. Pathology. 2003;35(6):484–91.
97. Jimenez RE, Keane TE, Hardy HT, Amin MB. pT1 urothelial carcinoma of the bladder: criteria for diagnosis, pitfalls, and clinical implications. Adv Anat Pathol. 2000;7(1):13–25.
98. Dhall D, Al-Ahmadie H, Olgac S. Nested variant of urothelial carcinoma. Arch Pathol Lab Med. 2007;131(11):1725–7.
99. Young RH, Zukerberg LR. Microcystic transitional cell carcinomas of the urinary bladder. A report of four cases. Am J Clin Pathol. 1991;96(5):635–9.
100. Drew PA, Furman J, Civantos F, Murphy WM. The nested variant of transitional cell carcinoma: an aggressive neoplasm with innocuous histology. Mod Pathol. 1996;9(10):989–94.
101. Younes M, Sussman J, True LD. The usefulness of the level of the muscularis mucosae in the staging of invasive transitional cell carcinoma of the urinary bladder. Cancer. 1990;66(3):543–8.
102. Holmang S, Hedelin H, Anderstrom C, Holmberg E, Johansson SL. The importance of the depth of

invasion in stage T1 bladder carcinoma: a prospective cohort study. J Urol. 1997;157(3):800–3; discussion 4.
103. Chan TY, Epstein JI. In situ adenocarcinoma of the bladder. Am J Surg Pathol. 2001;25(7):892–9.
104. Lim M, Adsay NV, Grignon D, Osunkoya AO. Urothelial carcinoma with villoglandular differentiation: a study of 14 cases. Mod Pathol. 2009;22(10):1280–6.
105. Miller JS, Epstein JI. Noninvasive urothelial carcinoma of the bladder with glandular differentiation: report of 24 cases. Am J Surg Pathol. 2009;33(8):1241–8.
106. Guo CC, Fine SW, Epstein JI. Noninvasive squamous lesions in the urinary bladder: a clinicopathologic analysis of 29 cases. Am J Surg Pathol. 2006;30(7):883–91.
107. Ahmad I, Barnetson RJ, Krishna NS. Keratinizing squamous metaplasia of the bladder: a review. Urol Int. 2008;81(3):247–51.
108. Nieder AM, Brausi M, Lamm D, O'Donnell M, Tomita K, Woo H, et al. Management of stage T1 tumors of the bladder: International Consensus Panel. Urology. 2005;66(6 Suppl 1):108–25.
109. Fujimoto N, Harada S, Terado M, Sato H, Matsumoto T. Multiple biopsies of normal-looking urothelium in patients with superficial bladder cancer: are they necessary? Int J Urol. 2003;10(12):631–5.
110. van der Meijden A, Oosterlinck W, Brausi M, Kurth KH, Sylvester R, de Balincourt C. Significance of bladder biopsies in Ta, T1 bladder tumors: a report from the EORTC Genito-Urinary Tract Cancer Cooperative Group. EORTC-GU Group Superficial Bladder Committee. Eur Urol. 1999;35(4):267–71.
111. Miladi M, Peyromaure M, Zerbib M, Saighi D, Debre B. The value of a second transurethral resection in evaluating patients with bladder tumours. Eur Urol. 2003;43(3):241–5.
112. Herr HW. The value of a second transurethral resection in evaluating patients with bladder tumors. J Urol. 1999;162(1):74–6.
113. Schwaibold HE, Sivalingam S, May F, Hartung R. The value of a second transurethral resection for T1 bladder cancer. BJU Int. 2006;97(6):1199–201.
114. Dutta SC, Smith Jr JA, Shappell SB, Coffey CS, Chang SS, Cookson MS. Clinical under staging of high risk non-muscle invasive urothelial carcinoma treated with radical cystectomy. J Urol. 2001;166(2):490–3.
115. Herr HW, Donat SM, Dalbagni G. Can restaging transurethral resection of T1 bladder cancer select patients for immediate cystectomy? J Urol. 2007;177(1):75–9; discussion 9.
116. Herr HW. Restaging transurethral resection of high risk superficial bladder cancer improves the initial response to bacillus Calmette-Guerin therapy. J Urol. 2005;174(6):2134–7.
117. Lee CT, Dunn RL, Ingold C, Montie JE, Wood Jr DP. Early-stage bladder cancer surveillance does not improve survival if high-risk patients are permitted to progress to muscle invasion. Urology. 2007;69(6):1068–72.
118. Wasco MJ, Daignault S, Zhang Y, Kunju LP, Kinnaman M, Braun T, et al. Urothelial carcinoma with divergent histologic differentiation (mixed histologic features) predicts the presence of locally advanced bladder cancer when detected at transurethral resection. Urology. 2007;70(1):69–74.
119. Kamat AM, Gee JR, Dinney CP, Grossman HB, Swanson DA, Millikan RE, et al. The case for early cystectomy in the treatment of non-muscle invasive micropapillary bladder carcinoma. J Urol. 2006;175(3 Pt 1):881–5.
120. Lin O, Cardillo M, Dalbagni G, Linkov I, Hutchinson B, Reuter VE. Nested variant of urothelial carcinoma: a clinicopathologic and immunohistochemical study of 12 cases. Mod Pathol. 2003;16(12):1289–98.
121. Dahm P, Gschwend JE. Malignant non-urothelial neoplasms of the urinary bladder: a review. Eur Urol. 2003;44(6):672–81.
122. Rogers CG, Palapattu GS, Shariat SF, Karakiewicz PI, Bastian PJ, Lotan Y, et al. Clinical outcomes following radical cystectomy for primary nontransitional cell carcinoma of the bladder compared to transitional cell carcinoma of the bladder. J Urol. 2006;175(6):2048–53; discussion 53.
123. Nigwekar P, Tamboli P, Amin MB, Osunkoya AO, Ben-Dor D, Amin MB. Plasmacytoid urothelial carcinoma: detailed analysis of morphology with clinicopathologic correlation in 17 cases. Am J Surg Pathol. 2009;33(3):417–24.
124. Siefker-Radtke AO, Dinney CP, Abrahams NA, Moran C, Shen Y, Pisters LL, et al. Evidence supporting preoperative chemotherapy for small cell carcinoma of the bladder: a retrospective review of the MD. Anderson cancer experience. J Urol. 2004;172(2):481–4.
125. Siefker-Radtke AO, Kamat AM, Grossman HB, Williams DL, Qiao W, Thall PF, et al. Phase II clinical trial of neoadjuvant alternating doublet chemotherapy with ifosfamide/doxorubicin and etoposide/cisplatin in small-cell urothelial cancer. J Clin Oncol. 2009;27(16):2592–7.
126. Bohle A, Leyh H, Frei C, Kuhn M, Tschada R, Pottek T, et al. Single postoperative instillation of gemcitabine in patients with non-muscle-invasive transitional cell carcinoma of the bladder: a randomised, double-blind, placebo-controlled phase III multicentre study. Eur Urol. 2009;56(3):495–503.
127. Lamm DL, Riggs DR, Traynelis CL, Nseyo UO. Apparent failure of current intravesical chemotherapy prophylaxis to influence the long-term course of superficial transitional cell carcinoma of the bladder. J Urol. 1995;153(5):1444–50.
128. O'Donnell MA. Practical applications of intravesical chemotherapy and immunotherapy in high-risk patients with superficial bladder cancer. Urol Clin North Am. 2005;32(2):121–31.

129. Portillo J, Martin B, Hernandez R, Correas M, Gutierrez J, Del Valle J, et al. Results at 43 months' follow-up of a double-blind, randomized, prospective clinical trial using intravesical interferon alpha-2b in the prophylaxis of stage pT1 transitional cell carcinoma of the bladder. Urology. 1997;49(2):187–90.
130. Sylvester RJ, Oosterlinck W, van der Meijden AP. A single immediate postoperative instillation of chemotherapy decreases the risk of recurrence in patients with stage Ta T1 bladder cancer: a meta-analysis of published results of randomized clinical trials. J Urol. 2004;171(6 Pt 1):2186–90, quiz 435.
131. Bohle A, Jocham D, Bock PR. Intravesical bacillus Calmette-Guerin versus mitomycin C for superficial bladder cancer: a formal meta-analysis of comparative studies on recurrence and toxicity. J Urol. 2003;169(1):90–5.
132. Coplen DE, Marcus MD, Myers JA, Ratliff TL, Catalona WJ. Long-term followup of patients treated with 1 or 2, 6-week courses of intravesical bacillus Calmette-Guerin: analysis of possible predictors of response free of tumor. J Urol. 1990;144(3):652–7.
133. Hudson MA, Herr HW. Carcinoma in situ of the bladder. J Urol. 1995;153(3 Pt 1):564–72.
134. Herr HW, Wartinger DD, Fair WR, Oettgen HF. Bacillus Calmette-Guerin therapy for superficial bladder cancer: a 10-year followup. J Urol. 1992;147(4):1020–3.
135. Han RF, Pan JG. Can intravesical bacillus Calmette-Guerin reduce recurrence in patients with superficial bladder cancer? A meta-analysis of randomized trials. Urology. 2006;67(6):1216–23.
136. Lamm DL, Blumenstein BA, Crissman JD, Montie JE, Gottesman JE, Lowe BA, et al. Maintenance bacillus Calmette-Guerin immunotherapy for recurrent TA, T1 and carcinoma in situ transitional cell carcinoma of the bladder: a randomized Southwest Oncology Group Study. J Urol. 2000;163(4):1124–9.
137. Bohle A, Bock PR. Intravesical bacille Calmette-Guerin versus mitomycin C in superficial bladder cancer: formal meta-analysis of comparative studies on tumor progression. Urology. 2004;63(4):682–6; discussion 6–7.
138. Belldegrun AS, Franklin JR, O'Donnell MA, Gomella LG, Klein E, Neri R, et al. Superficial bladder cancer: the role of interferon-alpha. J Urol. 1998;159(6):1793–801.
139. Joudi FN, Smith BJ, O'Donnell MA. Final results from a national multicenter phase II trial of combination bacillus Calmette-Guerin plus interferon alpha-2B for reducing recurrence of superficial bladder cancer. Urol Oncol. 2006;24(4):344–8.
140. Lamm DL. Bacillus Calmette-Guerin immunotherapy of superficial bladder cancer. Nippon Hinyokika Gakkai Zasshi. 1995;86(1):9–10.
141. Lamm DL. Efficacy and safety of bacille Calmette-Guerin immunotherapy in superficial bladder cancer. Clin Infect Dis. 2000;31 Suppl 3:S86–90.
142. Lamm DL, Blumenstein BA, David Crawford E, Crissman JD, Lowe BA, Smith JA, et al. Randomized intergroup comparison of bacillus calmette-guerin immunotherapy and mitomycin C chemotherapy prophylaxis in superficial transitional cell carcinoma of the bladder a southwest oncology group study. Urol Oncol. 1995;1(3):119–26.
143. van der Meijden AP, Sylvester RJ, Oosterlinck W, Hoeltl W, Bono AV, EG-UTC.Group. Maintenance Bacillus Calmette-Guerin for Ta T1 bladder tumors is not associated with increased toxicity: results from a European Organisation for Research and Treatment of Cancer Genito-Urinary Group Phase III Trial. Eur Urol. 2003;44(4):429–34.
144. Martínez-Piñeiro JA, Flores N, Isorna S, Solsona E, Sebastián JL, Pertusa C, et al. Long-term follow-up of a randomized prospective trial comparing a standard 81 mg dose of intravesical bacille Calmette-Guérin with a reduced dose of 27 mg in superficial bladder cancer. BJU Int. 2002;89(7):671–80.
145. Ojea A, Nogueira JL, Solsona E, Flores N, Gómez JMF, Molina JR, et al. A multicentre, randomised prospective trial comparing three intravesical adjuvant therapies for intermediate-risk superficial bladder cancer: low-dose bacillus Calmette-Guerin (27 mg) versus very low-dose bacillus Calmette-Guerin (13.5 mg) versus mitomycin C. Eur Urol. 2007;52(5):1398–406.
146. Bassi P, Spinadin R, Carando R, Balta G, Pagano F. Modified induction course: a solution to side-effects? Eur Urol. 2000;37 Suppl 1:31–2.
147. Shelley MD, Wilt TJ, Court J, Coles B, Kynaston H, Mason MD. Intravesical bacillus Calmette-Guerin is superior to mitomycin C in reducing tumour recurrence in high-risk superficial bladder cancer: a meta-analysis of randomized trials. BJU Int. 2004;93(4):485–90.
148. Sylvester RJ, van der Meijden AP, Witjes JA, Kurth K. Bacillus calmette-guerin versus chemotherapy for the intravesical treatment of patients with carcinoma in situ of the bladder: a meta-analysis of the published results of randomized clinical trials. J Urol. 2005;174(1):86–91; discussion–2.
149. Sylvester RJ, van der Meijden AP, Oosterlinck W, Witjes JA, Bouffioux C, Denis L, et al. Predicting recurrence and progression in individual patients with stage Ta T1 bladder cancer using EORTC risk tables: a combined analysis of 2596 patients from seven EORTC trials. Eur Urol. 2006;49(3):466–5; discussion 75–7.
150. Huang GJ, Hamilton AS, Lo M, Stein JP, Penson DF. Predictors of intravesical therapy for non-muscle invasive bladder cancer: results from the surveillance, epidemiology and end results program 2003 patterns of care project. J Urol. 2008;180(2):520–4; discussion 4.
151. Babjuk M, Oosterlinck W, Sylvester R, Kaasinen E, Bohle A, Palou-Redorta J. EAU guidelines on

non-muscle-invasive urothelial carcinoma of the bladder. Eur Urol. 2008;54(2):303–14.
152. Thompson Jr RA, Campbell Jr EW, Kramer HC, Jacobs SC, Naslund MJ. Late invasive recurrence despite long-term surveillance for superficial bladder cancer. J Urol. 1993;149(5):1010–1.
153. Holmang S, Johansson SL. Stage Ta-T1 bladder cancer: the relationship between findings at first followup cystoscopy and subsequent recurrence and progression. J Urol. 2002;167(4):1634–7.
154. Holmang S, Hedelin H, Anderstrom C, Johansson SL. The relationship among multiple recurrences, progression and prognosis of patients with stages Ta and T1 transitional cell cancer of the bladder followed for at least 20 years. J Urol. 1995;153(6):1823–6; discussion 6–7.
155. Soloway MS, Bruck DS, Kim SS. Expectant management of small, recurrent, noninvasive papillary bladder tumors. J Urol. 2003;170(2 Pt 1):438–41.
156. Donat SM, North A, Dalbagni G, Herr HW. Efficacy of office fulguration for recurrent low grade papillary bladder tumors less than 0.5 cm. J Urol. 2004;171(2 Pt 1):636–9.
157. Herr HW, Dalbagni G. Defining bacillus Calmette-Guerin refractory superficial bladder tumors. J Urol. 2003;169(5):1706–8.
158. Witjes JA. Management of BCG failures in superficial bladder cancer: a review. Eur Urol. 2006;49(5): 790–7.
159. Malmstrom PU, Wijkstrom H, Lundholm C, Wester K, Busch C, Norlen BJ. 5-year followup of a randomized prospective study comparing mitomycin C and bacillus Calmette-Guerin in patients with superficial bladder carcinoma. Swedish-Norwegian Bladder Cancer Study Group. J Urol. 1999;161(4): 1124–7.
160. Steinberg G, Bahnson R, Brosman S, Middleton R, Wajsman Z, Wehle M. Efficacy and safety of valrubicin for the treatment of Bacillus Calmette-Guerin refractory carcinoma in situ of the bladder. The Valrubicin Study Group. J Urol. 2000;163(3): 761–7.
161. O'Donnell MA, Boehle A. Treatment options for BCG failures. World J Urol. 2006;24(5):481–7.
162. Dalbagni G, Russo P, Bochner B, Ben-Porat L, Sheinfeld J, Sogani P, et al. Phase II trial of intravesical gemcitabine in bacille Calmette-Guerin-refractory transitional cell carcinoma of the bladder. J Clin Oncol. 2006;24(18):2729–34.
163. Davis JW, Sheth SI, Doviak MJ, Schellhammer PF. Superficial bladder carcinoma treated with bacillus Calmette-Guerin: progression-free and disease specific survival with minimum 10-year followup. J Urol. 2002;167(2 Pt 1):494–500; discussion 1.
164. Herr HW. Timing of cystectomy for superficial bladder tumors. Urol Oncol. 2000;5(4):162–5.
165. Herr HW, Sogani PC. Does early cystectomy improve the survival of patients with high risk superficial bladder tumors? J Urol. 2001;166(4): 1296–9.
166. Huguet J, Crego M, Sabate S, Salvador J, Palou J, Villavicencio H. Cystectomy in patients with high risk superficial bladder tumors who fail intravesical BCG therapy: pre-cystectomy prostate involvement as a prognostic factor. Eur Urol. 2005;48(1):53–9; discussion 9.
167. Cookson MS, Herr HW, Zhang ZF, Soloway S, Sogani PC, Fair WR. The treated natural history of high risk superficial bladder cancer: 15-year outcome. J Urol. 1997;158(1):62–7.
168. Leblanc B, Duclos AJ, Benard F, Cote J, Valiquette L, Paquin JM, et al. Long-term followup of initial Ta grade 1 transitional cell carcinoma of the bladder. J Urol. 1999;162(6):1946–50.
169. Cheng L, Neumann RM, Bostwick DG. Papillary urothelial neoplasms of low malignant potential. Clinical and biologic implications. Cancer. 1999;86(10):2102–8.
170. Koss LG. Bladder cancer from a perspective of 40 years. J Cell Biochem Suppl. 1992;16I:23–9.
171. Dreicer R, Li H, Stein M, DiPaola R, Eleff M, Roth BJ, et al. Phase 2 trial of sorafenib in patients with advanced urothelial cancer: a trial of the Eastern Cooperative Oncology Group. Cancer. 2009;115(18):4090–5.

Muscle-Invasive Urothelial Carcinoma: Conventional and Variant Subtypes

7

Jennifer M. Taylor, Bernard Bochner, Mahul B. Amin, and Donna E. Hansel

Introduction

Urothelial carcinoma can be subdivided primarily into conventional and nonconventional subtypes. Conventional urothelial carcinoma comprises the vast majority (>90%) of all forms of urinary tract cancer and arises from either papillary or flat in situ lesions. In contrast, nonconventional carcinoma of the urinary tract includes squamous cell carcinoma, adenocarcinoma, and small cell carcinoma, which are discussed in individual chapters within the text.

Urothelial carcinoma also presents as a variety of "variants" [1]. These variants are generally considered to represent a derivative of conventional urothelial carcinoma. Histologic variants comprise up to 40% of carcinomas of the renal pelvis [2], although exact numbers from the bladder are not available. Aside from the interesting pathologic features associated with these variants, differences in prognosis and treatment are becoming apparent. A listing of currently recognized variants is presented in Table 7.1. An overview of all variants will be provided, with the exception of micropapillary carcinoma, which is discussed in a separate chapter.

In general, variant morphology is treated in a similar fashion to conventional urothelial carcinoma, with few exceptions—micropapillary carcinoma being the most critical of these. Although variants may occur in pure form, they are often admixed with conventional urothelial carcinoma. The importance in recognizing these variants is highlighted in small biopsy specimens, in which conventional urothelial carcinoma may be lacking and the differential diagnosis may include either benign entities or carcinomas arising from other sites.

Clinical Presentation

Approximately 20–30% of newly diagnosed patients present with muscle-invasive or advanced disease while the majority of new tumors are nonmuscle-invasive. Although in general the clinical behavior of noninvasive disease proceeds along a more benign course, up to a third of

J.M. Taylor (✉)
University of Pittsburgh Medical Center, 300 Halket St, Pittsburgh, PA 15232, USA
e-mail: taylorjm2@upmc.edu

B. Bochner
Department of Surgery, Memorial Sloan Kettering Cancer Center, Kimmel Center for Prostate and Urologic Cancers, 353 E. 68th Street, New York, NY 10065, USA
e-mail: bochnerb@mskcc.org

M.B. Amin
Department of Pathology and Laboratory Medicine, Cedars-Sinai Medical Center, 8700 Beverly Boulevard, South Tower, Suite 8709, Los Angeles, CA 90048, USA
e-mail: mahul.amin@cshs.org

D.E. Hansel
Department of Pathology, Cleveland Clinic, 9500 Euclid Avenue Desk L25, Cleveland, OH 44195, USA
e-mail: Hanseld@ccf.org

D.E. Hansel et al. (eds.), *The Urinary Tract: A Comprehensive Guide to Patient Diagnosis and Management*, DOI 10.1007/978-1-4614-5320-8_7, © Springer Science+Business Media New York 2012

Table 7.1 Urothelial carcinoma variants

Urothelial carcinoma variants
Urothelial carcinoma with squamous and/or glandular differentiation ("divergent differentiation")
Benign-appearing features
Nested
Small tubular/glandular
Microcystic
Carcinoma with distinguishing cytoplasmic features
Clear cell/glycogen rich
Plasmacytoid
Rhabdoid
Lipoid rich
Micropapillary
Urothelial carcinoma with trophoblastic differentiation
Lymphoepithelioma-like carcinoma
Sarcomatoid
Carcinoma with stromal-associated features
Pseudosarcomatous stroma
Stromal osseous/cartilaginous metaplasia
Osteoclast-type giant cells
Undifferentiated/poorly differentiated carcinoma
Osteoclast-rich undifferentiated carcinoma
Giant cell undifferentiated carcinoma

patients with nonmuscle-invasive disease progress to muscle-invasive disease [3, 4].

The most common presenting symptom for patients with urothelial carcinoma is hematuria. This may be microscopic or gross hematuria, and up to 90–95% of patients with bladder cancer have detectable hematuria, particularly when tested serially. Hematuria tends to be painless and intermittent, prompting many patients to ignore their initial symptoms. The bleeding may stop for weeks before returning, which may then lead to patients to seek medical attention. Most patients who report an episode of gross hematuria will be referred to a urologist; however, fewer than 40% of people found to have microhematuria by dipstick evaluation are referred for further workup [5, 6]. Microscopic hematuria is present in up to 15% of the general population; however, the incidence of bladder cancer overall is less than 1%. There is often a delay in referral for a definitive evaluation as initial treatment for alternative diagnoses, such as cystitis or benign prostatic hyperplasia. This delay may lead to more extensive disease in patients with high-risk disease. Additional presenting symptoms include irritative voiding symptoms, including frequency and urgency, particularly when concomitant carcinoma in situ (CIS) is present. Tumors may present with voiding obstruction particularly if lesions are located at the bladder neck or urethra. Muscle-invasive tumors may compress or obstruct a ureter, leading to hydronephrosis and flank pain. Many times, slowly developing obstruction can develop without symptoms. Distant disease can present with bone pain, hemoptysis, or jaundice.

Upon referral to urology, the typical workup includes labs such as complete blood count, metabolic panel (including creatinine) and coagulation studies, urine cytology, cystoscopy, and axial imaging (computed tomography (CT) or magnetic resonance imaging (MRI)) to evaluate the upper tracts. The presence of tumor in the bladder then will prompt surgical management with transurethral resection of bladder tumor, for histologic diagnosis, including depth of invasion. If muscle is not present in the initial resection specimen, re-resection is indicated to conclusively diagnose muscle-invasion. The diagnosis of muscle-invasive disease then initiates planning for definitive therapy, as described as follows.

Pathology

Conventional Urothelial Carcinoma

Invasive urothelial carcinoma generally arises from well-recognized precursor lesions, including high-grade papillary urothelial carcinoma or flat urothelial carcinoma in situ. Urothelial carcinoma can vary in appearance, but is generally characterized by nests or sheets of atypical urothelial cells surrounded by retraction artifact (Fig. 7.1). Occasionally, individual cells may be present. Carcinoma cells are usually medium to large in size and the cytoplasm is often pale to eosinophilic in color. Nuclear atypia varies from minimal to marked, with some tumors displaying prominent pleomorphism. Nucleoli are generally rare. Angiolymphatic invasion may be present in a subset of tumors, although it is often challenging

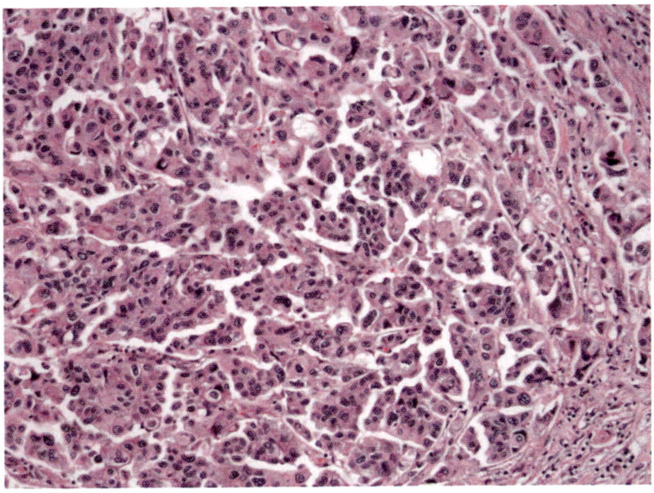

Fig. 7.1 Conventional urothelial carcinoma

Table 7.2 Immunohistochemical markers in conventional urothelial carcinoma

Marker	Function	Localization	Urothelial carcinoma positive (%)
p63	p53 homologue	Nucleus	70–80
High-molecular-weight cytokeratin	Intermediate keratin filament	Cytoplasm	90–100
Cytokeratin 7	Intermediate filament protein	Cytoplasm	100
Cytokeratin 20	Type I keratin	Cytoplasm	50–60
Thrombomodulin	Glycoprotein	Cytoplasm	80–90
Uroplakin III	Glycoprotein	Cytoplasm	25–40
GATA-3	T-cell enhancer binding protein	Nuclear	70–80
S100-P	Calcium-binding protein	Cytoplasm and/or nucleus	70–80
p53	Tumor suppressor	Nucleus (mutated)	80–90

to distinguish this finding from retraction artifact, unless large vessels or the periphery of the lesion is involved.

In diagnostically challenging cases, immunohistochemical stains may be used to determine the urothelial nature of the lesion, especially in metastatic sites (Table 7.2). The most common immunohistochemical stains include p63, high-molecular-weight cytokeratin, cytokeratin 7, cytokeratin 20, uroplakin III, p53, and thrombomodulin. Recent work suggests that additional markers including GATA-3 and S100-P may also prove beneficial in determining site of origin [7]. However, no panel of markers appears to be entirely specific and thus metastatic lesions often are presented in light of a differential diagnosis.

Urothelial Carcinoma with Squamous and/or Glandular Differentiation ("Divergent Differentiation")

The most common variant forms of urothelial carcinoma are those with glandular and/or squamous differentiation. The reported frequency of these forms of urothelial carcinoma varies, but approximately 60% of urothelial carcinomas demonstrate squamous differentiation and up to 10% of carcinomas demonstrate glandular differentiation [8].

Squamous differentiation consists of recognizable squamous morphology—including eosinophilic, glassy cytoplasm, keratin formation, and intercellular bridges (Fig. 7.2a).

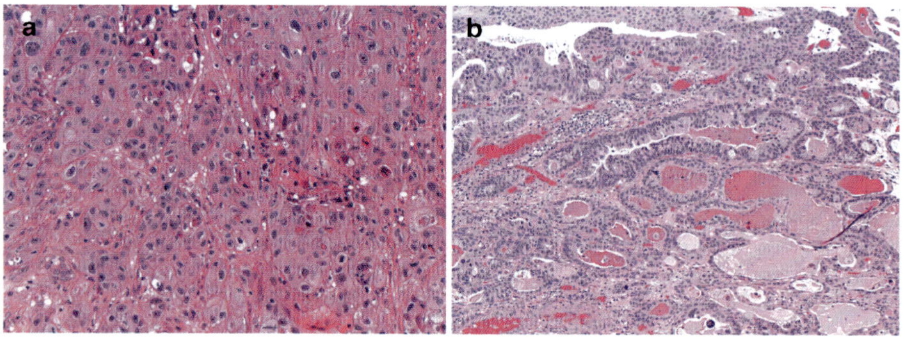

Fig. 7.2 Urothelial carcinoma with divergent differentiation may show (**a**) squamous differentiation, (**b**) glandular differentiation, or both

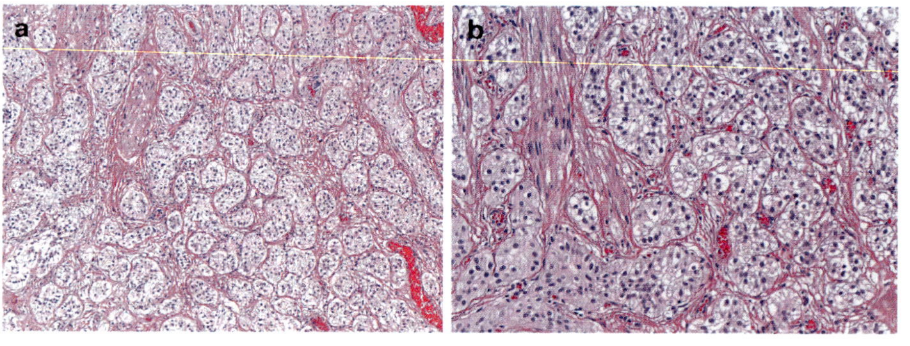

Fig. 7.3 (**a**, **b**)Nested urothelial carcinoma

Glandular differentiation may have a spectrum of appearances, including colonic-type glands, glands with abundant mucin production or signet ring cells (Fig. 7.2b). Historically, carcinomas with glandular and/or squamous differentiation (also termed "divergent" differentiation) have been considered to have worse outcomes, relative to conventional urothelial carcinoma [9–12]. However, these carcinomas appear to present at a higher stage and stage-for-stage comparisons suggest no difference in outcomes. No studies have specifically evaluated the role of histological variants in the response to adjuvant therapy, although response to neoadjuvant therapy appears to be impacted [13]. Specifically, patients with squamous or glandular differentiation appear to have improved survival following neoadjuvant therapy with methotrexate, vinblastine, doxorubicin, and cisplatin (MVAC).

Nested Variant

Less than 100 cases of nested urothelial carcinoma have been reported [14–19]. This variant represents one of the most diagnostically challenging variants—the carcinoma is defined by nests of extraordinarily bland urothelial cells that closely mirror normal urothelium (Fig. 7.3a). However, irregular nests and haphazard growth can occasionally provide clues as to the diagnosis. On superficial biopsy, this entity is especially treacherous, as it can closely mimic von Brunn nest proliferations (Fig. 7.3b). Deeper specimens will often reveal an infiltrative pattern with occasional invasion into the underlying muscularis propria. Cellular atypia is also often recognized in this deeper portion of the lesion. Immunohistochemical analysis reveals similar patterns to conventional urothelial carcinoma,

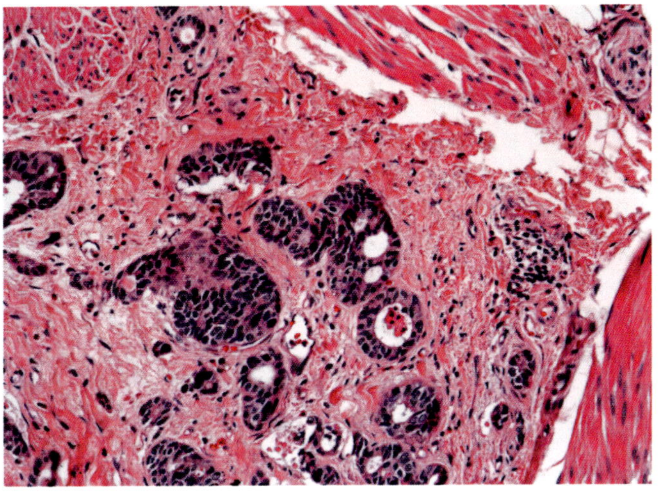

Fig. 7.4 Urothelial carcinoma with small tubules

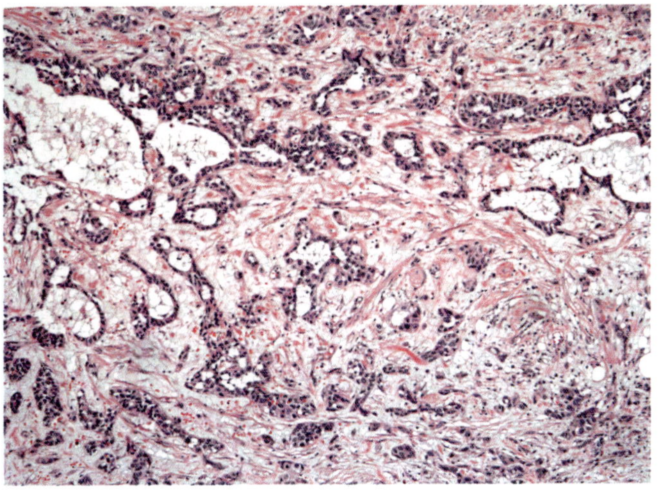

Fig. 7.5 Microcystic urothelial carcinoma

including strong nuclear p53 staining. Despite the small number of reported cases, this variant appears to carry a poor prognosis, with progressive disease and metastases occurring frequently [14–19]. In light of this, early diagnosis and caution on superficial biopsies by the pathologist is especially important.

Small Tubular/Glandular Variant

This variant of urothelial carcinoma consists primarily of small- to medium-sized tubules lined by attenuated urothelial cells with minimal atypia (Fig. 7.4). This variant is highly invasive and often presents at a high stage. Diagnostic challenges abound on superficial biopsy and may potentially contribute to the poor outcomes associated with this variant [20, 21]. The differential diagnosis includes benign entities such as nephrogenic adenoma and cystitis cystica.

Microcystic Variant

Less than 20 cases of this variant have been reported [22–24]. Comprised of small cystically dilated tubules, the microcystic variant is also diagnostically challenging and can mimic cystitis cystica (Fig. 7.5). Evidence of its malignant

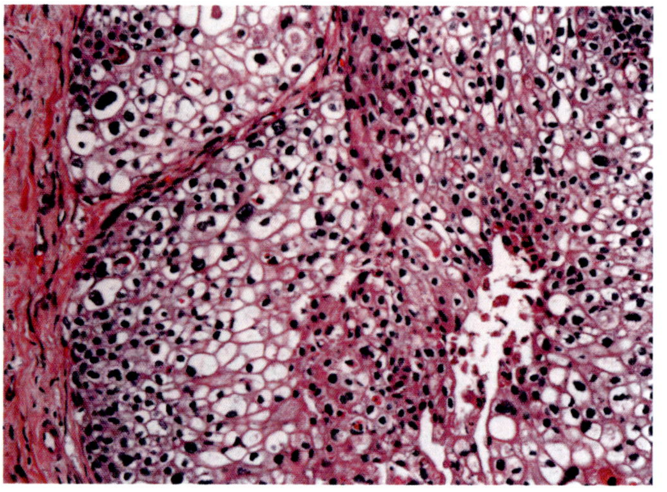

Fig. 7.6 Clear cell/glycogen-rich variant (image courtesy of Dr. Jonathan Epstein, Johns Hopkins Hospital)

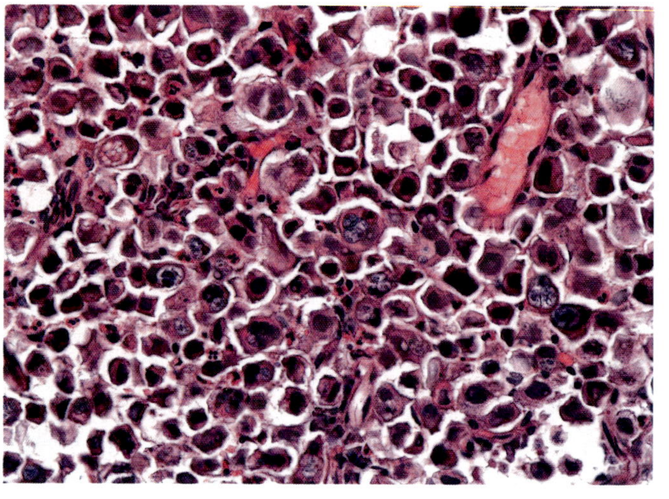

Fig. 7.7 Urothelial carcinoma with plasmacytoid differentiation

nature is reflected in the haphazard, infiltrative pattern of the tubules and the variation in tubules size. Additional histologic features include a urothelial and glandular lining of the tubules, which may be flattened, as well as secretions that may become inspissated and appear targetoid or calcified. In general, outcomes are comparable to conventional urothelial carcinoma.

Clear Cell/Glycogen-Rich Variant

This variant has been primarily described in case reports and is characterized by a combination of morphologic patterns that include solid, papillary, or tubulocystic architecture [25–29]. Defining features include glycogen-rich, clear cytoplasm and high-grade cytologic features (Fig. 7.6), which raises the differential diagnosis of metastatic clear cell renal cell carcinoma and clear cell adenocarcinoma. Due to the low number of reported cases, no consensus regarding outcomes can be made.

Plasmacytoid Variant

The plasmacytoid variant demonstrates discohesive, single cells—which mimic plasma cells—within a loose, myxoid stroma (Fig. 7.7) [30–42].

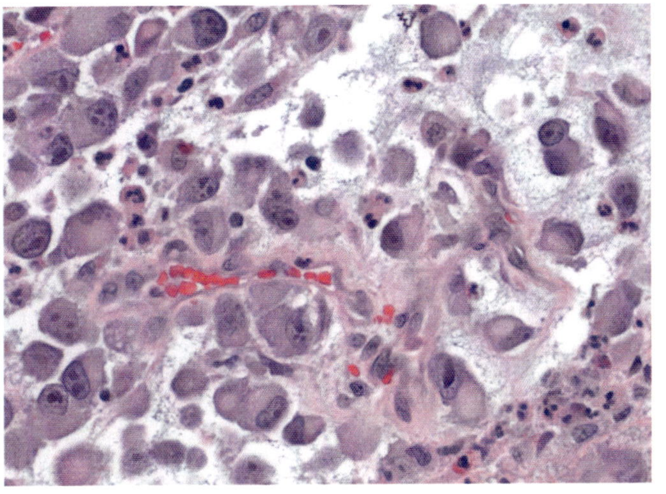

Fig. 7.8 Urothelial carcinoma with rhabdoid differentiation (image courtesy of Dr. Jonathan Epstein, Johns Hopkins Hospital)

High-grade nuclear features are common and raise the differential of lymphoma, plasmacytoma, gastric carcinoma, lobular breast cancer, malignant melanoma, and rhabdomyosarcoma, among others. The diagnosis of carcinoma is made by immunohistochemistry for cytokeratin in combination with immunostains of exclusion for other entities. As CD138—a plasma cell marker—may be positive in this variant, this stain should not be used in isolation. Most patients with this diagnosis present at an advanced stage, often with metastases.

Rhabdoid Variant

This variant is defined by large, discohesive cells with prominent cell borders and large vesicular nuclei (Fig. 7.8) [43, 44]. Eosinophilic cytoplasmic inclusions are frequently identified. To distinguish these variant carcinomas from true extrarenal rhabdoid tumors (which generally occur in the pediatric population), additional analysis of the INI1 gene should be performed. As fewer than ten cases have been reported in the literature, outcome data are sparse.

Lymphoepithelioma-Like Carcinoma

This variant derives its name from its histologic similarity to lymphoepithelioma of the upper aerodigestive tract. In contrast to this entity, however, lymphoepithelioma-like carcinoma (LELC) is not associated with Epstein Barr virus (EBV) [45, 46]. Fewer than 75 cases of this entity have been reported in the literature [45–51]. The epithelial component of this tumor demonstrates syncytial-like growth, with cells containing large, vesicular nuclei and prominent nucleoli (Fig. 7.9). This tumor is associated with a prominent lymphoid infiltrate that primarily consists of nonclonal B and T cells. Some studies have suggested that LELC in pure form is exquisitely sensitive to chemotherapy as a primary therapy [48, 50]. Carcinomas with a predominant LELC component appear to have a more favorable prognosis than urothelial carcinoma. For lesions that contain an admixture of urothelial carcinoma and LELC, the outcomes are primarily associated with the pathologic stage of urothelial carcinoma. LELC treated by cystectomy showed a 5-year actuarial survival rate of 59%, similar to that of conventional, muscle-invasive urothelial carcinoma [46].

Lipoid Rich Variant

This variant derives its name from the large, multivacuolated carcinoma cells that contain clear cytoplasm and, as such, resemble lipoblasts (Fig. 7.10) [52]. However, in contrast to true

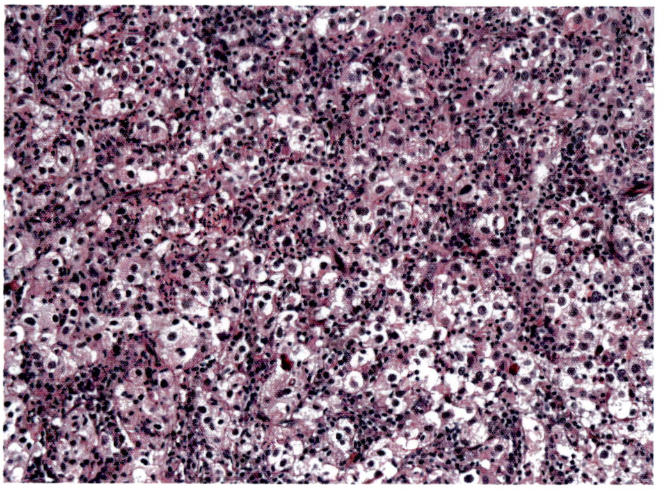

Fig. 7.9 Lymphoepithelioma-like carcinoma

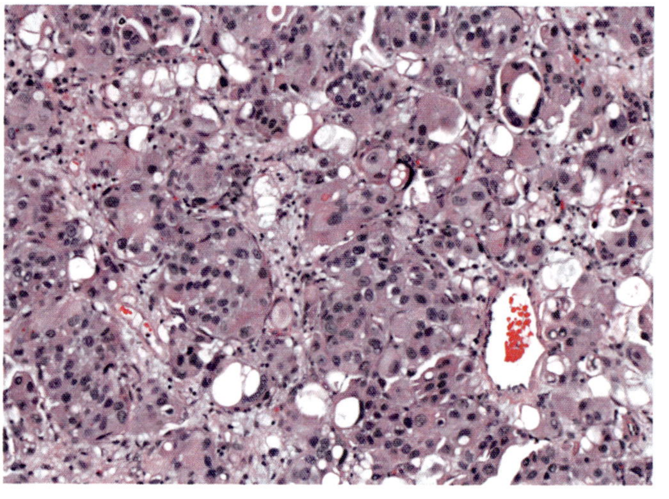

Fig. 7.10 Urothelial carcinoma with lipoid differentiation

lipoblasts, true lipid is lacking by special stains and the cells are S100 negative, hence "lipoid" variant [53]. This variant is generally not found in pure form, but may comprise up to 50% of an invasive urothelial carcinoma. The outcomes associated with this variant are unknown due to the low number of cases reported in the literature (<10).

Urothelial Carcinoma with Trophoblastic Differentiation

The majority of cases of this variant consist of invasive high-grade urothelial carcinoma admixed with trophoblastic cells (Fig. 7.11a) [54–58]. In general, this variant spans a spectrum—from cases with few trophoblastic cells to those with distinct foci of choriocarcinomatous differentiation to rare cases that resemble true choriocarcinoma. Also included in this category is otherwise conventional urothelial carcinoma with beta-HCG immunoreactivity (Fig. 7.11b), which may include up to 33% of urothelial carcinomas [30]. A subset of these lesions can demonstrate increased human chorionic gonadotropin secretion and may be associated with gynecomastia [54–58]. The presence of syncytiotrophoblasts is associated

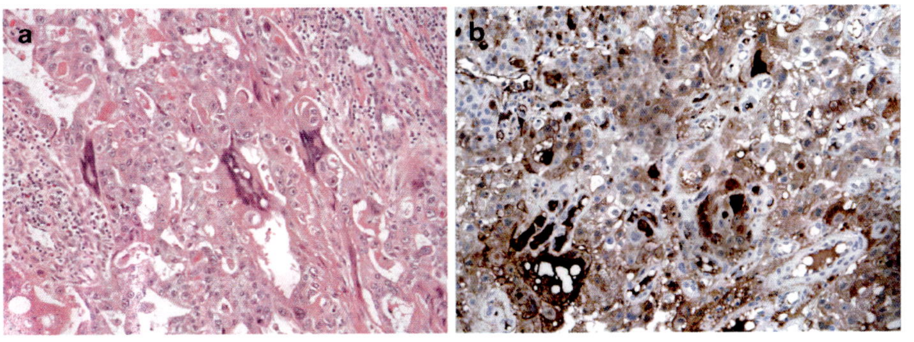

Fig. 7.11 Urothelial carcinoma with trophoblastic differentiation showing (**a**) prominent syncytiotrophoblastic cells and (**b**) beta-HCG immunoreactivity

Fig. 7.12 Sarcomatoid urothelial carcinoma

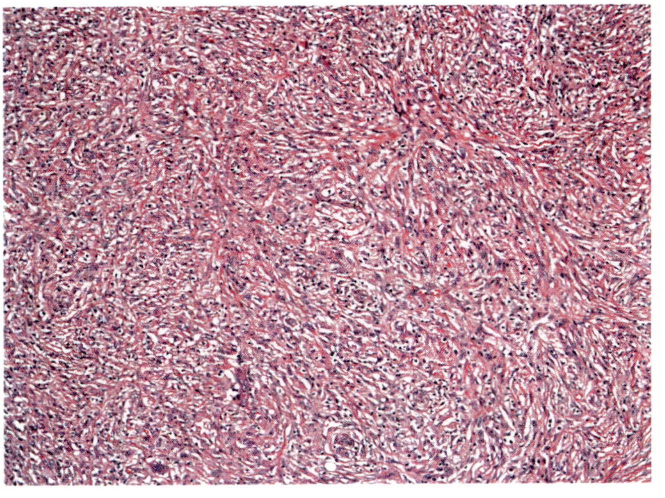

with poor outcomes, with the majority of patients progressing to death within 1 year of diagnosis.

Sarcomatoid Carcinoma ("Carcinosarcoma")

Sarcomatoid carcinoma comprises <1% of all bladder cancers and is defined by its spindled morphology that may readily mimic a sarcoma under light microscopy (Fig. 7.12) [59–68]. Risk factors for this variant include external beam radiation for prostate cancer and intravescial cyclophosphamide treatment [69]. Sarcomatoid carcinoma (or differentiation) may occur in conjunction with any form of bladder cancer; often, residual background cancer may be identified, although the sarcomatoid component may ultimately overrun the entire lesion. Molecular analyses have demonstrated the clonal relationship between sarcomatoid carcinoma and background bladder cancer, supporting the epithelial derivation of the sarcomatoid component [61, 70]. Heterologous elements such as osteosarcoma, chondrosarcoma, rhabdomyosarcoma, and other sarcoma histologies may be present. Sarcomatoid carcinoma is often positive for pancytokeratin, and it has been suggested that a panel of immunomarkers that include pancytokeratin, smooth muscle actin, desmin, Alk-1, p63, and high-molecular-weight cytokeratin may differentiate these lesions from true sarcomas [71].

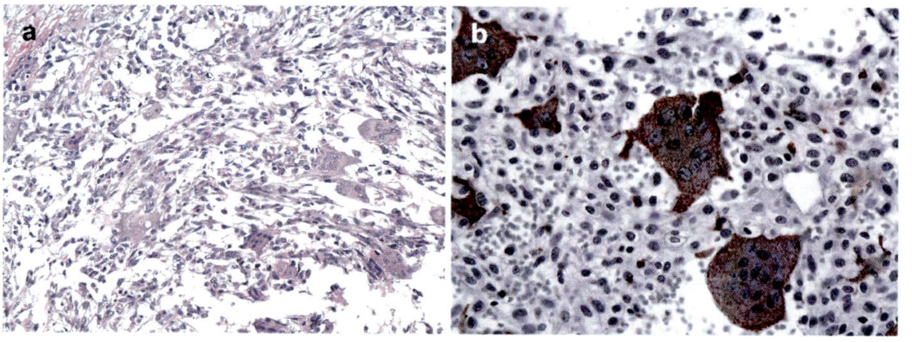

Fig. 7.13 Osteoclast-rich undifferentiated carcinoma showing (**a**) prominent multinucleated cells and (**b**) CD68 immunoreactivity

Fig. 7.14 Giant cell undifferentiated urothelial carcinoma

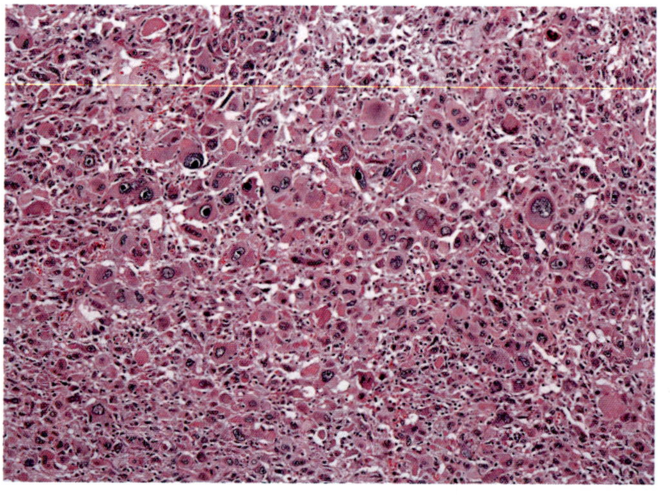

Most sarcomatoid carcinomas present at high stage and are often associated with lymph node and distant metastases. Prognosis is poor, with 70% of patients dying within 2 years of diagnosis [5, 59–74].

Osteoclast-Rich Undifferentiated Carcinoma

This lesion is defined by a prominent stromal reaction to the invasive carcinoma with occasional large atypical mesenchymal cells that may appear osteoclastic or undifferentiated in nature [75–77]. Fewer than 20 cases of osteoclast-rich undifferentiated bladder carcinoma have been reported [78, 79]. These lesions typically contain three components: (1) osteoclast-like giant cells positive for immunomarkers CD68, CD51, and CD54 (Fig. 7.13a, b); (2) mononuclear cells that show reactivity for epithelial markers; and (3) otherwise recognizable urothelial carcinoma. These carcinomas are considered high-grade, aggressive cancers. In the largest series of 6 cases, 4 out of 5 patients with this diagnosis died of disease [79]. Similar results have been identified in the remainder of published cases, with metastatic spread common.

Giant Cell Undifferentiated Carcinoma

In contrast to other forms of bladder cancer with large "giant" cells, this variant is characterized by an abundance of pleomorphic, anaplastic giant cells that are loosely cohesive and may be multinucleated (Fig. 7.14) [80–82]. To date, studies on outcomes are limited, but no significant difference in outcomes between this variant and conventional urothelial carcinoma has been described.

Surgical Management

Radical Cystectomy

The mainstay of therapy for invasive, nonmetastatic bladder cancer is radical cystectomy (RC) with a thorough pelvic lymph node dissection (PLND). Radical surgical techniques were developed based on an understanding of the natural history of the progressive pathways of invasive bladder cancer, which include local extension through the bladder wall into the perivesical tissues and subsequent regional dissemination. Resection of these tissues to include the regional pelvic lymphatics provides a potential curative treatment for those patients without distant spread. Radical cystectomy is the treatment of choice for the majority of organ-confined, locally invasive tumors, but select cases of nonmuscle-invasive cancers, regionally metastatic lesions, and even some select advanced tumors may also be optimally managed with radical cystectomy [81–89].

Surgical Resection

Radical cystectomy is defined as removal of the bladder and surrounding structures and must be combined with a regional lymphadenectomy. In men, this entails the en bloc removal of the bladder, urachus, prostate, and seminal vesicles. In women, completion of an anterior exenteration with removal of the bladder, uterus, fallopian tubes, ovaries, and anterior vaginal wall is completed. A thorough pelvic lymph node dissection should be performed in men and women with invasive bladder cancer undergoing either procedure.

Perioperative systemic chemotherapy plays a role in the overall management of patients with invasive bladder cancer undergoing radical cystectomy but does not alter the surgical approach. Perioperative radiation therapy, however, may change the surgical approach particularly with respect to the extent of the pelvic lymph node dissection. Patients that have previously received definitive pelvic radiation for either bladder cancer or another pelvic malignancy are likely to have developed a fibrotic reaction along the lymphatics and vascular structures within the pelvis. An extended pelvic lymph node dissection in this setting is associated with an increased risk of vascular and nerve damage as well as long-term lymphedema of the lower extremities.

Based on the classic wide excision of the bladder and prostate, virtually all men are rendered impotent following radical cystectomy; however, preservation of the cavernosal nerves is surgically feasible and, when oncologically reasonable, can be successfully completed. Based on the descriptions of Walsh and Donker, a clear understanding of the anatomic relationships between the cavernosal nerve bundles and the bladder and prostate exists [90]. The course of the neurovascular structures from the pelvic plexus, to the lateral tips of the seminal vesicles and posterior lateral aspect of the prostate gland, lends itself to careful preservation when no evidence of tumor is present in these regions. Initial reports in 1987 described the technique for neurovascular bundle preservation at radical cystectomy, which included identification of the bundles lateral to the seminal vesicle tips and careful dissection of the bundles away from the lateral aspect of the prostate [91]. This allowed for ligation of the posterior vascular pedicles to the bladder while preserving the neurovascular structures as they coursed to the corpora cavernosal from the pelvic plexus. Patient selection is important to minimize the risk of local tumor recurrence in the region of the nerve bundles. In addition to excluding patients with poor preoperative erectile function, the exclusion of any patient with tumor extension in the region of the posterior pedicles or evidence of invasion of the prostate is critical to ensure complete tumor resection. In properly selected patients, at least 45% of patients should be expected to maintain potency postoperatively [92, 93].

Excision of the urethra is dictated by preoperative endoscopic and histologic information and the planned type of urinary diversion. Overt involvement of high-grade tumor of the membranous or penile urethra mandates urethrectomy. In women, the urethra is typically removed en bloc with the specimen unless orthotopic diversion is anticipated. Preoperative endoscopic evaluation is necessary to rule out overt urethral involvement and full thickness frozen section of the urethral margin at the time of cystectomy is used to histologically confirm the negative status of the urethral margin. Using these evaluation criteria, urethral recurrence risk is low and women can safely be offered orthotopic reconstruction with appropriate selection. Select centers perform prostate-sparing cystectomy in men, with the intention to maximize preservation of the neurovascular structures that control erectile functions; this modality remains investigative at this time [94, 95].

Lymph Node Dissection

Early identification of the pathways for progression of invasive bladder cancer identified that the regional pelvic lymph nodes served as an early site of involvement. Associations between the extent of tumor invasion into the bladder wall and the risk for regional pelvic lymph node involvement were elucidated from early autopsy studies of patients with invasive tumors and it is from this information that our current staging system is based [96–98]. Early surgical approaches to invasive disease neglected the regional pelvic lymphatics when the bladder was resected. As a result, initial reports detailing outcomes after cystectomy were associated with a very high pelvic recurrence rate, which in many cases likely represented progressive disease in involved pelvic lymph nodes. It became clear that surgical approaches to the management of invasive tumors would require a more aggressive technique that included extirpation of the pelvic lymphatics draining the bladder [99].

Anatomic studies delineated the lymphatic drainage pathways of the bladder and provided the necessary information for establishing a pelvic lymph node dissection as a part of the radical cystectomy procedure. The primary drainage of the bladder forms a partial ring of pelvic lymphatics that includes the hypogastric, obturator, external iliac, and presacral regions. The primary pelvic lymphatics drain into the common iliac lymphatics and then into the more proximal retroperitoneal nodes. These descriptions mirrored the drainage of the other pelvic organs and provided guidance to pelvic surgeons treating a variety of pelvic malignancies towards establishing a rational surgical approach to the regional lymphatics of the pelvis [100].

Following the incorporation of a PLND with the removal of the bladder and perivesical tissues (radical cystectomy), initial reported outcomes in patients with node-positive disease demonstrated a very poor overall survival and a high rate of pelvic recurrences. However, in more contemporary radical cystectomy series that incorporate a thorough pelvic lymph node dissection, approximately one-third of all node-positive patients are rendered disease free [101]. Subsets of node-positive patients demonstrate a more favorable outcome and are characterized by earlier stage primary tumors (≤ pT2) and lower volume disease at the nodal level (fewer positive nodes, absence of extracapsular extension) [102–105].

Debate continues on the extent of the PLND necessary to maximize patient outcome. Various anatomic zones have been championed as the "standard" dissection to be included at RC. Dissections range from a limited (obturator and hypogastic regions), "standard" (obturator, hypogastric, and external iliac) and extended (obturator, hypogastric, external iliac, common iliac, lower retroperitoneal nodes to base of inferior mesenteric artery). Mapping studies have detailed the location of the involved pelvic lymph nodes associated with invasive bladder tumors [106–108]. Extensive evidence demonstrates a progressive pattern of spread with initial primary lymphatic zone involvement followed by more proximal zones. Although typically not seen in the absence of primary region involvement, secondary drainage region involvement has been identified in relatively early stage disease. As depth of invasion by the primary tumor increases, so does the risk of secondary regional nodal involvement. A 290-patient multicenter RC and extended PLND surgical mapping study noted that 74% of all involved pelvic lymph nodes (444/599 positive lymph nodes) lay outside of a limited template (obturator/hypogastric regions) [106].

Such studies suggest that extended dissections would be needed in most invasive tumors to maximize a complete resection of potentially involved nodes. Indeed series have noted an association between the number of lymph nodes removed (used as surrogate for the completeness of resection) and disease control as measured by overall or disease-specific survival. To date no level 1 evidence exists establishing the superiority of the extended PLND over a lesser dissection; however, given the available data, it is the authors' recommendation that a more extensive dissection should be included routinely to optimize staging and provide any potential therapeutic advantage associated with a more thorough dissection. Current American Joint Committee on Cancer (AJCC) guidelines suggest that a minimum of 12 lymph nodes be evaluated to properly stage the regional lymphatics [109]. However this is currently only a recommendation, does not address the potential therapeutic benefits of a more extensive LN dissection, and is not included in the staging system.

Morbidity and Mortality Associated with Radical Cystectomy

Preoperative counseling should include a discussion of the perioperative complications that may occur after such a complex operation. Using a standardized reporting system of all outcomes within 90 days of cystectomy, data collected on 1,142 patients in a high-volume tertiary-level center documented a 64% overall complication rate [110]. Notably, 58% of those complications occurred after hospital discharge, highlighting the need for morbidity tracking beyond discharge and even beyond 30 days postoperatively. Of the complications, 87% were low grade (grade 0–2), emphasizing that major complications impact only a minority of patients who undergo RC.

Donat et al. recently compared these outcomes by age and found that older patients (≥80 years old) had a nonsignificantly higher rate of complications after RC compared to younger patients (<80 years old), with 55% minor complications vs. 50% and 17% major complications vs. 13% ($p=0.15$) [111]. The risk for major complications appeared to plateau beyond age 65. Age alone should not be an exclusion criterion for offering RC.

Given the current shift in the treatment paradigm toward integrated surgical and systemic therapy, a closer examination of the complications in the aforementioned cohort was undertaken in that context. Approximately 30% of the patients experienced complications that could interfere with the timely administration of adjuvant chemotherapy [112], suggesting that the integration of chemotherapy should be considered and discussed at the time of diagnosis and treatment disposition.

Minimally Invasive Approaches

Laparoscopy and minimally invasive surgery offer an alternative to open surgery, but oncologic efficacy and overall safety for radical cystectomy and urinary diversion have not yet been completely elucidated. Laparoscopic cystectomy has not gained in popularity, but robotic-assisted surgery has gained traction despite a lack of adequate oncologic efficacy data. Individual series have reported the potential advantages of decreased operative time, decreased blood loss, decreased incidence of postoperative bowel effects, and shortened length of hospital stay [113–116]. Thus far, early surgeon experience and short duration of follow-up limit the conclusions that can be drawn [117]. The extent of lymph node dissection and the technical steps involved in urinary diversion also present unique challenges for robotic-assisted approaches.

Multimodal Therapy

The modern treatment paradigm integrates the use of systemic chemotherapy in patients with clinically localized muscle-invasive urothelial cancer who are appropriate candidates for definitive surgical resection, with a category 1 recommendation for consideration in the most current guidelines from the National Comprehensive Cancer Network (NCCN) [118].

The natural history of muscle-invasive urothelial cancer is characterized by progressive local invasion, dissemination to the regional pelvic lymph nodes followed by distant organ involvement. Involvement of the pelvic lymph nodes and the development of micrometastatic disease can occur early in the invasive process [101, 119, 120]. Surgery alone cures up to 80% of patients with organ-confined disease, 60% of patients with extravesical LN negative tumors, and about 30% of those with lymph node-positive disease. Based on the risk of early dissemination, the paradigm of primary surgical management had shifted to include a multimodal approach, comprised of surgical resection and perioperative chemotherapy, either in a neoadjuvant or in a adjuvant fashion. Neoadjuvant chemotherapy has been shown to confer a significant survival advantage when compared to RC alone [121–123]. The International Collaboration of Trialists randomized 976 patients with cT2-T4a, N0-Nx, M0 bladder cancer to three cycles of cisplatin, methotrexate, and vinblastine or no chemotherapy prior to definitive treatment by RC, radiotherapy (RT), or both [122]. There was a 6% absolute survival benefit at 7.4 years for those patients who received neoadjuvant chemotherapy. A meta-analysis of 2,688 patients in ten randomized trials established a 5% absolute survival benefit at 5 years [124] and a 13% reduction in risk of death (HR 0.87; 0.78, 0.97; $p=0.016$). The benefit was across all muscle-invasive stages and was seen only with cisplatin-based regimens. There has a been a notable difference in tumor downstaging across multiple trials, with pT0 rates of 32.5% and 38% after chemotherapy vs. 12.3% and 15%, respectively, in the control arms of the two largest randomized trials [121, 122]. Complete pathologic response at cystectomy is associated with improved long-term survival [125, 126].

The evidence in support of adjuvant chemotherapy is less robust, but patients with adverse pathologic features at the time of cystectomy, including nodal involvement, extravesical disease (pT3/T4), or lymphovascular invasion, should undergo a discussion of the options. A meta-analysis of the six randomized trials using adjuvant chemotherapy in 491 patients showed a 25% relative reduction in the risk of death with adjuvant chemotherapy (HR 0.75; 95% CI 0.6, 0.96; $p=0.019$) with a clear call for further trials [125]. These analyzed trials were limited by methodological shortcomings and small numbers and led the authors of the meta-analysis to conclude that power to determine the efficacy of adjuvant chemotherapy is lacking. Current trials are ongoing to address this question and compare immediate adjuvant chemotherapy with chemotherapy at the time of recurrence. Poor accrual to many of the recent adjuvant chemotherapy studies in both Europe and the USA has led to their early closure.

The timing of chemotherapy administration and surgery is also important to bear in mind. Evidence suggests a negative impact on patient outcome if there is a delay from time of diagnosis to cystectomy greater than 12 weeks, including a delay due to chemotherapy administration or tolerance [117, 127–130]. As described previously, potential morbidity from surgery may interfere with the ability to administer adjuvant chemotherapy [113] and the potential benefit of the chemotherapy may be compromised. Patients with muscle-invasive disease should be counseled on the risks and benefits of integrated treatment prior to beginning any treatment. The decision to administer chemotherapy must consider patient and disease factors, such as age, comorbidities, and adverse clinical features.

Bladder Preservation

Proper selection of patients for bladder-preserving strategies requires consideration of multiple factors. A distinction must be made between those for whom cystectomy would offer curative intent and those for whom cystectomy would be inadequate, due to the presence of metastatic disease at presentation. This discussion will focus on those patients without metastatic disease who are candidates for a bladder-preserving strategy due to patient choice or comorbidities.

Partial Cystectomy

Partial removal of the tumor-bearing portion of the bladder has long been discussed as an option for managing select invasive tumors. The advantages of partial cystectomy include preserving overall bladder function (storage and emptying), preservation of sexual function, and a decreased morbidity compared to radical cystectomy and urinary diversion. The procedure should include a full thickness excision of the affected bladder wall, perivesical fat, overlying peritoneum, and bilateral pelvic lymph nodes. Initial attempts at partial cystectomy were associated with high rates of both local and distant failures significantly curtailing interest in the procedure [131–133]. Strict inclusion criteria were instituted as selection criteria for partial cystectomy were refined and outcomes improved; however, using these criteria, only 3–10% of patients presenting with invasive disease may be considered eligible for this approach [134–136]. SEER data, however, would suggest that a more broad use of partial cystectomy occurs [137].

Previously observed high local recurrence rates following partial cystectomy prompted the adoption of very strict selection criteria for appropriate patients. Solitary tumors with no associated carcinoma in situ and no previous history of bladder cancer may be considered as eligible candidates. The tumors must be amenable to resection with a 2 cm margin of normal tissue, limiting the optimal tumor location to regions away from the bladder neck and trigone. Low-lying tumors that would require excision of the ureteral orifice and ureteral reimplantation are not absolute contraindications for partial cystectomy, but this does increase the technical challenges and potential complications associated with the procedure.

Evaluation prior to partial cystectomy includes a thorough cystoscopic examination and mapping biopsies of the tumor and surrounding bladder. Location, size, and histology of the primary tumor are obtained. In addition bladder biopsies can help to identify the clear margins around the tumor so that intraoperatively the clear resection site can be visible. During the procedure the pelvis is properly toweled off so as to minimize seeding of tumor cells into the pelvic cavity. Full thickness of excision of the bladder wall, perivesical tissues, and overlying peritoneum must be achieved. A bilateral pelvic lymph node dissection should be included with the same limits of dissection required for a radical cystectomy. Bilateral dissection is necessary based on mapping data that have identified a high rate of crossover nodal involvement even with strictly unilaterally located invasive tumors. The bladder is repaired in multiple layers to complete a watertight closure.

Early experience with partial cystectomy noted a very high bladder recurrence rate of 29–78% [132, 138], including a 50% risk of developing a subsequent muscle-invasive tumor [139]. Seeding of the wound with subsequent recurrence within the incision site was also an observed complication (3–40%). For patients that relapse within the bladder, salvage cystectomy can be performed. Survival after salvage radical cystectomy is related to the final pathology of the bladder tumor (approximate 5-year survival: 75% Ta-T1, 40% T2, 20% T3, <10% T4). In contrast, with careful selection criteria and strict patient follow-up, more contemporary series have demonstrated improved outcomes after partial cystectomy. Local recurrence within the bladder ranges from 17 to 57%, with a similar risk of muscle-invasive recurrences noted. About one-fourth of cases that recurred within the bladder required salvage radical cystectomy in these series and those patients demonstrated a nearly 70% 5-year survival. Improved techniques that included carefully packing the pelvis and wound led to a dramatic improvement in the devastating complication of wound recurrences. Overall, approximately two-thirds of patients in these contemporary series survived with their bladders intact [134–136]. Importantly, CIS and positive resection margins are predictors of severe recurrences and poor overall survival. These factors highlight the importance of proper patient selection and optimal tumor characteristics associated with disease-free outcome.

Trimodality Therapy for Bladder Preservation

Radiotherapy (RT) and the combined chemoradiation therapy (CRT) have been studied as therapies with bladder preservation. RT as monotherapy has demonstrated inferior long term survival when compared to RC [140]. The combination of RT and chemotherapy as definitive treatment has been studied in varying regimens with similar overall survival to overall patient cohorts undergoing standard surgical therapy [141].

The only prospective randomized trial to report the comparison of radiotherapy with and without cisplatin-based chemotherapy [142] showed a decreased pelvic relapse rate after combined therapy, with 67% achieving pelvic control vs. 47% with RT alone ($p=0.36$). This study, with a small sample size of 99 patients, did not show improved survival or rate of metastatic disease. The experience with bladder-preserving strategies over nearly 25 years at Erlangen University shows an improvement in 5-year overall survival from 40% with RT alone to 60–80% with multimodal therapy utilizing transurethral resection and CRT [143].

At the time of transurethral resection (TUR), complete resection is imperative to maximize outcome to combined chemotherapy and bladder radiation. Incomplete resection has been shown to have a dramatic effect on survival, with 10-year overall survival rates of 50% with complete resection vs. 18% for patients with macroscopically residual disease prior to CRT [144]. In a report of 415 patients treated with radiotherapy or radiochemotherapy, resection status after TUR was independently predictive on multivariable analysis of complete remission after definitive bladder-preserving treatment. Long-term data on 348 patients treated over 16 years at Massachusetts General Hospital (MGH) demonstrate a complete response to CRT in 79% of patients with a complete TUR vs. 56% of patients with an incomplete TUR ($p<0.001$) [141]. Up to 80% of patients treated with bladder preservation strategies are able to maintain their bladder long-term, and prospective data from the MGH experience using trimodal therapy have shown similar survival between those who underwent immediate cystectomy for incomplete response and delayed cystectomy for recurrent disease [145].

Another imperative step is a cystoscopic surveillance and biopsy at a set timepoint after CRT, generally at 6 weeks following the end of therapy. Long-term close follow-up is imperative, due to the risk for relapse in the bladder. Across numerous contemporary studies, salvage cystectomy for recurrence is required in approximately one-quarter of patients [146]. The local toxicity effects have greatly diminished with refinements to the treatment modalities. From a center with more than 20 years of experience with bladder-preserving strategies, Efstathiou et al. report a 7% rate of late pelvic toxicity from radiation among 285 patients [147], and Zietman et al. found that 78% of patients have compliant bladders by urodynamics and fewer than 25% report irritative genitourinary or gastrointestinal symptoms [148].

References

1. Mahul MB. Histological variants of urothelial carcinoma: diagnostic, therapeutic and prognostic implications. Mod Pathol. 2009;22 Suppl 2:S96–118.
2. Perez-Montiel D, Hes O, Michal M, Suster S. Micropapillary urothelial carcinoma of the upper urinary tract: clinicopathologic study of five cases. Am J Clin Pathol. 2006;126(1):86–92.
3. Chou R, Dana T. Screening adults for bladder cancer: a review of the evidence for the U.S. preventive services task force. Ann Intern Med. 2010;153(7):461–8.
4. Kaufman DS, Shipley WU, Feldman AS. Bladder cancer. Lancet. 2009;374(9685):239–49.
5. Nieder AM, Lotan Y, Nuss GR, Langston JP, Vyas S, Manoharan M, et al. Are patients with hematuria appropriately referred to urology? A multi-institutional questionnaire based survey. Urol Oncol. 2010;28(5):500–3.

6. Johnson EK, Daignault S, Zhang Y, Lee CT. Patterns of hematuria referral to urologists: does a gender disparity exist? Urology. 2008;72(3):498–502.
7. Gruver AM, Westfall D, Farver CF, Luthringer DJ, Osunkoya AO, McKenney JK, et al. Selective immunohistochemical markers to distinguish between metastatic high grade urothelial carcinoma to the lung and primary poorly differentiated invasive squamous carcinoma. Abstract 823. San Antonio, Texas:United States and Canadian Academy of Pathology;2011.
8. Black PC, Brown GA, Dinney CP. The impact of variant histology on the outcome of bladder cancer treated with curative intent. Urol Oncol. 2009; 27(1):3–7.
9. Zhai QJ, Black J, Ayala AG, Ro JY. Histologic variants of infiltrating urothelial carcinoma. Arch Pathol Lab Med. 2007;131(8):1244–56.
10. Budia Alba A, Queipo Zaragoza JA, Perez Ebri ML, et al. Comparative study of pure epidermoid carcinoma of the bladder and transitional cell carcinoma with squamous or mixed differentiated foci. Actas Urol Esp. 1999;23(2):111–8.
11. Hong JY, Choi MK, Uhm JE, et al. Palliative chemotherapy for non-transitional cell carcinomas of the urothelial tract. Med Oncol. 2009;26(2):186–92.
12. Lopez-Beltran A, Martin J, Garcia J, Toro M. Squamous and glandular differentiation in urothelial bladder carcinomas. Histopathology, histochemistry and immunohistochemical expression of carcinoembryonic antigen. Histol Histopathol. 1988;3(1):63–8.
13. Scosyrev E, Ely BW, Messing EM, Speights VO, Grossman HB, Wood DP, et al. Do mixed histological features affect survival benefit from neoadjuvant platinum-based combination chemotherapy in patients with locally advanced bladder cancer? A secondary analysis of Southwest Oncology Group-Directed Intergroup Study (S8710). BJU Int. 2011;108(5):693–9.
14. Dhall D, Al-Ahmadie H, Olgac S. Nested variant of urothelial carcinoma. Arch Pathol Lab Med. 2007;131(11):1725–7.
15. Drew PA, Furman J, Civantos F, Murphy WM. The nested variant of transitional cell carcinoma: an aggressive neoplasm with innocuous histology. Mod Pathol. 1996;9(10):989–94.
16. Holmang S, Johansson SL. The nested variant of transitional cell carcinoma–a rare neoplasm with poor prognosis. Scand J Urol Nephrol. 2001;35(2):102–5.
17. Lin O, Cardillo M, Dalbagni G, et al. Nested variant of urothelial carcinoma: a clinicopathologic and immunohistochemical study of 12 cases. Mod Pathol. 2003;16(12):1289–98.
18. Murphy WM, Deana DG. The nested variant of transitional cell carcinoma: a neoplasm resembling proliferation of Brunn's nests. Mod Pathol. 1992;5(3): 240–3.
19. Nese N, Kandiloglu AR, Atesci YZ. Nested variant of transitional cell carcinoma with osseous metaplasia of the urinary bladder: a case report and review of published reports. Int J Urol. 2007;14(4):365–7.
20. Ro J, Lapham R, Amin M. Deceptively bland transitional cell carcinoma of the urinary bladder-further characterization of subtle and diagnostically tracherous patterns of invasion in urothelial neoplasia. Adv Anat Pathol. 1997;4:244–51.
21. Young RH, Oliva E. Transitional cell carcinomas of the urinary bladder that may be underdiagnosed. A report of four invasive cases exemplifying the homology between neoplastic and non-neoplastic transitional cell lesions. Am J Surg Pathol. 1996;20(12): 1448–54.
22. Leroy X, Leteurtre E, De La Taille A, et al. Microcystic transitional cell carcinoma: a report of 2 cases arising in the renal pelvis. Arch Pathol Lab Med. 2002;126(7):859–61.
23. Young RH, Zukerberg LR. Microcystic transitional cell carcinomas of the urinary bladder. A report of four cases. Am J Clin Pathol. 1991;96(5):635–9.
24. Sari A, Uyaroglu MA, Ermete M, et al. Microcystic urothelial carcinoma of the urinary bladder metastatic to the penis. Pathol Oncol Res. 2007;13(2): 170–3.
25. Gilcrease MZ, Delgado R, Vuitch F, Albores-Saavedra J. Clear cell adenocarcinoma and nephrogenic adenoma of the urethra and urinary bladder: a histopathologic and immunohistochemical comparison. Hum Pathol. 1998;29(12):1451–6.
26. Kotliar SN, Wood CG, Schaeffer AJ, Oyasu R. Transitional cell carcinoma exhibiting clear cell features. A differential diagnosis for clear cell adenocarcinoma of the urinary tract. Arch Pathol Lab Med. 1995;119(1):79–81.
27. Oliva E, Amin MB, Jimenez R, Young RH. Clear cell carcinoma of the urinary bladder: a report and comparison of four tumors of mullerian origin and nine of probable urothelial origin with discussion of histogenesis and diagnostic problems. Am J Surg Pathol. 2002;26(2):190–7.
28. Sun K, Huan Y, Unger PD. Clear cell adenocarcinoma of urinary bladder and urethra: another urinary tract lesion immunoreactive for P504S. Arch Pathol Lab Med. 2008;132(9):1417–22.
29. Sung MT, Zhang S, MacLennan GT, et al. Histogenesis of clear cell adenocarcinoma in the urinary tract: evidence of urothelial origin. Clin Cancer Res. 2008;14(7):1947–55.
30. Shimada K, Nakamura M, Ishida E, Konishi N. Urothelial carcinoma with plasmacytoid variants producing both human chorionic gonadotropin and carbohydrate antigen 19-9. Urology. 2006;68(4):891 e7–10.
31. Coyne JD, Sim E. Urothelial neoplasia with plasmacytoid morphology. Histopathology. 2006;48(2): 200–1.
32. Fritsche HM, Burger M, Denzinger S, et al. Plasmacytoid urothelial carcinoma of the bladder: histological and clinical features of 5 cases. J Urol. 2008;180(5):1923–7.

33. Gaafar A, Garmendia M, de Miguel E, et al. Plasmacytoid urothelial carcinoma of the urinary bladder. A study of 7 cases. Actas Urol Esp. 2008;32(8):806–10.
34. Kohno T, Kitamura M, Akai H, et al. Plasmacytoid urothelial carcinoma of the bladder. Int J Urol. 2006;13(4):485–6.
35. Mai KT, Park PC, Yazdi HM, et al. Plasmacytoid urothelial carcinoma of the urinary bladder report of seven new cases. Eur Urol. 2006;50(5):1111–4.
36. Nigwekar P, Tamboli P, Amin MB, Osunkoya AO, Ben-Dor D. Plasmacytoid urothelial carcinoma: detailed analysis of morphology with clinicopathologic correlation in 17 cases. Am J Surg Pathol. 2009;33(3):417–24.
37. Ro JY, Shen SS, Lee HI, et al. Plasmacytoid transitional cell carcinoma of urinary bladder: a clinicopathologic study of 9 cases. Am J Surg Pathol. 2008;32(5):752–7.
38. Sahin AA, Myhre M, Ro JY, et al. Plasmacytoid transitional cell carcinoma. Report of a case with initial presentation mimicking multiple myeloma. Acta Cytol. 1991;35(3):277–80.
39. Sato K, Ueda Y, Kawamura K, Aihara K, Katsuda S. Plasmacytoid urothelial carcinoma of the urinary bladder: a case report and immunohistochemical study. Pathol Res Pract. 2009;205(3):189–94.
40. Soylu A, Aydin NE, Yilmaz U, Kutlu R, Gunes A. Urothelial carcinoma featuring lipid cell and plasmacytoid morphology with poor prognostic outcome. Urology. 2005;65(4):797.
41. Zhang XM, Elhosseiny A, Melamed MR. Plasmacytoid urothelial carcinoma of the bladder. A case report and the first description of urinary cytology. Acta Cytol. 2002;46(2):412–6.
42. Baldwin L, Lee AH, Al-Talib RK, Theaker JM. Transitional cell carcinoma of the bladder mimicking lobular carcinoma of the breast: a discohesive variant of urothelial carcinoma. Histopathology. 2005;46(1):50–6.
43. Kumar S, Kumar D, Cowan DF. Transitional cell carcinoma with rhabdoid features. Am J Surg Pathol. 1992;16(5):515–21.
44. Parwani AV, Herawi M, Volmar K, Tsay SH, Epstein JI. Urothelial carcinoma with rhabdoid features: report of 6 cases. Hum Pathol. 2006; 37(2):168–72.
45. Gulley ML, Amin MB, Nicholls JM, et al. Epstein-Barr virus is detected in undifferentiated nasopharyngeal carcinoma but not in lymphoepithelioma-like carcinoma of the urinary bladder. Hum Pathol. 1995;26(11):1207–14.
46. Tamas EF, Nielsen ME, Schoenberg MP, Epstein JI. Lymphoepithelioma-like carcinoma of the urinary tract: a clinicopathological study of 30 pure and mixed cases. Mod Pathol. 2007;20(8):828–34.
47. Nigwekar P, Amin MB. The many faces of urothelial carcinoma: an update with an emphasis on recently described variants. Adv Anat Pathol. 2008;15(4): 218–33.
48. Holmang S, Borghede G, Johansson SL. Bladder carcinoma with lymphoepithelioma-like differentiation: a report of 9 cases. J Urol. 1998;159(3): 779–82.
49. Dinney CP, Ro JY, Babaian RJ, Johnson DE. Lymphoepithelioma of the bladder: a clinicopathological study of 3 cases. J Urol. 1993;149(4):840–1.
50. Amin MB, Ro JY, Lee KM, et al. Lymphoepithelioma-like carcinoma of the urinary bladder. Am J Surg Pathol. 1994;18(5):466–73.
51. Lopez-Beltran A, Luque RJ, Vicioso L, et al. Lymphoepithelioma-like carcinoma of the urinary bladder: a clinicopathologic study of 13 cases. Virchows Arch. 2001;438(6):552–7.
52. Eble JN, Epstein JI, Sesterhenn IA, editors. Pathology & genetics of tumors of the urinary system and male genital organs. Lyon, France: IARC; 2004.
53. Leroy X, Gonzalez S, Zini L, Aubert S. Lipoid-cell variant of urothelial carcinoma: a clinicopathologic and immunohistochemical study of five cases. Am J Surg Pathol. 2007;31(5):770–3.
54. Dirnhofer S, Koessler P, Ensinger C, et al. Production of trophoblastic hormones by transitional cell carcinoma of the bladder: association to tumor stage and grade. Hum Pathol. 1998;29(4):377–82.
55. Iles RK, Chard T. Human chorionic gonadotropin expression by bladder cancers: biology and clinical potential. J Urol. 1991;145(3):453–8.
56. Iles RK, Jenkins BJ, Oliver RT, Blandy JP, Chard T. Beta human chorionic gonadotrophin in serum and urine. A marker for metastatic urothelial cancer. Br J Urol. 1989;64(3):241–4.
57. Martin JE, Jenkins BJ, Zuk RJ, Oliver RT, Baithun SI. Human chorionic gonadotrophin expression and histological findings as predictors of response to radiotherapy in carcinoma of the bladder. Virchows Arch A Pathol Anat Histopathol. 1989;414(3): 273–7.
58. Sievert K, Weber EA, Herwig R, et al. Pure primary choriocarcinoma of the urinary bladder with long-term survival. Urology. 2000;56(5):856.
59. Lopez-Beltran A, Pacelli A, Rothenberg HJ, et al. Carcinosarcoma and sarcomatoid carcinoma of the bladder: clinicopathological study of 41 cases. J Urol. 1998;159(5):1497–503.
60. Wright JL, Black PC, Brown GA, et al. Differences in survival among patients with sarcomatoid carcinoma, carcinosarcoma and urothelial carcinoma of the bladder. J Urol. 2007;178(6):2302–6; discussion 7.
61. Sung MT, Wang M, MacLennan GT, et al. Histogenesis of sarcomatoid urothelial carcinoma of the urinary bladder: evidence for a common clonal origin with divergent differentiation. J Pathol. 2007;211(4):420–30.
62. Jones EC, Young RH. Myxoid and sclerosing sarcomatoid transitional cell carcinoma of the urinary bladder: a clinicopathologic and immunohistochemical study of 25 cases. Mod Pathol. 1997;10(9):908–16.
63. Acikalin MF, Kabukcuoglu S, Can C. Sarcomatoid carcinoma of the renal pelvis with giant cell tumor-like

features: case report with immunohistochemical findings. Int J Urol. 2005;12(2):199–203.
64. Young RH, Wick MR, Mills SE. Sarcomatoid carcinoma of the urinary bladder. A clinicopathologic analysis of 12 cases and review of the literature. Am J Clin Pathol. 1988;90(6):653–61.
65. Torenbeek R, Blomjous CE, de Bruin PC, Newling DW, Meijer CJ. Sarcomatoid carcinoma of the urinary bladder. Clinicopathologic analysis of 18 cases with immunohistochemical and electron microscopic findings. Am J Surg Pathol. 1994;18(3):241–9.
66. Ikegami H, Iwasaki H, Ohjimi Y, et al. Sarcomatoid carcinoma of the urinary bladder: a clinicopathologic and immunohistochemical analysis of 14 patients. Hum Pathol. 2000;31(3):332–40.
67. Reuter VE. Sarcomatoid lesions of the urogenital tract. Semin Diagn Pathol. 1993;10(2):188–201.
68. Young RH, Wick MR. Transitional cell carcinoma of the urinary bladder with pseudosarcomatous stroma. Am J Clin Pathol. 1988;90(2):216–9.
69. Shah SK, Lui PD, Baldwin DD, Ruckle HC. Urothelial carcinoma after external beam radiation therapy for prostate cancer. J Urol. 2006;175(6):2063–6.
70. Armstrong AB, Wang M, Eble JN, et al. TP53 mutational analysis supports monoclonal origin of biphasic sarcomatoid urothelial carcinoma (carcinosarcoma) of the urinary bladder. Mod Pathol. 2009;22(1):113–8.
71. Westfall DE, Folpe AL, Paner GP, et al. Utility of a comprehensive immunohistochemical panel in the differential diagnosis of spindle cell lesions of the urinary bladder. Am J Surg Pathol. 2009;33(1): 99–105.
72. Harik LR, Merino C, Coindre JM, et al. Pseudosarcomatous myofibroblastic proliferations of the bladder: a clinicopathologic study of 42 cases. Am J Surg Pathol. 2006;30(7):787–94.
73. Mahadevia PS, Alexander JE, Rojas-Corona R, Koss LG. Pseudosarcomatous stromal reaction in primary and metastatic urothelial carcinoma. A source of diagnostic difficulty. Am J Surg Pathol. 1989;13(9):782–90.
74. Young RH. Spindle cell lesions of the urinary bladder. Histol Histopathol. 1990;5(4):505–12.
75. Amir G, Rosenmann E. Osteoclast-like giant cell tumour of the urinary bladder. Histopathology. 1990;17(5):413–8.
76. Garcia Garcia F, Garcia Ligero J, Martinez Diaz F, et al. Bladder carcinoma with osteoclast-type giant cells. A case with a rare presentation. Review of the literature. Actas Urol Esp. 2003;27(4):317–20.
77. Kruger S, Johannisson R, Kausch I, Feller AC. Papillary urothelial bladder carcinoma associated with osteoclast-like giant cells. Int Urol Nephrol. 2005;37(1):61–4.
78. Zukerberg LR, Armin AR, Pisharodi L, Young RH. Transitional cell carcinoma of the urinary bladder with osteoclast-type giant cells: a report of two cases and review of the literature. Histopathology. 1990; 17(5):407–11.
79. Baydar D, Amin MB, Epstein JI. Osteoclast-rich undifferentiated carcinomas of the urinary tract. Mod Pathol. 2006;19(2):161–71.
80. Eble JN, Young RH. Carcinoma of the urinary bladder: a review of its diverse morphology. Semin Diagn Pathol. 1997;14(2):98–108.
81. Young RH, Eble JN. Unusual forms of carcinoma of the urinary bladder. Hum Pathol. 1991;22(10):948–65.
82. Stein JP. Indications for early cystectomy. Urology. 2003;62(4):591–5.
83. Chang SS, Cookson MS. Radical cystectomy for bladder cancer: the case for early intervention. Urol Clin North Am. 2005;32(2):147–55.
84. Montgomery JS, Weizer AZ, Montie JE. T1 bladder cancer: advocating early cystectomy to improve oncologic control. Urol Oncol. 2010;28(5):466–8.
85. Herr HW, Donat SM. Outcome of patients with grossly node positive bladder cancer after pelvic lymph node dissection and radical cystectomy. J Urol. 2001;165(1):62–4; discussion 64.
86. Sweeney P, Millikan R, Donat M, et al. Is there a therapeutic role for post-chemotherapy retroperitoneal lymph node dissection in metastatic transitional cell carcinoma of the bladder? J Urol. 2003; 169(6):2113–7.
87. Dodd PM, McCaffrey JA, Herr H, et al. Outcome of postchemotherapy surgery after treatment with methotrexate, vinblastine, doxorubicin, and cisplatin in patients with unresectable or metastatic transitional cell carcinoma. J Clin Oncol. 1999;17(8): 2546–52.
88. Skinner DG. Management of invasive bladder cancer: a meticulous pelvic node dissection can make a difference. J Urol. 1982;128(1):34–6.
89. Herr HW. Surgical factors in bladder cancer: more (nodes) + more (pathology) = less (mortality). BJU Int. 2003;92(3):187–8.
90. Walsh PC, Donker PJ. Impotence following radical prostatectomy: insight into etiology and prevention. J Urol. 1982;128(3):492–7.
91. Schlegel PN, Walsh PC. Neuroanatomical approach to radical cystoprostatectomy with preservation of sexual function. J Urol. 1987;138(6):1402–6.
92. Kessler TM, Burkhard FC, Studer UE. Clinical indications and outcomes with nerve-sparing cystectomy in patients with bladder cancer. Urol Clin North Am. 2005;32(2):165–75.
93. Schoenberg MP, Walsh PC, Breakzeale DR, Marshall FF, Mostwin JL, Brendler CB. Local recurrence and survival following nerve sparing radical cystoprostatectomy for bladder cancer: 10-year followup. J Urol. 1996;155(2):490–4.
94. Hautmann RE, Stein JP. Neobladder with prostatic capsule and seminal-sparing cystectomy for bladder cancer: a step in the wrong direction. Urol Clin North Am. 2005;32(2):177–85.
95. Richards KA, Parks GE, Badlani GH, Kader AK, Hemal AK, Pettus JA. Developing selection criteria for prostate-sparing cystectomy: a review of

cystoprostatectomy specimens. Urology. 2010; 75(5):1116–20.
96. Cunningham J. Tumors of the bladder. J Urol. 1931;25:559.
97. Colston J, Leadbetter WF. Infiltrating carcinoma of the bladder. J Urol. 1936;36:669.
98. Jewett H, Strong G. Infiltrating carcinoma of the bladder: relation of depth of penetration of the bladder wall to incidence of local extension and metastases. J Urol. 1946;55:366–72.
99. Marshall VF, Whitmore Jr WF. Simple cystectomy for cancer of the urinary bladder; 100 consecutive cases; 2 years later. J Urol. 1950;63(2):232–41.
100. Brunschwig A. Complete excision of pelvic viscera for advanced carcinoma; a one-stage abdominoperineal operation with end colostomy and bilateral ureteral implantation into the colon above the colostomy. Cancer. 1948;1(2):177–83.
101. International Bladder Cancer Nomogram Consortium, Bochner BH, Kattan MW, Vora KC. Postoperative nomogram predicting risk of recurrence after radical cystectomy for bladder cancer. J Clin Oncol. 2006;24(24):3967–72.
102. Stein JP, Cai J, Groshen S, Skinner DG. Risk factors for patients with pelvic lymph node metastases following radical cystectomy with en bloc pelvic lymphadenectomy: concept of lymph node density. J Urol. 2003;170(1):35–41.
103. Herr HW. Superiority of ratio based lymph node staging for bladder cancer. J Urol. 2003;169(3): 943–5.
104. Karl A, Carroll PR, Gschwend JE, et al. The impact of lymphadenectomy and lymph node metastasis on the outcomes of radical cystectomy for bladder cancer. Eur Urol. 2009;55(4):826–35.
105. Fleischmann A, Thalmann GN, Markwalder R, Studer UE. Extracapsular extension of pelvic lymph node metastases from urothelial carcinoma of the bladder is an independent prognostic factor. J Clin Oncol. 2005;23(10):2358–65.
106. Leissner J, Ghoneim MA, Abol-Enein H, et al. Extended radical lymphadenectomy in patients with urothelial bladder cancer: results of a prospective multicenter study. J Urol. 2004;171(1):139–44.
107. Vazina A, Dugi D, Shariat SF, Evans J, Link R, Lerner SP. Stage specific lymph node metastasis mapping in radical cystectomy specimens. J Urol. 2004;171(5):1830–4.
108. Bochner BH, Cho D, Herr HW, Donat M, Kattan MW, Dalbagni G. Prospectively packaged lymph node dissections with radical cystectomy: evaluation of node count variability and node mapping. J Urol. 2004;172(4 Pt 1):1286–90.
109. AJCC. Urinary bladder. In: Edge SB, Byrd DR, Compton CC, editors. AJCC cancer staging manual. 7th ed. New York, NY: Springer; 2010.
110. Shabsigh A, Korets R, Vora KC, et al. Defining early morbidity of radical cystectomy for patients with bladder cancer using a standardized reporting methodology. Eur Urol. 2009;55(1):164–74.
111. Donat SM, Siegrist T, Cronin A, Savage C, Milowsky MI, Herr HW. Radical cystectomy in octogenarians–does morbidity outweigh the potential survival benefits? J Urol. 2010;183(6):2171–7.
112. Donat SM, Shabsigh A, Savage C, et al. Potential impact of postoperative early complications on the timing of adjuvant chemotherapy in patients undergoing radical cystectomy: a high-volume tertiary cancer center experience. Eur Urol. 2009;55(1): 177–85.
113. Hellenthal NJ, Hussain A, Andrews PE, et al. Surgical margin status after robot assisted radical cystectomy: results from the International Robotic Cystectomy Consortium. J Urol. 2010;184(1): 87–91.
114. Haber GP, Crouzet S, Gill IS. Laparoscopic and robotic assisted radical cystectomy for bladder cancer: a critical analysis. Eur Urol. 2008;54(1):54–62.
115. Pruthi RS, Nielsen ME, Nix J, Smith A, Schultz H, Wallen EM. Robotic radical cystectomy for bladder cancer: surgical and pathological outcomes in 100 consecutive cases. J Urol. 2009;183(2):510–4.
116. Ng CK, Kauffman EC, Lee MM, et al. A comparison of postoperative complications in open versus robotic cystectomy. Eur Urol. 2009;57(2):274–81.
117. Chade DC, Laudone VP, Bochner BH, Parra RO. Oncological outcomes after radical cystectomy for bladder cancer: open versus minimally invasive approaches. J Urol. 2010;183(3):862–9.
118. Montie JE, NCCN Guidelines Panel Members. NCCN clinical practice guidelines in oncology: bladder cancer. N.C.C. Network: Editor; 2011.
119. Ghoneim MA, el-Mekresh MM, el-Baz MA, et al. Radical cystectomy for carcinoma of the bladder: critical evaluation of the results in 1,026 cases. J Urol. 1997;158(2):393–9.
120. Leissner J, Hohenfellner R, Thuroff JW, Wolf HK, et al. Lymphadenectomy in patients with transitional cell carcinoma of the urinary bladder; significance for staging and prognosis. BJU Int. 2000;85(7): 817–23.
121. Grossman HB, Natale RB, Tangen CM, et al. Neoadjuvant chemotherapy plus cystectomy compared with cystectomy alone for locally advanced bladder cancer. N Engl J Med. 2003;349(9):859–66.
122. International collaboration of trialists on behalf of the Medical Research Council, Advanced Bladder Cancer Working Party, EORTC Genito-Urinary Group, Australian Bladder Cancer Study Group, National Cancer Institute of Canada Clinical Trials Group. Finnbladder, Norwegian Bladder Cancer Study Group, Club Urologico Espanol de Tratamiento Oncologico (CUETO) group. Neoadjuvant cisplatin, methotrexate, and vinblastine chemotherapy for muscle-invasive bladder cancer: a randomised controlled trial. International collaboration of trialists. Lancet. 1999;354(9178):533–40.
123. Hall RR. Updated results of a randomised controlled trial of neoadjuvant cisplatin (C), methotrexate (M) and vinblastine (V) chemotherapy for muscle-inva-

sive bladder cancer. Proc Am Soc Clin Oncol. 2002;21:abstr 710.

124. Collaboration. A.B.C.M.-a.neoadjuvant chemotherapy in invasive bladder cancer: a systematic review and meta-analysis. Lancet. 2003;361(9373):1927–34.
125. Advanced Bladder Cancer Meta-Analysis Collaboration. Adjuvant chemotherapy for invasive bladder cancer (individual patient data). Cochrane Database Syst Rev. 2006(2): CD006018.
126. Isbarn H, Karakiewicz PI, Shariat SF, et al. Residual pathological stage at radical cystectomy significantly impacts outcomes for initial T2N0 bladder cancer. J Urol. 2009;182(2):459–65; discussion 465.
127. Sanchez-Ortiz RF, Huang WC, Mick R, Van Arsdalen KN, Wein AJ, Malkowicz SB. An interval longer than 12 weeks between the diagnosis of muscle invasion and cystectomy is associated with worse outcome in bladder carcinoma. J Urol. 2003;169(1): 110–5; discussion 115.
128. Mahmud SM, Fong B, Fahmy N, Tanguay S, Aprikian AG. Effect of preoperative delay on survival in patients with bladder cancer undergoing cystectomy in Quebec: a population based study. J Urol. 2006;175(1):78–83; discussion 83.
129. Weight CJ, Garcia JA, Hansel DE, et al. Lack of pathologic down-staging with neoadjuvant chemotherapy for muscle-invasive urothelial carcinoma of the bladder: a contemporary series. Cancer. 2009; 115(4):792–9.
130. Gore JL, Lai J, Setodij CM, Litwin MS, Saigal CS. Urologic Diseases in America Project. Mortality increases when radical cystectomy is delayed more than 12 weeks: results from a Surveillance, Epidemiology, and End Results-Medicare analysis. Cancer. 2009;115(5):988–96.
131. Pontes JE, Lopez R. Tumor recurrence following partial cystectomy. Prog Clin Biol Res. 1984; 162A:387–92.
132. Faysal MH, Freiha FS. Evaluation of partial cystectomy for carcinoma of bladder. Urology. 1979;14(4): 352–6.
133. Long RT, Grummon RA, Spratt JS, Perez-Mesa C. Carcinoma of the urinary bladder. (Comparison with radical, simple, and partial cystectomy and intravesical formalin. Cancer. 1972;29(1):98–105.
134. Holzbeierlein JM, Lopez-Corona E, Bochner BH, et al. Partial cystectomy: a contemporary review of the Memorial Sloan-Kettering Cancer Center experience and recommendations for patient selection. J Urol. 2004;172(3):878–81.
135. Smaldone MC, Jacobs BL, Smaldone AM, Hrebinko RL. Long-term results of selective partial cystectomy for invasive urothelial bladder carcinoma. Urology. 2008;72(3):613–6.
136. Kassouf W, Swanson D, Kamat AM, et al. Partial cystectomy for muscle invasive urothelial carcinoma of the bladder: a contemporary review of the M. D. Anderson Cancer Center experience. J Urol. 2006; 175(6):2058–62.
137. Hollenbeck BK, Taub DA, Dunn RL, Wei JT. Quality of care: partial cystectomy for bladder cancer—a case of inappropriate use? J Urol. 2005;174(3):1050–4; discussion 1054.
138. Merrell RW, Brown HE, Rose JF. Bladder carcinoma treated by partial cystectomy: a review of 54 cases. J Urol. 1979;122(4):471–2.
139. Dandekar NP, Tongaonkar HB, Dalal AV, Kulkarni JN, Kamat MR. Partial cystectomy for invasive bladder cancer. J Surg Oncol. 1995;60(1):24–9.
140. Shelley MD, Barber J, Wilt T, Mason MD. Surgery versus radiotherapy for muscle invasive bladder cancer. Cochrane Database Syst Rev. 2002;1(1): CD002079.
141. Shipley WU, Kaufman DS, Zehr E, et al. Selective bladder preservation by combined modality protocol treatment: long-term outcomes of 190 patients with invasive bladder cancer. Urology. 2002;60(1):62–7; discussion 67–8.
142. Coppin CM, Gospodarowicz MK, James K, et al. Improved local control of invasive bladder cancer by concurrent cisplatin and preoperative or definitive radiation. The National Cancer Institute of Canada Clinical Trials Group. J Clin Oncol. 1996;14(11): 2901–7.
143. Ott OJ, Rodel C, Weiss C, et al. Radiochemotherapy for bladder cancer. Clin Oncol (R Coll Radiol). 2009;21(7):557–65.
144. Rodel C, Grabenbauer GG, Kuhn R, et al. Combined-modality treatment and selective organ preservation in invasive bladder cancer: long-term results. J Clin Oncol. 2002;20(14):3061–71.
145. Efstathiou JA, Coen J, Spiegel DY, et al.15-year outcomes of selective bladder preservation for invasive bladder cancer: the Massachusetts General Hospital experience, in 2010 Genitourinary Cancers Symposium 2010: San Francisco, CA.
146. Rodel C, Weiss C, Sauer R. Trimodality treatment and selective organ preservation for bladder cancer. J Clin Oncol. 2006;24(35):5536–44.
147. Efstathiou JA, Bae K, Shipley WU, et al. Late pelvic toxicity after bladder-sparing therapy in patients with invasive bladder cancer: RTOG 89-03, 95-06, 97-06, 99-06. J Clin Oncol. 2009;27(25):4055–61.
148. Zietman AL, Sacco D, Skowronski U, et al. Organ conservation in invasive bladder cancer by transurethral resection, chemotherapy and radiation: results of a urodynamic and quality of life study on long-term survivors. J Urol. 2003;170(5):1772–6.

Micropapillary Carcinoma

8

Joseph C. Klink, Andrew J. Stephenson, and Jesse K. McKenney

Introduction

Micropapillary carcinoma of the urothelial tract (MPC) was described by Amin et al. in 1994 as a morphologic variant of urothelial carcinoma that closely resembles the histologic appearance of ovarian serous carcinoma [1]. They reported frequent presentation with high stage disease, extensive vascular invasion, and lymph node metastasis. Numerous other clinicopathologic series of MPC within the genitourinary tract have been published, and it has become increasingly well recognized as a unique and aggressive carcinoma variant. To date, 358 cases of MPC have been reported in retrospective case series in the literature [1–19]. No prospective series or randomized trials have been published about this uncommon variant. These case series are not reported in a standardized fashion, so drawing firm conclusions from the available literature is difficult.

J.C. Klink (✉) • A.J. Stephenson
Section of Urologic Oncology, Glickman Urologic and Kidney Institute, Cleveland Clinic, 9500 Euclid Avenue, Cleveland, OH 44195, USA
e-mail: klinkj@ccf.org; stephea2@ccf.org

J.K. McKenney
Department of Pathology, Stanford University Medical Center, 300 Pasteur Drive, H2110, Stanford, CA 94025, USA
e-mail: jmck@stanford.edu

The incidence of MPC in urothelial carcinoma of the bladder is 2.6% overall, with a reported range of 0.7–8% [1–4, 7, 9, 14]. In our personal experience, at least focal areas with a micropapillary pattern are seen at cystectomy in 3–5% of invasive urothelial carcinomas (unpublished data). The male predominance is striking (approximate 7:1 male:female ratio). MPC has also been reported in the upper tract in 42 patients (26 in the renal pelvis, two in the ureteropelvic junction, 12 in the ureter, three in the both the ureter and the renal pelvis) with a male:female ratio of 2.2:1 and an overall incidence of 2.6% (range 2.3–2.8%) [4, 6, 8, 15]. For MPC in any location, the mean age of diagnosis is close to 68 years old in most series. The youngest patient was 22 years old [6] and the oldest patients were 92 years old [2, 14, 15].

MPC has been diagnosed in all stages of urothelial carcinoma, but inconsistent reporting makes summarizing the stage of presentation difficult. The majority of bladder MPCs appear clinically localized at diagnosis with 38% ≤cT1 (superficial), 31% cT2 (muscle invasive but confined to the bladder), 17% cT3 (invasion of perivesicle fat), and 14% cT4 (invading other organs) or node positive or metastatic [1–4, 9, 11, 14, 19]. This is in contrast to upper tract MPC which, based on a very limited number of patients, usually presents at somewhat more advanced stages with 10% ≤cT1, 6% cT2, 65% cT3, and 19% cT4 [8, 15]. It should be noted that the actual distribution of stage at presentation in the general population may be

D.E. Hansel et al. (eds.), *The Urinary Tract: A Comprehensive Guide to Patient Diagnosis and Management*,
DOI 10.1007/978-1-4614-5320-8_8, © Springer Science+Business Media New York 2012

significantly different than what is reported in several of these series that identified only patients who had removal of the entire organ (bladder or kidney/ureter), an approach which often overlooks cases of superficial disease as well as cases of metastatic disease.

Pathogenesis

No reliable information is available on the pathogenesis of MPC because of its rarity. Since MPC usually arises on a background of high-grade urothelial carcinoma, standard risk factors for urothelial carcinoma such as cigarette smoking may play a role. A possible etiology is mentioned for only 16 patients out of the 358 published cases [7, 8]. Possible etiologies included tobacco smoking ($n=13$), phenacetin abuse ($n=2$), and external beam radiation 15 years prior ($n=1$), but no definite causation can be established from this small number of cases. The pathogenesis of MPC needs to be studied in a systematic and controlled manner.

Clinical Presentation

Gross hematuria is the most common presenting symptom of MPC in both the bladder and the upper tracts. Bladder MPC can also present with microscopic hematuria, urinary obstruction, dysuria, suprapubic pain, urgency, frequency, recurrent urinary tract infections, or suspicious findings on surveillance cystoscopy for prior urothelial carcinoma [1, 4, 9, 14]. Upper tract MPC can present with flank pain, microscopic hematuria, hydronephrosis, or abnormal urine cytology [6, 8]. Two patients presented with metastatic disease and were diagnosed by biopsy of an enlarged left supraclavicular node [4] or cervical node [8].

Cystoscopic/Clinical Examination Findings

The diagnosis of MPC is made almost exclusively on pathologic examination of a surgical specimen. No findings on cystoscopic or clinical examination are pathognomonic for MPC. On cystoscopy, MPC may appear as an exophytic papillary tumor not appreciably different from standard urothelial carcinoma. In some cases, MPC may spread within the lamina propria and be undetectable by cystoscopy because the overlying bladder mucosa appears normal, even after the disease becomes metastatic [14]. This tendency toward submucosal spread may partially explain the high progression rates with bladder preservation strategies. If the urologist is misled by a normal cystoscopy, he may recommend continued surveillance for patients that actually have extensive submucosal spread of disease. Because this pattern of spread occasionally exists, we recommend against surveillance by cystoscopy only in patients with a history of MPC. These patients should undergo random bladder biopsies for surveillance, even with normal-appearing bladders.

Clinical evaluation of MPC should be similar to typical urothelial carcinoma. Once the pathologic diagnosis of MPC has been made on a specimen from transurethral resection of a bladder tumor (TURBT), the patient should receive a comprehensive evaluation for signs of local invasion or metastatic disease. Creatinine, electrolytes, liver enzymes, and lactate dehydrogenase should be checked for signs of organ dysfunction or paraneoplastic syndromes. A three-phase CT of the abdomen and pelvis should be obtained with special attention given to the excretory phase to rule out upper tract tumors. We recommend routine chest CT instead of chest X-ray on initial evaluation for metastatic disease after the diagnosis of MPC because of the aggressive nature and rapid spread of this entity. The results of these evaluations may demonstrate that curative surgery is not possible. Unfortunately, metastatic disease is frequently identified pathologically after surgery even in the absence of identifiable disease spread by these testing modalities.

Pathology

Establishing a minimal threshold for classification of a urothelial carcinoma as micropapillary type is the most significant problem in the pathologic

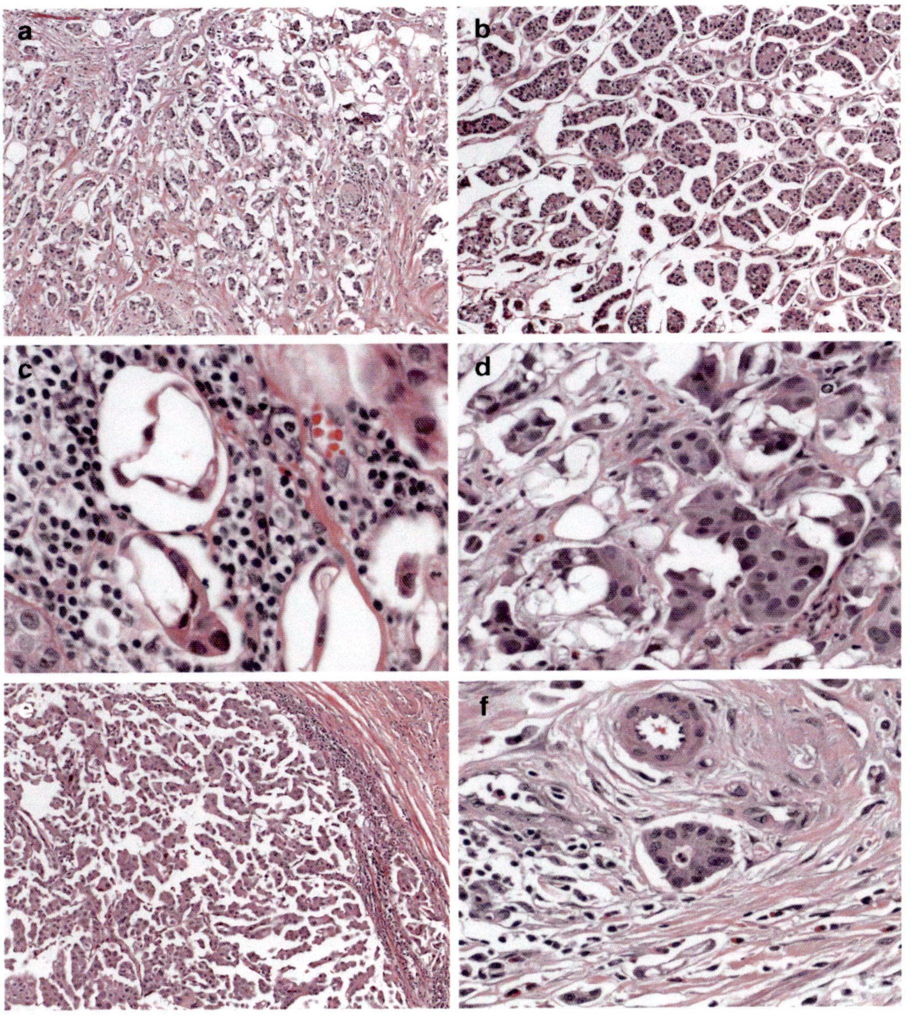

Fig. 8.1 Histologic features of micropapillary carcinoma. (**a**) Back-to-back, confluent lacunar spaces. (**b**) Multiple tumor nests in the same lacunar space. (**c**) Epithelial ring forms. (**d**) Intracytoplasmic vacuoles. (**e**) Elongated papillae. (**f**) Peripheral orientation of nuclei

diagnosis of MPC. One of the histologic hallmarks of MPC is the presence of stromal retraction spaces surrounding the nests of carcinoma cells (Fig. 8.1a–f). Unfortunately, this feature is not entirely specific as many invasive urothelial carcinomas of no special type share this feature (Fig. 8.2a, b) [18, 20]. The cellular nests of MPC are typically quite small, but there is a wide spectrum of nest sizes that may be encountered in urothelial carcinomas, making the establishment of definitive criteria based entirely on size problematic. In a recent interobserver reproducibility study by Sangoi et al., a set of restrictive criteria were proposed that allowed for a greater degree of agreement (Table 8.1) [20]. These restrictive criteria identify a group of more prototypical MPCs that include cases with small tumor cell nests within stromal retraction spaces, which are often back-to-back and often contain multiple tumor cell nests within each single retraction space (see Fig. 8.1a, b). Other secondary features that are frequently seen include epithelial ring forms, intracytoplasmic vacuolization, elongated epithelial nests (i.e., micropapillae), and peripherally

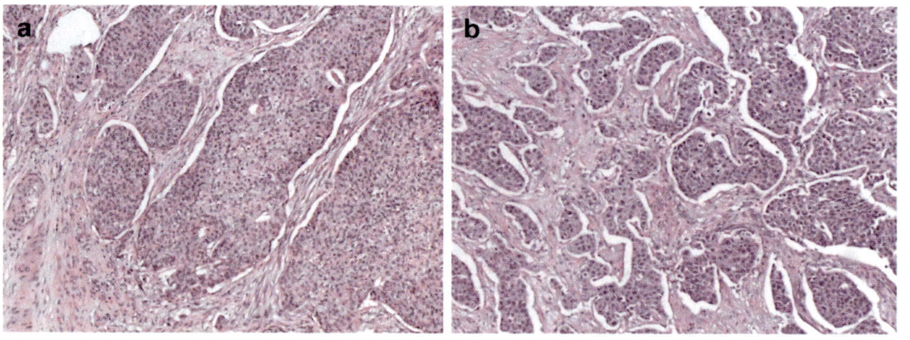

Fig. 8.2 Histologic features of typical urothelial carcinoma with retraction (non-micropapillary). (**a**) Large epithelial nests (>5 cells across narrowest width). (**b**) Confluent and branching epithelial growth

Table 8.1 Recommended histologic features for micropapillary vs. non-micropapillary carcinoma

Restrictive criteria for micropapillary carcinoma	Features of typical (non-micropapillary) urothelial carcinoma with retraction
Primary features	Primary features
Multiple small nests in single retraction space	Large nest size (≥5 nuclei across the narrowest width of the nest)
Often back-to-back lacunar spaces	Large branching or confluent aggregates of neoplastic epithelium
Secondary features frequently present	Secondary features frequently present
Epithelial ring forms	Individual single nests in a retraction space
Intracytoplasmic vacuolization Peripherally oriented nuclei	Individual lacunar spaces widely separated by stroma

oriented nuclei (see Fig. 8.1c–f). Microscopic features suggesting that a urothelial carcinoma should not be classified as micropapillary include large nest size (generally greater than 5 or more nuclei across the narrowest width of the nest) and large branching aggregates or epithelial confluence of the tumor cell aggregates (see Fig. 8.2a, b).

Noninvasive patterns of micropapillary carcinoma are also seen and are characterized by thin elongated filiform processes of neoplastic cells arising from the main papillary stalk (Fig. 8.3a–c) [1]. These "micropapillae" in the noninvasive component typically have a longer length than width. In our experience, these micropapillary patterns in noninvasive urothelial carcinomas are often admixed with histologic patterns previously described as glandular or villoglandular [21, 22] The distinction between noninvasive carcinomas with villo/glandular and micropapillary features, and any potential clinical significance to this distinction, has not been evaluated.

Several studies have proposed the potential utility of adjunctive immunohistochemical markers in the diagnosis of MPC. A "reverse polarity" pattern of immunoreactivity with the MUC1 antibody, whereby the stroma-facing (basal) cell surfaces acquire apical secretory properties, has been previously reported as typical of MPC [23–26]. Similarly, immunohistochemical expression of CA125 and Her2Neu has been reported as distinctive for MPC [9, 17, 27, 28]; however, Sangoi et al. have previously reported that these markers are not entirely specific for MPC when compared specifically to invasive urothelial carcinomas with prominent stromal retraction (specificity: MUC1 37%, CA125 87%, and Her2Neu 92%) [18]. As such, these markers lack reliable diagnostic utility in challenging cases, especially

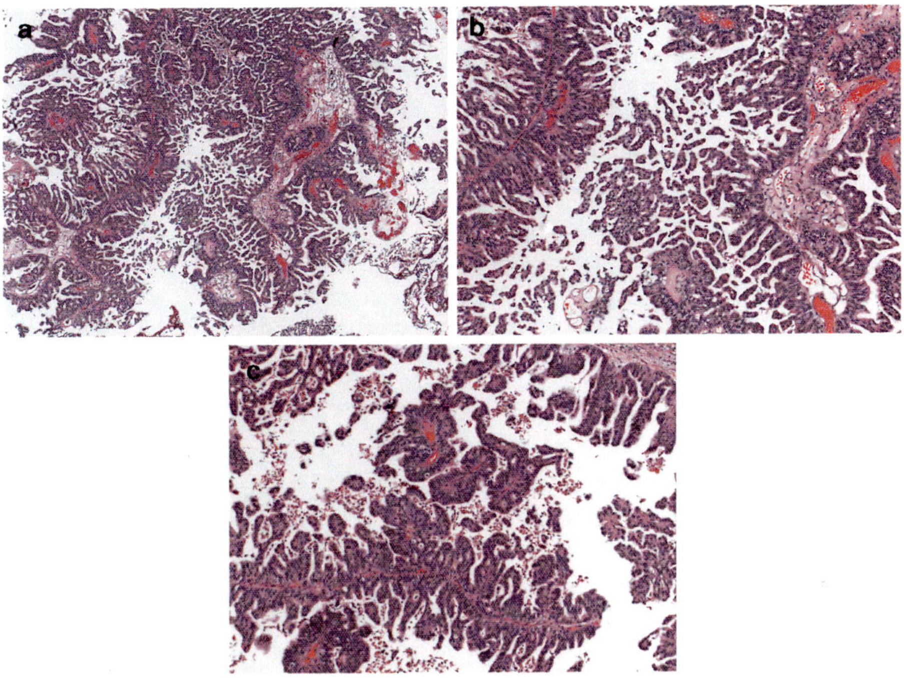

Fig. 8.3 Noninvasive papillary urothelial carcinoma with micropapillary features. (**a**, **b**) Elongated slender micropapillae arising from the papillary core (the length of the elongated epithelial structures is generally greater than the width). (**c**) In some cases, there is an admixture of tumor with features previously described as noninvasive papillary urothelial carcinoma with glandular/villoglandular differentiation. This combination is frequent in our experience, and the distinction between glandular/villoglandular and micropapillary may be very difficult in a subset of cases

since it is our experience that invasive urothelial carcinoma with associated stromal retraction is much more common than MPC. Although KL-6 is another antibody that has recently been reported as a sensitive marker of urothelial MPC, further studies are needed to compare specificity versus invasive urothelial carcinoma with prominent stromal retraction [29]. At present, we would recommend that the diagnosis of MPC should be based on histologic features, and we suggest use of the restrictive criteria proposed by Sangoi et al. given the potential therapeutic impact of the diagnosis (see Table 8.1) [20].

In cases presenting with metastatic disease, the most problematic pathologic issue is establishing the anatomic site of origin, since many parenchymal organs may give rise to carcinomas with an identical micropapillary appearance. In general, carcinomas with a micropapillary pattern maintain the expected immunophenotypic findings of more histologically typical carcinomas of similar anatomic origin [23].

Management

The management of MPC is determined by its aggressive nature with immediate cystectomy being the preferred treatment for nearly all stages. Since understaging is very common, the management of pTa and pT1 disease is difficult and remains somewhat controversial. In the largest published series, 75% of patients who underwent immediate cystectomy for clinically localized disease had a pathologic stage that was higher than their clinical stage, and 38% had pathologically positive nodes [11]. The overall survival of the 44 patients who presented with nonmuscle invasive disease was no better than the 37 who presented with invasive but resectable disease. In another series of 34 patients with ≤T1 on TURBT and CT, 71% were ≥T2 and 26% were T4 at cystectomy [2]. Even the patients with the lowest stage (cTa) had a 25% mortality rate from metastatic disease at a mean survival of 33 months. A low percentage of MPC also should not dissuade one from aggressive surgical management as metastasis and death have been reported even in patients with less than 10% MPC [2, 3].

Retrospective studies suggest that intravesical Bacillus Calmette Guérin (BCG) therapy is ineffective in patients with MPC. BCG is attenuated live *Mycobacterium bovis* which can be instilled in the bladder to prevent progression and recurrence of nonmuscle invasive bladder cancer. In the sentinel article on BCG in MPC, Kamat et al. reviewed the records of 44 patients with nonmuscle invasive MPC, of whom 27 received BCG [12]. Of these 27 patients, 18 (67%) progressed to ≥T2 and 6 (22%) developed metastatic disease during treatment. Only 5 (19%) were cancer free without cystectomy at 30 months median follow-up. The median cancer-specific survival for patients who had a cystectomy only after BCG failed was 62 months compared with more than 10 years for those who had immediate cystectomy without BCG. In another study, all 7 patients who were treated initially with BCG were ≥T3a at cystectomy, and all but one had lymph node metastases [19]. These dismal results suggest that conservative management with BCG should not be offered to patients with invasive MPC.

No prospective trials of chemotherapy for MPC have been performed, but the limited available retrospective data suggest minimal benefit. The choice of chemotherapy regimens seems to have been driven by the urothelial component of the disease with most patients receiving either MVAC (methotrexate, vinblastine, doxorubicin, and cisplatin) or GC (gemcitabine and cisplatin). Response rates were poor overall with many patients progressing and dying of their disease. In the largest series, 23 of 100 patients received neoadjuvant chemotherapy for surgically resectable disease [11]. At cystectomy, those who received neoadjuvant chemotherapy were more likely to have ≥pT3 (68.7%) than those who underwent immediate cystectomy (34.8%). The 5-year overall survival was no better for neoadjuvant chemotherapy patients (63%) than for immediate cystectomy patient (71%). In the same series, of 19 patients who received chemotherapy for unresectable disease, 10 patients had an objective response and were then able to undergo cystectomy, but their median overall survival was 28 months. In the series by Ghoneim et al. [19], all three patients that received neoadjuvant GC had extensive residual disease (≥pT3 or pN+) at cystectomy. The one patient who received MVAC never reached cystectomy because he died of febrile neutropenia. Three series reported follow-up for a combined total of 31 patients who received adjuvant chemotherapy, mostly for node-positive histology at cystectomy [7, 11, 19]. Of these patients, only 6 (19%) were alive at last follow-up, and the median survival in the one study reporting it was 40 months with a 40% 5-year overall survival [19]. Several other studies reported small numbers of patients receiving chemotherapy as neoadjuvant, adjuvant, or primary treatment, and most of these patients experienced progression or death [1, 6, 8, 9, 14].

MPC tumors likely do not respond to radiation therapy, based on very limited data. Only 14 patients have been reported who received radiation with or without chemotherapy for MPC in the absence of cystectomy or nephroureterectomy and have follow-up available. All of these patients died of their disease except one who was alive with disease at only 6 months of follow-up [1, 7, 9, 14]. A few patients have received radiation after cystectomy or nephroureterectomy, but the reporting of these patients is too inconsistent to draw any conclusions. More data are necessary before any firm conclusions can be drawn about the efficacy of radiation therapy for MPC.

Immediate cystectomy is generally the treatment of choice for all invasive MPC. This recommendation comes from the apparent lack of efficacy of BCG, chemotherapy, and radiation therapy, the frequent understaging observed at TURBT, and two retrospective studies showing improved survival from immediate cystectomy vs. other treatment modalities [11, 19]. Patients with noninvasive papillary urothelial carcinoma showing micropapillary features (pTa disease) should be aggressively restaged to ensure adequate evaluation and followed very closely for recurrence/progression. Although some studies have included a few cases of pTa micropapillary carcinoma, it has not been adequately shown that these cases have a higher progression compared to otherwise typical noninvasive high-grade papillary urothelial carcinoma. Importantly, there has not been sufficient study of the appropriate histologic criteria for a diagnosis as noninvasive micropapillary carcinoma to warrant its use for changing the current standard clinical management for pTa disease. In our experience, classifying a noninvasive papillary carcinoma as micropapillary can be difficult and is subject to significant intraobserver variability, especially when the histologic changes are present only focally. There would seem to be a much greater risk of overtreatment in this group of noninvasive tumors.

Lymph node dissection at the time of cystectomy is important for prognostication, but there is no evidence for or against a lymph node dissection being therapeutic in these patients. Lymph node metastases are frequently missed on imaging in this population. In the studies reporting results from lymph node dissections for clinically node negative disease, 54 (52%) of 103 patients had positive lymph nodes [7, 11, 19]. This significantly changes the treatment options and prognosis for patients otherwise thought to be curable with or without bladder sparing.

Outcomes

The overall 5-year survival was approximately 38% across all studies reporting this outcome (248 patients). This was improved to 70% overall 5 year survival and 52% overall 10-year survival for those who had immediate cystectomy for resectable disease in one study [11]. Delaying cystectomy for other treatments was associated with decreased overall survival (OS). The 5-year cancer-specific survival for patients who presented with ≤cT1 and had cystectomy after failed BCG was 60% (median survival 62 months) versus 72% (median survival not reached) for those who underwent an immediate cystectomy. Median OS for ≥cT2 but resectable disease was 62 months with neoadjuvant chemotherapy and more than 180 months for those who had initial cystectomy in one study [11], and 23 vs. 46 months in another study [19]. Higher stage at presentation, as expected, led to decreased survival [2]. The median OS was 17 months for those with unresectable disease [11].

A greater percent of the tumor made up of MPC portended a worse prognosis in several studies [1–4, 9]. Patients are usually grouped into <10% MPC, 10–50% MPC, and >50% MPC. Those with >50% MPC typically fare the worst, but the association is weak and does not stand up to multivariate analysis [2].

Metastases are found most commonly in the lung, followed by liver and bone. They have also been described in the peritoneum, mesentery, sigmoid colon, brain, ureters, chest wall, scrotum, and nodes of the pelvis, retroperitoneum, paraaortic, inguinal, and supraclavicular areas [4, 6–9, 14, 15, 30].

Micropapillary carcinoma is an aggressive variant of urothelial carcinoma of the bladder or upper tracts. The limited studies published to date suggest that immediate radical surgery is the safest treatment choice for attempting to achieve long-term survival for these patients. Randomized controlled trials are needed to definitively answer many remaining questions about this rare entity.

References

1. Amin MB, Ro JY, el-Sharkawy T, Lee KM, Troncoso P, Silva EG, et al. Micropapillary variant of transitional cell carcinoma of the urinary bladder. Histologic pattern resembling ovarian papillary serous carcinoma. Am J Surg Pathol. 1994;18:1224–32.
2. Comperat E, Roupret M, Yaxley J, Reynolds J, Varinot J, Ouzaid I, et al. Micropapillary urothelial carcinoma of the urinary bladder: a clinicopathological analysis of 72 cases. Pathology. 2010;42:650–4.
3. Alkibay T, Sozen S, Gurocak S, Isik Gonul I, Poyraz A, Ure I. Micropapillary pattern in urothelial carcinoma: a clinicopathological analysis. Urol Int. 2009; 83:300–5.

4. Alvarado-Cabrero I, Sierra-Santiesteban FI, Mantilla-Morales A, Hernandez-Hernandez DM. Micropapillary carcinoma of the urothelial tract. A clinicopathologic study of 38 cases. Ann Diagn Pathol. 2005;9:1–5.
5. Domanowska E, Jozwicki W, Domaniewski J, Golda R, Skok Z, Wisniewska H, et al. Muscle-invasive urothelial cell carcinoma of the human bladder: multidirectional differentiation and ability to metastasize. Hum Pathol. 2007;38:741–6.
6. Guo CC, Tamboli P, Czerniak B. Micropapillary variant of urothelial carcinoma in the upper urinary tract: a clinicopathologic study of 11 cases. Arch Pathol Lab Med. 2009;133:62–6.
7. Heudel P, El Karak F, Ismaili N, Droz JP, Flechon A. Micropapillary bladder cancer: a review of Leon Berard Cancer Center experience. BMC Urol. 2009;9:5.
8. Holmang S, Thomsen J, Johansson SL. Micropapillary carcinoma of the renal pelvis and ureter. J Urol. 2006;175:463–6; discussion 6–7.
9. Johansson SL, Borghede G, Holmang S. Micropapillary bladder carcinoma: a clinicopathological study of 20 cases. J Urol. 1999;161:1798–802.
10. Jozwicki W, Domaniewski J, Skok Z, Wolski Z, Domanowska E, Jozwicka G. Usefulness of histologic homogeneity estimation of muscle-invasive urinary bladder cancer in an individual prognosis: a mapping study. Urology. 2005;66:1122–6.
11. Kamat AM, Dinney CP, Gee JR, Grossman HB, Siefker-Radtke AO, Tamboli P, et al. Micropapillary bladder cancer: a review of the University of Texas M. D. Anderson Cancer Center experience with 100 consecutive patients. Cancer. 2007;110:62–7.
12. Kamat AM, Gee JR, Dinney CP, Grossman HB, Swanson DA, Millikan RE, et al. The case for early cystectomy in the treatment of nonmuscle invasive micropapillary bladder carcinoma. J Urol. 2006;175:881–5.
13. Lopez-Beltran A, Montironi R, Blanca A, Cheng L. Invasive micropapillary urothelial carcinoma of the bladder. Hum Pathol. 2010;41(8):1159–64.
14. Maranchie JK, Bouyounes BT, Zhang PL, O'Donnell MA, Summerhayes IC, DeWolf WC. Clinical and pathological characteristics of micropapillary transitional cell carcinoma: a highly aggressive variant. J Urol. 2000;163:748–51.
15. Perez-Montiel D, Hes O, Michal M, Suster S. Micropapillary urothelial carcinoma of the upper urinary tract: clinicopathologic study of five cases. Am J Clin Pathol. 2006;126:86–92.
16. Perez-Montiel D, Wakely PE, Hes O, Michal M, Suster S. High-grade urothelial carcinoma of the renal pelvis: clinicopathologic study of 108 cases with emphasis on unusual morphologic variants. Mod Pathol. 2006;19:494–503.
17. Samaratunga H, Khoo K. Micropapillary variant of urothelial carcinoma of the urinary bladder; a clinicopathological and immunohistochemical study. Histopathology. 2004;45:55–64.
18. Sangoi AR, Higgins JP, Rouse RV, Schneider AG, McKenney JK. Immunohistochemical comparison of MUC1, CA125, and Her2Neu in invasive micropapillary carcinoma of the urinary tract and typical invasive urothelial carcinoma with retraction artifact. Mod Pathol. 2009;22:660–7.
19. Ghoneim IA, Miocinovic R, Stephenson AJ, Garcia JA, Gong MC, Campbell SC, et al. Neoadjuvant systemic therapy or early cystectomy? single-center analysis of outcomes after therapy for patients with clinically localized micropapillary urothelial carcinoma of the bladder. Urology. 2011;77:867–70.
20. Sangoi AR, Beck AH, Amin MB, Cheng L, Epstein JI, Hansel DE, et al. Interobserver reproducibility in the diagnosis of invasive micropapillary carcinoma of the urinary tract among urologic pathologists. Am J Surg Pathol. 2010;34:1367–76.
21. Lim M, Adsay NV, Grignon D, Osunkoya AO. Urothelial carcinoma with villoglandular differentiation: a study of 14 cases. Mod Pathol. 2009; 22(10):1280–6. Epub 2009 Jul 10. PubMed PMID: 19593329.
22. Miller JS, Epstein JI. Noninvasive urothelial carcinoma of the bladder with glandular differentiation: report of 24 cases. Am J Surg Pathol. 2009;33(8):1241–8. PubMed PMID: 19440144).
23. Lotan TL, Ye H, Melamed J, Wu XR, Shih Ie M, Epstein JI. Immunohistochemical panel to identify the primary site of invasive micropapillary carcinoma. Am J Surg Pathol. 2009;33:1037–41.
24. Munakata S, Tahara H, Kojima K, Kishimoto T. Micropapillary urothelial carcinoma of the renal pelvis: report of a case and review of the literature. Med Sci Monit. 2007;13:CS47–52.
25. Nassar H, Pansare V, Zhang H, Che M, Sakr W, Ali-Fehmi R, et al. Pathogenesis of invasive micropapillary carcinoma: role of MUC1 glycoprotein. Mod Pathol. 2004;17:1045–50.
26. Ohtsuki Y, Ochi K, Okada Y, Kato M, Lee GH, Furihata M. Micropapillary component of urothelial carcinoma detected in transurethral resection of bladder tumor (TUR-BT) tissues: a case report. Med Mol Morphol. 2008;41:113–6.
27. Kuroda N, Tamura M, Ohara M, Hirouchi T, Mizuno K, Miyazaki E. Invasive micropapillary carcinoma of the urinary bladder: an immunohistochemical study of neoplastic and stromal cells. Int J Urol. 2006; 13:1015–8.
28. Zhang H, Ali-Fehmi R, Bianco F. Characteristic immunohistochemical profiles and aggressive behavior of micropapillary and other histological variants and subtypes of urothelial carcinoma. Mod Pathol. 2004;17(Suppl 1):186A (782).
29. Ohtsuki Y, Kuroda N, Umeoka T, Watanabe R, Ochi K, Okada Y, et al. KL-6 is another useful marker in assessing a micropapillary pattern in carcinomas of the breast and urinary bladder, but not the colon. Med Mol Morphol. 2009;42:123–7.
30. Amin MB. Histological variants of urothelial carcinoma: diagnostic, therapeutic and prognostic implications. Mod Pathol. 2009;22 Suppl 2:S96–118.

Small Cell Urothelial Carcinoma

9

Anil Parwani, Colin Dinney, and Arlene Siefker-Radtke

Introduction

Small cell urothelial cancer is a rare form of bladder cancer for which there is no standard therapy. The majority of available literature, mostly in the form of small retrospective reviews, encompasses a range of treatment from surgery, radiation, and chemotherapy, given in a variety of sequences and combinations. As a result, surgery has been considered by many to be the de facto standard in the setting of surgically resectable disease [1, 2]. While occasional long-term survivors have been reported with these approaches, the universally poor outcomes typically observed have left many to consider it a disease where treatment is futile [3]. However, more recently published data, including the first clinical trial in small cell urothelial cancer, are providing new-found hope, with the potential for improved outcomes using neoadjuvant chemotherapy followed by surgery [4–6].

A. Parwani (✉)
University of Pittsburgh Medical Center Shadyside, 5230 Centre Avenue, West Wing Ground Floor, Room 07, Pittsburgh, PA 15232, USA
e-mail: parwaniav@upmc.edu

C. Dinney
Department of Urology, The University of Texas M.D. Anderson Cancer Center, 1515 Holcombe Boulevard, Unit 1373, Houston, TX 77030, USA
e-mail: cdinney@mdanderson.org

A. Siefker-Radtke
Department of Genitourinary Medical Oncology, The University of Texas M.D. Anderson Cancer Center, 1155 Herman Pressler, Unit 1374, Houston, TX 77030, USA
e-mail: asiefker@mdanderson.org

Clinical Presentation

The presentation of small cell urothelial cancer is virtually indistinguishable from the more traditional transitional cell urothelial cancer. Most patients present with hematuria and irritative voiding symptoms including dysuria, frequency, and, depending upon its location, urinary obstruction and renal insufficiency [2]. Since this variant, like small cell tumors of the lung and prostate, typically is associated with a rapid rate of proliferation, symptoms can progress quite rapidly. Therefore, it is imperative that the patient evaluation proceeds quickly in order to initiate therapy, thereby avoiding the development of complications and/or metastases.

Pathogenesis

As with urothelial carcinoma (UC) small cell carcinoma can occur anywhere along the urinary tract. However, the majority of tumors occur in the bladder with only rare occurrences in the ureter [5]. Care should be made to distinguish tumors occurring along the urethra from small cell carcinoma of the prostate gland. Since many small cell carcinomas arise in the setting of urothelial

D.E. Hansel et al. (eds.), *The Urinary Tract: A Comprehensive Guide to Patient Diagnosis and Management*,
DOI 10.1007/978-1-4614-5320-8_9, © Springer Science+Business Media New York 2012

carcinoma, abnormalities of the urothelium, including papillary urothelial carcinoma and urothelial carcinoma in situ (CIS), support the diagnosis of urothelial origin [4, 7, 8]. Likewise, small cell carcinomas of the prostate often arise in the setting of prostate cancer with associated elevation in prostate-specific antigen (PSA). However, elevations in PSA can be seen with urethral tumors invading the prostate, so an abnormal PSA alone, without supportive pathology, should be interpreted with caution.

Though the origin of small cell carcinoma of the urothelial tract is not definitively known, many theories regarding the development of these tumors have been proposed [9–12]. The presence of neuroendocrine markers and neurosecretory granules has been used to support a theory that small cell tumors arise from the malignant transformation of neuroendocrine cells found sporadically in the bladder mucosa next to the basal lamina. Similarly, a second theory postulates that these tumors arise from metaplasia of the urothelial epithelium, with small cell carcinoma representing a high-grade form of divergent differentiation. In an additional attempt to explain the coexistence of small cell carcinoma with urothelial tumors, a third theory hypothesizes the origin from a multipotential stem cell capable of differentiating along multiple lineages. Loss of heterozygosity studies in a small series of small cell carcinomas coexisting with urothelial carcinoma suggest their origination from a common, clonal precursor [13]. Though a consensus may not be reached regarding the histogenesis of small cell carcinomas, once present, they display an extremely aggressive biology, similar to small cell carcinomas of other organs.

Clinical Evaluation and Cystoscopy

The clinical evaluation is, again, similar to that for traditional urothelial tumors. Diagnosis is typically made only after the pathology is reviewed from cystoscopic resection. Since recent data suggest an increased risk of brain metastases in patients with ≥stage 3 small cell carcinoma (≥cT3b, N^+, or M^+) [5], it is important to complete staging prior to beginning therapy. In addition to the traditional radiographic imaging with computed tomography (CT) or magnetic resonance imaging (MRI) of the abdomen and pelvis, as well as imaging of the chest (CT, MRI, or chest X-ray), the authors would advocate for a thorough transurethral resection of tumor, followed by an exam under anesthesia (EUA) to document the potential risk for tumor invading beyond the wall of the bladder or adherence to the pelvic sidewall. A baseline CT or MRI of the brain in patients with stage 3 or greater small cell urothelial cancer is also recommended.

Pathology

Gross Pathology

Most of the small cell carcinomas of the urinary tract arise in the urinary bladder with only rare reports of small cell carcinoma in other areas of the urothelial tract [4, 5]. They usually present as large mass lesions and may arise in all regions of the bladder, including bladder diverticula [14]. There are no distinguishing characteristics between small cell urothelial cancer and the more traditional urothelial carcinomas on gross pathology. Grossly, the tumor may appear ulcerated, nodular (Fig. 9.1), infiltrative, sessile, or solid [14, 15].

Microscopic Pathology

Consistent with their pulmonary counterparts, the diagnosis of small cell urothelial cancer is typically made on the basis of morphology [8, 11]. However, the bladder tumors often have one or more other types of tumor components such as urothelial carcinoma, squamous cell carcinoma, adenocarcinoma, or sarcomatoid carcinomas [8, 11, 15]. A component of urothelial CIS may be present, which is helpful to confirm urothelial origin [5, 7, 14–16] (Fig. 9.2).

At low magnification, the tumor has a diffuse growth of small to intermediate sized round blue cells with hyperchromatic nuclei. Rarely, the

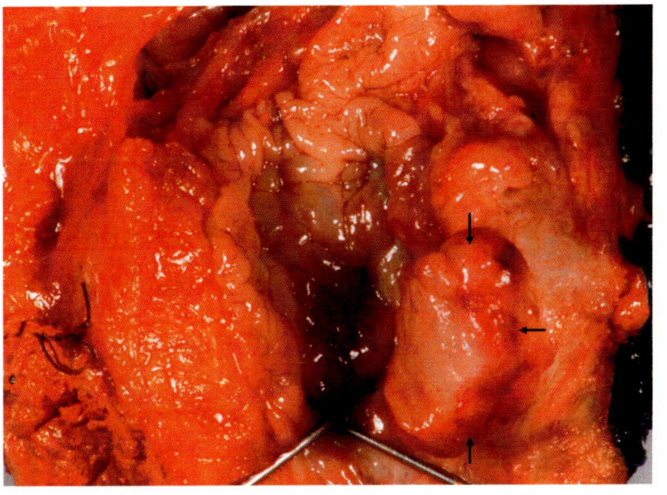

Fig. 9.1 Gross appearance of a pure small cell carcinoma of the urinary bladder. The tumor was a pedunculated exophytic mass located in the left anterior wall of the bladder and grossly and microscopically involved the detrusor muscle (*arrows*)

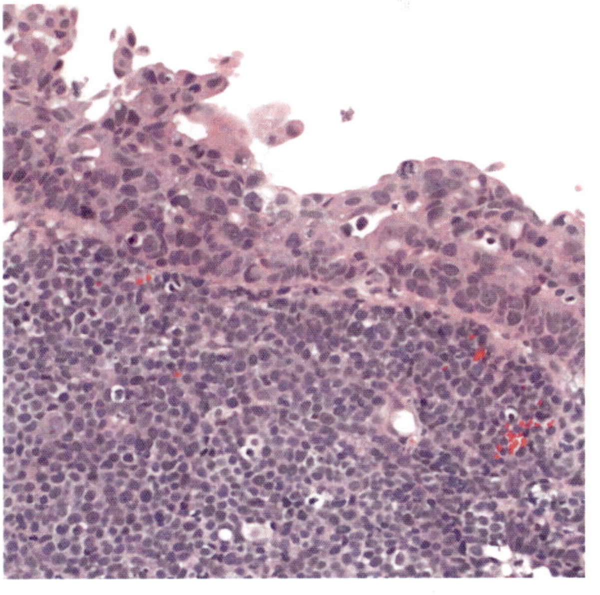

Fig. 9.2 Small cell carcinoma with associated flat urothelial carcinoma in situ (CIS). In this case, small cell carcinoma was the only component present, making the identification of flat CIS an important diagnostic feature. Note the enlarged nuclei and cells with high nuclear to cytoplasmic ratio in the CIS component

tumors show a nested or organoid growth pattern. On higher magnification, small, uniform cells with nuclear molding and scant cytoplasm are present (Figs. 9.2 and 9.3). The nuclei contain evenly dispersed finely stippled chromatin and inconspicuous nucleoli. Mitoses and apoptotic debris are easily seen and usually frequent. Occasionally, scattered larger pleomorphic cells may be present. Necrosis, crush artifact, and vascular invasion are also commonly seen. DNA encrustation of blood vessel walls may be present (Azzopardi phenomenon) [8, 11, 15–17]. The majority of the tumors also show detrusor muscle (muscularis propria) invasion [2, 4, 5, 7].

The neuroendocrine origin may be demonstrated in a number of ways, including the use of electron microscopy or histochemical stains to show the presence of neuroendocrine granules. However, the most commonly employed method is by performing immunohistochemistry (IHC)

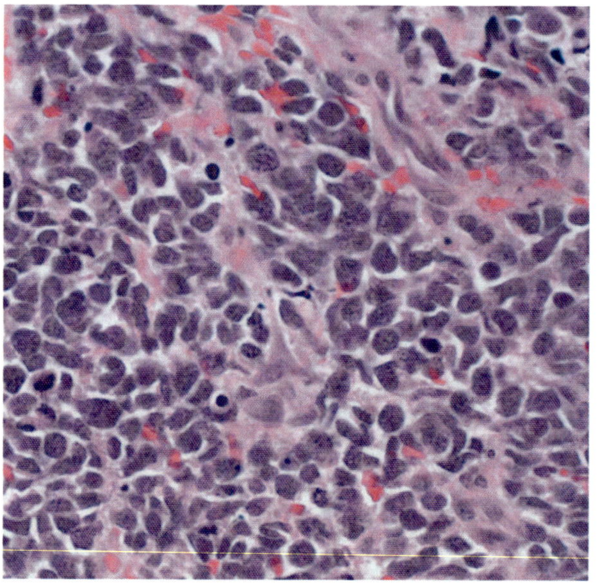

Fig. 9.3 Small cell carcinoma with an infiltrative appearance and with uniform cells with scant cytoplasm and showing characteristic nuclear molding

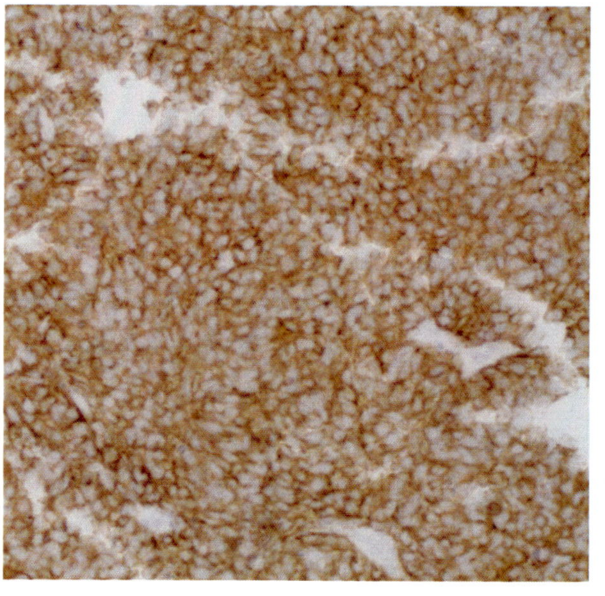

Fig. 9.4 Synaptophysin immunohistochemistry shows strong and diffuse staining in a case of bladder small cell carcinoma

for chromogranin, synaptophysin (Fig. 9.4), and cytokeratin (dot-like staining) (Fig. 9.5) [8, 9, 11, 16]. Recent studies suggest that P16 and P63 IHC may be useful in distinguishing small cell carcinomas from poorly differentiated urothelial carcinomas with P16 expression higher in small cell carcinomas of the bladder (92.8%) compared to high-grade urothelial carcinomas (43.7%). In contrast, P63 was positive in the majority of urothelial carcinomas (81.3%) and negative in small cell carcinomas [18].

Large cell neuroendocrine carcinomas have also been described in the urinary bladder. It is not uncommon for areas with more abundant cytoplasm and prominent nucleoli (Fig. 9.6), which would meet the definition for large cell neuroendocrine carcinoma in the lung, to be admixed with typical small cell carcinoma. This

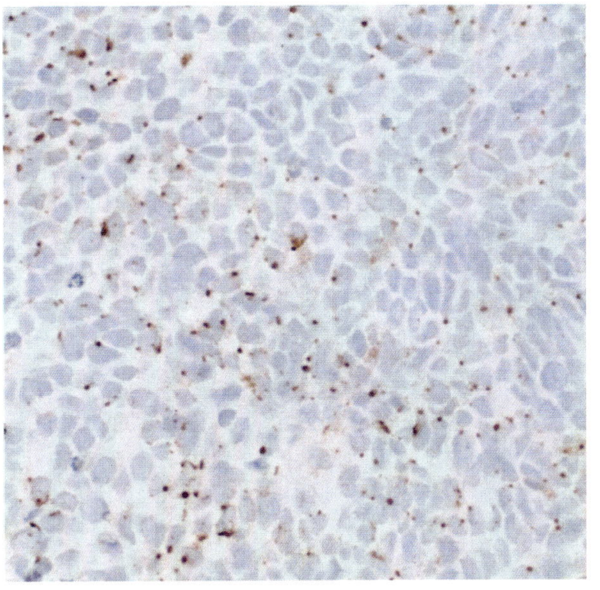

Fig. 9.5 Cytokeratin immunohistochemistry shows "dot-like" positivity in a case of bladder small cell carcinoma

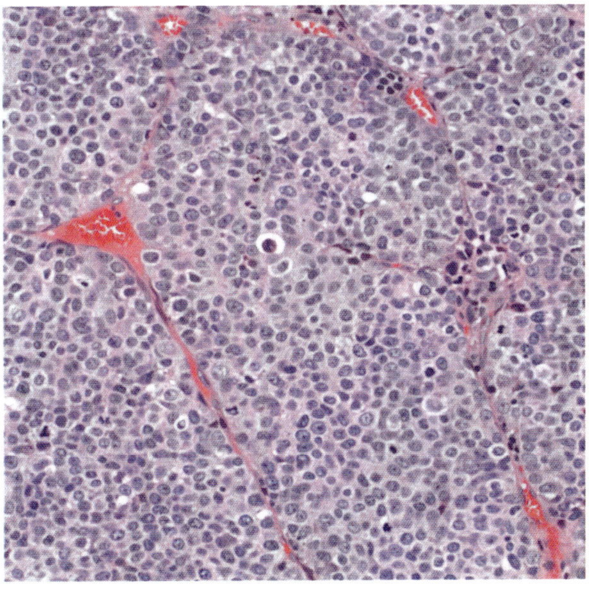

Fig. 9.6 Large cell neuroendocrine carcinoma of the urinary bladder. Compared to small cell carcinoma, the large cell neuroendocrine carcinomas may have distinct architecture such as a nested or an organoid growth pattern. The cells have more abundant cytoplasm and the nuclei, as seen in this case, are more prominent

distinction is not critical in the bladder as treatment remains the same, and there has been no notable survival difference observed when large cell neuroendocrine histology is present [7].

Differential Diagnosis

The differential diagnosis of small cell carcinomas is broad and includes entities such as malignant lymphoma, lymphoepithelioma-like carcinoma, poorly differentiated urothelial carcinoma, plasmacytoid variant of urothelial carcinoma, or, more infrequently, metastatic small cell carcinoma from other sites such as the lung [15, 16]. Usually a patient's history and clinical information, including radiographic imaging, are sufficient to determine if a metastasis to the bladder is a consideration. The presence of a concurrent urothelial component or even the presence of urothelial CIS helps to confirm a urothelial origin. Overall, knowledge of the clinical information, history, and appropriate use of ancillary studies including immunohistochemical stains can be extremely helpful in the diagnostic process.

Management

While the treatment for metastatic small cell carcinoma generally has focused on systemic chemotherapy, the treatment for surgically resectable disease has been evolving. In recognition that surgery alone led to few long-term disease specific survivors, many institutions began incorporating multimodality treatment regimens combining systemic therapy with radiation and surgery. Recent evidence suggests that neoadjuvant chemotherapy followed by surgery may be the optimal treatment paradigm, at least as compared with historical data.

Surgically Resectable Disease

Historically, radical cystectomy was considered the de facto treatment for patients with surgically resectable disease [1]. However, since many patients treated with this strategy died within 1 year of diagnosis, the prognosis, even in the setting of surgically resectable disease, was invariably poor. Clinical understaging of the primary tumor is often the rule. In one large series, the pathologic stage was higher than expected in 56% of patients treated with initial cystectomy [4]. Furthermore, surgery was aborted in the operating room in 20% of those deemed surgical candidates, despite a median time of 24 days from diagnosis to surgery [4]. Other groups report only a 10–16% 5-year survival with cystectomy [3, 7], with up to 76% of patients with surgically resectable small cell carcinomas having metastases at the time of cystectomy [7]. Furthermore, Cheng et al. reported no difference in survival between those who did or did not undergo cystectomy for surgically resectable disease [3]. It is extremely likely that the rapid growth rates and high likelihood of microscopic metastases associated with small cell carcinoma contribute to the observed clinical understaging typically associated with this malignancy.

In contrast to the poor outcomes with initial surgery observed by other centers, a recent report from the Mayo Clinic advocates for surgery alone in the setting of surgically resectable small cell urothelial cancer [2]. They report a 3-year OS of 63.6% in 12 patients with stage 2 small cell urothelial cancer; however, half of these patients experienced a relapse. It is not altogether clear how many patients were upstaged at surgery; 73% of the reported patients had stage 3 or 4 disease at surgery with uniformly poor outcomes in this stage. While it remains an unanswered question whether there is a benefit from adjuvant treatment in a patient with an incidental finding of pT2N0M0 small cell cancer at cystectomy, the preponderance of literature currently reports the significant risk of pathologic upstaging at cystectomy that inevitably leads to poor outcomes when following an approach of surgery alone.

As a result of the poor outcomes observed with cystectomy alone, investigators began to integrate and combine chemotherapy with surgery. Early reports suggested a median survival of 21.1 months after incorporating adjuvant chemotherapy [19], with another suggesting 4 of 5 survivors (of 19 total patients) when cystectomy was followed by adjuvant chemotherapy [11]. However, despite an improved overall and recurrence-free survival with multimodality therapy as compared to cystectomy alone, 5-year survival remained around 10% [7]. Likewise, there was no difference in survival reported by the M. D. Anderson Cancer Center (MDACC) with the addition of adjuvant chemotherapy [4]. However, it should be noted that the lack of uniformity in treatment, especially regarding the choice of chemotherapy regimens, could impact the reported utility of adjuvant chemotherapy. As a result, and in light of the poor prognosis from surgery alone, many investigators continue to offer adjuvant chemotherapy, especially when small cell carcinoma is diagnosed at cystectomy.

With the knowledge that small cell cancer can be a chemosensitive disease and after observing the rapid tumor growth rates leading to aborted cystectomy, investigators at the MDACC altered their strategy. Neoadjuvant chemotherapy became the strategy of choice [4]. The benefits of this, in retrospect, seem quite obvious. Systemic chemotherapy can typically be initiated quickly, providing timely control of this rapidly proliferating tumor and hopefully resulting in tumor downstaging and negative margins at surgery. This strategy may also provide valuable prognostic information; the MDACC series suggests no tumor-related deaths in those ≤pT2N0M0 following neoadjuvant chemotherapy [4].

In another report of neoadjuvant chemotherapy, Walther et al. reported 5 of 7 patients alive and cancer free more than 36 months after combined modality treatment; of these 7 patients, 5 were treated with preoperative chemotherapy [6]. Additional promising results were reported by the MDACC. In this review of 46 patients, neoadjuvant chemotherapy was associated with an improved survival, with a 5-year disease-specific survival of 78%, as compared to 36% 5-year disease-specific survival in those treated with initial surgery ($p=0.03$) [4]. While many different chemotherapy combinations were used in this retrospectively treated group of patients, there was a sense that chemotherapy combinations directed to the small cell phenotype, such as etoposide with cisplatin, and ifosfamide with adriamycin, were more likely to eradicate the small cell carcinoma component.

Recently, investigators at the MDACC published results from the first clinical trial in small cell urothelial cancer [5]. Patients with surgically resectable small cell urothelial cancer (≤cT4aN0M0) received four cycles of neoadjuvant chemotherapy with ifosfamide and adriamycin alternating with etoposide and cisplatin. Of 18 patients receiving neoadjuvant treatment, 13 (72%) remain alive and cancer free with a median overall survival of 58 months. Pathologic downstaging to <pT1N0M0 occurred in 14 of 18 patients (78%). Patients with cT2N0M0 tumors fared much better than those with cT3b-4aN0M0 disease. Since the majority of patients with cT3b-4aN0M0 tumors still had viable small cell cancer remaining at the time of surgery, it is not certain whether this reflects aggressive biology in the setting of a larger tumor burden, or an inadequate course of chemotherapy. Currently, the authors are recommending four cycles neoadjuvant chemotherapy with a small cell carcinoma-directed regimen in cT2N0M0 disease, and two cycles beyond maximal response (typically closer to six cycles chemotherapy) in patients with cT3b-4aN0M0 small cell urothelial cancer.

Drawing upon the experience of small cell lung cancer, investigators have employed radiation therapy as a focal consolidative measure in patients with localized disease. Some small series have reported long-term survivors with chemotherapy followed by radiation to the pelvis [20–22]; however, the median overall survival reported is on the order of 17–20 months [21, 22]. One of the most promising reports observed a median survival of 41 months with a 70% disease-specific survival in 10 patients with localized disease treated with chemoradiation [23]. However, 60% of their long-term survivors developed recurrent local disease and required further treatment, including cystectomy. A similar scenario, with additional localized relapses, has been reported in other series [21, 22]. This supports the growing observation that many small cell carcinomas of the urinary bladder arise in the setting of urothelial carcinoma with urothelial carcinoma in situ (CIS) reported in anywhere from 56 to 76% of patients [5, 7]. With concern for the long-term risk of recurrent localized cancer in those with intact, irradiated bladders, the authors currently advocate for cystectomy (after neoadjuvant chemotherapy) as the localized therapy of choice. However, in a setting where surgery is associated with unacceptable risk to the patient, the authors would recommend consolidation (after neoadjuvant chemotherapy) with radiation.

Metastatic Disease

Unfortunately, the prognosis in the setting of metastatic disease remains poor with few long-term survivors. The median survival in the metastatic setting closely reflects that reported with small cell lung cancer, and small cell tumors of other organs, like the prostate [24], with a median life expectancy ranging from 7.5 to 15 months [4, 5, 19]. Some long-term survivors have been reported, mostly in the setting of patients with lymph node metastases who respond completely to chemotherapy and undergo surgical consolidation with cystectomy and node dissection [4, 5]. The authors' current strategy is to treat to two cycles beyond maximal response using a small cell chemotherapy regimen such as etoposide and cisplatin and then offer surgical consolidation for those who wish to take an aggressive approach with node-only disease and have a clinically complete response to chemotherapy.

Brain Metastases and Prophylactic Cranial Irradiation

Brain metastases have been only rarely reported in the setting of small cell urothelial cancer. While this could indicate a lack of awareness or monitoring for this possibility, it is equally likely that with the historically poor outcomes, patients typically did not live long enough to develop symptomatic brain metastases. Interestingly, in the recently reported small cell urothelial cancer clinical trial, investigators noted an incidence of symptomatic brain metastases on the order of 50% in the subset of patients with stage 3 or 4 urothelial cancer [5]. None of the patients with stage 2 disease developed brain metastases. Furthermore, 88% of those developing brain metastases had no progressive tumor elsewhere. This may reflect the close follow-up associated with a clinical trial, and the routine use of a small cell chemotherapy regimen that may better control the tumor in other metastatic sites. As a result, investigators at MDACC are now offering prophylactic cranial irradiation on a clinical trial to the subset of patients with stage 3 or 4 small cell urothelial cancer.

Conclusion

Small cell urothelial cancer is a rare tumor of the bladder whose diagnosis can be made based upon morphologic features with adjunctive immunohistochemical studies, including chromogranin and synaptophysin. Currently, there is no standard therapy for the treatment of small cell urothelial cancer. Recently published data from the first phase II clinical trial in this rare tumor suggest that for patients with surgically resectable disease (≤cT4aN0M0) neoadjuvant chemotherapy followed by cystectomy/cystoprostatectomy provides a higher likelihood of survival as compared with historical data. Use of a chemotherapy regimen directed toward the small cell cancer component, such as etoposide with cisplatin, is recommended. Chemotherapy followed by local consolidation with radiation may be a reasonable alternative, especially in patients who are not surgical candidates. However, the frequent presence of CIS and higher relapse rates, including local failure in the bladder, suggest that consolidation with surgery may provide more optimal control. The prognosis in the setting of metastatic small cell urothelial cancer remains poor, with few long-term survivors. The higher incidence of brain metastases observed in the setting of stage 3–4 disease suggests a subset of patients for whom prophylactic cranial irradiation may be considered. Substantial work is required in this rare tumor to optimize chemotherapy, local consolidation, and determine the role for radiation.

References

1. Sternberg CN, Swanson DA. Non-transitional cell bladder cancer. In: Raghavan D, Scher HI, Leiber SA, Lange P, editors. Principles and practice of genitourinary oncology. Philadelphia: Lippincott - Raven Publishers; 1997. p. 322–3.
2. Choong NW, Quevedo JF, Kaur JS. Small cell carcinoma of the urinary bladder. The Mayo Clinic experience. Cancer. 2005;103(6):1172–8.
3. Cheng L, Pan CX, Yang XJ, Lopez-Beltran A, MacLennan GT, Lin H, et al. Small cell carcinoma of the urinary bladder: a clinicopathologic analysis of 64 patients. Cancer. 2004;101(5):957–62.
4. Siefker-Radtke AO, Dinney CP, Abrahams NA, Moran C, Shen Y, Pisters LL, et al. Evidence supporting preoperative chemotherapy for small cell carcinoma of the bladder: a retrospective review of the M. D. Anderson cancer experience. J Urol. 2004;172(2):481–4.
5. Siefker-Radtke AO, Kamat AM, Grossman HB, Williams DL, Qiao W, Thall PF, et al. Phase II clinical

trial of neoadjuvant alternating doublet chemotherapy with ifosfamide/doxorubicin and etoposide/cisplatin in small-cell urothelial cancer. J Clin Oncol. 2009; 27(16):2592–7.

6. Walther PJ. Adjuvant/neo-adjuvant etoposide/cisplatin and cystectomy for management of invasive small cell carcinoma of the bladder. J Urol. 2002;167(4):285.
7. Quek ML, Nichols PW, Yamzon J, Daneshmand S, Miranda G, Cai J, et al. Radical cystectomy for primary neuroendocrine tumors of the bladder: the university of southern california experience. J Urol. 2005;174(1):93–6.
8. Abrahams NA, Moran C, Reyes AO, Siefker-Radtke A, Ayala AG. Small cell carcinoma of the bladder: a contemporary clinicopathological study of 51 cases. Histopathology. 2005;46(1):57–63.
9. Blomjous CE, Vos W, De Voogt HJ, Van der Valk P, Meijer CJ. Department of Pathology FUHATN. Small cell carcinoma of the urinary bladder. A clinicopathologic, morphometric, immunohistochemical, and ultrastructural study of 18 cases. Cancer. 1989;64(6): 1347–57.
10. Sved P, Gomez P, Manoharan M, Civantos F, Soloway MS. Small cell carcinoma of the bladder. BJU Int. 2004;94(1):12–7.
11. Grignon DJ, Ro JY, Ayala AG, Shum DT, Ordâoänez NG, Logothetis CJ, et al. Small cell carcinoma of the urinary bladder. A clinicopathologic analysis of 22 cases. Cancer. 1992;69(2):527–36.
12. Christopher ME, Seftel AD, Sorenson K, Resnick MI. Small cell carcinoma of the genitourinary tract: an immunohistochemical, electron microscopic and clinicopathological study. J Urol. 1991;146(2):382–8.
13. Cheng L, Jones TD, McCarthy RP, Eble JN, Wang M, MacLennan GT, et al. Molecular genetic evidence for a common clonal origin of urinary bladder small cell carcinoma and coexisting urothelial carcinoma. Am J Pathol. 2005;166(5):1533–9.
14. Tamas EF, Stephenson AJ, Campbell SC, Montague DK, Trusty DC, Hansel DE. Histopathologic features and clinical outcomes in 71 cases of bladder diverticula. Arch Pathol Lab Med. 2009;133(5):791–6.
15. Amin MB. Histological variants of urothelial carcinoma: diagnostic, therapeutic and prognostic implications. Mod Pathol. 2009;22 Suppl 2:S96–118.
16. Pant-Purohit M, Lopez-Beltran A, Montironi R, MacLennan GT, Cheng L. Small cell carcinoma of the urinary bladder. Histol Histopathol. 2010;25(2): 217–21.
17. Ismaili N, Arifi S, Flechon A, El Mesbahi O, Blay JY, Droz JP, et al. Small cell cancer of the bladder: pathology, diagnosis, treatment and prognosis. Bull Cancer. 2009;96(6):E30–44.
18. Buza N, Cohen PJ, Pei H, Parkash V. Inverse p16 and p63 expression in small cell carcinoma and high-grade urothelial cell carcinoma of the urinary bladder. Int J Surg Pathol. 2010;18(2):94–102.
19. Abbas F, Civantos F, Benedetto P. Small cell carcinoma of the bladder and prostate. Urology. 1995;46(5):617–30.
20. Bastâus R, Caballero JM, Gonzâalez G, Borrat P, Casalots J, Gomez de Segura G. Small cell carcinoma of the urinary bladder treated with chemotherapy and radiotherapy: results in five cases. Eur Urol. 1999; 35(4):323–6.
21. Bex A, de Vries R, Pos F, Kerst M, Horenblas S. Long-term survival after sequential chemoradiation for limited disease small cell carcinoma of the bladder. World J Urol. 2009;27(1):101–6.
22. Asmis TR, Reaume MN, Dahrouge S, Malone S. Genitourinary small cell carcinoma: a retrospective review of treatment and survival patterns at the Ottawa Hospital Regional Cancer Center. BJU Int. 2006; 97(4):711–5.
23. Lohrisch C, Murray N, Pickles T, Sullivan L, British Columbia Cancer Agency VBCC. Small cell carcinoma of the bladder: long term outcome with integrated chemoradiation. Cancer. 1999;86(11): 2346–52.
24. Papandreou CN, Daliani DD, Thall PF, Tu SM, Wang X, Reyes A, et al. Results of a phase II study with doxorubicin, etoposide, and cisplatin in patients with fully characterized small-cell carcinoma of the prostate. J Clin Oncol. 2002;20(14):3072–80.

10 Squamous Cell Carcinoma

Donna E. Hansel and Amr Fergany

Introduction

In addition to urothelial carcinoma, adenocarcinoma, and small cell carcinoma, squamous cell carcinoma represents a major morphologic subtype of bladder cancer that harbors unique pathogenetic and molecular alterations. In the United States, squamous cell carcinoma affects less than 5% of all bladder cancer patients, with primary risk factors that include tobacco smoke, long-term catheterization, urinary tract calculi, and a nonfunctioning bladder [1]. A male predominance is common (approximate 3:1 male:female ratio) and patients tend to be older (>60 years of age). Squamous cell carcinoma may also occur in the upper tract, with this form of carcinoma representing up to 10% of all renal pelvis carcinomas and also likely incited by chronic inflammatory conditions [2–4]. In contrast to the bladder, upper tract squamous cell carcinoma tends to have a roughly equal proportion of men and women affected by the disease [3].

D.E. Hansel (✉)
Department of Pathology, Cleveland Clinic, 9500 Euclid Avenue Desk L25, Cleveland, OH 44195, USA
e-mail: Hanseld@ccf.org

A. Fergany
Sections of Oncology, Laparoscopy and Robotics, Cleveland Clinic, Glickman Urological and Kidney Institute, 9500 Euclid Avenue, Q10, Cleveland, OH 44195, USA
e-mail: Fergana@ccf.org

In other regions of the world—such as Africa and portions of the Middle East—squamous cell carcinoma occurs at a much higher frequency and affects a larger proportion of bladder cancer patients. In Egypt, bladder cancer represents approximately 30% of all cancers and is the leading cancer cause in males and the second leading cancer cause in females [5]. A primary risk factor in these locations includes infection with the *Schistosoma* ("bilharzial") parasite, whose eggs lodge in the bladder wall and are believed to represent a source of chronic bladder inflammation that ultimately leads to the development of carcinoma. Patients with schistosomal-derived squamous carcinoma are generally younger (46.7 years) and have a slightly higher male:female ratio (5:1) [6]. Current estimates from the National Cancer Institute in Egypt suggest that there has been a reduction in schistosomal-associated bladder cancer between the years 1977 and 2007, with bladder cancer frequency declining from 27.6 to 11.7% and schistosomal-associated bladder cancer declining from 82.4 to 55.3% [7]. This likely reflects improved control over schistosomal infection in rural populations; however, squamous cell carcinoma remains the most common type of bladder cancer in these regions.

Squamous cell carcinoma of the urinary tract thus reflects two distinct etiologies—infectious and noninfectious—that ultimately share similar morphological features, albeit varied clinical presentations. Despite these differing etiologies, overall patient management for this disease

D.E. Hansel et al. (eds.), *The Urinary Tract: A Comprehensive Guide to Patient Diagnosis and Management*, DOI 10.1007/978-1-4614-5320-8_10, © Springer Science+Business Media New York 2012

remains similar, although more information is available for cancers arising within the bladder.

Pathogenesis

A variety of factors can incite the development of squamous cell carcinoma of the bladder, with a common element including the ability to induce chronic irritation and inflammation of the bladder wall and upper tract (Table 10.1). Additionally, upper tract squamous cell carcinoma has been associated with analgesic abuse with phenacetin [2].

Tobacco smoke—a common risk factor for all forms of urinary tract cancer—has been estimated to increase the risk of squamous cell carcinoma by fivefold over that of nonsmokers [8], with increasing risk associated with increasing duration of exposure [9]. Although the direct molecular alterations associated with tobacco smoke and squamous cell carcinoma development are unknown, the carcinogenic properties of tobacco and its metabolites are well recognized for all forms of bladder cancer. Patients with nonfunctional bladders or those who undergo chronic catheterization are at increased risk for the development of carcinoma likely due to the presence of urinary stasis and resultant injury and inflammation of the surrounding bladder wall, which may result in increased cell turnover and subsequent genetic alterations. This hypothesis appears similar to that proposed for the increased risk of squamous cell carcinoma arising within bladder diverticula [10].

Human papillomavirus (HPV) infection has been well studied in bladder squamous cell carcinoma [11–14]. Analysis of both low- and high-risk HPV subtypes in large series of non-schistosomal squamous cancers has yielded few positive cases and HPV is generally not considered to be a primary pathogenic mechanism of disease, although very few upper tract cancers have been evaluated [15]. Despite these findings, a handful of patients with extensive, recurrent condylomata of the urinary tract have been reported to develop squamous cell carcinoma at various sites along the urinary tract [12, 16].

Perhaps one of the best studied risk factors in the development of squamous cell carcinoma of the bladder is infection with the schistosomal parasite, including *Schistosoma haematobium*, *Schistosoma mansoni*, and *Schistosoma japonicum*, with *S. haematobium* most commonly associated with the development of bladder cancer. The schistosomal parasite is a trematode worm that circulates in the bloodstream, resulting in portal hypertension and deposition of parasitic eggs within the mucosa and submucosa of the bladder (Fig. 10.1). These eggs ultimately become calcified and can incite an inflammatory reaction characterized by granulomas, as well as associated neutrophils, eosinophils, and lymphocytes.

Schistosomal infection has been present in Egypt since at least 1900 BCE, with the finding of calcified eggs in Egyptian mummies and historical documentation of hematuria within the population since this time [17]. An increased prevalence of infection occurred after the building of dams (in the southern part of Egypt) to control seasonal flooding of the Nile. The Aswan dam was built in the early part of the twentieth century, and a second larger dam, the High Dam, was concluded in 1971. These irrigation projects were intended primarily to provide a sustained predictable source of irrigation water to the fertile soil of the Nile Valley, and avoid the destruction caused by annual flooding, as well as droughts and poor crops during low flood years. As a result of the absence of flooding, the critical intermediate host for bilharzial worm (*Bulinus* sp. snails) was now in a year-round permanent irrigation system and proliferated during the dry season. Permanent and stagnant water also increased aquatic plant life, which provided a habitat for these snails.

Several recent studies have focused on the role of schistosomal antigens in inducing squamous carcinoma of the bladder. Total antigen from *S. haematobium*, obtained by extraction of whole worms, was found to increase cell proliferation, prolong S-phase, decrease apoptosis, and promote migration of Chinese hamster ovary (CHO) cells [18, 19]. Furthermore, total antigen was found to downregulate the tumor suppressor p27 and increase the proapoptotic

Table 10.1 Risk factors in the development of squamous cell carcinoma of the bladder

Nonschistosomal	
Tobacco smoke	Risk factor for all forms of bladder cancer; carcinogenic effect
Nonfunctioning bladder	Well-recognized risk factor; likely results in carcinoma due to increased urinary stasis and inflammation
Chronic catheterization	Well-recognized risk factor; both chronic and intermittent catheterization have been associated with squamous carcinoma
Diverticula	Increased risk of developing squamous cell carcinoma, likely due to urinary stasis
Condyloma acuminatum	Rare; generally develops into invasive carcinoma in patients with extensive condylomata
Schistosomal (bilharzial)	
Schistosoma haematobium	Most commonly associated with squamous cell carcinoma
Schistosoma mansoni	Less commonly implicated
Schistosoma japonicum	Less commonly implicated

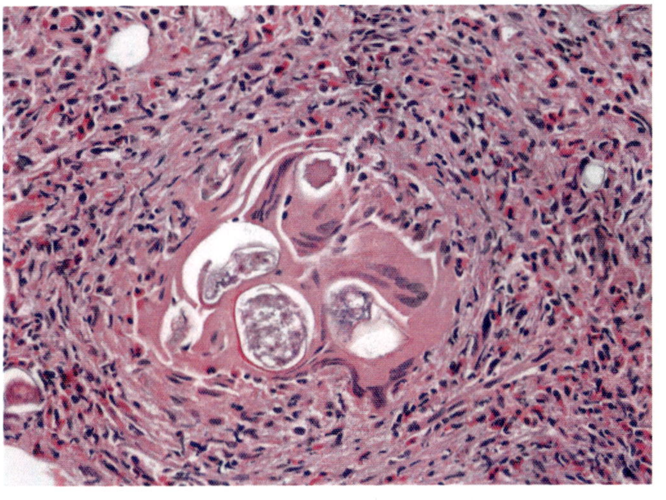

Fig. 10.1 Schistosomal infection of the bladder is often characterized by calcified eggs or portions of parasite that incite an inflammatory reaction consisting of giant cells and abundant eosinophils

Bcl-2 molecule [19]. Instillation of total antigen into the bladders of CD-1 mice appeared to promote urothelial inflammation and dysplasia [20], suggesting a direct link between antigen exposure and early tumorigenesis. The downstream mediators of total antigen, however, remain to be determined.

Clinical Presentation

The clinical presentation of patients with squamous cell carcinoma differs from that of patients with urothelial cancer. Most patients with squamous cancer present with severe, unrelenting symptoms associated with cystitis (frequency, urgency, dysuria, strangury), commonly described as an exacerbation of longstanding lower urinary symptoms. Lower abdominal or pelvic pain is common, and sometimes severe. Hematuria as the sole presenting symptom is uncommon, in contrast to urothelial cancers where the presenting symptom is usually painless gross hematuria. Patients with schistosomal squamous carcinoma occasionally present with necroturia, or the passage of whitish necrotic pieces of tumor, with urination. This presentation is more common in patients with verrucous carcinoma, where parts of the significantly necrotic bulk of the tumor shed into the urine.

Patients commonly present with a large, easily palpable pelvic or abdominal bladder mass. Such bladder masses are usually painful and tender, allowing easy clinical distinction from urothelial cancer, which is rarely, if ever, painful or tender on clinical evaluation. Most patients with squamous carcinoma present in advanced stages of disease, likely due to the long-standing nature of lower urinary symptoms making patients delay seeking medical attention. It is estimated that about 25% are inoperable at presentation [21], and the majority (80%) are T3 or higher at surgery [16, 22].

Cystoscopic/Clinical Examination Findings

Diagnostic and staging evaluation for squamous cell carcinoma is similar to urothelial tumors. Large pelvic/abdominal masses are more common in this disease and often noted on computed tomography (CT) scans or other sectional imaging. On plain abdominal films, irregular intraluminal calcification (on the surface of the tumor) suggests carcinoma, and an irregular filling defect is usually noted on cystography. Such findings are less commonly noted today, as these older tests have become superseded by more modern axial imaging. Metastatic lymphadenopathy is less common than in urothelial carcinoma—particularly when the bulky size of the primary tumor is considered—suggesting a more locally aggressive natural history for the disease.

Cystoscopy with biopsy remains the confirmatory diagnostic procedure. Squamous cell carcinoma, particularly the schistosomal variety, usually appears as a nodular fungating mass and less commonly as an ulcerative lesion. *Verrucous carcinoma* is a unique well-differentiated variety of schistosomal squamous cell carcinoma that appears as a whitish fibrillary mass due to extensive keratinization, and carries a more favorable prognosis [23]. Unlike urothelial carcinoma, deep biopsies to include bladder wall muscularis are generally not historically mandated when squamous cell carcinoma is suspected, as treatment options do not depend upon depth of bladder wall involvement, rather on the pathological diagnosis of the tumor alone. However, due to the concern of a urothelial carcinoma with extensive squamous differentiation on incomplete sampling and new staging guidelines recommending muscularis propria evaluation on bladder cancer staging, sampling of this layer of the bladder wall may be prudent.

Pathology

The diagnosis of primary squamous cell carcinoma of the urinary bladder is restricted to lesions whose invasive component consists purely of squamous cell carcinoma. Since urothelial carcinomas may show extensive squamous differentiation, this distinction may be difficult in a subset of cases, particularly in biopsy samples. The presence of associated noninvasive squamous lesions may assist in the classification of a lesion as squamous in nature; however, the acceptance of foci of noninvasive urothelial neoplasia—such as urothelial carcinoma in situ—in cases diagnosed as primary squamous cell carcinoma has recently been proposed and will be discussed in further detail later [16]. Ultimately, the distinction between pure squamous cell carcinoma and urothelial carcinoma with squamous differentiation on biopsy or transurethral resection (TUR) may not be possible. Although foci of conventional urothelial carcinoma admixed with squamous differentiation on biopsy or TUR favor a urothelial carcinoma with divergent differentiation, only complete sampling of a carcinoma at radical cystectomy can truly diagnose a pure squamous cell carcinoma.

On gross examination, squamous cell carcinoma may appear as an exophytic, white, flaky mass or as an ulcerated region involving the urinary tract lining. Squamous cell carcinoma is graded in a similar manner to squamous cancers at other sites: well, moderately, and poorly differentiated (Figs. 10.2a–c). Typically, the most poorly differentiated area of the lesion is considered when categorizing these lesions, with differentiation characterized by organization of the squamous nests and the formation of keratin

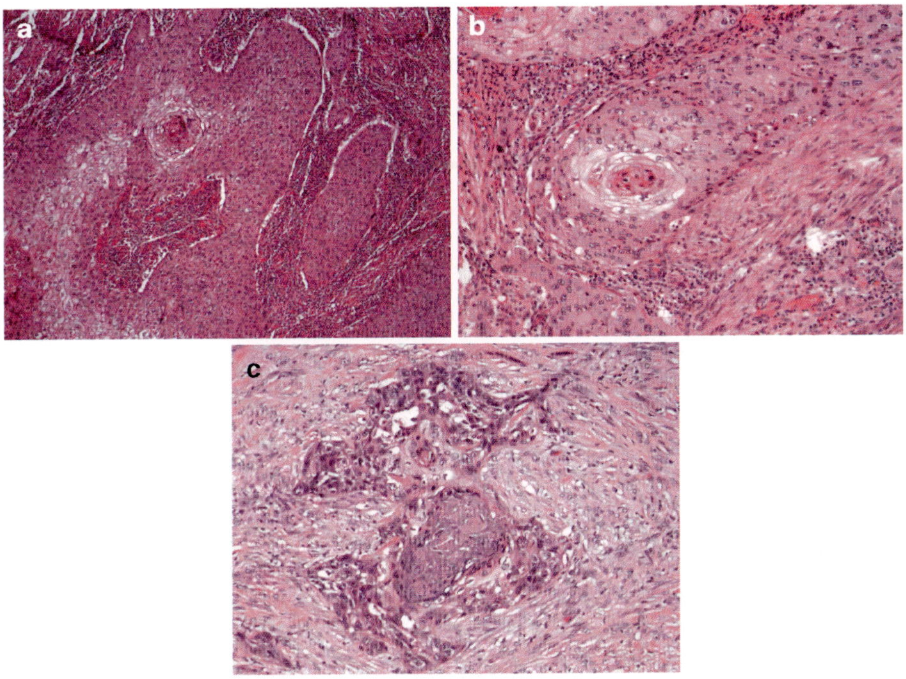

Fig. 10.2 (**a**) Well-differentiated squamous cell carcinoma demonstrates glassy eosinophilic cytoplasm, intercellular bridges, and abundant keratin. (**b**) The majority of bladder squamous carcinomas are considered moderately differentiated with variable keratin formation and atypia. (**c**) Poorly differentiated squamous cell carcinoma contains scant keratin and may be difficult to differentiate from poorly differentiated urothelial carcinoma

pearls. Approximately 60% of all carcinomas are moderately differentiated, with the remainder being poorly differentiated (30%) and few cases being well differentiated (10%). Regardless of the extent of differentiation, areas that have recognizable squamous differentiation can usually be identified and are defined by eosinophilic cytoplasm, intracellular desmosomes, and keratin formation. Additional histological findings associated with these carcinomas include necrosis, a desmoplastic tissue response (Fig. 10.3a), and a foreign-body giant cell reaction to keratin (Fig. 10.3b). Perineural invasion and angiolymphatic invasion occur in approximately 15–20% of cases. Rarely, squamous cell carcinomas may take on a more unusual appearance that includes bizarre atypia of the cancerous cells (Fig. 10.4a), a sarcomatoid or spindled appearance (Fig. 10.4b), the development of pseudocystic or "pseudoangiomatous" structures, large nest formation with central necrosis and clear cell features (Fig. 10.4c). Generally, however, areas that resemble more classical squamous cell carcinoma can be found within the specimen that ensures the correct diagnosis.

Verrucous carcinoma represents an uncommon but distinct variant of squamous cell carcinoma that commonly occurs in patients with schistosomal infection. At low magnification, the carcinoma demonstrates an exophytic, papillary appearance with the deep aspect demonstrating a rounded "pushing" appearance (Fig. 10.5). Overall, the carcinomas lack significant atypia at the architectural or cytologic level and have been suggested to carry a more favorable prognosis, although rigorous study of this form of bladder carcinoma has not been performed.

A variety of precursor lesions have been associated with the development of squamous cell carcinoma. Classic precursors include keratinizing squamous metaplasia, squamous dysplasia, and squamous cell carcinoma in situ (Fig. 10.6a, b).

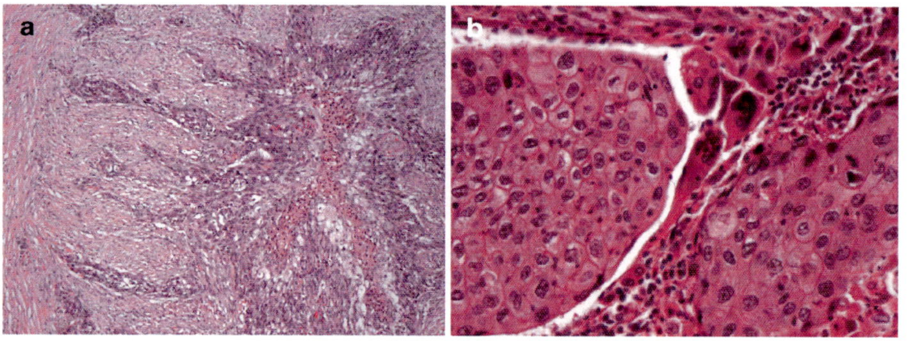

Fig. 10.3 (**a**) Desmoplasia is frequently associated with squamous cell carcinoma of the bladder. (**b**) A giant cell reaction to keratin may be readily identified in some tumors

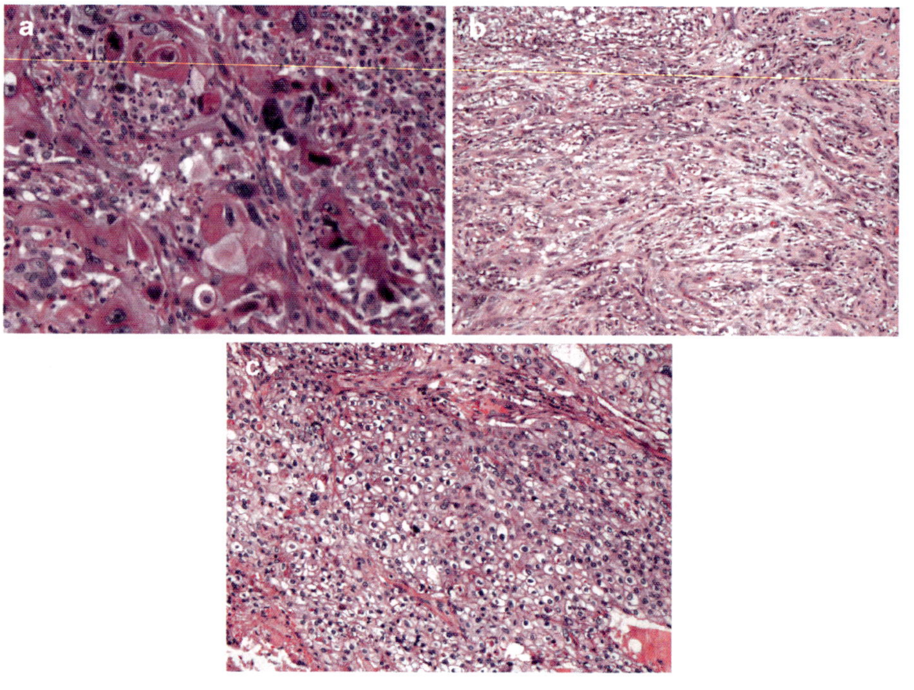

Fig. 10.4 (**a**) Bizarre atypia of squamous carcinoma cells is a rare, but distinctive feature, in a subset of cases. (**b**) Occasionally, squamous cell carcinoma may demonstrate a prominent spindled or sarcomatoid appearance. (**c**) Rarely, cytoplasmic clearing may give a squamous cell carcinoma an unusual microscopic appearance. The finding of intercellular bridges and keratin validates the diagnosis

Verrucous squamous hyperplasia, characterized by repetitive upward tenting of the bladder surface that contains squamous metaplasia with marked keratin formation, has been recently reported as associated with invasive squamous cell carcinoma (Fig. 10.7). Exophytic squamous lesions may also be identified and include both polypoid and papillary-like structures lined by atypical squamous epithelium. In rare instances, condyloma acuminatum may be associated with invasive squamous cell carcinoma, although this is generally an exception, with only a few cases reported in the literature. Similar to condylomata at other sites, lesions in the bladder are defined by exophytic papillary-

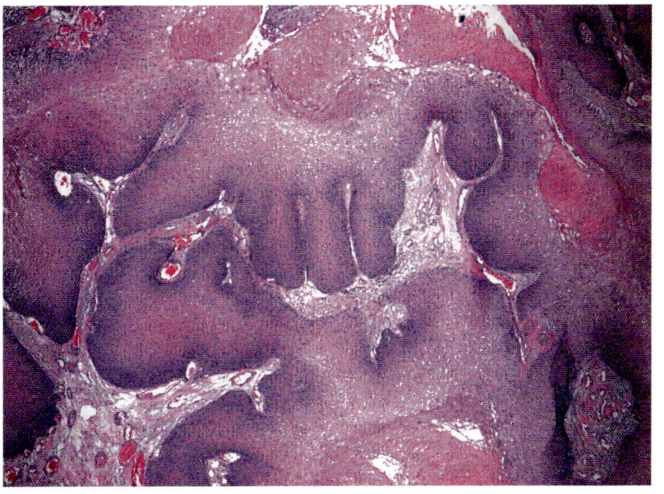

Fig. 10.5 Verrucous carcinoma is characterized by large, pushing invasive fronts associated with well-differentiated carcinoma

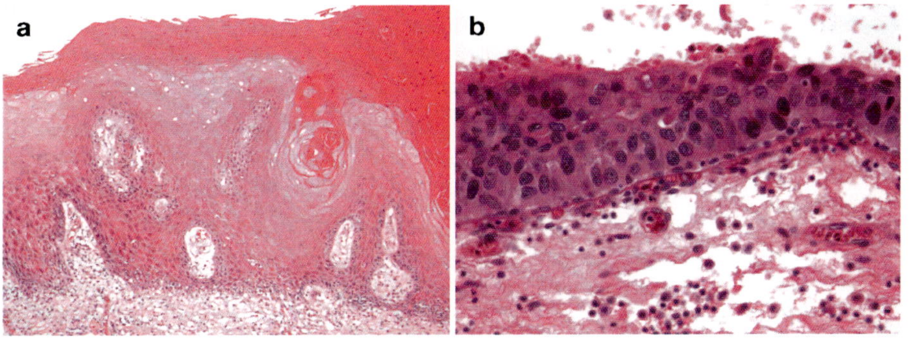

Fig. 10.6 (**a**) Keratinizing squamous metaplasia is commonly found in association with squamous cell carcinoma. (**b**) Squamous carcinoma in situ (high grade dysplasia) demonstrates marked nuclear atypia and disorganization of the epithelial layer. Prominent eosinophilic cytoplasm and defined cell–cell borders support a squamous morphology

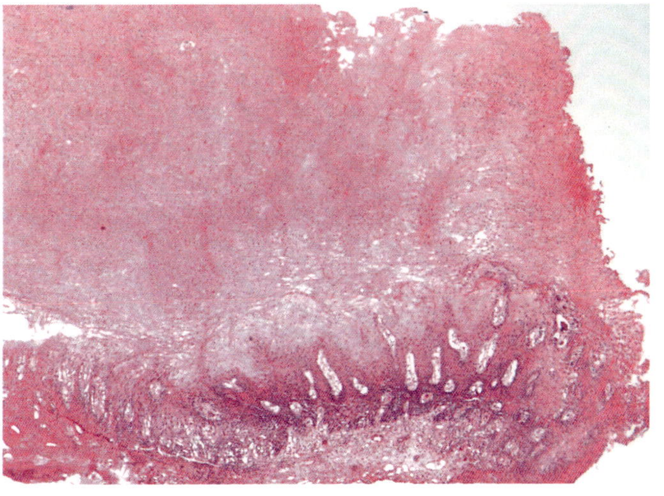

Fig. 10.7 Verrucous squamous hyperplasia is a recently described precursor to squamous carcinoma of the bladder and is characterized by repetitive upward tenting of the urothelium with prominent hyperkeratosis. By cystoscopy, this lesion would appear as a white plaque

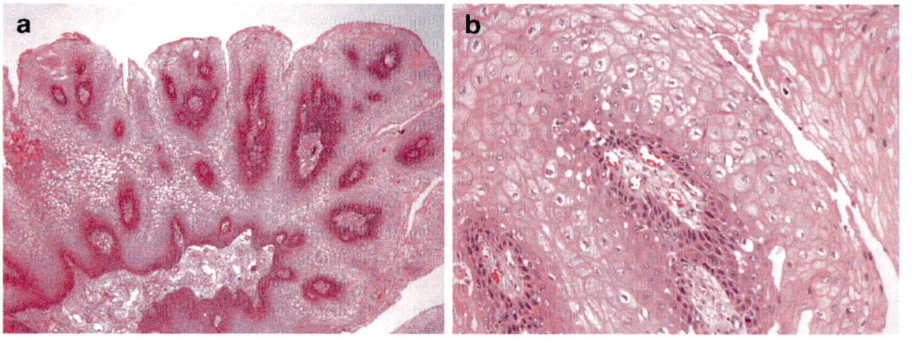

Fig. 10.8 (**a**) Condylomata are infrequently associated with invasive squamous carcinoma. (**b**) Higher magnification reveals prominent koilocytosis of the squamous nuclei, a characteristic feature of papillomavirus infection

like structures of variable thickness with typical viral koilocytosis (Fig. 10.8a, b).

Although prior doctrine stated that any component of urothelial carcinoma in situ would classify the lesion as "urothelial carcinoma with squamous differentiation," this concept has recently been contested [16]. Given the shared pathogenic factors of squamous and urothelial carcinomas, the presence of multiple separate in situ precursor lesions on extensive sampling of a bladder with otherwise typical squamous carcinoma is not surprising. In our experience, flat urothelial carcinoma in situ may also be associated with squamous cell carcinoma in a subset of cases and often coexists with the other squamous cell carcinoma precursors described previously. The prior suggestion that the presence of any flat urothelial carcinoma in situ should reclassify a bladder carcinoma as a urothelial carcinoma with divergent differentiation was based on a mapping study of only three bladders. Within our larger series of 45 cases, it became apparent that flat urothelial carcinoma in situ was only one of several in situ lesions that could coexist in a patient with otherwise typical squamous cell carcinoma.

Outcomes and Management

Management of squamous cell carcinoma of the bladder is influenced by several factors that differ from management of urothelial carcinoma. Squamous carcinoma is almost never diagnosed in superficial stage. Thus, diagnostic endeavors to accurately stage the tumor within the bladder, as well as attempts to develop treatment algorithms for superficial disease (TUR, intravesical Bacillus Calmette-Guérin (BCG), etc.), provide limited value. Response to definitive curative-intent radiotherapy is poor, and no meaningful systemic chemotherapy is available. These factors make radical surgery the only real therapeutic option for patients with squamous carcinoma of the bladder. To date, the chance of cure for patients with metastatic disease has remained minimal.

For non-schistosomal squamous carcinoma, the results of surgery are similar to the outcomes reported for urothelial carcinoma when compared stage for stage. Surgical failures die overwhelmingly from local pelvic recurrence with rare distant metastatic disease [16, 24, 25].

For schistosomal squamous carcinoma, radical surgery remains the mainstay of treatment with tumor stage, grade, and lymph node involvement affecting long-term outcome. An overall 5-year survival approximating 50% has been reported [16, 22]. Limited reports of benefit with neoadjuvant radiation treatment have not resulted in widespread adoption of this technique [26]. Due to the localized nature of schistosomal squamous carcinoma, partial cystectomy can be offered in select patients with smaller tumors preferably in the bladder dome and in patients whose tumors demonstrate a verrucous appearance. Conflicting reports of outcomes with this technique probably reflect patient selection differences [27]. Although more useful in schistosomal squamous carcinoma than in urothelial carcinoma, partial cystectomy remains a treatment option for a very small minority of carefully selected patients.

Additional Molecular Alterations

A handful of previous studies have attempted to address the molecular differences that underlie the development of bladder squamous cell carcinoma. One study using a proteomics-based approach identified an increase in galectin-7 and high-molecular-weight keratins in squamous cell carcinoma of the bladder, although these findings appeared to correlate best with tumor differentiation rather than subtype [28]. A second study examined gene expression differences between nine bladder cancer cell lines, using one squamous cancer cell line, SCaBER, and eight conventional urothelial carcinoma cell lines [29]. Results from this study identified a combined use of keratin 10 and caveolin-1 to stratify squamous and conventional urothelial carcinomas, although the validation of these results was performed primarily on a small number of *Schistosomiasis*-related squamous cell carcinomas, which have been previously demonstrated to contain a different molecular profile from non-*Schistosomiasis* squamous cell carcinoma of the bladder.

Several molecules identified in these and other studies hold promise as putative candidates in the development of bladder squamous cell carcinoma, especially if validated in a larger study of human bladder tumors. PTHrP is a molecule that is widely expressed throughout the body and functions to regulate smooth muscle tone, epithelial calcium transport, and cellular proliferation [30]. PTHrP can be expressed at high levels in several tumors, including lung and head and neck squamous cell carcinomas, and appears to mediate the paraneoplastic syndrome of "hypercalcemia of malignancy" [31]. Increased levels of serum PTHrP, as well as immunohistochemical reactivity for the PTHrP protein in bladder cancer specimens, have been occasionally reported in single patients [32]. In addition, increased expression of PTHrP has been identified in the urothelium of patients with spinal cord injury, a recognized risk factor in the development of bladder squamous cell carcinoma, but not in the urothelium of control patients [33]. PTHrP has been suggested to inhibit the apoptotic cascade and to mediate cellular proliferation by interacting with the epidermal growth factor (EGF) pathway [34]. Of note, increased expression of the EGF receptor has been well documented in noninvasive squamous cell lesions of the bladder [12], and interactions between PTHrP and EGF cascades may serve a role in mediating squamous cell carcinoma survival and proliferation in the bladder.

Another differentially expressed molecule that is upregulated in bladder squamous cell carcinoma is caveolin-1. Caveolin-1 is one of a subset of structural proteins that functions in cellular protein trafficking, cholesterol homeostasis, and signal transduction [35]. In caveolin-1 knockout mice, the bladder demonstrates alterations in smooth muscle function and voiding difficulties, suggesting a role for caveolin-1 in normal bladder function [36]. In addition, caveolin-1 appears to be upregulated in invasive bladder cancer and the extent of caveolin-1 expression correlates with the amount of squamous differentiation present within the tumor, although these findings were not validated in bladder squamous cell carcinomas [37]. In contrast, normal urothelium did not demonstrate any expression of the caveolin-1 protein.

Calcitonin receptor-like receptor (CALCRL) has also been described in the cited studies as being upregulated in bladder squamous cell carcinoma relative to conventional urothelial carcinoma. CALCRL is a cell surface receptor that interacts with either calcitonin or adrenomedullin, depending on the coexpression of a subset of interacting molecules termed RAMPs [38]. CALCRL, via interaction with adrenomedullin, has been proposed to mediate tumor-endothelial interaction, as well as trophoblastic cell line invasion, although the expression and function of these molecules have not been studied in the urothelial tract [39, 40]. Finally, members of the carbonic anhydrase (CA) family have been studied as mediators of the hypoxia transcriptome, which has also proven important in invasive bladder cancer [41]. Expression of one member of the CA family, CA9, appears to correlate with a reduced survival rate in patients with conventional urothelial carcinoma [42], although no studies have been performed on bladder cancer using CA2 specifically.

References

1. Shokeir AA. Squamous cell carcinoma of the bladder: pathology, diagnosis and treatment. BJU Int. 2004; 93(2):216–20.
2. Li MK, Cheung WL. Squamous cell carcinoma of the renal pelvis. J Urol. 1987;138(2):269–71.
3. Holmang S, Lele SM, Johansson SL. Squamous cell carcinoma of the renal pelvis and ureter: incidence, symptoms, treatment and outcome. J Urol. 2007; 178(1):51–6.
4. Bhandari A, Alassi O, Rogers C, MacLennan GT. Squamous cell carcinoma of the renal pelvis. J Urol. 2010;183(5):2023–4.
5. El-Sheikh SS, Madaan S, Alhasso A, Abel P, Stamp G, Lalani EN. Cyclooxygenase-2: a possible target in schistosoma-associated bladder cancer. BJU Int. 2001;88(9):921–7.
6. El-Bolkainy MN, Mokhtar NM, Ghoneim MA, Hussein MH. The impact of schistosomiasis on the pathology of bladder carcinoma. Cancer. 1981;48(12): 2643–8.
7. Gouda I, Mokhtar N, Bilal D, El-Bolkainy T, El-Bolkainy NM. Bilharziasis and bladder cancer: a time trend analysis of 9843 patients. J Egypt Natl Canc Inst. 2007;19(2):158–62.
8. Fortuny J, Kogevinas M, Chang-Claude J, Gonzalez CA, Hours M, Jockel KH, et al. Tobacco, occupation and non-transitional-cell carcinoma of the bladder: an international case-control study. Int J Cancer. 1999;80(1):44–6.
9. Kantor AF, Hartge P, Hoover RN, Fraumeni Jr JF. Epidemiological characteristics of squamous cell carcinoma and adenocarcinoma of the bladder. Cancer Res. 1988;48(13):3853–5.
10. Tamas EF, Stephenson AJ, Campbell SC, Montague DK, Trusty DC, Hansel DE. Histopathologic features and clinical outcomes in 71 cases of bladder diverticula. Arch Pathol Lab Med. 2009;133(5):791–6.
11. Del Mistro A, Koss LG, Braunstein J, Bennett B, Saccomano G, Simons KM. Condylomata acuminata of the urinary bladder. Natural history, viral typing, and DNA content. Am J Surg Pathol. 1988;12(3): 205–15.
12. Guo CC, Fine SW, Epstein JI. Noninvasive squamous lesions in the urinary bladder: a clinicopathologic analysis of 29 cases. Am J Surg Pathol. 2006;30(7): 883–91.
13. Mvula M, Iwasaka T, Iguchi A, Nakamura S, Masaki Z, Sugimori H. Do human papillomaviruses have a role in the pathogenesis of bladder carcinoma? J Urol. 1996;155(2):471–4.
14. Westenend PJ, Stoop JA, Hendriks JG. Human papillomaviruses 6/11, 16/18 and 31/33/51 are not associated with squamous cell carcinoma of the urinary bladder. BJU Int. 2001;88(3):198–201.
15. Amato NA, Moretti FS, Boscia FM, Mele F. Urinary bladder, urethral and renal condylomata, due to human papilloma virus (HPV) type 11 associated with transitional cell tumors in bladder, ureter and kidney: a case report. Minerva Ginecol. 2008;60(3):264–5.
16. Lagwinski N, Thomas A, Stephenson AJ, Campbell S, Hoschar AP, El-Gabry E, et al. Squamous cell carcinoma of the bladder: a clinicopathologic analysis of 45 cases. Am J Surg Pathol. 2007;31(12):1777–87.
17. Badr M. Schistosomiasis in ancient Egypt. In: E-Ba C, editor. Detection of bladder cancer associatd with schistosomiasis. Cairo, Egypt: Alahram Press; 1981. p. 1–8.
18. Botelho M, Oliveira P, Gomes J, Gartner F, Lopes C, da Costa JM, et al. Tumourigenic effect of Schistosoma haematobium total antigen in mammalian cells. Int J Exp Pathol. 2009;90(4):448–53.
19. Botelho M, Ferreira AC, Oliveira MJ, Domingues A, Machado JC, da Costa JM. Schistosoma haematobium total antigen induces increased proliferation, migration and invasion, and decreases apoptosis of normal epithelial cells. Int J Parasitol. 2009;39(10): 1083–91.
20. Botelho MC, Oliveira PA, Lopes C, Correia da Costa JM, Machado JC. Urothelial dysplasia and inflammation induced by Schistosoma haematobium total antigen instillation in mice normal urothelium. Urol Oncol. 2009.
21. el-Boulkany MN, Ghoneim MA, Mansour MA. Carcinoma of the bilharzial bladder in Egypt Clinical and pathological features. Br J Urol. 1972;44(5): 561–70.
22. Ghoneim MA, el-Mekresh MM, el-Baz MA, el-Attar IA, Ashamallah A. Radical cystectomy for carcinoma of the bladder: critical evaluation of the results in 1,026 cases. J Urol. 1997;158(2):393–9.
23. el-Sebai I, Sherif M, el-Bolkainy MN, Mansour MA, Ghoneim MA. Verrucose squamous carcinoma of bladder. Urology. 1974;4(4):407–10.
24. Rogers CG, Palapattu GS, Shariat SF, Karakiewicz PI, Bastian PJ, Lotan Y, et al. Clinical outcomes following radical cystectomy for primary nontransitional cell carcinoma of the bladder compared to transitional cell carcinoma of the bladder. J Urol. 2006;175(6): 2048–53; discussion 53.

25. Nishiyama H, Habuchi T, Watanabe J, Teramukai S, Tada H, Ono Y, et al. Clinical outcome of a large-scale multi-institutional retrospective study for locally advanced bladder cancer: a survey including 1131 patients treated during 1990-2000 in Japan. Eur Urol. 2004;45(2):176–81.
26. Awwad H, El-Baki HA, El-Bolkainy N, Burgers M, El-Badawy S, Mansour M, et al. Pre-operative irradiation of T3-carcinoma in bilharzial bladder: a comparison between hyperfractionation and conventional fractionation. Int J Radiat Oncol Biol Phys. 1979;5(6):787–94.
27. Omar A, Sherif M. Segmental resection for carcinoma of the bladder. J Egypt Med Assoc. 1969;52(11): 975–8.
28. Ostergaard M, Rasmussen HH, Nielsen HV, Vorum H, Orntoft TF, Wolf H, et al. Proteome profiling of bladder squamous cell carcinomas: identification of markers that define their degree of differentiation. Cancer Res. 1997;57(18):4111–7.
29. Sanchez-Carbayo M, Socci ND, Charytonowicz E, Lu M, Prystowsky M, Childs G, et al. Molecular profiling of bladder cancer using cDNA microarrays: defining histogenesis and biological phenotypes. Cancer Res. 2002;62(23):6973–80.
30. Philbrick WM, Wysolmerski JJ, Galbraith S, Holt E, Orloff JJ, Yang KH, et al. Defining the roles of parathyroid hormone-related protein in normal physiology. Physiol Rev. 1996;76(1):127–73.
31. Tsuchimochi M, Kameta A, Sue M, Katagiri M. Immunohistochemical localization of parathyroid hormone-related protein (PTHrP) and serum PTHrP in normocalcemic patients with oral squamous cell carcinoma. Odontology. 2005;93(1):61–71.
32. Chaudhary UB, Milling DL, Bissada NK. Transitional cell carcinoma of the bladder producing parathyroid hormone-related protein (PTHrP). Can J Urol. 2004;11(1):2136–8.
33. Vaidyanathan S, McCreavy DT, McDicken IW, Soni BM, Mansour P, Wlodarski B, et al. Immunohistochemical study of parathyroid hormone-related protein in vesical transitional epithelium of patients with spinal cord injury. Spinal Cord. 1999;37(11): 760–4.
34. Hastings RH, Araiza F, Burton DW, Bedley M, Deftos LJ. Parathyroid hormone-related protein regulates apoptosis in lung cancer cells through protein kinase A. Am J Physiol Cell Physiol. 2004;287(6): C1616–22.
35. Williams TM, Lisanti MP. The Caveolin genes: from cell biology to medicine. Ann Med. 2004;36(8): 584–95.
36. Woodman SE, Cheung MW, Tarr M, North AC, Schubert W, Lagaud G, et al. Urogenital alterations in aged male caveolin-1 knockout mice. J Urol. 2004;171(2 Pt 1):950–7.
37. Fong A, Garcia E, Gwynn L, Lisanti MP, Fazzari MJ, Li M. Expression of caveolin-1 and caveolin-2 in urothelial carcinoma of the urinary bladder correlates with tumor grade and squamous differentiation. Am J Clin Pathol. 2003;120(1):93–100.
38. Nikitenko LL, Blucher N, Fox SB, Bicknell R, Smith DM, Rees MC. Adrenomedullin and CGRP interact with endogenous calcitonin-receptor-like receptor in endothelial cells and induce its desensitisation by different mechanisms. J Cell Sci. 2006;119 (Pt 5):910–22.
39. Khodarev NN, Yu J, Labay E, Darga T, Brown CK, Mauceri HJ, et al. Tumour-endothelium interactions in co-culture: coordinated changes of gene expression profiles and phenotypic properties of endothelial cells. J Cell Sci. 2003;116(Pt 6):1013–22.
40. Zhang X, Green KE, Yallampalli C, Dong YL. Adrenomedullin enhances invasion by trophoblast cell lines. Biol Reprod. 2005;73(4):619–26.
41. Ord JJ, Streeter EH, Roberts IS, Cranston D, Harris AL. Comparison of hypoxia transcriptome in vitro with in vivo gene expression in human bladder cancer. Br J Cancer. 2005;93(3):346–54.
42. Hussain SA, Palmer DH, Ganesan R, Hiller L, Gregory J, Murray PG, et al. Carbonic anhydrase IX, a marker of hypoxia: correlation with clinical outcome in transitional cell carcinoma of the bladder. Oncol Rep. 2004;11(5):1005–10.

Adenocarcinoma of the Urinary Bladder

11

Gladell P. Paner and Wade J. Sexton

Introduction

Adenocarcinoma of the bladder is rare, accounting for up to 2% of bladder cancers in North America and Europe. Most adenocarcinomas arise from the bladder mucosa, although about a third arise from urachal remnants. While adenocarcinomas from these two sites are often lumped under the same category, relevant differences exist and—importantly—these are treated as two different tumors. Recognized risks of adenocarcinoma such as schistosomiasis, extrophy, bladder augmentation, or neurogenic bladder appear to induce a setting of chronic mucosal irritation. Intestinal metaplasia, when extensive, may be associated with adenocarcinoma, although its causal role in tumorigenesis is under debate. Typical manifestations are similar to the other more common bladder cancers, with the exception of occasional mucosuria and the presence of a gelatinous mass.

Most adenocarcinomas are invasive and may be associated with a limited number of preinvasive glandular lesions. Invasive adenocarcinoma shows a spectrum of morphologies, and it appears that mucinous histology behaves relatively better and signet-ring cell subtype poorer. Distinction from metastatic adenocarcinoma of other organ sites must be made, and pathological distinction is complicated by morphological and immunohistochemical overlap, particularly with colorectal adenocarcinoma. Correlation with clinical, radiographic, and endoscopic findings is often critical in this differential diagnosis.

Adenocarcinoma portends poorer survival than urothelial carcinoma, often due to the advanced stage at the time of diagnosis. Since data are limited to small, retrospective studies, multimodal treatment paradigms are poorly defined. The mainstay of treatment for adenocarcinoma of the bladder is radical and pelvic lymph node. Partial cystectomy with en-bloc resection of bladder dome, urachal ligament, and umbilicus is an accepted surgical intervention for urachal adenocarcinoma. Role of radiation therapy and chemotherapy remains unclear.

Clinical Presentation

Epidemiology and Risk Factors

Primary adenocarcinoma of the bladder comprises 0.5–2% of the bladder cancers diagnosed in Western countries [1] compared to nearly 10% of all bladder cancers identified in countries with

G.P. Paner (✉)
Department of Pathology and Section of Urology, Department of Surgery, The University of Chicago, 5841 S. Maryland Avenue, MC 6101 AMB Room S626, Chicago, IL 60637, USA
e-mail: gladell.paner@uchospitals.edu

W.J. Sexton
Moffitt Cancer Center, Genitourinary Oncology Program, 12902 Magnolia Drive, Tampa, FL 33612, USA
e-mail: wade.sexton@moffitt.org

D.E. Hansel et al. (eds.), *The Urinary Tract: A Comprehensive Guide to Patient Diagnosis and Management*, DOI 10.1007/978-1-4614-5320-8_11, © Springer Science+Business Media New York 2012

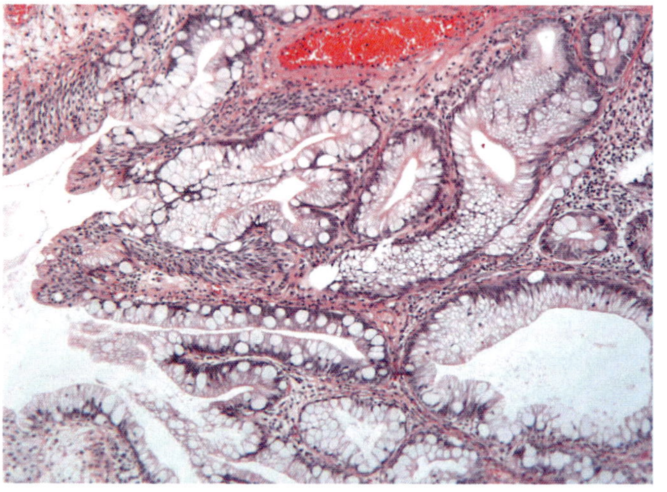

Fig. 11.1 Intestinal metaplasia with goblet cells of the urothelium representing a variant of cystitis glandularis

endemic schistosomiasis [2]. This striking difference is primarily due to different geographical risk factors. In North America and Europe, risk factors for primary bladder adenocarcinoma include bladder extrophy, bladder augmentation, chronic bladder irritation or infection, cystitis glandularis, and intestinal metaplasia [3].

Cystitis glandularis represents glandular metaplasia of von Brunn's nests resulting from chronic inflammation (Fig. 11.1). While some believe it to be a precursor of adenocarcinoma [4], others have debated its significance as a true bladder adenocarcinoma risk factor and report that cystitis cystica and cystitis glandularis can be seen in a variety of bladder inflammatory conditions and in normal bladder biopsies [5]. Long-term follow-up has not established this inflammatory pathological finding as a definitive premalignant lesion. Likewise, extensive intestinal metaplasia—seen alone or in patients with a history of bladder extrophy—has been reported as an adenocarcinoma risk factor. However, some studies of extrophy patients with long-term follow-up demonstrated no subsequent malignant transformation of intestinal metaplasia into adenocarcinoma [6, 7].

The most important risk factor for the development of nonurachal adenocarcinoma of the bladder is bilharzial infection with *Schistosoma haematobium*. Schistosomiasis is most strongly associated with squamous cell carcinoma of the bladder, but the endemic nature of this parasite also accounts for the larger numbers of Egyptian patients with adenocarcinoma histology compared to North American and European populations. There is an increased incidence of bilharzial bladder cancers particularly in younger men within endemic areas due to the increased exposure to schistosomes in agricultural work environments [8]. Similar to other bladder cancers such as urothelial and squamous cell carcinomas, most nonurachal adenocarcinomas occur in men.

It is estimated that urachal adenocarcinoma comprises less than 1% of all bladder cancers combined, yet accounts for 10–35% of primary bladder adenocarcinomas [9–12]. Urachal adenocarcinomas occur with equal frequency in men and women. The median age at diagnosis is 50–56 years, significantly younger than that reported for patients with nonurachal adenocarcinomas (median age at diagnosis 64–69 years) [12–14]. The urachus is a vestigial structure that develops during early embryogenesis and serves to connect the bladder to the allantois. As the bladder descends into the pelvis, the lumen of the allantois closes and becomes the urachus, which in adulthood serves no functional purpose. Following delivery, it becomes a fibrous cord known as the median umbilical ligament. Persistent remnants of the allantois or failure of the urachus to close might lead to the development of an urachal cyst, vesicourachal diverticulum, a patent urachus, or an epithelial neoplasm. Neoplasms potentially arise from any of three distinct tissue layers within the urachus: an epithelial canal lined by urothelium, submucosal connective tissue, or smooth muscle. In part due to the rarity of these tumors, there are no known risk factors for the development of urachal adenocarcinomas. In addition, autopsy series suggest that 70% of adults have an epithelialized canal in the urachus and 30% of the general population have some degree of a patent urachal tubular or cystic structure that connects anywhere along the midline of the bladder—most commonly to the dome but also to the midline posterior or anterior wall [15–17]. Obviously, many of these anomalies exist without ever having developed into urachal tumors.

Signs and Symptoms

Most patients with primary bladder adenocarcinoma present with symptoms similar to other carcinomas originating from the bladder urothelium, including gross hematuria and irritative lower urinary tract symptoms such as urinary frequency and urgency. Less common symptoms include those related to bladder outlet obstruction or to renal obstruction—either dependent upon tumor bulk or the presence of muscle-invasive disease obstructing the bladder neck or the ureteral orifices. A majority of patients with urachal adenocarcinomas have locally advanced disease at presentation. Clinically silent local and distant progression are common prior to the onset of symptoms due to the extraperitoneal and often extravesical location of the tumors. Nevertheless, some patients with urachal tumors report mucosuria due to the presence of enteric type tumor elements visualized pathologically. Additional signs and symptoms include suprapubic or umbilical pain, referred pain to the genitalia, umbilical discharge, or the presence of a suprapubic mass [18].

Adenocarcinomas Metastatic to Bladder

Nonurachal adenocarcinomas must be distinguished from metastatic bladder involvement from other sites. Metastasis to the bladder occurs on average 7 years following the diagnosis of the primary malignancy [19]. Metastatic lesions typically infiltrate the bladder wall, occasionally causing mucosal ulceration and urinary symptoms [20]. Although it is often difficult to distinguish primary bladder adenocarcinoma from metastatic disease, a high index of suspicion must be maintained for the possibility of metastatic disease particularly in patients with a known history of a separate primary malignancy. The most common sites of origin of metastatic disease to the bladder include: genitourinary cancers (kidney, prostate, testis, and seminal vesicles), gynecologic cancers (cervix, vulva, ovary, and uterus), colorectal carcinomas, melanomas, breast cancers, and gastric cancers. The majority of metastatic cancers involving the bladder are adenocarcinomas [21] and approximately half of the metastatic lesions involve the bladder neck or trigone [22]. Metastases to the bladder dome or to the bladder midline are rare.

Secondary adenocarcinomas arising from the genitourinary tract or from the lower gastrointestinal tract are more common than primary bladder adenocarcinomas and more often involve the bladder through direct contact and extension. Colon cancers for instance may erode directly into the bladder and on occasion will be associated with pneumaturia or fecaluria. Clinical history, radiographic evaluation, and endoscopic assessment confirm the expected diagnosis. In patients without direct extension, histology alone may not distinguish primary from metastatic lesions. A primary adenocarcinoma is supported by the presence of glandular change of the surface urothelium, including adenocarcinoma in situ on biopsy [21, 22].

When the diagnosis is uncertain—or when a patient's history, symptoms, or radiographic studies suggest an alternative primary site—examination of the breasts, prostate, colon and rectum should be performed (including stool for occult blood). Further consideration can be given towards colonoscopy, esophagogastroduodenoscopy, and mammography pending the results of the physical examination and radiographic evaluation. Immunohistochemical staining and other specialized tests may occasionally aid in distinguishing primary from metastatic bladder involvement [23, 24].

Diagnostic Evaluation and Staging

Evaluation typically includes cystoscopy, especially when patients present with lower urinary tract symptoms. A transurethral resection of the bladder tumor (TURBT) and an exam under anesthesia are required for clinical staging. If the patient has invasive disease, an exam under anesthesia is important to determine whether the tumor is resectable with negative surgical margins—especially when cross-sectional computed tomography (CT) scans or magnetic resonance imaging (MRI) scans suggest the possibility of locally advanced disease. Radiographic studies of the chest, abdomen, and pelvis require careful scrutiny as many patients present with regional or distant metastases. Cross-sectional imaging might reveal an extravesical primary tumor with metastatic involvement of the bladder. Occasionally, peritoneal carcinomatosis and pseudomyxoma peritonei are identified with abdominal imaging [11, 25]. Recent evidence suggests that positive Urovysion FISH results may be seen in up to 75% of primary and secondary bladder adenocarcinomas. There are significant overlapping chromosomal aberrations between adenocarcinomas and urothelial carcinomas accounting for the positive FISH assays. A positive FISH result in this setting would not distinguish between these tumor histologies and would need to be correlated with additional clinical and cytomorphologic assessments [26].

The TNM staging system is used for both clinical and pathological staging of primary bladder adenocarcinomas and is identical to the staging of other urothelial-derived bladder cancers, including urothelial carcinomas and squamous cell carcinomas. A different staging system is used for urachal adenocarcinomas as they often arise from the muscle wall or external to the bladder and grow towards the urothelium. Sheldon proposed the initial staging system in 1984 (Table 11.1) and to date this system has been the most widely adopted and utilized despite suggested modifications from other institutions [10, 27]. Most patients present with stage III or stage IV cancers due to the insidious onset of lower urinary tract or lower abdominal symptoms. Contrary to urachal tumors, most primary adenocarcinomas are heralded by gross hematuria, urinary frequency, or urinary urgency.

Table 11.1 Sheldon staging system for urachal adenocarcinoma [10]

Stage I—No invasion beyond the urachal mucosa
Stage II—Invasion confined to the urachus
Stage III—Local extension into:
Bladder (III-A)
Abdominal wall (III-B)
Peritoneum (III-C)
Stage IV—Metastases involving:
Regional lymph nodes (IV-A)
Distant sites (IV-B)

Pathology

By anatomic distribution, the vast majority of adenocarcinomas can be divided into those arising directly from bladder mucosa and those arising from urachal remnants. In rare instances, adenocarcinoma may arise from bladder extrophy and intestinal bladder augmentation or ileal conduit. Rarely, adenocarcinoma may arise from endometriosis involving the bladder.

Several criteria have been proposed for the diagnosis of an urachal adenocarcinoma [18]. Generally, these tumors are located in the bladder dome or elsewhere in the midline of the bladder and bladder involvement is not a requirement for the diagnosis. When the bladder mucosa is involved by tumor, there is often a characteristic sharp demarcation between tumor and normal bladder surface urothelium. Other supportive criteria include the absence of urothelial dysplasia,

Table 11.2 Pathologic characteristics of nonurachal and urachal adenocarcinoma

	Nonurachal adenocarcinoma	Urachal adenocarcinoma
Location	Most commonly trigone and bladder neck region	Dome, less commonly anterior wall or supravesical area
Focality	Uni- or multifocal	Unifocal
Growth	Solid	Solid or cystic
Endovesical mucosal mass	Present	Often discreet or absent
Histology	Mucinous<nonmucinous	Mucinous>nonmucinous
Surface epithelium overlying tumor	Malignant or dysplastic glandular epithelium	Benign urothelium or ulcerated by tumor
Cystitis cystica, cystitis glandularis, and intestinal metaplasia	Common	Rare
Urachal remnants	Absent or not associated with tumor if present	Occasionally seen admixed with tumor

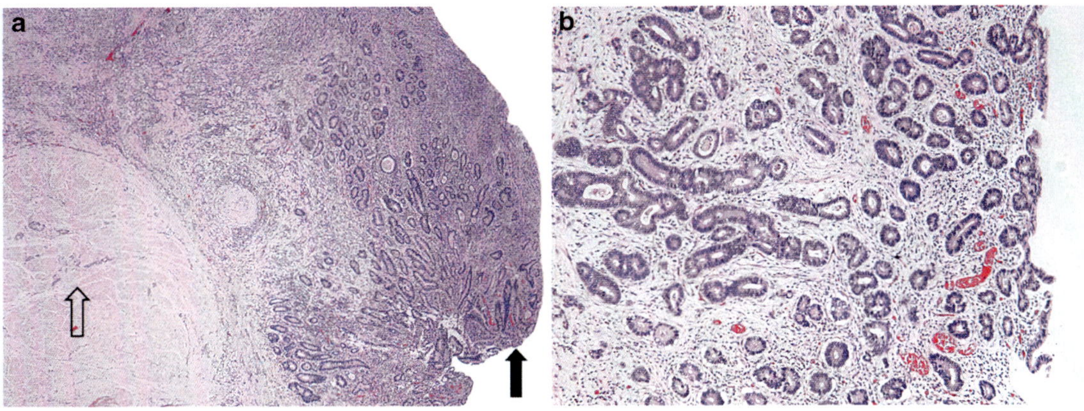

Fig. 11.2 (**a**) Bladder adenocarcinoma arising from dysplastic intestinal epithelium (*dark arrow*) and invading into deep muscle (*open arrow*). (**b**) Surface epithelium is completely replaced by dysplastic intestinal glands and shows transition to invasive carcinoma

absence of cystitis cystica or cystitis glandularis transitioning to the tumor, and absence of primary adenocarcinoma from another organ site. A cystic or solid lower midline mass without visible bladder involvement merits consideration of an urachal tumor until proven otherwise.

Several gross and histologic characteristics are helpful in distinguishing nonurachal from urachal adenocarcinoma (Table 11.2) (Figs. 11.2a, b and 11.3). However, most of these features are better appreciated only in large resection specimens, and histopathological distinction in limited tissue samples (e.g., biopsy, TURBT) can be challenging and may require clinical and radiologic correlations for diagnosis.

Gross Findings

Adenocarcinoma can occur at any sites of the bladder, and most commonly involves the trigone and ureteric insertion sites [7, 28–31]. The lesion is often solitary, although nonurachal adenocarcinoma can exhibit multifocality [30, 32, 33]. Urachal adenocarcinoma is typically located in bladder dome where the urachus is principally situated, but may also occur along the anterior wall near the bladder midline and supravesical part of urachus [7, 24]. Very rarely, adenocarcinoma may arise within a bladder diverticulum [32, 34, 35].

The gross appearance of bladder adenocarcinoma varies from sessile to nodular or papillary

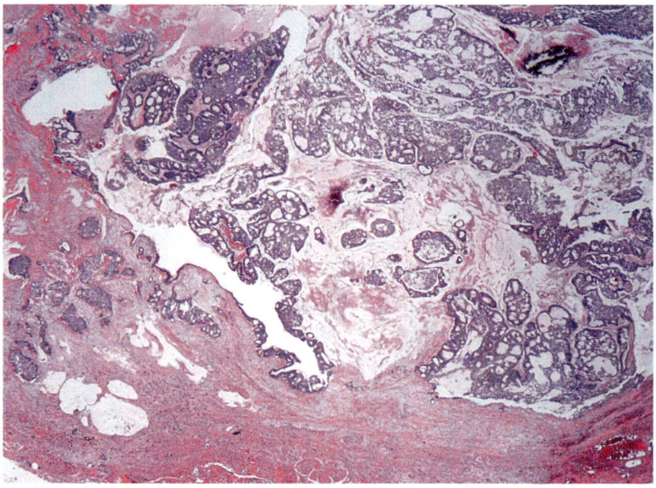

Fig. 11.3 Urachal adenocarcinoma. Tumor involves deep muscle, but surface epithelium is intact and lined by benign urothelium

with variably discernable infiltrative component, or that indistinguishable from invasive urothelial carcinoma [31, 33]. Mucoid material may be copious and produce a gelatinous appearance, a finding indicative of adenocarcinoma. Most tumors are large, about half greater than 4 cm, and can extensively involve the bladder wall [27, 28, 30]. Deep bladder wall invasion and extravesical extensions are common at presentation [14, 36, 37]. The signet-ring cell carcinoma subtype may extensively infiltrate the bladder without forming a distinct mass lesion [38–41]. The bladder wall appears diffusely thickened and firm due to carcinoma infiltration, resembling a "linitis plastica" appearance of gastric cancer. This pattern of widespread bladder infiltration has been described in both nonurachal and urachal signet-ring cell carcinomas [39], and indicates a poorer prognosis. Urachal adenocarcinoma often invades the bladder wall, perivesical or periurachal tissues, the abdominal wall, and can extend superiorly to involve the space of Retzius towards the umbilicus [42]. Early stage intramural or extravesical urachal adenocarcinoma often spares the bladder mucosa and is present without a visible mucosal lesion.

Histologic Features

NonInvasive Glandular Neoplasms

The vast majority of glandular tumors of the bladder are invasive tumors. Uncommonly, related noninvasive glandular neoplasms such as villous adenoma, urachal adenoma, and adenocarcinoma in situ may occur. The preinvasive tumor should have no invasive component confirmed by adequate sampling and must occur in pure glandular form (i.e., no mixed urothelial carcinoma component) to classify under these categories.

Villous Adenoma

This lesion contains villiform architecture similar to typical villous adenoma of the gastrointestinal tract [43–46]. Most villous adenomas occur in the bladder proper and may arise from metaplastic urothelium or, less commonly, from urachal remnants [45–47]. The tumor exhibits elongated finger-like fronds containing central fibrovascular cores that are lined by pseudostratified columnar epithelium with variable intracytoplasmic mucin and goblet cells (Fig. 11.4). The epithelial cells display nuclear

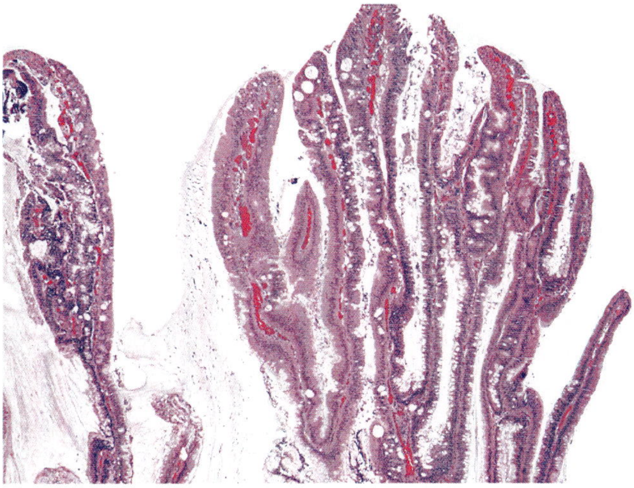

Fig. 11.4 Villous adenoma of the bladder

stratification, nuclear crowding, nuclear hyperchromasia, and mitoses. Extracellular mucin can be abundant and may dissect the underlying stromal tissue to mimic an invasive adenocarcinoma. Coexistent intestinal metaplasia, cystitis cystica, and cystitis glandularis are often present in adjacent bladder mucosa. Associated invasive adenocarcinoma is present in up to 53% of cases [45]. The morphology of the invasive adenocarcinoma component is often similar to that of villous adenoma. High-grade noninvasive foci—or adenocarcinoma in situ—is seen in up to 17% of villous adenomas that contain more complex architecture such as cribriform glands, severe nuclear atypia, and increased mitotic activity. Prognosis is excellent with a pure noninvasive villous adenoma [45, 46]. The presence of concomitant invasive adenocarcinoma may result in recurrence and metastasis, and thus requires more aggressive therapy. Villous adenomas should be completely sampled and examined histologically to ensure the absence of invasive adenocarcinoma component.

Urachal Adenoma (Mucinous Cystadenoma)

There are a few reports of low-grade tumors arising in the urachus, and these lesions present as mucous-filled cystic or multilocular lesions that lack an invasive carcinoma component [47–50]. Most of these tumors occur in the lower aspect of the urachus. The lesions are lined by cuboidal to columnar cells of enteric to mucinous type with occasional goblet cells (Fig. 11.5). Some authors proposed the term "mucinous cystic tumor of uncertain malignant potential" for noninvasive low-grade adenomatous cystic lesions exhibiting minimal pleomorphism, in a similar manner to appendiceal mucinous tumors, which harbor a better prognosis [48, 51]. High-grade foci, when present, are characterized by increased cellularity, stratification, and severe cytologic atypia. Invasive adenocarcinoma and pseudomyxoma peritonei can arise from urachal adenoma [52, 53]. Data are limited, but reported pure urachal adenomas behave favorably. Similar to villous adenoma, noninvasive urachal tumors should be extensively sampled and examined histologically to make certain the absence of an invasive carcinoma component.

Adenocarcinoma In Situ

Rarely, adenocarcinoma without associated villous architecture or an invasive component may arise from bladder mucosa [54]. Most adenocarcinoma in situ reported in the literature is often admixed with urothelial carcinoma, either insitu, papillary or invasive. Controversy exists in

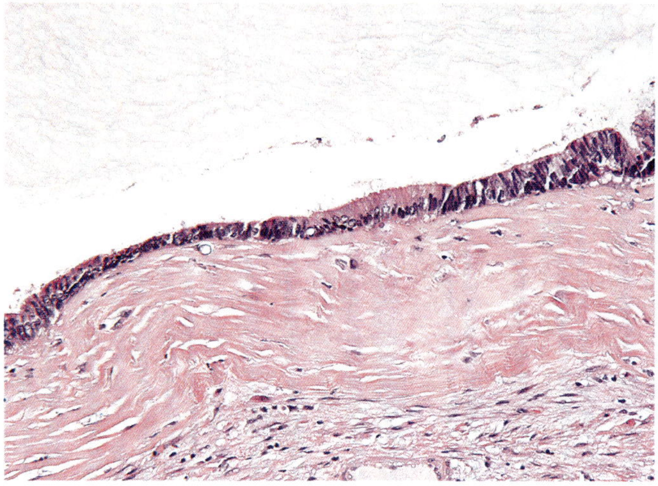

Fig. 11.5 Urachal cystadenoma. The cyst is lined by low-grade dysplastic intestinal epithelium with focal stratification and no stromal invasion

classifying these lesions, as some experts strictly require adenocarcinoma to be in pure form, and prefer to label mixed tumors as urothelial carcinoma with glandular differentiation [55]. However, pure glandular lesions do occur in 10% of adenocarcinoma in situ cases. Adenocarcinoma in situ can have a papillary, cribriform, or flat architecture and the bladder surface is lined by columnar cells with elongated nuclei and apical cytoplasm. The degree of cytological atypia is often moderate to severe and mitoses are frequent. The majority of patients with mixed and pure adenocarcinoma in situ have an associated invasive carcinoma either concurrently or subsequently that may include urothelial carcinoma (often micropapillary type) and small cell carcinoma. Progression to invasive adenocarcinoma, however, is not typical, at least in the reported cases [54]. Compared with urothelial carcinoma in situ, progression to invasive carcinoma is relatively higher in adenocarcinoma insitu (36% vs. 74%) [54].

Invasive Adenocarcinoma

Several morphological subtypes have been described for invasive adenocarcinoma and encompass both bladder and urachal tumors [9, 12, 28, 56]. Terminologies used have varied among authors [9, 12, 28, 56]. The nomenclature used by Grignon et al. [9] is the most widely recognized and includes mucinous, enteric, signet-ring cell, not-otherwise specified, and mixed subtypes (Fig. 11.6) [57, 58]. Admixture of these morphological patterns is common, and a 75% cut-off for a predominant pattern is used to consider a subtype distinct [9]. Rare variants, including clear cell and hepatoid adenocarcinomas, have been subsequently included into the classification scheme [59–63]. Distribution of morphological subtypes slightly varies between nonurachal and urachal adenocarcinomas [12]. Mucinous morphology is more often seen in urachal adenocarcinomas (48–50%), whereas nonmucinous subtypes are predominant in non-urachal adenocarcinomas (17–24%) [9, 12, 64]. The significance of morphological subtyping in adenocarcinoma is unclear, although the mucinous subtype is considered to be less aggressive, whereas the signet-ring cell subtype shows aggressive behavior [9, 16, 29]. The degree of tumor differentiation, however, has been shown to be an important prognostic variable, with low-grade or better differentiated tumors behaving relatively better [12, 27, 65].

Cystitis cystica, cystitis glandularis, and intestinal metaplasia are occasionally seen in the

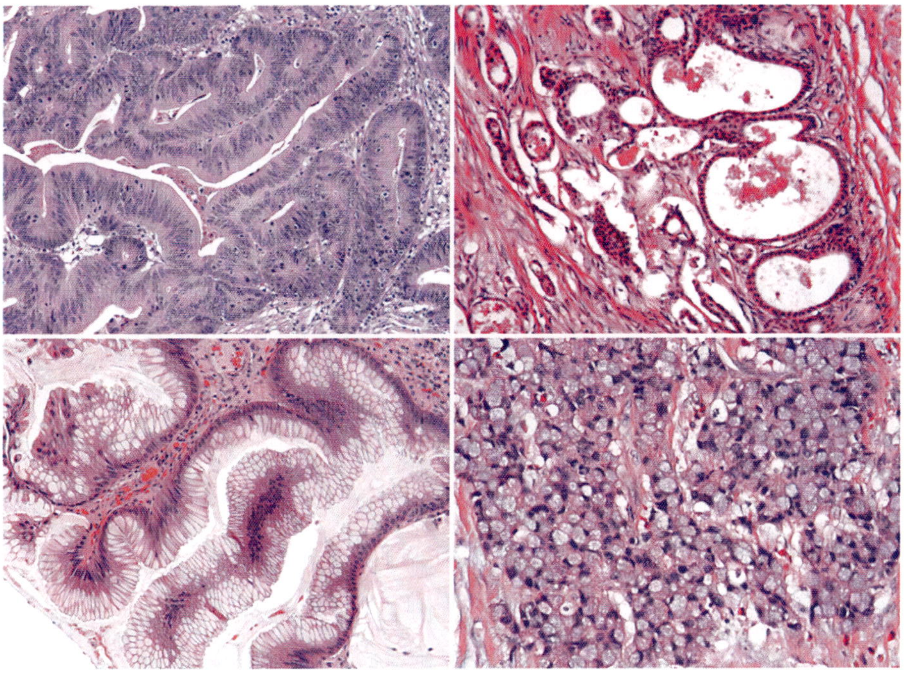

Fig. 11.6 Enteric, mucinous, signet-ring cell, and not-otherwise specified morphologic subtypes of adenocarcinoma (counterclockwise from *upper left*)

adjacent bladder mucosa associated with a nonurachal adenocarcinoma. However, cystitis cystica and cystitis glandularis may also be seen—albeit infrequently—in the mucosa of a bladder with urachal adenocarcinoma. Thus, the presence of these benign lesions does not preclude a diagnosis of an urachal primary [66]. Cystitis cystica is a von Brunn nest that acquired luminal space and became cystically dilated and sometimes contains eosinophilic secretions. Typical cystitis glandularis consists of glands with innermost lining composed of cuboidal or columnar cells surrounded peripherally by urothelial cells. Those that contain abundant mucin-secreting goblet cells are known as cystitis glandularis of intestinal type. Cystitis cystica and cystitis glandularis can be florid; the latter when extensive may mimic a well-differentiated adenocarcinoma.

Benign urachal remnants may be identified in up to 63% of urachal adenocarcinomas and are lined by either benign urothelial or glandular cells (Fig. 11.7) [66]. Adenomatous change may be seen in these epithelial remnants and demonstrate a morphological transition to invasive carcinoma.

Mucinous (Including Colloid)

Glands or nests of malignant mucinous epithelium in a background of variable amounts of extracellular mucin characterize this subtype. More often, mucin is copious and clusters of tumor cells appear to float in a mucinous pool, specifically referred to as *colloid type adenocarcinoma* (Fig. 11.8) [9, 43]. Carcinoma cells in nests, cords, or cribriform structures are seen within the mucinous pool. Occasionally, signet-ring cells are seen in mucinous lakes admixed with mucin-containing cells.

Enteric (Colonic)

The architecture and cytology of this subtype resemble typical primary intestinal adenocarcinoma [9, 28, 56, 66] and consist of irregular or cribriform glands lined by tall columnar cells

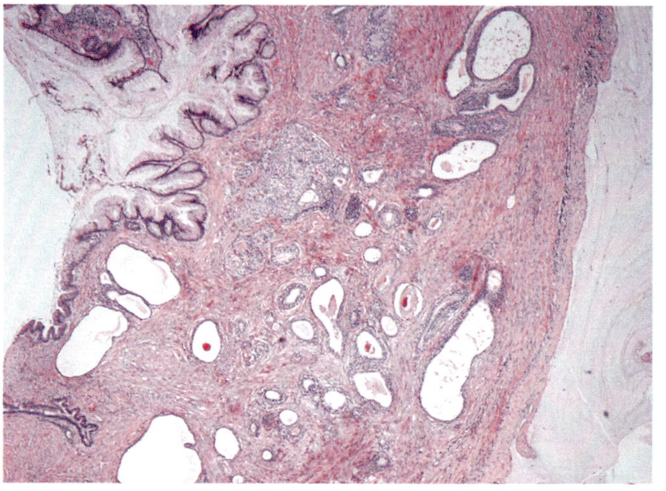

Fig. 11.7 Benign urachal remnants seen within urachal mucinous adenocarcinoma

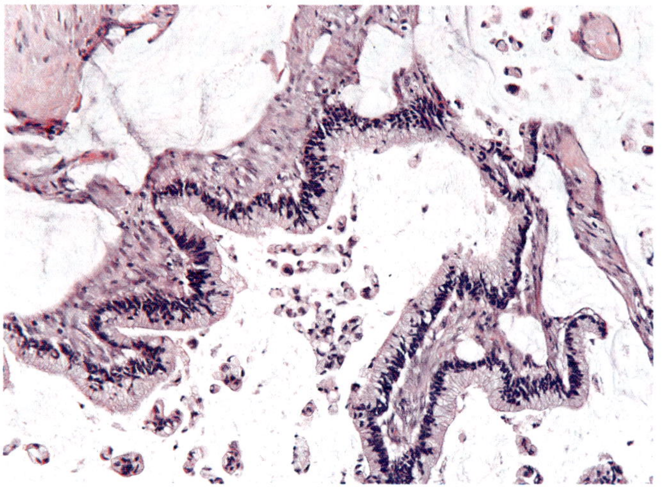

Fig. 11.8 Colloid adenocarcinoma with predominant mucinous epithelium. Occasional signet-ring cells are seen floating in mucinous pool

with basally situated elongated or pencil-shaped nuclei. This subtype is morphologically indistinguishable from an extension of colorectal carcinoma to the bladder. Extracellular mucin is typically not abundant, although the enteric subtype with copious mucin resembling colloid carcinoma does occur [66].

Signet-Ring Cell

These carcinoma cells contain intracytoplasmic mucin that peripherally displaces the nucleus [38, 40, 67]. Intracellular mucin may appear as a single clear vacuole or as foamy vesicular cytoplasm. Signet-ring cells occur either in pure form or may be variably admixed with other morphological subtypes [40, 66]. In urachal adenocarcinoma, signet-ring cells are often seen floating in mucinous pools [67]. The strict definition of signet-ring cell carcinoma requires tumors composed predominantly of signet-ring cells and lacking abundant extracellular mucin. This poorly differentiated carcinoma typically invades in a single cell pattern and tends to infiltrate the bladder wall diffusely, producing a "linitis plastica" appearance seen in gastric signet-ring cell carcinoma [68]. Prognosis is worse with pure diffuse signet-ring cells (versus those with mixed histology) and with nonurachal carcinomas (versus urachal signet-ring cell carcinoma) [40].

Not-Otherwise Specified Type

This subtype pertains to nonurothelial gland-forming carcinomas that do not conform to any of the described morphological types. This pattern is relatively more common in nonurachal than in urachal adenocarcinoma [9].

Mixed

Admixture of these patterns may occur, as long as none of the specific morphological subtypes comprising more than 75% of the tumor [9].

Unusual Variants

Clear Cell Adenocarcinoma

This distinctive type of bladder adenocarcinoma has a conspicuous component of cells with abundant clear cell cytoplasm and hobnail morphology, histologically similar to those occurring in the gynecologic tract [59–61]. The carcinoma cells have high-grade cytology and exhibit tubulocystic, papillary, or solid growth. The origin of this tumor is controversial and suggested to be Müllerian in nature because of its strong female preponderance and propensity to occur concomitantly with endometriosis of the bladder. However, its periodic admixture with urothelial carcinoma suggests an origin in the bladder urothelium. It is suggested that clear cell adenocarcinoma tends not to behave aggressively even when diagnosed at high stage [59].

Hepatoid Adenocarcinoma

This rarest subtype of bladder adenocarcinoma has a striking morphological, ultrastructural, and immunohistochemical resemblance to hepatocellular carcinoma, and includes cords or trabeculae of malignant polygonal cells with abundant cytoplasm, intracytoplasmic hyaline globules, bile canaliculi formation, and bile duct production resembling hepatocytic cells [62, 63]. This tumor also expresses markers of hepatocyte differentiation such as HepPar1, alpha-fetoprotein (AFP), and polyclonal carcinoma embryonic antigen (CEA) within a canalicular pattern [62, 63]. Knowledge of this unusual subtype is important and should not be mistaken as bladder involvement by metastatic hepatocellular carcinoma or yolk sac tumor with hepatoid morphology. Hepatoid adenocarcinoma is suggested to have an aggressive behavior. The exact histogenesis of this tumor is unclear.

Immunohistochemistry

The immunohistochemical staining profile of bladder adenocarcinoma closely resembles that of adenocarcinoma of the gastrointestinal tract. Bladder adenocarcinoma typically expresses the intestinal markers villin, CEA, and CDX2 [66, 69, 70], although some studies suggested expression to be less frequent than in colonic adenocarcinoma [23, 71, 72]. CK7 and CK20 staining is variable in bladder adenocarcinoma and overlaps with that seen in colorectal adenocarcinomas [23, 66, 69, 70, 72]. Among the epithelial markers, keratin 34BE12 is expressed in 66% of urachal carcinomas in contrast to only 11% of colonic adenocarcinoma [66]. Currently, nuclear β-catenin expression appears to be the most specific in distinguishing colonic from bladder adenocarcinoma (Fig. 11.9) [23, 66, 69]. Whereas the majority of colonic adenocarcinomas are nuclear β-catenin positive (81%), bladder adenocarcinoma is generally negative [23, 69]. Focal expression of nuclear β-catenin can be seen in 7% of urachal carcinomas [66]. β-catenin staining is ubiquitously present in the cytoplasm of both colonic and bladder adenocarcinomas and the background reaction may cause difficulty in the interpretation of nuclear staining. Thus, there is no absolute marker to distinguish bladder and colonic adenocarcinoma. However, diffuse nuclear β-catenin staining would argue against bladder adenocarcinoma and diffuse keratin β E12 staining would argue against colonic adenocarcinoma.

Similarly, bladder and gastrointestinal tract signet-ring cell carcinomas exhibit overlap in the expression of CK7, CK20, CDX2, and β-catenin, although the expression of intestinal

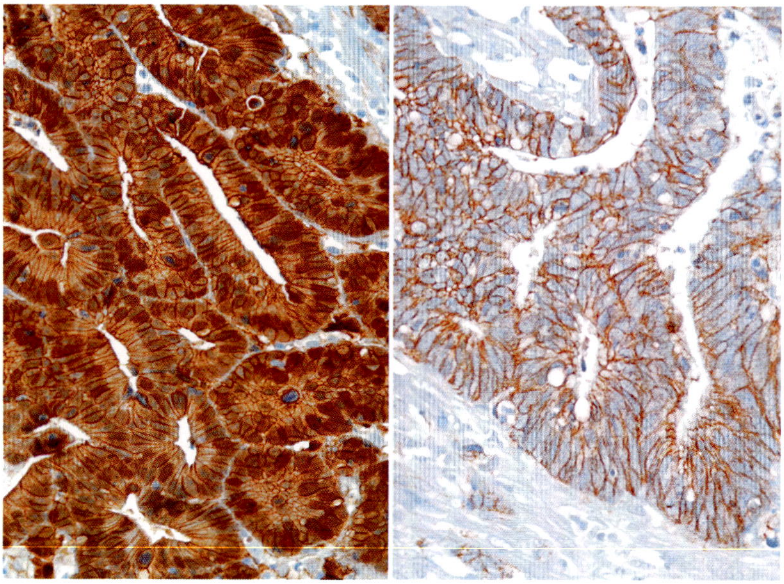

Fig. 11.9 β-catenin immunostain shows nuclear positivity in colonic adenocarcinoma (*left*) and nuclear negativity in bladder adenocarcinoma (*right*). Both tumors show cytoplasmic staining

markers seem to be lower in bladder signet-ring cell carcinoma [68]. The intestinal markers claudin-18 and REG-IV are considered to be specific for gastric signet-ring cell carcinoma (versus lung and breast signet-ring cell carcinomas); however, these are also expressed by bladder signet-ring cell carcinoma [69]. Thus, no marker can differentiate bladder from gastrointestinal signet-ring cell carcinoma. Distinction from signet-ring cell carcinomas of other organ sites such as lung or breast can be aided by their lack of expression of intestinal markers.

Bladder adenocarcinoma does not stain with the traditional prostate markers prostate-specific antigen (PSA) and prostate-specific acid phosphate (PSAP), although rare cross-reactivity with polyclonal antibody to PSAP can occur [9, 72, 73]. PSAP staining, when present in bladder adenocarcinoma, is only focal, whereas it is diffuse in prostate adenocarcinoma [9, 74]. The newer prostatic markers P501S (prostein) and prostate-specific membrane antigen (PSMA) are expressed in 11% of bladder adenocarcinomas, show moderate to diffuse staining, and thus should be interpreted with caution in the differential diagnosis with prostate adenocarcinoma [73]. Unlike bladder adenocarcinoma, prostate adenocarcinoma typically exhibits granular perinuclear P501S staining and apical membranous PSMA staining [73]. The prostate cancer selective marker α methylacyl coenzyme A racemase (AMACR) also stains bladder adenocarcinoma; hence, it is not useful in this differential diagnostic context [71]. Thus, PSA and monoclonal PSAP are the most specific markers in distinguishing prostate from bladder adenocarcinoma. However, poorly differentiated prostate carcinoma may lose PSA and PSAP expression in 15% and 5% of cases, respectively [73], and other prostate markers such as P501S and PSMA can be added in this scenario.

Other subtypes such as clear cell adenocarcinoma strongly express CA125 and hepatoid adenocarcinoma expresses hepPar1, AFP, α1-antitrypsin, and canalicular polyclonal CEA pattern, which are unique for these subtypes [59, 60, 62, 63].

Histological Differential Diagnosis

Cystitis glandularis of intestinal type—when extensive and with mucin extravasation—may histologically mimic a well-differentiated bladder adenocarcinoma [75, 76]. In contrast to bladder adenocarcinoma, cystitis glandularis lacks cytologic atypia and has few or absent mitoses. Cystitis glandularis has sharp underlying boundary and lacks destructive stromal infiltration, in contrast to the irregular infiltrative glands of bladder adenocarcinoma, which may deeply infiltrate the muscularis propria.

Glandular differentiation can be seen in 6% of invasive urothelial carcinomas [77] and is characterized by the presence of lumina lined by columnar epithelium with apical cytoplasm and variable mucin (true glands). Rarely, gland-like spaces may occur in urothelial carcinoma, in which the lumina are lined instead by urothelial cells. True glandular differentiation and gland-like lumina can be distinguished from pure bladder adenocarcinoma by the presence of an admixed, typical in situ, papillary, or invasive urothelial carcinoma component. Diagnosis can be challenging in limited tissue samples when the lesion is not appreciated in its entirety (i.e., biopsy). The clinical significance of true glandular differentiation in urothelial carcinoma is unclear, although pure bladder adenocarcinoma appears to behave more aggressively than urothelial carcinoma.

Secondary adenocarcinoma of the bladder can be due to a metastasis from other primary sites or more commonly from direct extension by prostate or colorectal adenocarcinoma. Metastases to bladder from other organ sites often occur at a late stage or with disseminated disease and thus uncommonly pose a clinicopathological diagnostic problem. Difficulty in diagnosis, however, may occur when adenocarcinoma is encountered at a metastatic site (e.g., lymph node biopsy). Colorectal adenocarcinoma resembles enteric type bladder adenocarcinoma and distinction is virtually impossible by morphology alone. Diagnosis can be aided by the use of immunohistochemistry (keratin βE12 and β-catenin) and with clinical, endoscopic, and radiological correlation. Secondary invasion by prostate adenocarcinoma to bladder is far more common than primary bladder adenocarcinoma. Morphological distinction from bladder adenocarcinoma of conventional (acinar) prostatic adenocarcinoma is less problematic, although the ductal adenocarcinoma and mucinous variants of prostatic adenocarcinoma can be a challenging differential diagnosis. Use of immunohistochemical stains including prostatic (PSA and monoclonal PSAP) and intestinal (CDX2, villin) markers is helpful in these situations. Distinction from adenocarcinomas of other sites such as breast and lung primaries can be aided by their lack of expression of CK20 and intestinal markers.

Clear cell adenocarcinoma can be mimicked by nephrogenic adenoma because of its clear and hobnailed cells. However, degree of atypia is more severe and mitosis is frequent in clear cell adenocarcinoma.

Clinical Features, Management, and Survival

Adenocarcinomas of the bladder appear more aggressive than urothelial carcinomas, largely due to the presence of advanced disease in patients at the time of diagnosis [14, 37]. Evidence suggests that overall survival is very much stage dependent [78]. However, when adjusting for tumor stage and grade, some reports reveal equivalent survival outcomes compared with the more predominant group of patients with urothelial cell histology [14]. A more favorable prognosis is recognized in patients with urachal and bilharzial adenocarcinomas compared to patients with primary adenocarcinomas [78].

Nonschistosomal-Associated Adenocarcinoma

The optimal multidisciplinary management strategy for nonbilharzial primary adenocarcinomas has been poorly defined due to the rare occurrence of this tumor and the resultant lack of evidence-based treatment paradigms. Nevertheless, the central component of multimodality therapy centers on surgical resection. A minority of patients present with nonmuscle-invasive tumors. Cystoscopy and transurethral resection of tumor alone are rarely sufficient. Most patients with adenocarcinoma confined to the urothelium (clinical stage Ta) or to the underlying lamina propria (clinical stage T1) would experience tumor recurrence or tumor progression with observation alone. Current intravesical therapies (i.e., BCG, mitomycin-C) have no proven efficacy in the management of nonmuscle invasive bladder adenocarcinoma. For primary adenocarcinomas, cystectomy (with or without adjuvant radiation therapy), pelvic lymph node dissection, and urinary diversion remain the standard of care. The goals of surgical therapy include a complete resection characterized by the prevention of tumor spillage, the achievement of negative surgical margins (R0), and a complete lymphadenectomy [79]. Primary radiation therapy is an option for otherwise unacceptable cystectomy candidates. Whether primary radiation therapy produces inferior, equivalent, or better results than surgery is unknown due to the limitations with experience in patients with this type of cancer.

Most experience with nonbilharzial primary bladder adenocarcinomas in North America is reported in the form of retrospective case series with limited numbers of patients often managed over decades [9, 13]. Five-year survival in these series ranges from 30 to 48%, inferior to the survival typically reported for patients with urothelial carcinoma of the bladder. Recently, Rogers et al. [37] evaluated patients undergoing cystectomy at three different academic institutions. Five-year cancer-specific survival for urothelial carcinoma and adenocarcinoma were 68% and 13%, respectively [37]. The survival difference was likely due to the significantly greater percentage of adenocarcinoma patients with pathologic stage T3–T4 disease (76% vs. 42%). Lughezzani and colleagues [14] examined 17 Surveillance, Epidemiology, and End Results registries for patients diagnosed with bladder adenocarcinoma over an 18-year period. While there were no differences in stage-specific survival amongst patients with adenocarcinoma compared to urothelial carcinoma, significantly greater percentages of adenocarcinoma patients had pathologic stage T3-T4 disease (61.4% vs. 47.3%) and lymph node positive disease (26.5% vs. 21.7%) [14]. The similar stage-specific survival suggests that there are biologic features common to other urothelial-derived malignancies. It is poorly understood why patients with adenocarcinoma present with more advanced disease. There are several different histologic subtypes of adenocarcinomas that might potentially impact tumor invasiveness and disease progression. The signet-ring cell subtype appears to be particularly aggressive. The presence of increasing tumor percentages of signet-ring cell differentiation has been associated with a poor prognosis. These patients have an increased rate of adverse pathologic features such as an unresectable primary tumor and lymph node metastases, both characteristics leading to decreased overall survival [7].

Schistosomal-Associated Adenocarcinoma

Most experience with bilharzial adenocarcinomas is derived from Egypt where schistosomiasis is endemic and where bladder cancer is the most common and the second most common cancer diagnosed amongst men and women, respectively [78]. A recent extensive surgical series update revealed that 9.6% of patients undergoing cystectomy had primary nonurachal adenocarcinoma (compared to 49.4% with squamous cell carcinoma and 36.4% with urothelial carcinoma). Of the patients with adenocarcinoma, 83% were found to harbor bilharzial eggs [2]. Contrary to the reported experience with nonbilharzial adenocarcinoma, approximately 20% of patients in this series had pT3 or pT4 cancer, approximately 20% had lymph node positive disease, and 5-year survival was 57.5%, a significant improvement in all pathologic and survival parameters over patients with nonbilharzial disease [2]. Differences in tumor grade between nonbilharzial and bilharzial adenocarcinomas likely affect the reported differences in pathologic findings and survival. The majority of tumors are lower grade tumors (grade I or grade II) in patients with bilharzial adenocarcinoma compared to a much greater incidence of high-grade tumors in patients with primary nonbilharzial adenocarcinoma and urothelial carcinoma [2, 14].

Urachal Adenocarcinoma

While partial cystectomy might be an option for highly selected patients with urothelial carcinomas, the routine surgical management of urachal adenocarcinomas involves the en-bloc resection of the bladder dome (or the midline portion of the bladder involved by tumor), the urachal ligament, and the umbilicus [11, 42, 66]. En-bloc resection is supported by recent observations that up to 7% of patients with urachal cancer have primary tumors that involve the umbilicus [10, 11] and relapse rates are higher in patients that do not undergo en-bloc resection [11, 27]. Minimally invasive surgical approaches for both cystectomy and partial cystectomy have been described, albeit with relatively short-term follow-up [80–82]. The advantages afforded to patients with minimally invasive approaches include less blood loss and more rapid convalescence. As most patients with adenocarcinomas have locally advanced disease, patients offered minimally invasive surgery will need to be selected carefully to maximize the therapeutic efficacy of surgery for these high-risk tumors.

The 5-year overall survival for patients with urachal adenocarcinoma is reported to be 27–61% [9, 11, 12, 83, 84]. Good prognostic factors for patients with urachal adenocarcinomas include negative surgical margins, en-bloc excision of the urachal tumor with the umbilicus (plus the portion of involved bladder), and the absence of lymph node metastases, distant metastases, and peritoneal carcinomatosis [11, 27, 85]. Patients with regional lymph node metastases have a clinical course similar to patients with distant metastases in that long-term survival is reportedly poor for both clinical scenarios [11].

Recent data reveal that patients with urachal adenocarcinoma have a better prognosis than patients with primary nonbilharzial adenocarcinoma, even though a significantly greater proportion of patients with urachal tumors present with distant metastases. On the contrary, urachal tumors are more likely to be well or moderately differentiated compared with nonurachal adenocarcinomas (65% vs. 34%). Urachal tumors are diagnosed at an earlier age of onset, likely in patients with fewer competing comorbidities compared to patients with primary bladder adenocarcinoma. In a review of available Surveillance, Epidemiology, and End Results (SEER) data, the 5-year overall survival was greater for patients with urachal tumors (48%) compared to those with nonurachal adenocarcinoma (35%), even after adjusting for stage, grade, age, histologic subtype, gender, surgical management, and the year of diagnosis. Median survival was demonstrated to be 58 and 29 months, respectively [12]. In the same SEER analysis, patients with localized disease had nonsignificant differences in survival. However, in patients with regional or distant disease, the risk of death was significantly less in those with urachal cancers [12].

Radiation Therapy and Chemotherapy

The role of both radiation and chemotherapy for bladder and urachal adenocarcinoma is poorly defined. Effective multimodality treatment strategies are desired given the high risk of local recurrence following cystectomy and the unfavorable survival implications associated with the development of both regional and distant metastatic diseases. At least in North America and in Europe, the incidence of adenocarcinoma is low. Accrual to clinical trials exploring new treatment paradigms would require many years and a concerted effort amongst major high-volume academic centers. As a result, experience with nonsurgical local or systemic therapies is limited to retrospective case series or anecdotal single-institutional reviews.

Most experience with neoadjuvant or adjuvant radiation stems from nations with endemic schistosomiasis. While adenocarcinoma accounts for a far greater percentage of patients with bladder cancer in these regions compared to Western countries, it still represents a smaller percentage of patients than those with squamous cell carcinoma or urothelial carcinoma. Neoadjuvant and adjuvant radiotherapy may be beneficial in patients with bilharzial cancers, particularly for patients with locally advanced tumors (pathologic stage T3 or T4) [86, 87]. Specifically in patients with bilharzial adenocarcinoma, a large retrospective review of cystectomy patients managed with postoperative adjuvant radiation revealed a significantly improved 5-year disease-free survival rate (61%) compared to patients managed with surgery alone (37%). Disease-free survival was likely impacted most by the improvement in local control, which was 53% in cystectomy alone patients compared to 96% for the postoperative radiotherapy patients [88]. Unfortunately, there are insufficient data to determine how radiation therapy should be integrated into the management of patients with nonbilharzial or urachal adenocarcinomas. The most common indication would include patients with positive surgical margins. Otherwise, experience is limited and recommendations are based on low level or anecdotal evidence.

Similar to experience with radiation therapy, there is little current evidence that systemic chemotherapy favorably impacts survival. Traditional cisplatin-based chemotherapy regimens used for urothelial carcinoma (i.e., MVAC) may have little impact on urachal and nonurachal adenocarcinomas. Physicians from the Mayo clinic evaluated their long-term experience in patients with urachal cancers. They identified no survival benefit in 39 patients who required salvage chemotherapy for advanced or for metastatic disease [27]. Other centers have reported limited response rates in patients treated for adenocarcinoma using the combination regimen of ifosfamide, paclitaxel, and cisplatin [89]. Urachal adenocarcinomas share a clinical course more typical of colorectal adenocarcinomas and may respond to perioperative 5-fluorouracil (5FU)-based regimens. A report from MD Anderson Cancer Center revealed a 33% response rate to the combination of 5FU and cisplatin [11]. Based on these encouraging findings, researchers have initiated a trial specifically for bladder adenocarcinoma and urachal adenocarcinoma patients using the regimen containing 5FU, leucovorin, gemcitabine, and cisplatin [11]. Currently, there are no standard recommendations regarding the use of neoadjuvant or adjuvant chemotherapy for adenocarcinoma although adjuvant treatment may be offered based on more recent experience with systemic therapies.

References

1. Lynch CF, Cohen MB. Urinary system. Cancer. 1995;75(1 Suppl):316–29.
2. Ghoneim MA, Abdel-Latif M, el-Mekresh M, et al. Radical cystectomy for carcinoma of the bladder: 2,720 consecutive cases 5 years later. J Urol. 2008; 180(1):121–7.
3. Filmer RB, Spencer JR. Malignancies in bladder augmentations and intestinal conduits. J Urol. 1990; 143:671–8.
4. Sözen S, Gürocak S, Uzüm N, Biri H, Memiş L, Bozkirli I. The importance of re-evaluation in patients with cystitis glandularis associated with pelvic lipomatosis: a case report. Urol Oncol. 2004;22(5): 428–30.
5. Smith AK, Hansel DE, Jones JS. Role of cystitis cystica et glandularis and intestinal metaplasia in development of bladder carcinoma. Urology. 2008;71(5): 915–8.
6. Corica FA, Husmann DA, Churchill BM, et al. Intestinal metaplasia is not a strong risk factor for bladder cancer: study of 53 cases with long-term follow-up. Urology. 1997;50(3):427–31.
7. Thomas DG, Ward AM, Williams JL. A study of 52 cases of adenocarcinoma of the bladder. Br J Urol. 1971;43(1):4–15.
8. Badawi AF, Mostafa MH, Probert A, O'Connor PJ. Role of schistosomiasis in human bladder cancer: evidence of association, aetiological factors, and basic mechanisms of carcinogenesis. Eur J Cancer Prev. 1995;4(1):45–59.
9. Grignon DJ, Ro JY, Ayala AG, Johnson DE, Ordóñez NG. Primary adenocarcinoma of the urinary bladder. A clinicopathologic analysis of 72 cases. Cancer. 1991;67(8):2165–72.
10. Sheldon CA, Clayman RV, Gonzalez R, Williams RD, Fraley EE. Malignant urachal lesions. J Urol. 1984;131(1):1–8.
11. Siefker-Radtke AO, Gee J, Shen Y, et al. Multimodality management of urachal carcinoma: the MD. Anderson Cancer Center experience. J Urol. 2003;169(4): 1295–8.

12. Wright JL, Porter MP, Li CI, Lange PH, Lin DW. Differences in survival among patients with urachal and nonurachal adenocarcinomas of the bladder. Cancer. 2006;107(4):721–8.
13. Dandekar NP, Dalal AV, Tongaonkar HB, Kamat MR. Adenocarcinoma of bladder. Eur J Surg Oncol. 1997;23(2):157–60.
14. Lughezzani G, Sun M, Jeldres C, et al. Adenocarcinoma versus urothelial carcinoma of the urinary bladder: comparison between pathologic stage at radical cystectomy and cancer-specific mortality. Urology. 2010;75(2):376–81.
15. D'Addessi A, Racioppi M, Fanasca A, La Rocca LM, Alcini E. Adenocarcinoma of the urachus: radical or conservative surgery? A report of a case and a review of the literature. Eur J Surg Oncol. 1998;24:131–3.
16. Santucci RA, True LD, Lange PH. Is partial cystectomy the treatment of choice for mucinous adenocarcinoma of the urachus? Urology. 1997;49:536–40.
17. Schubert GE, Pavkovic MB, Bethke-Bedürftig BA. Tubular urachal remnants in adult bladders. J Urol. 1982;127(1):40–2.
18. Siefker-Radtke A. Urachal carcinoma: surgical and chemotherapeutic options. Expert Rev Anticancer Ther. 2006;6(12):1715–21.
19. Feldman PA, Madeb R, Naroditsky I, Halachmi S, Nativ O. Metastatic breast cancer to the bladder: a diagnostic challenge and review of the literature. Urology. 2002;59(1):138.
20. Goldstein AG. Metastatic carcinoma to the bladder. J Urol. 1967;98(2):209–15.
21. Velcheti V, Govindan R. Metastatic cancer involving bladder: a review. Can J Urol. 2007;14(1):3443–8.
22. Bates AW, Baithun SI. Secondary neoplasms of the bladder are histological mimics of nontransitional cell primary tumours: clinicopathological and histological features of 282 cases. Histopathology. 2000; 36(1):32–40.
23. Raspollini MR, Nesi G, Baroni G, Girardi LR, Taddei GL. Immunohistochemistry in the differential diagnosis between primary and secondary intestinal adenocarcinoma of the urinary bladder. Appl Immunohistochem Mol Morphol. 2005;13(4):358–62.
24. Wang HL, Lu DW, Yerian LM, et al. Immunohistochemical distinction between primary adenocarcinoma of the bladder and secondary colorectal adenocarcinoma. Am J Surg Pathol. 2001;25(11):1380–7.
25. Takeuchi M, Matsuzaki K, Yoshida S, Nishitani H, Uehara H. Imaging findings of urachal mucinous cystadenocarcinoma associated with pseudomyxoma peritonei. Acta Radiol. 2004;45(3):348–50.
26. Reid-Nicholson MD, Ramalingam P, Adeagbo B, Cheng N, Peiper SC, Terris MK. The use of Urovysion fluorescence in situ hybridization in the diagnosis and surveillance of non-urothelial carcinoma of the bladder. Mod Pathol. 2009;22(1):119–27.
27. Ashley RA, Inman BA, Sebo TJ, et al. Urachal carcinoma: clinicopathologic features and long-term outcomes of an aggressive malignancy. Cancer. 2006;107(4):712–20.
28. Anderström C, Johansson SL, von Schultz L. Primary adenocarcinoma of the urinary bladder. A clinicopathologic and prognostic study. Cancer. 1983;52(7): 1273–80.
29. Burnett AL, Epstein JI, Marshall FF. Adenocarcinoma of urinary bladder: classification and management. Urology. 1991;37(4):315–21.
30. Kramer SA, Bredael J, Croker BP, Paulson DF, Glenn JF. Primary non-urachal adenocarcinoma of the bladder. J Urol. 1979;121(3):278–81.
31. Mostoffi FK, Thomson RV, Dean AL. Mucous adenocarcinoma of the urinary bladder. Cancer. 1955;8: 741–58.
32. Jacobo E, Loening S, Schmidt JD, Culp DA. Primary adenocarcinoma of the bladder: a retrospective study of 20 patients. J Urol. 1977;117(1):54–6.
33. Jones WA, Gibbons RP, Correa Jr RJ, Cummings KB, Mason JT. Primary adenocarcinoma of bladder. Urology. 1980;15(2):119–22.
34. Shigehara K, Taya T, Hisazumi H. Primary adenocarcinoma in the bladder diverticulum. Scand J Urol Nephrol. 2008;42(5):481–3.
35. Tamas EF, Stephenson AJ, Campbell SC, Montague DK, Trusty DC, Hansel DE. Histopathologic features and clinical outcomes in 71 cases of bladder diverticula. Arch Pathol Lab Med. 2009;133(5):791–6.
36. el-Mekresh MM, el-Baz MA, Abol-Enein H, Ghoneim MA. Primary adenocarcinoma of the urinary bladder: a report of 185 cases. Br J Urol. 1998;82(2):206–12.
37. Rogers CG, Palapattu GS, Shariat SF, et al. Clinical outcomes following radical cystectomy for primary nontransitional cell carcinoma of the bladder compared to transitional cell carcinoma of the bladder. J Urol. 2006;175(6):2048–53.
38. Blute ML, Engen DE, Travis WD, Kvols LK. Primary signet ring cell adenocarcinoma of the bladder. J Urol. 1989;141(1):17–21.
39. Gonzalez E, Fowler MR, Venable DD. Primary signet ring cell adenocarcinoma of the bladder (linitis plastica of the bladder): report of a case and review of the literature. J Urol. 1982;128(5):1027–30.
40. Grignon DJ, Ro JY, Ayala AG, Johnson DE. Primary signet-ring cell carcinoma of the urinary bladder. Am J Clin Pathol. 1991;95(1):13–20.
41. Poore TE, Egbert B, Jahnke R, Kraft JK. Signet ring cell adenocarcinoma of the bladder: linitis plastica variant. Arch Pathol Lab Med. 1981;105(4):203–4.
42. Herr HW. Urachal carcinoma: the case for extended partial cystectomy. J Urol. 1994;151(2):365–6.
43. Adegboyega PA, Adesokan A. Tubulovillous adenoma of the urinary bladder. Mod Pathol. 1999;12(7): 735–8.
44. Channer JL, Williams JL, Henry L. Villous adenoma of the bladder. J Clin Pathol. 1993;46(5):450–2.
45. Cheng L, Montironi R, Bostwick DG. Villous adenoma of the urinary tract: a report of 23 cases, including 8 with coexistent adenocarcinoma. Am J Surg Pathol. 1999;23(7):764–71.
46. Seibel JL, Prasad S, Weiss RE, Bancila E, Epstein JI. Villous adenoma of the urinary tract: a lesion

frequently associated with malignancy. Hum Pathol. 2002;33(2):236–41.

47. Eble JN, Hull MT, Rowland RG, Hostetter M. Villous adenoma of the urachus with mucusuria: a light and electron microscopic study. J Urol. 1986;135(6):1240–4.
48. Choi WWL, Amin MB, Tamboli P, Eble JN, Youn RH. Glandular neoplasms of the urachus: clinicopathologic and immunohistochemical analysis of 43 cases with special emphasis on low-grade mucinous cystic tumors. Mod Pathol. 2005;9:134A.
49. Hull MT, Warfel KA. Urachal cystadenoma with abundant glycogen: ultrastructural study. Ultrastruct Pathol. 1994;18(5):499–502.
50. Schell AJ, Nickel CJ, Isotalo PA. Complex mucinous cystadenoma of undetermined malignant potential of the urachus. Can Urol Assoc J. 2009;3(4):E39–41.
51. Carr NJ, McLean AD. A mucinous tumour of the urachus: adenoma or low grade mucinous cystic tumour of uncertain malignant potential? Adv Clin Path. 2001;5(3):93–7.
52. Ng KJ, Newman P, Price-Thomas JM. Carcinoma of the urachus associated with urachal adenoma. Br J Urol. 1991;67(2):215–6.
53. Stenhouse G, McRae D, Pollock AM. Urachal adenocarcinoma in situ with pseudomyxoma peritonei: a case report. J Clin Pathol. 2003;56(2):152–3.
54. Chan TY, Epstein JI. In situ adenocarcinoma of the bladder. Am J Surg Pathol. 2001;25(7):892–9.
55. Miller JS, Epstein JI. Noninvasive urothelial carcinoma of the bladder with glandular differentiation: report of 24 cases. Am J Surg Pathol. 2009;33(8):1241–8.
56. Abenoza P, Manivel C, Fraley EE. Primary adenocarcinoma of urinary bladder. Clinicopathologic study of 16 cases. Urology. 1987;29:9–14.
57. Ayala AG, Tamboli P. Urachal carcinoma. In: Eble JN, Sauter G, Epstein JI, Sesterhenn IA, editors. World Health Organization classification of tumours. Pathology & genetics. Tumours of the urinary system and male genital organs. Lyon, France: IARC Press; 2004. p. 131–2.
58. Ayala AG, Tamboli P, El-Bolkainy MN, et al. Adenocarcinoma. In: Eble JN, Sauter G, Epstein JI, Sesterhenn IA, editors. World Health Organization classification of tumours. Pathology & genetics. Tumours of the urinary system and male genital organs. Lyon, France: IARC Press; 2004. p. 128–30.
59. Drew PA, Murphy WM, Civantos F, Speights VO. The histogenesis of clear cell adenocarcinoma of the lower urinary tract. Case series and review of the literature. Hum Pathol. 1996;27(3):248–52.
60. Oliva E, Amin MB, Jimenez R, Young RH. Clear cell carcinoma of the urinary bladder: a report and comparison of four tumors of mullerian origin and nine of probable urothelial origin with discussion of histogenesis and diagnostic problems. Am J Surg Pathol. 2002;26(2):190–7.
61. Young RH, Scully RE. Clear cell adenocarcinoma of the bladder and urethra. A report of three cases and review of the literature. Am J Surg Pathol. 1985; 9(11):816–26.
62. Burgués O, Ferrer J, Navarro S, Ramos D, Botella E, Llombart-Bosch A. Hepatoid adenocarcinoma of the urinary bladder. An unusual neoplasm. Virchows Arch. 1999;435(1):71–5.
63. Lopez-Beltran A, Luque RJ, Quintero A, Requena MJ, Montironi R. Hepatoid adenocarcinoma of the urinary bladder. Virchows Arch. 2003;442(4): 381–7.
64. Molina JR, Quevedo JF, Furth AF, et al. Predictors of survival from urachal cancer: a Mayo Clinic study of 49 cases. Cancer. 2007;110(11):2434–40.
65. Herr HW, Bochner BH, Sharp D, Dalbagni G, Reuter VE. Urachal carcinoma: contemporary surgical outcomes. J Urol. 2007;178(1):74–8.
66. Gopalan A, Sharp DS, Fine SW, et al. Urachal carcinoma: a clinicopathologic analysis of 24 cases with outcome correlation. Am J Surg Pathol. 2009;33(5): 659–68.
67. Egevad L, Håkansson U, Grabe M, Ehrnstrom R. Urachal signet-cell adenocarcinoma. Scand J Urol Nephrol. 2009;43(1):88–91.
68. Thomas AA, Stephenson AJ, Campbell SC, Jones JS, Hansel DE. Clinicopathologic features and utility of immunohistochemical markers in signet-ring cell adenocarcinoma of the bladder. Hum Pathol. 2009; 40(1):108–16.
69. Paner GP, McKenney JK, Yao JL, Frankerl WL, Shen SS, Jimenez RE. Immunohistochemical analysis of urachal carcinoma with emphasis on its morphologic types and their differential diagnosis with metastatic colonic adenocarcinoma: diagnostic role of traditional and novel markers. Mod Pathol. 2009;22:188A.
70. Tamboli P, Mohsin SK, Hailemariam S, Amin MB. Colonic adenocarcinoma metastatic to the urinary tract versus primary tumors of the urinary tract with glandular differentiation: a report of 7 cases and investigation using a limited immunohistochemical panel. Arch Pathol Lab Med. 2002;126(9):1057–63.
71. Suh N, Yang XJ, Tretiakova MS, Humphrey PA, Wang HL. Value of CDX2, villin, and alpha-methylacyl coenzyme A racemase immunostains in the distinction between primary adenocarcinoma of the bladder and secondary colorectal adenocarcinoma. Mod Pathol. 2005;18(9):1217–22.
72. Torenbeek R, Lagendijk JH, Van Diest PJ, Bril H, van de Molengraft FJ, Meijer CJ. Value of a panel of antibodies to identify the primary origin of adenocarcinomas presenting as bladder carcinoma. Histopathology. 1998;32(1):20–7.
73. Lane Z, Hansel DE, Epstein JI. Immunohistochemical expression of prostatic antigens in adenocarcinoma and villous adenoma of the urinary bladder. Am J Surg Pathol. 2008;32(9):1322–6.
74. Epstein JI, Kuhajda FP, Lieberman PH. Prostate-specific acid phosphatase immunoreactivity in adenocarcinomas of the urinary bladder. Hum Pathol. 1986;17(9):939–42.
75. Jacobs LB, Brooks JD, Epstein JI. Differentiation of colonic metaplasia from adenocarcinoma of urinary bladder. Hum Pathol. 1997;28(10):1152–7.

76. Young RH, Bostwick DG. Florid cystitis glandularis of intestinal type with mucin extravasation: a mimic of adenocarcinoma. Am J Surg Pathol. 1996; 20(12):1462–8.
77. López-Beltrán A, Martín J, García J, Toro M. Squamous and glandular differentiation in urothelial bladder carcinomas. Histopathology, histochemistry and immunohistochemical expression of carcinoembryonic antigen. Histol Histopathol. 1988;3(1): 63–8.
78. Gilligan T, Dreicer R. The atypical urothelial cancer patient: management of bladder cancers of non-transitional cell histology and cancers of the ureters and renal pelvis. Semin Oncol. 2007;34(2):145–53.
79. Skinner EC, Stein JP, Skinner DG. Surgical benchmarks for the treatment of invasive bladder cancer. Urol Oncol. 2007;25(1):66–71.
80. Correa JJ, Hakky TS, Spiess PE, Chuang T, Sexton WJ. Robotic assisted partial cystectomy with en-bloc excision of the urachus and the umbilicus for urachal adenocarcinoma. J Robotic Surg. 2010;3:235–8.
81. Pruthi RS, Nielsen ME, Nix J, Smith A, Schultz H, Wallen EM. Robotic radical cystectomy for bladder cancer: surgical and pathological outcomes in 100 consecutive cases. J Urol. 2010;183(2):510–4.
82. Wadhwa P, Kolla SB, Hemal AK. Laparoscopic en bloc partial cystectomy with bilateral pelvic lymphadenectomy for urachal adenocarcinoma. Urology. 2006;67:837–43.
83. Henly DR, Farrow GM, Zincke H. Urachal cancer: role of conservative surgery. Urology. 1993;42(6):635–9.
84. Wilson TG, Pritchett TR, Lieskovsky G, Warner NE, Skinner DG. Primary adenocarcinoma of bladder. Urology. 1991;38(3):223–6.
85. Pinthus JH, Haddad R, Trachtenberg J, et al. Population based survival data on urachal tumors. J Urol. 2006;175(6):2042–7.
86. Ghoneim MA, Ashamallah AK, Awaad HK, Whitmore Jr WF. Randomized trial of cystectomy with or without preoperative radiotherapy for carcinoma of the bilharzial bladder. J Urol. 1985;134(2):266–8.
87. Zaghloul MS, Awwad HK, Akoush HH, Omar S, Soliman O, el Attar I. Postoperative radiotherapy of carcinoma in bilharzial bladder: improved disease free survival through improving local control. Int J Radiat Oncol Biol Phys. 1992;23(3):511–7.
88. Zaghloul MS, Nouh A, Nazmy M, et al. Long-term results of primary adenocarcinoma of the urinary bladder: a report on 192 patients. Urol Oncol. 2006;24(1):13–20.
89. Galsky MD, Iasonos A, Mironov S, et al. Prospective trial of ifosfamide, paclitaxel, and cisplatin in patients with advanced non-transitional cell carcinoma of the urothelial tract. Urology. 2007;69(2):255–9.

12 Mesenchymal Lesions of the Urinary Bladder

Jesse K. McKenney and Mark L. Gonzalgo

Introduction

Proliferations of mesenchymal cells, which are mesoderm-derived cells that form connective tissues, are uncommon in the urinary bladder. The majority of these lesions are comprised of cells with myofibroblastic, smooth muscle, or skeletal muscle lineage. Urothelial carcinomas may also rarely have a spindle cell histology that closely mimic mesenchymal cells, and in some cases specific lines of true mesenchymal differentiation such as chondrosarcoma may be present (i.e., carcinosarcoma). This spectrum of mesenchymal lesions may be diagnostically challenging for pathologists due to the degree of histologic overlap between clinically benign and malignant lesions. In some instances, the number of different diagnostic terms that have been applied to the same lesion has added unnecessary confusion for urologists and pathologists alike. Finally, given the rarity of this spectrum of lesions, there are often little data available to help guide therapeutic decision-making. We discuss these diagnostic and treatment issues related to mesenchymal lesions of the urinary bladder in this chapter.

J.K. McKenney (✉) • M.L. Gonzalgo
Department of Pathology, Stanford University Medical Center, 300 Pasteur Drive, H2110, Stanford, CA 94025, USA
e-mail: jmck@stanford.ed; gonzalgo@stanford.edu

Myofibroblastic Proliferations

Identical myofibroblastic proliferations of the urinary bladder have been described under a variety of names, which include postoperative spindle cell nodule, inflammatory pseudotumor, pseudosarcomatous fibromyxoid tumor, pseudosarcomatous myofibroblastic proliferation, pseudosarcomatous spindle cell proliferation, and inflammatory myofibroblastic tumor (IMT) [1–16]. Myofibroblastic lesions are commonly divided into three diagnostic categories based on the (1) presence or (2) absence of a prior history of bladder instrumentation or (3) an association with overlying urothelial carcinoma [17, 18]. It should be emphasized that, for practical purposes, these three lesions are histologically indistinguishable, a finding that has led some authors to combine them under one diagnostic term "pseudosarcomatous myofibroblastic proliferation/tumor" [3, 6, 14, 19, 20]. These myofibroblastic proliferations of the urinary bladder most commonly occur in the second to fourth decade of life, but they may also occur in children [3, 6, 21]. The most common presenting symptom is gross hematuria, but abdominal pain and irritative or obstructive voiding symptoms have also been described.

Postoperative spindle cell nodules, by definition, occur after trauma, typically following bladder instrumentation. The time interval between instrumentation and development of a cellular proliferation is typically a few weeks to months; however, some authors have suggested

D.E. Hansel et al. (eds.), *The Urinary Tract: A Comprehensive Guide to Patient Diagnosis and Management*, DOI 10.1007/978-1-4614-5320-8_12, © Springer Science+Business Media New York 2012

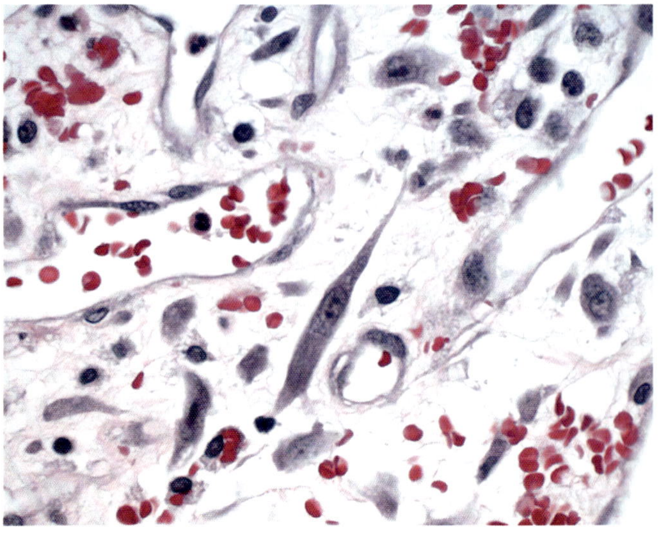

Fig. 12.1 Myofibroblasts have elongated cytoplasmic processes, fine nuclear chromatin, and variable nucleoli. Multiple nucleoli should not be taken as evidence of malignancy

that rare cases may occur a year or more after the initial insult. These post-instrumentation proliferations are usually small and rarely exceed 1 cm.

Pseudosarcomatous myofibroblastic proliferations (also called IMTs) are indistinguishable from trauma-induced postoperative spindle cell nodules; however, these lesions are typically larger in size (usually 2–8 cm, but over 30 cm reported). The recurrence rate for lesions in the urinary bladder has ranged from 0 to 19% and no metastases have been reported. One patient death secondary to urinary obstruction from local mass effect of an unresected vesical pseudosarcomatous myofibroblastic proliferation has been reported [9]. There is controversy regarding diagnostic terminology for these lesions, which can be confirmed by a survey of the nomenclature employed in current textbooks. Some authors suggest that vesical myofibroblastic proliferations are distinct from IMTs and should be combined under the term "pseudosarcomatous myofibroblastic proliferations," but this concept is still debated [11, 13].

Myofibroblastic proliferations have also been described in association with urothelial carcinoma (i.e., pseudosarcomatous stromal reaction associated with carcinoma) [17, 18]. These myofibroblastic proliferations may be intimately admixed with carcinoma or form a separate tumor-like nodule. In addition, patients with urothelial carcinoma may develop an otherwise typical postoperative spindle cell nodule secondary to prior transurethral resection. Because of the biphasic appearance, the main differential diagnosis for pathologists in this scenario is a sarcomatoid urothelial carcinoma. The distinction from malignant spindle cell lesions (e.g., leiomyosarcoma or sarcomatoid urothelial carcinoma) is the most clinically relevant task for the pathologist.

Pathology of Myofibroblastic Proliferations

Myofibroblastic proliferations have a characteristic cytology and low power architecture. Cytologically, the individual cells may appear spindled or stellate; the ends of the cells are usually tapered with elongated cytoplasmic processes identifiable at high power examination (Fig. 12.1). The cytoplasm varies from eosinophilic to more amphophilic. Nuclei have tapered or blunted ends with bland, noncondensed nuclear chromatin, and may show one or more small nucleoli. In some cases, the degree of variation in the size of

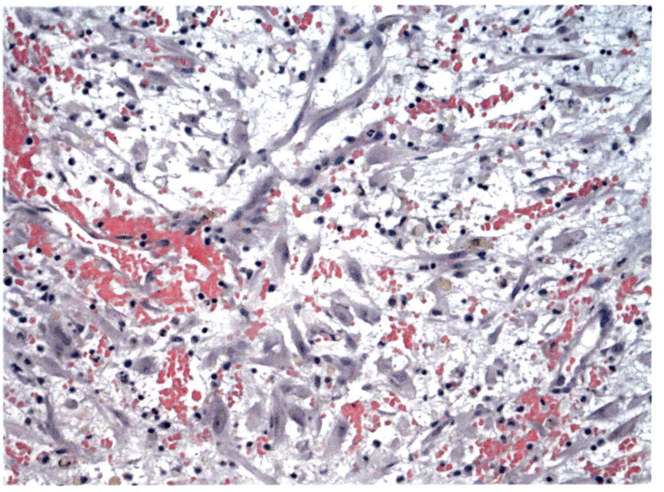

Fig. 12.2 Myofibroblastic proliferations often have myxoid stroma and a variable admixture of inflammatory cells

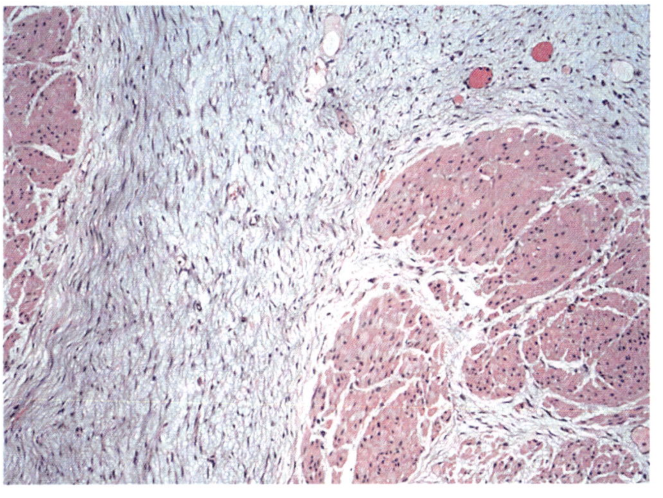

Fig. 12.3 Large myofibroblastic proliferations may involve the muscularis propria. This feature does not denote malignancy

individual cells may be pronounced, and scattered cells may have prominent macronucleoli. Despite these unusual features, however, the nuclear chromatin remains evenly distributed.

The most common pattern in the urinary bladder is myxoid that is characterized by a very loose, disorganized appearance (Fig. 12.2). There is often an associated mixed chronic inflammatory infiltrate and an irregular network of poorly organized small blood vessels. The lesional myofibroblastic cells frequently infiltrate the muscularis propria, but this should not be regarded as a sign of malignancy (Fig. 12.3).

Recent studies of vesical myofibroblastic proliferations have documented both ALK-1 (anaplastic lymphoma kinase) expression by immunohistochemistry and ALK gene rearrangements by FISH analysis in a subset of cases, findings typical of IMT in other anatomic sites [12, 22–25]. Whether the presence or absence of ALK-1 immunoreactivity/rearrangement has any clinical significance or defines subsets of myofibroblastic lesions in the bladder remains to be determined.

The immunophenotype of myofibroblastic proliferations in the urinary bladder is somewhat

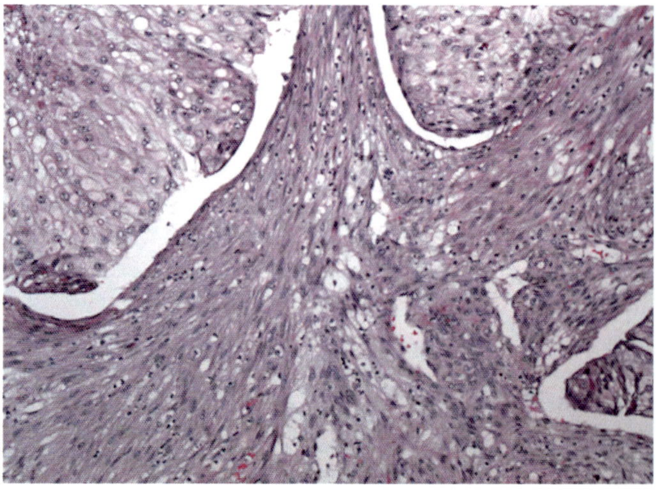

Fig. 12.4 Some invasive urothelial carcinomas may be associated with a florid myofibroblastic proliferation. In this example, large islands of carcinoma are surrounded by a myofibroblastic stromal response

different than that reported at other anatomic sites. Cytokeratin reactivity is frequently observed in myofibroblastic proliferations of the bladder (up to 84% in some series) [26] and most cases show reactivity for smooth muscle actin, while desmin expression is variable. Strong coexpression of smooth muscle actin and cytokeratin is characteristic of vesical myofibroblasts. Although h-caldesmon was initially touted as a specific marker of smooth muscle with utility in the distinction from myofibroblasts [27], h-caldesmon immunoreactivity was reported in 57–66% of vesical myofibroblastic lesions examined in two subsequent studies [13, 23].

Recent series have documented ALK-1 expression in 38–89% of cases [11–13, 23]. Tsuzuki et al. also performed ALK-1 immunostains on a series of eight sarcomatoid urothelial carcinomas and five genitourinary leiomyosarcomas (LMS) which were all negative, leading the authors to suggest the utility of ALK-1 in the distinction of myofibroblastic lesions from its mimics [24]. ALK-1 expression, however, is not entirely specific for IMT and is reported in other mesenchymal neoplasms (e.g., up to 20% of rhabdomyosarcoma (RMS)) [28].

Carcinomas associated with myofibroblastic proliferations may have histological overlap with sarcomatoid carcinoma. The cells of reactive myofibroblastic proliferations maintain relatively fine nuclear chromatin, while sarcomatoid carcinomas contain malignant spindle cells with coarse, clumpy chromatin in many areas. Invasive urothelial carcinomas with associated myofibroblastic proliferations may also pose staging problems if the spindle cells are mistaken for involvement of muscularis propria (Fig. 12.4). In general, the associated stroma has a more myxoid appearance compared to the muscularis propria (Fig. 12.5). Immunostains with the anti-smoothelin antibody typically show diffuse immunoreactivity in the smooth muscle cells of the muscularis propria, but not in myofibroblasts [29]. In addition, smooth muscle cells generally show strong and diffuse immunoreactivity with desmin, which is not entirely specific; however, this pattern is much less common in myofibroblasts.

Treatment of Myofibroblastic Proliferations

Endoscopic treatment with transurethral resection of bladder tumor (TURBT) is typically the first therapeutic intervention for myofibroblastic proliferations. The tumor mass is usually soft and amenable to transurethral resection because of smaller size at presentation (<5 cm). In one study,

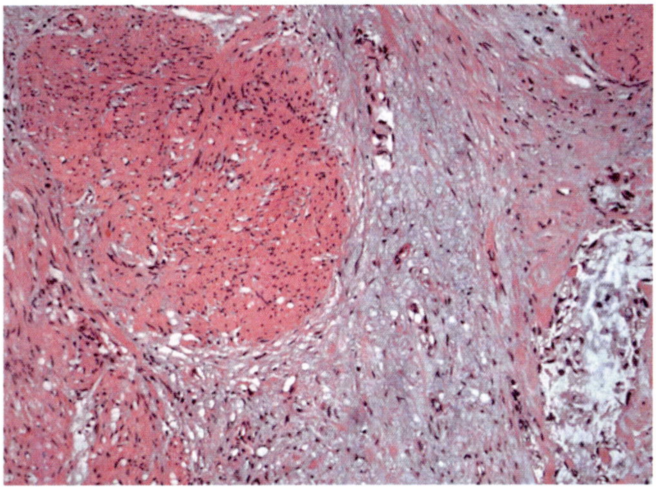

Fig. 12.5 Myofibroblastic proliferations (such as the one associated with invasive carcinoma in this example) maintain relatively fine nuclear chromatin; the stroma has a more myxoid appearance compared to the muscularis propria

no tumors recurred after transurethral resection or partial cystectomy [9]. One patient presented 5 months after TURBT with a histologically identical lesion that was considered to be incompletely resected tumor. Although there is no absolute size threshold that would prevent TURBT of myofibroblastic proliferations, partial cystectomy may be indicated for larger lesions that are not amenable to endoscopic management or for tumors located in proximity to the dome of the bladder.

Smooth Muscle Neoplasms

Smooth muscle neoplasms of the urinary bladder are rare, but are divided into two main categories: leiomyoma and leiomyosarcoma.

Pathology of Smooth Muscle Tumors

Leiomyomas represent the most common mesenchymal neoplasms of the urinary bladder [30–34]. They occur over a large age range, but there is a female predilection. Presenting symptoms include obstruction, irritative voiding symptoms, and hematuria. Most leiomyomas are small well circumscribed mass lesions, typically 2 cm or less; however, tumors up to 25 cm are reported. They have the same morphologic features as in other anatomic locations and are characterized by intersecting fascicles of spindle cells with abundant eosinophilic cytoplasm (Fig. 12.6). The cytoplasm is generally tapered and the nuclei are oval or elongated with blunted ends.

In the vast majority of leiomyomas, no significant nuclear atypia (i.e., no hyperchromasia or pleomorphism) is present. In addition, the lesions are well-circumscribed with no irregular infiltration into the surrounding muscularis propria. Coagulative tumor cell necrosis is not found in leiomyomas when strict rules are followed. Myxoid and/or epithelioid change is relatively uncommon in leiomyomas of the urinary bladder [34, 35]. A few cases of leiomyoma with degenerative type nuclear atypia (i.e. symplastic or atypical leiomyoma) were recently described; however, clinical follow-up data are limited at present [34]. A diagnosis of symplastic leiomyoma should be made with great caution and the presence of mitotic activity should prompt careful consideration of leiomyosarcoma.

Although LMSs are rare, they represent the most common primary vesical sarcoma [9, 33, 36–38]. They also occur over a broad age range; in contrast to leiomyoma, there is a male predominance.

LMS are rare in children, but are reported [39]. The mean size is 7 cm, and patients typically

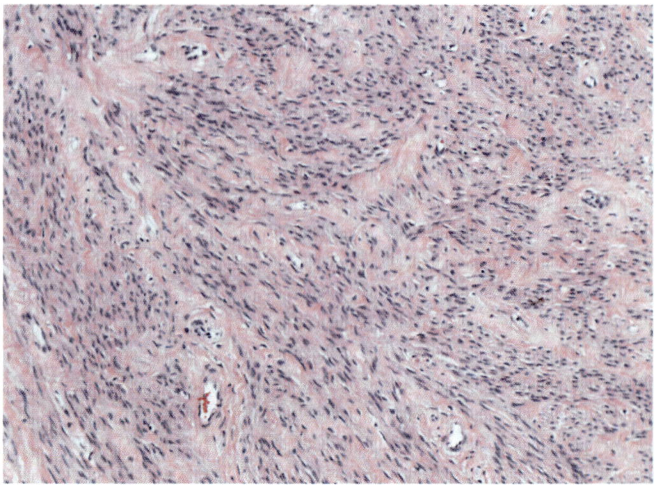

Fig. 12.6 Leiomyomas of the urinary bladder are cytologically bland, similar to their more common counterparts in the uterus

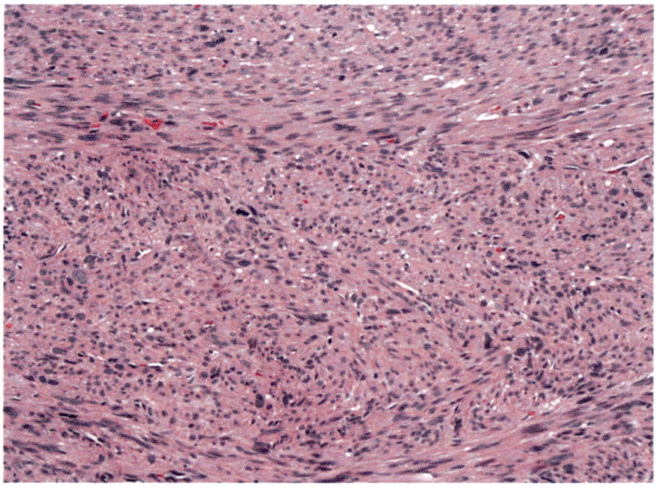

Fig. 12.7 Leiomyosarcomas may have a fascicular growth pattern and they often retain their eosinophilic appearance. The degree of cytologic atypia is greater than that seen in leiomyoma

present with hematuria and voiding symptoms. A subset of vesical LMS may be associated with prior chemotherapy, most commonly cyclophosphamide [39–44].

The typical histologic appearance is a cellular proliferation of spindle cells with prominent eosinophilic cytoplasm arranged into well-formed, intersecting fascicles (Fig. 12.7). Stromal myxoid change is frequently present, but epithelioid variants are exceedingly rare in the bladder. The following findings are typical for a diagnosis of malignancy in a true smooth muscle neoplasm of the bladder: significant nuclear pleomorphism with hyperchromasia (Fig. 12.8) and irregular nuclear membranes (which are usually readily identifiable at low power), coagulative tumor cell necrosis, increased mitotic activity, and infiltration of the muscularis propria.

Studies have used slightly different criteria for separating LMS into low- and high-grade groups, but it is suggested that tumors with significant nuclear atypia, mitotic activity (>5 mitotic figures/10 HPF), and coagulative necrosis have a high risk for recurrence, metastasis, and death due to disease, while tumors with less severe degrees of nuclear atypia, <5 mitotic figures/10 HPF, and no necrosis have a much smaller risk of aggressive behavior [9, 34, 36, 37]. These studies

Fig. 12.8 Leiomyosarcomas should have enlarged atypical cells and easily identified mitotic activity

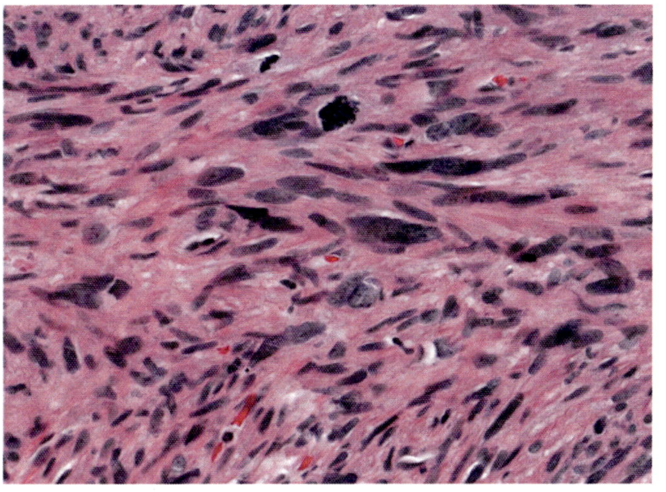

suggest that many, but not all patients with low-grade tumors have had long-term disease-free survival; however, a recent study suggests that most vesical LMS are aggressive high-grade sarcomas [38].

Most leiomyomas show diffuse immunoreactivity for actin, desmin, and h-caldesmon [27], but are nonreactive for cytokeratin [26]. Published series of LMSs have reported more variable staining with actin (43–100%) and desmin (0–60%). Some LMSs may also express cytokeratin (approximately 30% in one series, but 10% overall) or rarely EMA (approximately 5% overall). Cytoplasmic staining with epithelial markers is typically focal, and is generally restricted to low molecular weight keratin. Immunostains for ALK-1 have been negative in LMS [25, 26].

Treatment of Smooth Muscle Neoplasms

Leiomyomas that are smaller in size (< 5 cm) may be treated with transurethral resection alone. If the lesion is larger, but localized to certain areas within the bladder (i.e., dome), these tumors may be managed by partial cystectomy. Local excision or enucleation of bladder leiomyomas either by open or laparoscopic approaches has also been described. Leiomyosarcoma of the bladder is considered to be highly aggressive and would therefore be more appropriately treated with partial cystectomy (in select cases) or more commonly with radical cystectomy in combination with adjuvant therapy. Careful attention should be given to proper surgical technique when treating these tumors. Wide excision should be performed in order to achieve negative margin status and minimize the possibility of local recurrence. Leiomyosarcoma of the urinary bladder is a rare disease entity with a limited number of cases reported in the literature. In one study involving 34 cases, a total of 52% of patients developed metastatic disease following surgical treatment with the lungs being the most common site of recurrence [38]. Adverse outcomes were documented in 64% of cases.

Partial cystectomy has been reported for treatment of small tumors. In one case series, 4 out of 10 patients with bladder leiomyosarcoma treated with partial cystectomy remained free of disease at 5, 6, 6, and 9 years, respectively [36]. Radical cystectomy with urinary diversion (ileal conduit, catheterizable stoma, orthotopic neobladder) should be considered for patients with larger tumors or tumors located in areas of the bladder that would not permit partial cystectomy. The decision regarding which urinary diversion to perform should take into consideration patient performance status, renal function, and likelihood of receiving adjuvant or salvage therapy. A combined modality treatment approach with perioperative external beam radiotherapy, surgery, and intraoperative radiation therapy for locally advanced or recurrent uterine sarcomas has demonstrated good local disease control with acceptable toxicity [45]. While these results are promising for treatment of uterine sarcomas, the utility of adjuvant radiation therapy for treatment of bladder leiomyosarcoma is much less defined.

Skeletal Muscle Neoplasms

Children and adolescents may occasionally undergo biopsies for bladder masses. The most common urinary bladder tumor in this age group is the botryoid type of embryonal RMS. Rarely, vesical RMS may occur in adults.

Pathology of Rhabdomyosarcoma

RMS is subclassified primarily into embryonal and alveolar subtypes. Embryonal RMS may be further classified as botryoid, spindle cell, anaplastic, or not otherwise specified (NOS).

Embryonal Rhabdomyosarcoma, Botryoid Type

Botryoid RMS is by far the most frequently encountered neoplasm in pediatric bladder biopsies and responds well to current treatment protocols [46–50]. Grossly, these tumors present as polypoid, predominantly intraluminal bladder masses, and the clinical diagnosis is usually straightforward. Morphologically, the definitive feature is the "cambium layer," a proliferation of spindle cells condensed underneath and abutting the surface urothelial or squamous lining, typically forming an exophytic, polypoid growth pattern (Fig. 12.9). The spindle cells show varying degrees of differentiation ranging from undifferentiated mesenchymal cells to fully developed rhabdomyoblasts with prominent eosinophilic cytoplasm and cytoplasmic cross-striations. The botryoid type typically has areas with an abundant, loose myxoid stroma and relatively bland spindle cells (Fig. 12.10). If these bland foci are the only areas represented in the biopsy, one must have a high index of suspicion based on the clinical setting and seek immunohistochemical confirmation of skeletal muscle differentiation. RMSs may rarely contain foci of cartilage (Fig. 12.11), and this should not be used as evidence of a sarcomatoid carcinoma, or prevent patient enrollment into a RMS protocol.

Alveolar Rhabdomyosarcoma

Although rare, alveolar RMS may occur in the urinary bladder [51, 52]. This is an important distinction, because the prognosis for pediatric patients with alveolar RMS is much worse than embryonal, and a more aggressive chemotherapeutic regimen is required.

Morphologically, alveolar RMS may show a mixed classic alveolar or solid growth. All histologic patterns of alveolar RMS share the same cytology: the neoplastic cells resemble lymphoma with high nuclear-to-cytoplasmic ratios, round nuclear contours, and condensed nuclear chromatin. Focal areas may suggest myogenic differentiation and multinucleated rhabdomyoblasts may be present. However, alveolar RMSs frequently appear completely undifferentiated and mimic other malignant small round cell neoplasms.

In the classic pattern, the low power architecture is characteristic with fibrovascular septa dividing the neoplasm into separate nests. The neoplastic cells located centrally in the nests are typically discohesive, but residual cells line the septa in a hobnail or "picket fence" pattern. The discohesive cells may show considerable crush-like artifact and appear homogeneously "hyperchromatic." The solid type of alveolar RMS loses the low power nested architecture, and grows in confluent sheets (Fig. 12.12); however, the cytology of the neoplastic cells is identical to that described above. In morphologically ambiguous cases, diffuse myogenin immunoreactivity or PAX translocations are often used as surrogate markers of the alveolar subtype [53–58].

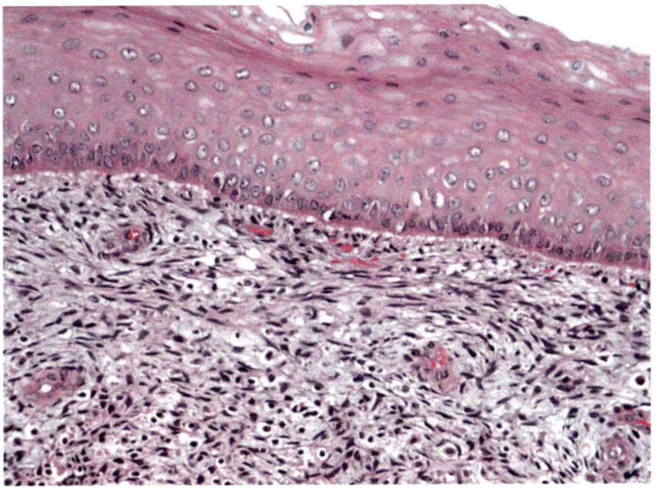

Fig. 12.9 The botryoid type of embryonal rhabdomyosarcoma is often characterized by a condensation of neoplastic spindle cells beneath the epithelium (i.e., the cambium layer)

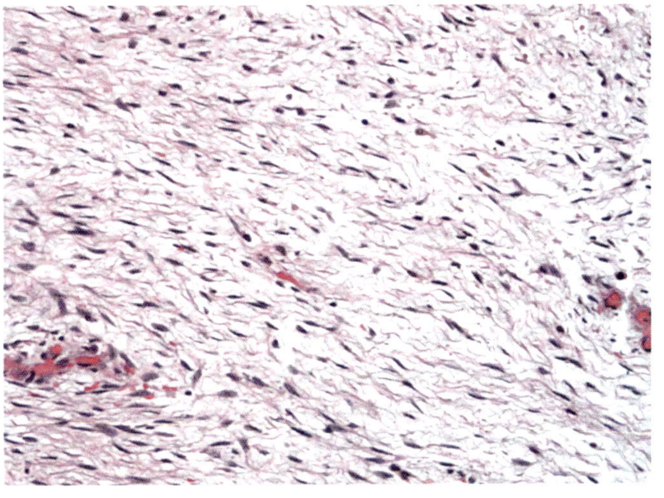

Fig. 12.10 Embryonal rhabdomyosarcoma may be deceptively benign appearing in some foci. In children, there should be a high index of suspicion for rhabdomyosarcoma with an appropriate immunohistochemical workup

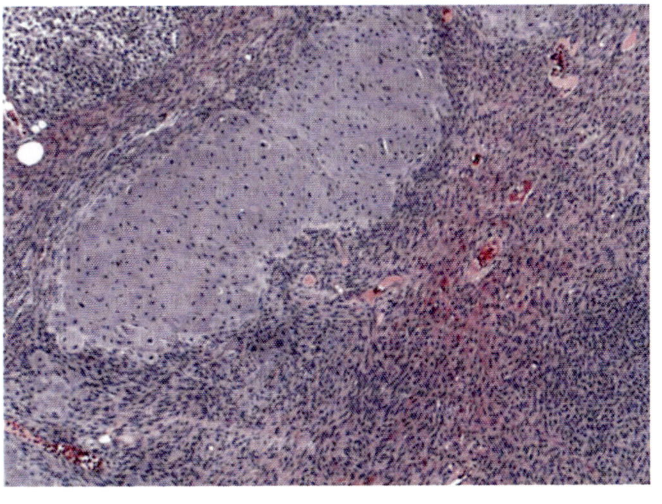

Fig. 12.11 Rhabdomyosarcoma may contain foci of cartilage, and this should not alter the diagnosis or therapy

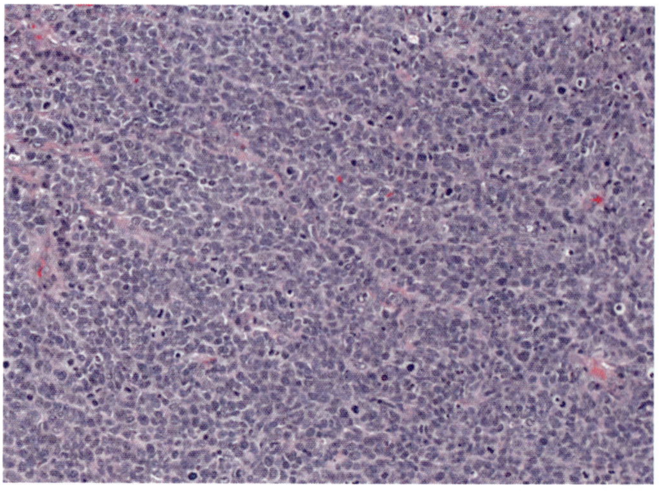

Fig. 12.12 Alveolar rhabdomyosarcoma generally has a round cell appearance that may mimic lymphoma or other round cell malignancy (e.g., small cell carcinoma)

In adult patients, the alveolar type or unusual unclassified patterns of RMS, commonly with anaplasia, are most common [59]. Primary RMS should be carefully distinguished from a carcinosarcoma with heterologous differentiation in adults. Additional tissue sampling to identify a carcinomatous component is often warranted. In adults, RMS may closely mimic small cell carcinoma because of the histologic appearance and the frequent immunoreactivity of RMS with synaptophysin [60]; however, RMS is generally keratin negative.

Immunohistochemistry of Rhabdomyosarcoma

Because of the consistent immunophenotype and the therapeutic implications, the diagnosis of RMS should generally be confirmed by immunohistochemistry. RMS usually shows strong cytoplasmic immunoreactivity for desmin and nuclear reactivity for either/both MyoD1 and myogenin. MyoD1 and myogenin are very specific markers of skeletal muscle differentiation and can help to avoid confusion with other neoplasms expressing desmin such as leiomyosarcoma or desmoplastic small round cell tumor.

Treatment of Rhabdomyosarcoma

RMS is the most common soft tissue sarcoma in children with approximately 350 cases reported annually in the USA. Approximately 20% of all RMSs involve the genitourinary system [61]. Pediatric patients are typically stratified according to risk of disease (prognostic groups: excellent, very good, good, poor), which consider tumor location, histologic, and surgical parameters. Low-risk patients have the best prognosis, while intermediate-risk or high-risk patients have an increased risk of relapse and incurable disease. Because relapses often occur at the site of the primary tumor, adequate local control is essential. Chemotherapy alone can be effective for achieving local control in some patients who have a complete response of the primary tumor. However, surgery and/or radiation therapy may be required for local control of residual disease.

Pediatric RMS may be treated with chemotherapy and/or radiation therapy before or after surgery. Surgical management of RMS varies depending on the location of the tumor; however, bladder-sparing approaches are frequently utilized in children. Partial cystectomy (wide excision) can be performed for tumors that are located at the dome of the bladder. For tumors located in other areas of the bladder, chemotherapy and radiation therapy are given first to shrink the tumor. Biopsies can be performed after initial therapy to determine if there is persistent disease that may require additional procedures. If cancer cells are present, surgery may be indicated to remove all or part of the bladder. Surgical guidelines for management of pediatric RMS can be found in the protocols of the Children's Oncology Group Soft Tissue Sarcoma Committee (formerly, Intergroup Rhabdomyosarcoma Study Group (IRSG)). Bladder preservation has been a primary goal of treatment for the pediatric population. Treatment of pediatric RMS involves a multidisciplinary approach using both chemotherapy and radiation before surgical resection. Approximately 60% of patients retained a functional bladder at 4 years from diagnosis and overall survival has been reported to be >85% [62, 63] (Hays et al. 1995).

Intergroup rhabdomyosarcoma study V (IRS-V) conducted several studies from 1997 to 2007. Most patients with bladder/prostate RMS (intermediate risk) were enrolled in a phase III randomized study of vincristine, dactinomycin, and cyclophosphamide (VAC) vs. VAC alternating with vincristine, topotecan, and cyclophosphamide. This regimen did not demonstrate improved outcomes compared with IRS-IV [64]. In IRS-IV (1991–1997), the role of hypofractionated radiation therapy and the use of ifosfamide and etoposide were examined. Approximately 82% of patients with nonmetastatic bladder/prostate RMS on IRS-IV survived at least 6 years. Local therapy included radiation and second-look operations following radiation therapy [64].

Adult bladder RMS is extremely rare with limited information regarding contemporary management. Most case reports in the literature have cited radical cystectomy followed by adjuvant chemotherapy as treatment for this condition in the adult population, but prognosis is generally poor. Given the paucity of data for bladder sarcomas, it is worthwhile to discuss combined-modality treatment approaches for retroperitoneal sarcomas. Surgical resection of localized tumor with gross and microscopically negative margins remains the standard of care [65]. Complete resection rates for retroperitoneal sarcomas range from 43 to 86%. Overall survival rates range from 36 to 63% at 5 years and 14–50% at 10 years [65]. The primary pattern of treatment failure after resection of a retroperitoneal sarcoma is local recurrence.

High relapse rates following surgery alone have led to the use of combined modality therapy for treatment of retroperitoneal sarcomas. Results from phase III clinical trials suggest that patients with extremity and trunk sarcomas have improved local control when treated with surgery plus radiation compared to surgery alone [66]. There are also data to support the use of surgery plus systemic chemotherapy for treatment of retroperitoneal sarcomas [67, 68]. The utility of radiation therapy (preoperative, intraoperative, postoperative) has also been explored for the treatment of retroperitoneal sarcomas. One of the only prospective, controlled trials treating patients with retroperitoneal sarcomas randomized 35 patients with resectable disease to receive postoperative external beam radiation therapy with or without intraoperative therapy [69]. At a median follow-up of 8 years, there was a significantly lower in-field local recurrence rate for patients treated with intraoperative and postoperative radiation (20%) compared to the external beam radiation therapy control group (80%). Other combined modality approaches for the treatment of patients with intermediate- or high-grade retroperitoneal sarcomas have utilized preoperative doxorubicin and ifosfamide followed by preoperative EBRT and surgical resection with intra- or postoperative radiation boost.

Sarcomatoid Urothelial Carcinoma

As in any anatomic site, carcinomas of the urinary bladder can "dedifferentiate" into a spindle cell neoplasm that histologically resembles a sarcoma. These carcinomas with a sarcomatous appearance have been reported under a variety of names including sarcomatoid carcinoma, metaplastic carcinoma, carcinosarcoma, malignant mixed mesodermal tumor, and spindle and giant cell carcinoma [70–77].

Pathology of Sarcomatoid Carcinoma

Sarcomatoid urothelial carcinoma may be biphasic with both a spindle cell and more conventional

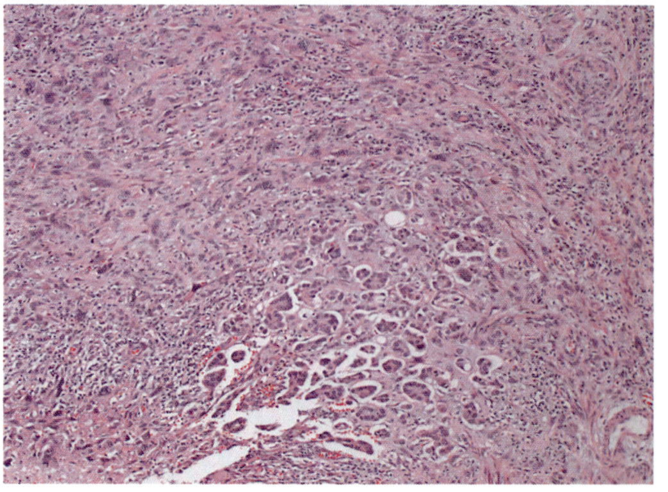

Fig. 12.13 This example of sarcomatoid carcinoma of the bladder shows an invasive micropapillary component adjacent to an undifferentiated sarcomatoid component. The diagnosis is rather straightforward when a carcinomatous component is present

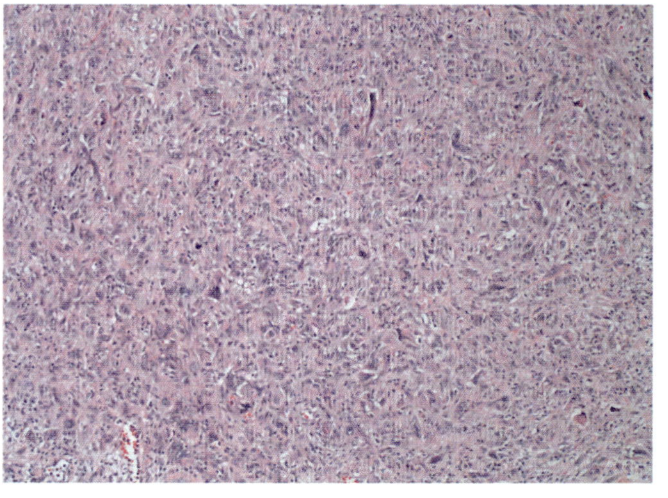

Fig. 12.14 In this example of sarcomatoid carcinoma, only the undifferentiated sarcomatoid component is present, which is indistinguishable from a primary sarcoma. In such cases, immunohistochemistry is needed to make the distinction

epithelial component or may have a completely sarcomatoid morphology [73, 75–80]. The epithelial component may be a papillary urothelial carcinoma, invasive urothelial carcinoma, urothelial carcinoma in situ, squamous cell carcinoma, adenocarcinoma, or small cell carcinoma (Fig. 12.13). Extensive tissue sampling may be required to identify minor foci of obvious epithelial differentiation. The spindle cell or "sarcomatoid" component typically shows marked nuclear pleomorphism and hyperchromasia, and usually has the appearance of an undifferentiated malignant spindle cell tumor (Fig. 12.14) or may acquire a specific line of heterologous differentiation (carcinosarcoma) that is histologically identical to subtypes of known sarcomas (Fig. 12.15). The prognostic significance of heterologous differentiation (e.g., chondrosarcoma, osteosarcoma, RMS) has been debated, but these tumors are usually high grade and high stage. One series has described sarcomatoid urothelial carcinomas with "myxoid and sclerosing" features that may closely mimic an IMT [81].

The immunoprofile of sarcomatoid urothelial carcinoma is variable. Although cytokeratin and EMA immunoreactivity is reported in 67–100% of cases, the spindle cell component may have only focal reactivity or may be completely

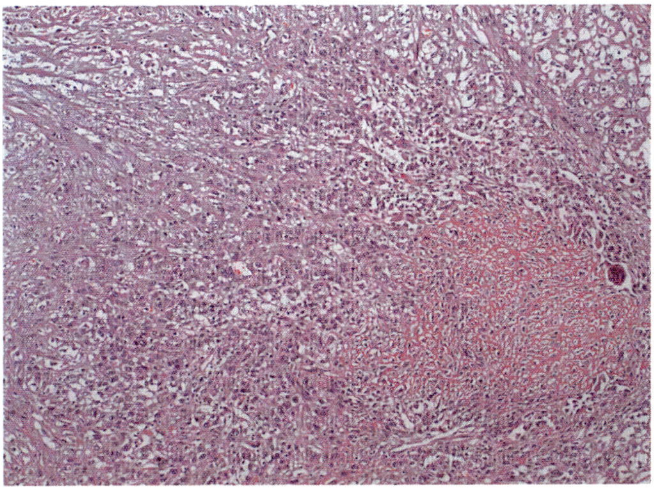

Fig. 12.15 A subset of sarcomatoid carcinomas show heterologous differentiation, which has been referred to as carcinosarcoma. This example shows a focus of osteosarcomatous differentiation in the *lower right*

negative. The spindle cell component may also variably express actin (15–80%) and/or desmin (0–40%), which may be diffuse in cases with myogenous differentiation. Cases showing a specific line of heterologous differentiation typically have the expected immunoprofile for that tissue type. Sarcomatoid carcinoma is generally managed in a fashion similar to aggressive urothelial carcinomas.

Other Mesenchymal Neoplasms

Rarely, mesenchymal neoplasms that are more common to other anatomic sites are seen in the bladder as primary tumors. A discussion of these extremely rare neoplasms is beyond the scope of this chapter, but the list of case reports and small series includes: solitary fibrous tumor/hemangiopericytoma [82, 83], neurofibroma, malignant fibrous histiocytoma/pleomorphic undifferentiated sarcoma [84], angiosarcoma [85, 86], liposarcoma [87, 88] granular cell tumor, clear cell sarcoma, Ewing's sarcoma/PNET, schwannoma, and angiomyolipoma/PEComa [89].

Because of the rarity of primary vesical sarcomas, one should exercise extreme caution in rendering a primary sarcoma diagnosis in the urinary bladder. The possibility of secondary involvement should be excluded clinically before the diagnosis of an unusual primary sarcoma is accepted. The exact method/site of biopsy is essential to the pathologic evaluation; therefore, the specimen label should clearly state whether a "bladder" biopsy is taken by transurethral route or from the peritoneum. For peritoneal biopsies, nonvesical sarcomas would be even more strongly considered. In addition, the possibility of heterologous differentiation within a sarcomatoid carcinoma should be considered and ruled out by extensive tissue sampling, clinical history, and immunohistochemistry. Tumors with specific lines of mesenchymal differentiation in patients with a past history of urothelial carcinoma (especially high-grade carcinomas) most likely represent heterologous sarcomatoid carcinoma even when an associated carcinomatous component cannot be demonstrated. One extremely rare caveat to this rule is encountered in patients with a history of radiation therapy and a possible radiation-induced sarcoma, but there is typically a long symptom-free latent period that may approach 10 years.

References

1. Proppe KH, Scully RE, Rosai J. Postoperative spindle cell nodules of genitourinary tract resembling sarcomas. A report of eight cases. Am J Surg Pathol. 1984;8(2):101–8.
2. Ro JY, Ayala AG, Ordonez NG, Swanson DA, Babaian RJ. Pseudosarcomatous fibromyxoid tumor of the urinary bladder. Am J Clin Pathol. 1986;86(5):583–90.

3. Albores-Saavedra J, Manivel JC, Essenfeld H, Dehner LP, Drut R, Gould E, et al. Pseudosarcomatous myofibroblastic proliferations in the urinary bladder of children. Cancer. 1990;66(6):1234–41.
4. Huang WL, Ro JY, Grignon DJ, Swanson D, Ordonez NG, Ayala AG. Postoperative spindle cell nodule of the prostate and bladder. J Urol. 1990;143(4):824–6.
5. Ro JY, el-Naggar AK, Amin MB, Sahin AA, Ordonez NG, Ayala AG. Pseudosarcomatous fibromyxoid tumor of the urinary bladder and prostate: immunohistochemical, ultrastructural, and DNA flow cytometric analyses of nine cases. Hum Pathol. 1993;24(11):1203–10.
6. Hojo H, Newton Jr WA, Hamoudi AB, Qualman SJ, Wakasa H, Suzuki S, et al. Pseudosarcomatous myofibroblastic tumor of the urinary bladder in children: a study of 11 cases with review of the literature. An Intergroup Rhabdomyosarcoma Study. Am J Surg Pathol. 1995;19(11):1224–36.
7. Lopez-Beltran A, Lopez-Ruiz J, Vicioso L. Inflammatory pseudotumor of the urinary bladder. A clinicopathological analysis of two cases. Urol Int. 1995;55(3):173–6.
8. Biyani CS, Sharma N, Nicol A, Heal MR. Postoperative spindle cell nodule of the bladder: a diagnostic problem. Urol Int. 1996;56(2):119–21.
9. Iczkowski KA, Shanks JH, Gadaleanu V, Cheng L, Jones EC, Neumann R, et al. Inflammatory pseudotumor and sarcoma of urinary bladder: differential diagnosis and outcome in thirty-eight spindle cell neoplasms. Mod Pathol. 2001;14(10):1043–51.
10. Poon KS, Moreira O, Jones EC, Treissman S, Gleave ME. Inflammatory pseudotumor of the urinary bladder: a report of five cases and review of the literature. Can J Urol. 2001;8(6):1409–15.
11. Harik LR, Merino C, Coindre JM, Amin MB, Pedeutour F, Weiss SW. Pseudosarcomatous myofibroblastic proliferations of the bladder: a clinicopathologic study of 42 cases. Am J Surg Pathol. 2006;30(7):787–94.
12. Hirsch MS, Dal Cin P, Fletcher CD. ALK expression in pseudosarcomatous myofibroblastic proliferations of the genitourinary tract. Histopathology. 2006; 48(5):569–78.
13. Montgomery EA, Shuster DD, Burkart AL, Esteban JM, Sgrignoli A, Elwood L, et al. Inflammatory myofibroblastic tumors of the urinary tract: a clinicopathologic study of 46 cases, including a malignant example inflammatory fibrosarcoma and a subset associated with high-grade urothelial carcinoma. Am J Surg Pathol. 2006;30(12):1502–12.
14. Houben CH. Pseudosarcomatous myofibroblastic proliferations of the bladder: a clinicopathologic study of 42 cases. Am J Surg Pathol. 2007;31(4):642; author reply.
15. Spiess PE, Tuziak T, Tibbs RF, Bassett R, Tamboli P, Brown GA, et al. Pseudosarcomatous and sarcomatous proliferations of the bladder. Hum Pathol. 2007;38(5):753–61.
16. Cheng L, Foster SR, MacLennan GT, Lopez-Beltran A, Zhang S, Montironi R. Inflammatory myofibroblastic tumors of the genitourinary tract–single entity or continuum? J Urol. 2008;180(4): 1235–40.
17. Young RH, Wick MR. Transitional cell carcinoma of the urinary bladder with pseudosarcomatous stroma. Am J Clin Pathol. 1988;90(2):216–9.
18. Mahadevia PS, Alexander JE, Rojas-Corona R, Koss LG. Pseudosarcomatous stromal reaction in primary and metastatic urothelial carcinoma. A source of diagnostic difficulty. Am J Surg Pathol. 1989;13(9): 782–90.
19. Lakshmanan Y, Wills ML, Gearhart JP. Inflammatory (pseudosarcomatous) myofibroblastic tumor of the bladder. Urology. 1997;50(2):285–8.
20. Karam JA, Kabbani W, Sagalowsky AI. Pseudosarcomatous fibromyxoid tumor of the bladder. Urol Oncol. 2008;26(3):291–4.
21. Mergan F, Jaubert F, Sauvat F, Hartmann O, Lortat-Jacob S, Revillon Y, et al. Inflammatory myofibroblastic tumor in children: clinical review with anaplastic lymphoma kinase, Epstein-Barr virus, and human herpesvirus 8 detection analysis. J Pediatr Surg. 2005; 40(10):1581–6.
22. Debiec-Rychter M, Marynen P, Hagemeijer A, Pauwels P. ALK-ATIC fusion in urinary bladder inflammatory myofibroblastic tumor. Genes Chromosomes Cancer. 2003;38(2):187–90.
23. Freeman A, Geddes N, Munson P, Joseph J, Ramani P, Sandison A, et al. Anaplastic lymphoma kinase (ALK 1) staining and molecular analysis in inflammatory myofibroblastic tumours of the bladder: a preliminary clinicopathological study of nine cases and review of the literature. Mod Pathol. 2004;17(7):765–71.
24. Tsuzuki T, Magi-Galluzzi C, Epstein JI. ALK-1 expression in inflammatory myofibroblastic tumor of the urinary bladder. Am J Surg Pathol. 2004; 28(12):1609–14.
25. Sukov WR, Cheville JC, Carlson AW, Shearer BM, Piatigorsky EJ, Grogg KL, et al. Utility of ALK-1 protein expression and ALK rearrangements in distinguishing inflammatory myofibroblastic tumor from malignant spindle cell lesions of the urinary bladder. Mod Pathol. 2007;20(5):592–603.
26. Westfall DE, Folpe AL, Paner GP, Oliva E, Goldstein L, Alsabeh R, et al. Utility of a comprehensive immunohistochemical panel in the differential diagnosis of spindle cell lesions of the urinary bladder. Am J Surg Pathol. 2009;33(1):99–105.
27. Watanabe K, Kusakabe T, Hoshi N, Saito A, Suzuki T. h-Caldesmon in leiomyosarcoma and tumors with smooth muscle cell-like differentiation: its specific expression in the smooth muscle cell tumor. Hum Pathol. 1999;30(4):392–6.
28. Cessna MH, Zhou H, Sanger WG, Perkins SL, Tripp S, Pickering D, et al. Expression of ALK1 and p80 in inflammatory myofibroblastic tumor and its mesenchymal mimics: a study of 135 cases. Mod Pathol. 2002;15(9):931–8.
29. Council L, Hameed O. Differential expression of immunohistochemical markers in bladder smooth

muscle and myofibroblasts, and the potential utility of desmin, smoothelin, and vimentin in staging of bladder carcinoma. Mod Pathol. 2009;22(5):639–50.
30. Lake MH, Kossow AS, Bokinsky G. Leiomyoma of the bladder and urethra. J Urol. 1981;125(5):742–3.
31. Luttwak Z, Koren R, Veltman V, Halpern M, Manes A, Lask D, et al. Leiomyoma of the urinary bladder. Pathol Oncol Res. 1998;4(4):308–9.
32. Yusim IE, Neulander EZ, Eidelberg I, Lismer LJ, Kaneti J. Leiomyoma of the genitourinary tract. Scand J Urol Nephrol. 2001;35(4):295–9.
33. Martin SA, Sears DL, Sebo TJ, Lohse CM, Cheville JC. Smooth muscle neoplasms of the urinary bladder: a clinicopathologic comparison of leiomyoma and leiomyosarcoma. Am J Surg Pathol. 2002;26(3):292–300.
34. Lee TK, Miyamoto H, Osunkoya AO, Guo CC, Weiss SW, Epstein JI. Smooth muscle neoplasms of the urinary bladder: a clinicopathologic study of 51 cases. Am J Surg Pathol. 2010;34(4):502–9.
35. Soloway D, Simon MA, Milikowski C, Soloway MS. Epithelioid leiomyoma of the bladder: an unusual cause of voiding symptoms. Urology. 1998;51(6):1037–9.
36. Swartz DA, Johnson DE, Ayala AG, Watkins DL. Bladder leiomyosarcoma: a review of 10 cases with 5-year followup. J Urol. 1985;133(2):200–2.
37. Mills SE, Bova GS, Wick MR, Young RH. Leiomyosarcoma of the urinary bladder. A clinicopathologic and immunohistochemical study of 15 cases. Am J Surg Pathol. 1989;13(6):480–9.
38. Lindberg MR, Fisher C, Thway K, Cao D, Cheville JC, Folpe AL. Leiomyosarcoma of the urinary bladder: a clinicopathological study of 34 cases. J Clin Pathol. 2010;63(8):708–13.
39. Lack EE. Leiomyosarcomas in childhood: a clinical and pathologic study of 10 cases. Pediatr Pathol. 1986;6(2–3):181–97.
40. Thrasher JB, Miller GJ, Wettlaufer JN. Bladder leiomyosarcoma following cyclophosphamide therapy for lupus nephritis. J Urol. 1990;143(1):119–21.
41. Motta L, Porcaro AB, Ficarra V, D'Amico A, Piubello Q, Comunale L. Leiomyosarcoma of the bladder fourteen years after cyclophosphamide therapy for retinoblastoma. Scand J Urol Nephrol. 2001;35(3):248–9.
42. Parekh DJ, Jung C, O'Conner J, Dutta S, Smith Jr ER. Leiomyosarcoma in urinary bladder after cyclophosphamide therapy for retinoblastoma and review of bladder sarcomas. Urology. 2002;60(1):164.
43. Bleoo SL, Godbout R, Rayner D, Tamimi Y, Moore RB. Leiomyosarcoma of the bladder in a retinoblastoma patient. Urol Int. 2003;71(1):118–21.
44. Tanguay C, Harvey I, Houde M, Srigley JR, Tetu B. Leiomyosarcoma of urinary bladder following cyclophosphamide therapy: report of two cases. Mod Pathol. 2003;16(5):512–4.
45. Barney BM, Petersen IA, Dowdy SC, Bakkum-Gamez JN, Haddock MG. Long-term outcomes with intraoperative radiotherapy as a component of treatment for locally advanced or recurrent uterine sarcoma. Int J Radiat Oncol Biol Phys. 2012;83(1):191-7. Epub 2011 Oct 8.
46. Donaldson SS, Meza J, Breneman JC, Crist WM, Laurie F, Qualman SJ, et al. Results from the IRS-IV randomized trial of hyperfractionated radiotherapy in children with rhabdomyosarcoma–a report from the IRSG. Int J Radiat Oncol Biol Phys. 2001;51(3):718–28.
47. Raney RB, Maurer HM, Anderson JR, Andrassy RJ, Donaldson SS, Qualman SJ, et al. The Intergroup Rhabdomyosarcoma Study Group (IRSG): major lessons from the IRS-I through IRS-IV studies as background for the current IRS-V treatment protocols. Sarcoma. 2001;5(1):9–15.
48. Ashlock R, Johnstone PA. Treatment modalities of bladder/prostate rhabdomyosarcoma: a review. Prostate Cancer Prostatic Dis. 2003;6(2):112–20.
49. Ferrer FA, Isakoff M, Koyle MA. Bladder/prostate rhabdomyosarcoma: past, present and future. J Urol. 2006;176(4 Pt 1):1283–91.
50. Seitz G, Dantonello TM, Int-Veen C, Blumenstock G, Godzinski J, Klingebiel T, et al. Treatment efficiency, outcome and surgical treatment problems in patients suffering from localized embryonal bladder/prostate rhabdomyosarcoma: a report from the Cooperative Soft Tissue Sarcoma trial CWS-96. Pediatr Blood Cancer. 2011;56(5):718–24.
51. Leuschner I, Harms D, Mattke A, Koscielniak E, Treuner J. Rhabdomyosarcoma of the urinary bladder and vagina: a clinicopathologic study with emphasis on recurrent disease: a report from the Kiel Pediatric Tumor Registry and the German CWS Study. Am J Surg Pathol. 2001;25(7):856–64.
52. Zaidi TS, Mushtaq I, Sebire N. Alveolar rhabdomyosarcoma of the bladder in a child. Pediatr Surg Int. 2006;22(5):474–6.
53. Barr FG. Gene fusions involving PAX and FOX family members in alveolar rhabdomyosarcoma. Oncogene. 2001;20(40):5736–46.
54. Davicioni E, Finckenstein FG, Shahbazian V, Buckley JD, Triche TJ, Anderson MJ. Identification of a PAX-FKHR gene expression signature that defines molecular classes and determines the prognosis of alveolar rhabdomyosarcomas. Cancer Res. 2006;66(14):6936–46.
55. Mercado GE, Barr FG. Fusions involving PAX and FOX genes in the molecular pathogenesis of alveolar rhabdomyosarcoma: recent advances. Curr Mol Med. 2007;7(1):47–61.
56. Parham DM, Qualman SJ, Teot L, Barr FG, Morotti R, Sorensen PH, et al. Correlation between histology and PAX/FKHR fusion status in alveolar rhabdomyosarcoma: a report from the Children's Oncology Group. Am J Surg Pathol. 2007;31(6):895–901.
57. Heerema-McKenney A, Wijnaendts LC, Pulliam JF, Lopez-Terrada D, McKenney JK, Zhu S, et al. Diffuse myogenin expression by immunohistochemistry is an independent marker of poor survival in pediatric rhabdomyosarcoma: a tissue microarray study of 71 primary tumors including correlation with molecular phenotype. Am J Surg Pathol. 2008;32(10):1513–22.

58. Stegmaier S, Poremba C, Schaefer KL, Leuschner I, Kazanowska B, Bekassy AN, et al. Prognostic value of PAX-FKHR fusion status in alveolar rhabdomyosarcoma: a report from the cooperative soft tissue sarcoma study group (CWS). Pediatr Blood Cancer. 2011;57(3):406–14.
59. Paner GP, McKenney JK, Epstein JI, Amin MB. Rhabdomyosarcoma of the urinary bladder in adults: predilection for alveolar morphology with anaplasia and significant morphologic overlap with small cell carcinoma. Am J Surg Pathol. 2008;32(7):1022–8.
60. Bahrami A, Gown AM, Baird GS, Hicks MJ, Folpe AL. Aberrant expression of epithelial and neuroendocrine markers in alveolar rhabdomyosarcoma: a potentially serious diagnostic pitfall. Mod Pathol. 2008;21(7):795–806.
61. Crist WM, Anderson JR, Meza JL, Fryer C, Raney RB, Ruymann FB, et al. Intergroup rhabdomyosarcoma study-IV: results for patients with nonmetastatic disease. J Clin Oncol. 2001;19(12):3091–102.
62. Corpron CA, Andrassy RJ, Hays DM, Raney RB, Wiener ES, Lawrence W, et al. Conservative management of uterine pediatric rhabdomyosarcoma: a report from the Intergroup Rhabdomyosarcoma Study III and IV pilot. J Pediatr Surg. 1995;30(7):942–4.
63. Andrassy RJ, Hays DM, Raney RB, Wiener ES, Lawrence W, Lobe TE et al. Conservative surgical management of vaginal and vulvar pediatric rhabdomyosarcoma: a report from the Intergroup Rhabdomyosarcoma Study III. J Pediatr Surg. 1995;30(7):1034-6; discussion 1036-7.
64. Arndt C, Rodeberg D, Breitfeld PP, Raney RB, Ullrich F, Donaldson S. Does bladder preservation (as a surgical principle) lead to retaining bladder function in bladder/prostate rhabdomyosarcoma? Results from intergroup rhabdomyosarcoma study IV. J Urol. 2004;171(6 Pt 1):2396–403.
65. Raut CP, Pisters PWT. Retroperitoneal sarcomas: combined-modality treatment approaches. J Surg Oncol. 2006;94(1):81–7.
66. Yang JC, Chang AE, Baker AR, Sindelar WF, Danforth DN, Topalian SL, et al. Randomized prospective study of the benefit of adjuvant radiation therapy in the treatment of soft tissue sarcomas of the extremity. J Clin Oncol. 1998;16(1):197–203.
67. Frustaci S, Gherlinzoni F. Adjuvant chemotherapy for adult soft tissue sarcomas of the extremities and girdles: results of the Italian randomized cooperative trial. J Clin Oncol. 2001;19(5):1238–47.
68. Tierney JF, Mosseri V, Stewart LA, Souhami RL, Parmar MK. Adjuvant chemotherapy for soft-tissue sarcoma: review and meta-analysis of the published results of randomized clinical trials. Br J Cancer. 1995;72(2):469–75.
69. Sindelar WF, Kinsella TJ, Chen PW, DeLaney TF, Tepper JE, Rosenberg SA, et al. Intraoperative radiotherapy in retroperitoneal sarcomas. Final results of a prospective, randomized, clinical trial. Arch Surg. 1993;128(4):402–10.
70. Komatsu H, Kinoshita K, Mikata N, Honma Y. Spindle and giant cell carcinoma of the bladder. Report of 3 cases. Eur Urol. 1985;11(2):141–4.
71. Bloxham CA, Bennett MK, Robinson MC. Bladder carcinosarcomas: three cases with diverse histogenesis. Histopathology. 1990;16(1):63–7.
72. Serio G, Zampatti C, Ceppi M. Spindle and giant cell carcinoma of the urinary bladder: a clinicopathological light microscopic and immunohistochemical study. Br J Urol. 1995;75(2):167–72.
73. Lopez-Beltran A, Pacelli A, Rothenberg HJ, Wollan PC, Zincke H, Blute ML, et al. Carcinosarcoma and sarcomatoid carcinoma of the bladder: clinicopathological study of 41 cases. J Urol. 1998;159(5): 1497–503.
74. Baschinsky DY, Chen JH, Vadmal MS, Lucas JG, Bahnson RR, Niemann TH. Carcinosarcoma of the urinary bladder–an aggressive tumor with diverse histogenesis. A clinicopathologic study of 4 cases and review of the literature. Arch Pathol Lab Med. 2000;124(8):1172–8.
75. Ikegami H, Iwasaki H, Ohjimi Y, Takeuchi T, Ariyoshi A, Kikuchi M. Sarcomatoid carcinoma of the urinary bladder: a clinicopathologic and immunohistochemical analysis of 14 patients. Hum Pathol. 2000;31(3):332–40.
76. Wright JL, Black PC, Brown GA, Porter MP, Kamat AM, Dinney CP, et al. Differences in survival among patients with sarcomatoid carcinoma, carcinosarcoma and urothelial carcinoma of the bladder. J Urol. 2007;178(6):2302-6; discussion 7.
77. Wang J, Wang FW, Lagrange CA, Hemstreet Iii GP, Kessinger A. Clinical features of sarcomatoid carcinoma (carcinosarcoma) of the urinary bladder: analysis of 221 cases. Sarcoma. 2010;2010. Pii:454792. Epub 2010 Jul 18. Pubmed PMID: 20706685 Pubmed Central PMCID: PMC2913791.
78. Ro JY, Ayala AG, Wishnow K. Sarcomatoid bladder carcinoma: clinicopathological and immunohisrtochemical study of 44 cases. Surg Pathol. 1988;1:359.
79. Young RH, Wick MR, Mills SE. Sarcomatoid carcinoma of the urinary bladder. A clinicopathologic analysis of 12 cases and review of the literature. Am J Clin Pathol. 1988;90(6):653–61.
80. Torenbeek R, Blomjous CE, de Bruin PC, Newling DW, Meijer CJ. Sarcomatoid carcinoma of the urinary bladder. Clinicopathologic analysis of 18 cases with immunohistochemical and electron microscopic findings. Am J Surg Pathol. 1994;18(3):241–9.
81. Jones EC, Young RH. Myxoid and sclerosing sarcomatoid transitional cell carcinoma of the urinary bladder: a clinicopathologic and immunohistochemical study of 25 cases. Mod Pathol. 1997;10(9):908–16.
82. Mentzel T, Bainbridge TC, Katenkamp D. Solitary fibrous tumour: clinicopathological, immunohistochemical, and ultrastructural analysis of 12 cases arising in soft tissues, nasal cavity and nasopharynx, urinary bladder and prostate. Virchows Arch. 1997;430(6):445–53.

83. Westra WH, Grenko RT, Epstein J. Solitary fibrous tumor of the lower urogenital tract: a report of five cases involving the seminal vesicles, urinary bladder, and prostate. Hum Pathol. 2000;31(1):63–8.
84. Oesterling JE, Epstein JI, Brendler CB. Myxoid malignant fibrous histiocytoma of the bladder. Cancer. 1990;66(8):1836–42.
85. Spiess PE, Kassouf W, Steinberg JR, Tuziak T, Hernandez M, Tibbs RF, et al. Review of the M.D. Anderson experience in the treatment of bladder sarcoma. Urol Oncol. 2007;25(1):38–45.
86. Tavora F, Montgomery E, Epstein JI. A series of vascular tumors and tumorlike lesions of the bladder. Am J Surg Pathol. 2008;32(8):1213–9.
87. Widdison AD, Feneley RC. Liposarcoma of the bladder. Br J Urol. 1989;64(6):655–6.
88. Biernat W, Salska Z, Biernat S. Myxoid liposarcoma of the urinary bladder. Pol J Pathol. 1996;47(1):41–3.
89. Sukov WR, Cheville JC, Amin MB, Gupta R, Folpe AL. Perivascular epithelioid cell tumor (PEComa) of the urinary bladder: report of 3 cases and review of the literature. Am J Surg Pathol. 2009;33(2):304–8.

Part IV

Urethral Disease

Nonneoplastic and Neoplastic Urethral Disease

13

Hadley Wood, Kenneth Angermeier, and Adeboye O. Osunkoya

Introduction

The urethra, which carries urine from the urinary bladder to the external urethral orifice for excretion and provides the conduit for semen in males, may be involved by a broad spectrum of both neoplastic and nonneoplastic diseases, which may produce very similar clinical symptoms. This chapter reviews the clinical and pathologic features of urethral diseases organized by clinical setting: urethral stricture, male urethral cancer, female urethral cancer, and female urethral diverticulum.

Urethral Stricture

Urethral strictures may be classified based upon their location. Anterior strictures involve the penile and bulbar urethra, whereas posterior strictures or stenoses occur in the membranous and prostatic urethra. The etiology of anterior urethral strictures has changed over time. Gonococcal urethritis was a common cause in the past, but prompt and effective antibiotic treatment and a growing acceptance of safe sexual practices has decreased the incidence of strictures related to this condition. Currently the most common etiology is traumatic injury, either external or iatrogenic. Anterior strictures have a bimodal presentation. Isolated bulbar strictures commonly present in younger men, presumably due to remote straddle injuries, although many cannot recall a specific event in childhood. Older patients tend to present with strictures related to iatrogeny or inflammation, predominantly lichen sclerosis (LS). Meatal and distal anterior strictures in particular are more likely to be seen in this latter population. Hypospadias and complications related to prior hypospadias repair may present at any point in life and typically involve the distal anterior urethra [1].

The most common etiology of posterior urethral stricture or stenosis continues to be pelvic fracture-related urethral injury. However, increased utilization of radiation and other ablative technologies for prostate cancer and benign prostatic hyperplasia (BPH) has led to an increase in iatrogenic posterior urethral stricture. Posterior urethral strictures associated with radiation present a particular challenge to the reconstructive urologist because they often involve both the prostatic and membranous urethra and may be associated with significant local tissue injury, fistula,

H. Wood
Cleveland Clinic, Glickman Urological and Kidney Institute, 9500 Euclid Avenue, Q10, Cleveland, OH 44195, USA
e-mail: woodh@ccf.org

K. Angermeier
Center for Genitourinary Reconstruction, Cleveland Clinic, Glickman Urological and Kidney Institute, 9500 Euclid Avenue, Cleveland, OH 44195, USA
e-mail: angermk@ccf.org

A.O. Osunkoya (✉)
Department of Pathology and Urology, Emory School of Medicine, 1364 Clifton Road NE, Room H-174, Atlanta, GA 30322, USA
e-mail: adeboye.osunkoya@emory.edu

D.E. Hansel et al. (eds.), *The Urinary Tract: A Comprehensive Guide to Patient Diagnosis and Management*, DOI 10.1007/978-1-4614-5320-8_13, © Springer Science+Business Media New York 2012

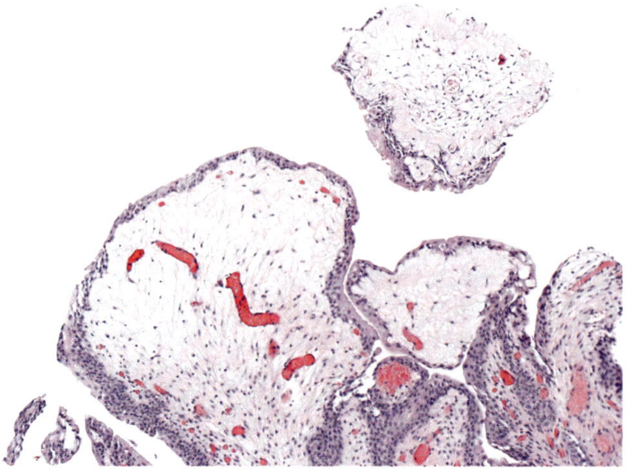

Fig. 13.1 Polypoid urethritis with edematous lamina propria

and are more likely to result in compromise of the urinary sphincter mechanism during surgical reconstruction.

Clinical Presentation

Urethral strictures typically present with progressive lower urinary tract symptoms, or less often urinary retention. Recurrent urinary tract infections, prostatitis, urethralgia, terminal hematuria, ejaculatory complaints, infertility, and urethral abscess or fistula represent other less common presentations. Patients may report a high degree of variability of urinary symptoms prior to developing urinary retention, with many reporting little or no urinary problems. In older men, long-standing lower urinary tract symptoms are often attributed to BPH, and urethral strictures are not uncommonly identified incidentally at the time of diagnostic cystoscopy or during attempted catheterization for another medical or surgical procedure. A history of prior urethral instrumentation, perineal trauma, sexually transmitted diseases, recurrent balanitis, or problems following circumcision should be elicited. Baseline sexual function, including the presence or absence of erectile curvature, should be assessed and documented. Physical examination should include assessment of body habitus to identify patients at risk for problems related to positioning at the time of surgery. The urethral meatus and glans penis are examined for the presence of inflammatory lesions such as LS or vitiligo, and for available normal hairless skin that may be used at the time of urethral reconstruction. The urethra is palpated to identify induration, abscess, or fistula that may be associated with advanced strictures or long-standing obstruction.

Pathogenesis

A urethral stricture is a scar resulting from an injury. Wound contraction is one of the basic mechanisms by which the body heals. Because the urethra is a circular structure, scar contraction occurs circumferentially and results in narrowing of the urethral lumen. In anterior strictures, the density of a stricture and its ultimate management depend not only upon the scarring of the urethral mucosa, but also the depth of the fibrosis involving the associated corpus spongiosum (spongiofibrosis). The posterior urethra is not surrounded by the corpus spongiosum. Strictures in the posterior urethra result from urethral distraction, tissue destruction, and ischemia resulting from pelvic fracture, radiotherapy, previous surgery, or a combination thereof.

Catheterization and other forms of instrumentation/procedures may also lead to polypoid urethritis (Fig. 13.1) and subsequent stricture

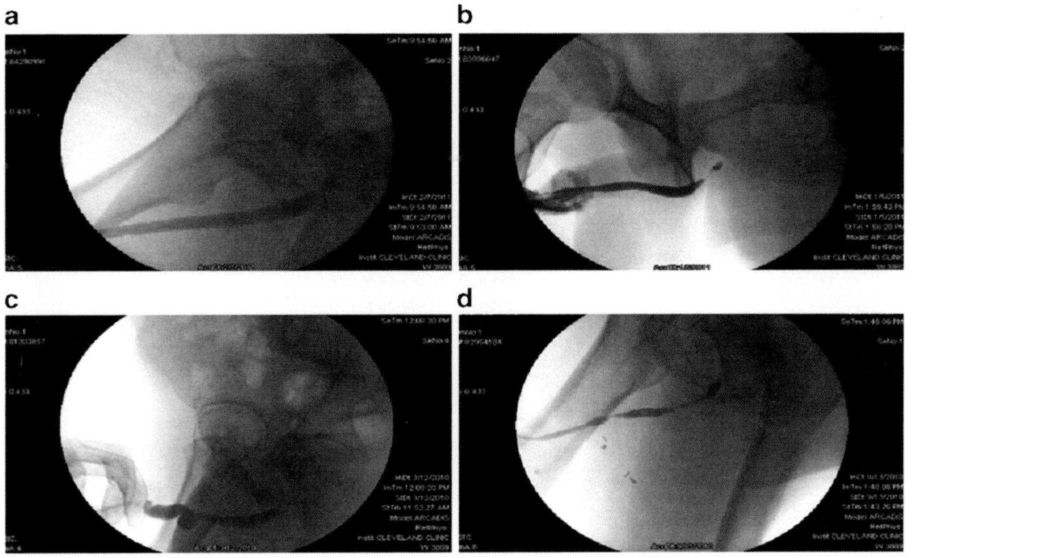

Fig. 13.2 Retrograde urethrogram findings. (**a**) Normal retrograde urethrogram. (**b**) Bulbar urethral injury from prior straddle injury. (**c**) RUG demonstrating penile urethral stricture and proximal diverticulum from prior hypospadias reconstruction. (**d**) RUG demonstrating panurethral stricture secondary to lichen sclerosis

formation. Strictures due to trauma are usually focal, while those due to infection may be multifocal. There are no specific histologic features; however, most strictures tend be associated with a host inflammatory response, fibrosis, and reactive epithelial changes.

Clinical Findings

The most common method used to diagnose a urethral stricture is flexible cystoscopy, usually performed for the evaluation of urinary symptoms. However, the optimal study to evaluate the extent and location of a stricture prior to surgical management is the retrograde urethrogram (RUG) (Fig. 13.2). If further evaluation is necessary, patients with or without an indwelling suprapubic catheter also undergo a voiding cystourethrogram (VCUG), which nicely complements the RUG to better evaluate the segment of the urethra proximal to the stricture. In the setting of posterior urethral stricture or stenosis, antegrade cystoscopy is also helpful to characterize the status of the proximal urethra and bladder neck. Concurrent antegrade flexible cystoscopy and RUG allow identification of the length of the urethral defect following pelvic fracture-related urethral distraction when other means are not able to do so (Fig. 13.3). Visualization of the bladder neck is also important in this setting, since scar and fixation of the anterior bladder neck may increase the risk of urinary incontinence following urethral reconstruction. Additionally, this technique is valuable in patients with posterior urethral obstructions following radiotherapy.

It is our practice to avoid urethral instrumentation for approximately 3 months prior to urethral reconstruction in order to allow full maturation of the scar for clear intraoperative determination of the extent of the urethral abnormality. This is important also because squamous metaplasia of the mucosa is not uncommon in the urethra proximal to a stricture (Fig. 13.4a, b), and it is otherwise difficult to know whether this area is destined to narrow down after relief of high pressure hydrodistention and correspondingly whether it should be included in the repair at the time of surgery. If necessary, preoperative cystoscopy can be performed using a pediatric cystoscope or a

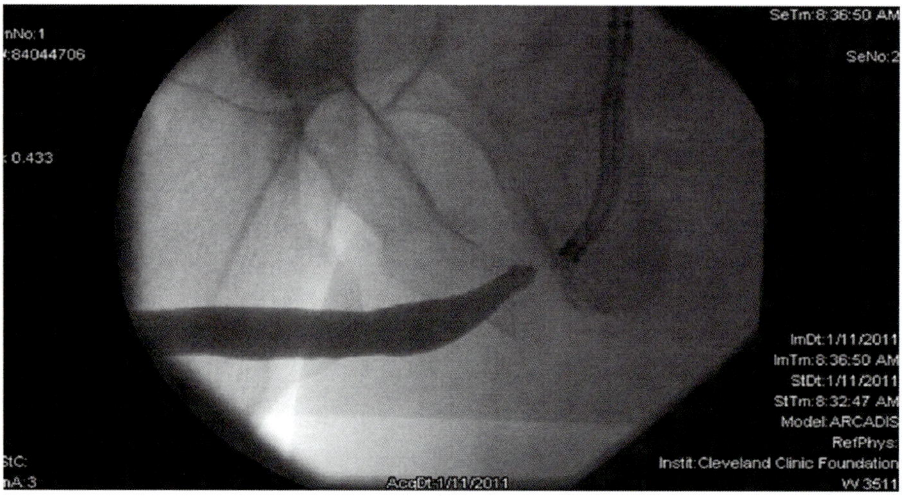

Fig. 13.3 Antegrade cystoscopy with concurrent RUG. Cystoscope tip demonstrates proximal extent of structure with the contrast from retrograde urethrography demonstrating the distal extent of the stricture

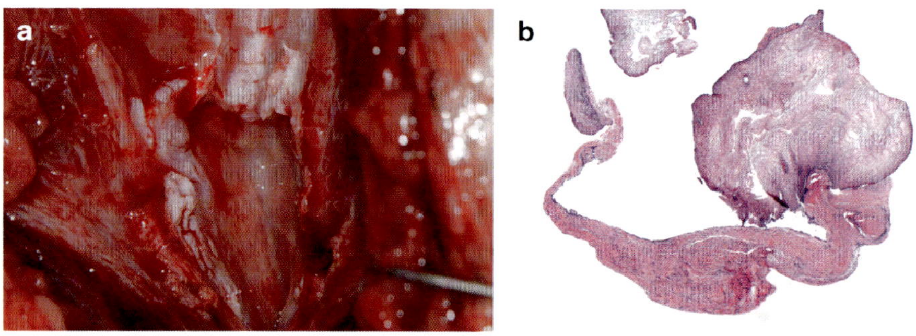

Fig. 13.4 (**a**, **b**) Urethral squamous metaplasia.

small-caliber flexible scope prior to procedure as long as the strictured segment is not dilated.

Management

Management of a urethral stricture is dictated by the etiology, location, length, depth of associated spongiofibrosis, and medical comorbidities. Urethral dilation is considered a management tool or temporizing measure, and is rarely curative. Direct vision internal urethrotomy (DVIU) is probably the most commonly used surgical procedure for urethral stricture and may be done using a cold knife or laser. DVIU is often used as a first-line treatment following diagnosis of an anterior urethral stricture. Success rates with this procedure have been reported at 50–70% for a relatively short bulbar stricture [2], but a more recent report suggests that this may be an overestimate [3]. Anterior strictures that are multiple, of long length, of narrow caliber with dense spongiofibrosis, or located within the penile urethra have decreased success following DVIU [2]. In most cases, if an initial attempt at DVIU is unsuccessful it is not helpful in the long term to repeat the procedure. Patients in this category who are medically fit for surgery have a much higher long-term cure rate with urethral reconstruction and should generally be guided in this direction if feasible. Posterior urethral strictures and stenoses infrequently demonstrate durable patency following conservative procedures, and open surgical reconstruction is warranted in the majority of cases.

Short bulbar urethral strictures that have failed or are not a candidate for DVIU may be managed with anastomotic urethroplasty. In this procedure, the strictured segment is excised, the urethra mobilized, and a primary anastomosis performed. Although typical candidates for this procedure have strictures 2–3 cm in length, it is technically easier to bridge longer strictures when they are located within the bulbar urethra proximally as opposed to distally. Anterior strictures within the penile or penobulbar urethra, or those too long for an anastomotic repair, are treated with substitution urethroplasty. The strictured segment is opened along the ventral or dorsal aspect, and then expanded using an onlay graft or flap. The most common tissue graft currently in use for this purpose is buccal mucosa; however, lingual mucosa, full thickness skin grafts (preferably genital), and colonic mucosa have also been used [4–6]. Substitution urethroplasty may also be performed using a penile or penoscrotal skin island based on a dartos fascia pedicle for the onlay. Penile strictures, particularly those related to LS or previous surgery for hypospadias, are often more reliably managed with staged buccal graft urethroplasty. The urethra is opened ventrally and buccal mucosa is sutured into place adjacent to the urethral plate and allowed to heal for 4–6 months. At the second operation, the well-healed buccal mucosa is tubularized to complete the reconstruction.

Patients with a posterior urethral distraction defect related to pelvic fracture typically undergo urethral reconstruction with a high rate of success. This is almost always performed with excision of the associated scar defect and a primary urethral anastomosis using a progressive perineal approach [7]. Preservation of the external sphincter is variable, and postoperative continence may be dependent on the bladder neck either totally or in part. Obliterative membranous strictures following brachytherapy for prostate cancer require the same type of surgical procedure, although there may be a somewhat higher risk of subsequent incontinence. Stenosis or obliteration of the prostatomembranous urethra may be associated with tissue necrosis, calcification, or fistula. Although highly complex, a percentage of these patients can be repaired using advanced reconstructive techniques. However, in some cases urinary diversion is the only reasonable option in the form of an indwelling suprapubic catheter, continent catheterizable channel with bladder augmentation, or ileal conduit.

Urethral Cancer: Male

Carcinoma of the male urethra is rare. When discussing urethral cancer, the bulbous, membranous, and prostatic segments are generally classified together as the posterior urethra, and the penile urethra is referred to as the anterior urethra. The bulbomembranous urethra is involved most frequently (60%), followed by the penile urethra (30%) and the prostatic urethra (10%). The histological subtype of urethral cancer varies and depends on location. Carcinomas of the prostatic urethra are urothelial in 90% and squamous cell in 10%. Within the bulbomembranous urethra, squamous cell carcinoma is most common and responsible for 90% of cases, followed by urothelial carcinoma in 10% and adenocarcinoma or undifferentiated in 10%. Similarly, penile urethral cancer is of squamous cell origin in 90% and urothelial in 10%. Overall, 80% of male urethral cancers are squamous cell carcinoma, 15% are urothelial carcinoma, and 5% are adenocarcinoma, melanoma, lymphoma, paraganglioma, sarcoma, or undifferentiated tumor [8]. Patient survival rates depend upon tumor location and grade. Overall survival rates for low-stage and high-stage tumors, respectively, are 83% and 36%. Anterior urethral cancer is associated with a survival rate of 69% and posterior urethral cancer 26% [9].

Clinical Presentation

The most common presenting symptoms are urethral bleeding, urethral discharge, urethral pain or dysuria, obstructive voiding symptoms, or a palpable urethral mass. Diagnosis may be delayed because the onset of symptoms is often insidious, and therefore a high index of clinical suspicion is required to diagnose these tumors expediently.

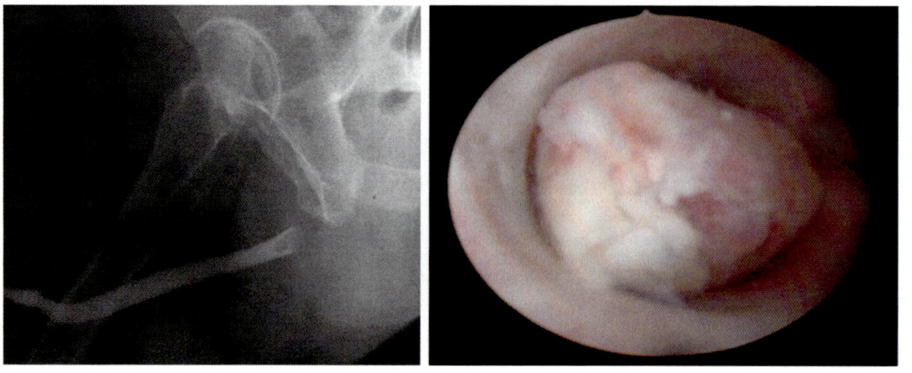

Fig. 13.5 Retrograde urethrogram and cystoscopic findings demonstrating a bulbar urethral cancer

Pathogenesis

Chronic inflammation due to sexually transmitted diseases, urethritis, and/or urethral stricture is the most common etiologic factor. There may also be a causal role for human papillomavirus (HPV) 16 in squamous cell carcinoma of the urethra [10, 11].

Clinical Findings

RUG may identify a filling defect in the urethra, or demonstrate a stricture with irregular borders. Cystoscopy with urethral biopsy confirms pathological diagnosis (Fig. 13.5). Patients who have undergone prior cystoprostatectomy and cutaneous diversion are known to be at risk for later development of urethral carcinoma with an incidence of 2.1–11.1% [12–14]. Urethral wash cytology can identify urethral cancer before it becomes clinically apparent. In the setting of an orthotopic neobladder, the risk of urethral recurrence is less than after some form of cutaneous diversion, with rates ranging from 0.5 to 4% [12–15]. Voided urine cytology is used to monitor these patients. Clinical evaluation of patients with known urethral carcinoma should include thorough examination of the entire urethra for the presence of firmness, induration, or fixation, rectal examination, and careful palpation of the groins to assess for lymphadenopathy. Lymphatics from the anterior urethra drain into the superficial and deep inguinal lymph nodes and occasionally into the external iliac lymph nodes. Tumors of the posterior urethra most commonly spread to the pelvic lymph nodes. Palpable inguinal lymph nodes occur in about 20% of cases and almost always represent metastatic disease, in contrast to penile cancer, in which a significant percentage of palpable nodes may be inflammatory.

Pathology

Carcinomas of the male urethra may present as carcinoma in situ (squamous or urothelial), non-invasive papillary urothelial carcinoma (low grade or high grade), invasive urothelial carcinomas, or invasive squamous cell carcinoma.

Carcinoma In Situ

Urothelial carcinoma in situ of the urethra may be primary (Fig. 13.6) or due to spread from an adjacent urinary bladder primary [16–19]. Urothelial carcinoma in situ has the identical morphologic spectrum as that seen in the bladder. Squamous cell carcinoma in situ shows full thickness basaloid atypia similar to that seen in the uterine cervix, often with some degree of keratinization in adjacent epithelium. One may also see varying levels of associated squamous dysplasia, or condylomatous changes in cases associated with HPV infection. Urothelial carcinoma in situ often extends into periurethral ducts and glands along the entire length of the urethra as well as into prostatic ducts (Fig. 13.7). It is critical to distinguish colonization of prostatic glands/

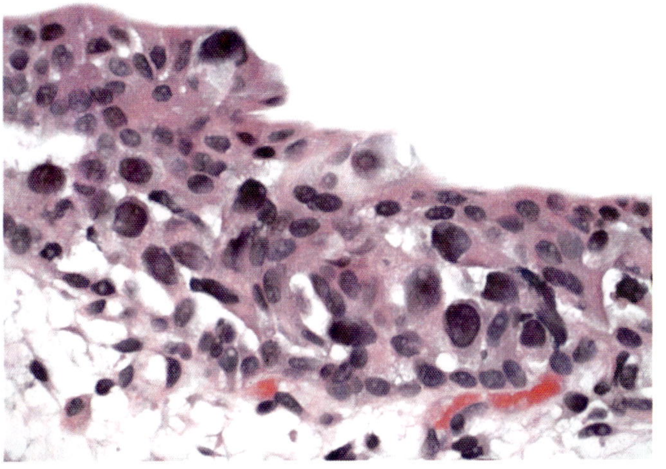

Fig. 13.6 Urothelial carcinoma in situ involving the prostatic urethra

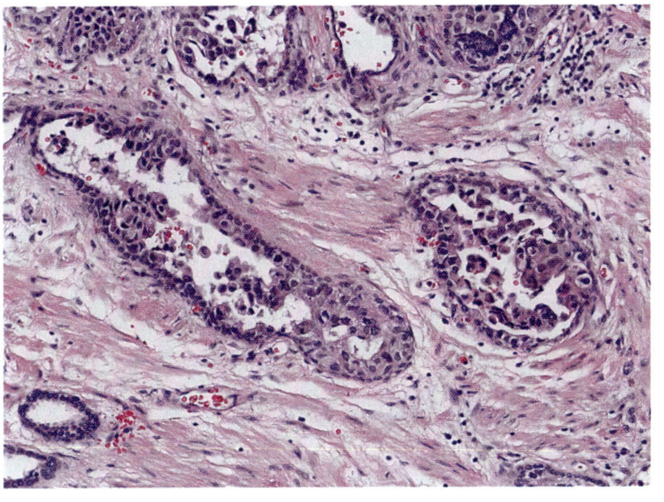

Fig. 13.7 Urothelial carcinoma of the prostatic urethra with colonization of the prostatic ducts and acini

ducts from true prostatic stromal invasion (Fig. 13.8) in view of the higher stage and associated poor prognosis. Noninvasive colonization of glands by carcinoma in situ maintains the rounded contours of prostate glands, and admixed prostatic secretory epithelial cells may be seen. In contrast, prostatic stromal invasion is characterized by irregular jagged nests of carcinoma, stromal retraction, or stromal desmoplasia [20].

Noninvasive Papillary Urothelial Carcinoma

Noninvasive papillary urothelial carcinoma of the urethra has a morphology identical to those in the urinary bladder as discussed in Chap. 6.

Invasive Carcinoma

Urothelial carcinoma: The full spectrum of invasive urothelial carcinoma, including variant forms, may be seen in the urethra. They are identical to those seen in the urinary bladder.

Squamous Cell Carcinoma

Squamous cell carcinomas may range from the very well-differentiated verrucous carcinomas to poorly differentiated squamous cell carcinomas. However, most cases are invasive moderately differentiated carcinomas at presentation (Fig. 13.9). Keratin pearls, abundant eosinophilic cytoplasm, and intercellular bridges usually allow recogni-

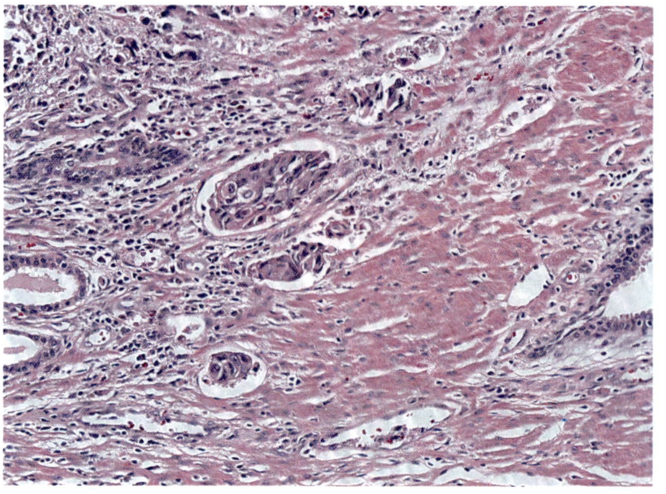

Fig. 13.8 Urothelial carcinoma of the prostatic urethra with stromal invasion

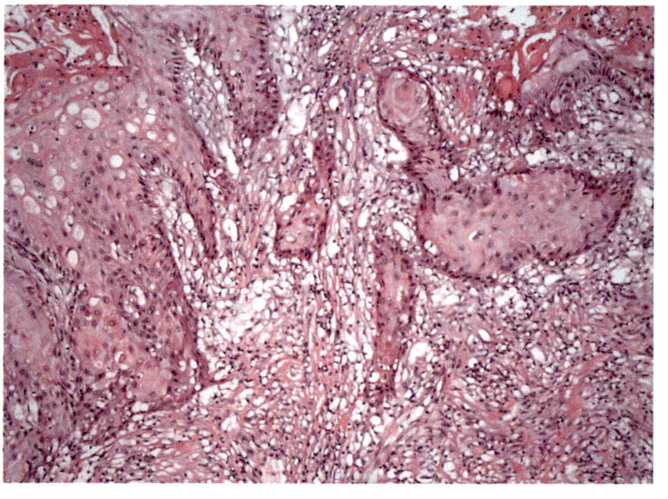

Fig. 13.9 Invasive moderately differentiated squamous cell cancer of the urethra

tion as squamous type. In a subset of cases, it may be difficult to distinguish primary squamous cell carcinoma of the urethra from urothelial carcinoma with extensive squamous differentiation. This issue is discussed fully in the chapter on squamous cell carcinoma of the bladder.

Adenocarcinoma

Adenocarcinomas of the urethra arise from the periurethral glands or through glandular metaplasia of the overlying urothelium. These are typically divided into nonclear cell and clear cell adenocarcinomas. Clear cell carcinoma is more frequently seen in female patients, but cases do occur in male patients [21, 22]. There are isolated reports of adenocarcinoma arising in Littre and Cowper's glands. Tumors arising in Cowper's glands are typically located in the bulbomembranous region, while those arising from Littré glands are typically located in the distal portion of the penile urethra (Fig. 13.10), though they may occasionally arise proximally. The so-called "primary mucin-producing urothelial type adenocarcinoma" is a rare tumor that also arises from the urothelium lining the prostatic urethra, resulting in adenocarcinoma identical to its more common counterpart seen in the urinary bladder (Fig. 13.11) [23]. Prostatic duct adenocarcinoma

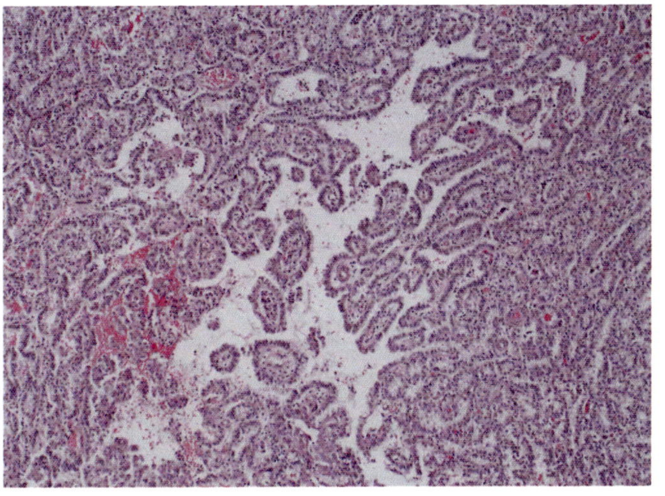

Fig. 13.10 Adenocarcinoma of the glands of Littré

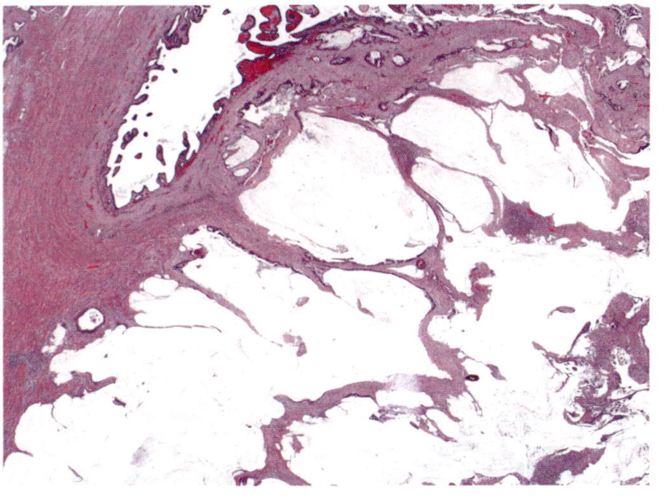

Fig. 13.11 Primary mucin-producing urothelial type adenocarcinoma

or usual type high-grade prostatic adenocarcinoma may present primarily as a urethral mass (Fig. 13.12). A significant number of prostatic duct adenocarcinomas arise from the periurethral region and are characterized by papillae with variable degree of complexity lined by tumor cells ranging from a single layer to multiple layers of stratified columnar epithelial cells with prominent nucleoli [24]. Patients may present with urinary obstruction, hematuria, and a papillary tumor that appears to arise from the urethra closely mimicking a urothelial origin. In some cases, the histologic distinction between high-grade urothelial and prostatic carcinoma may require adjunctive immunohistochemical testing. Prostatic adenocarcinomas typically express prostate-specific antigen (PSA) and prostate-specific acid phosphatase (PSAP), while they are negative with the urothelial markers uroplakin, thrombomodulin, p63, and high molecular weight cytokeratin.

Management

The primary form of treatment for men with urethral carcinoma is surgical excision (Fig. 13.13). In general, anterior urethral carcinoma is more amenable to surgical control, and the prognosis is better than that of posterior

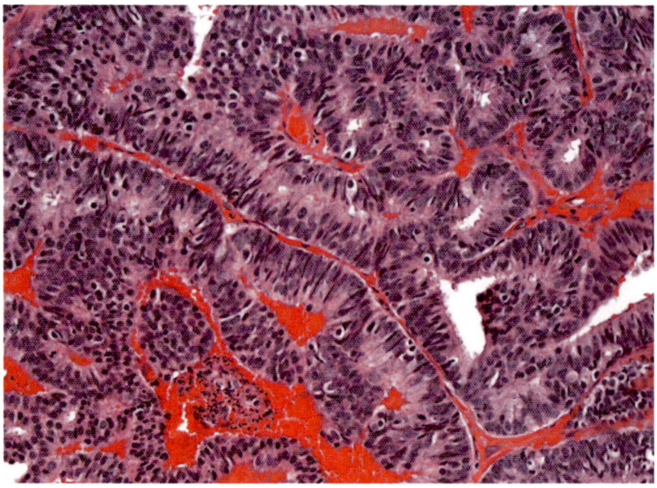

Fig. 13.12 Prostatic duct adenocarcinoma and usual type high grade prostatic adenocarcinoma presenting as a urethral mass

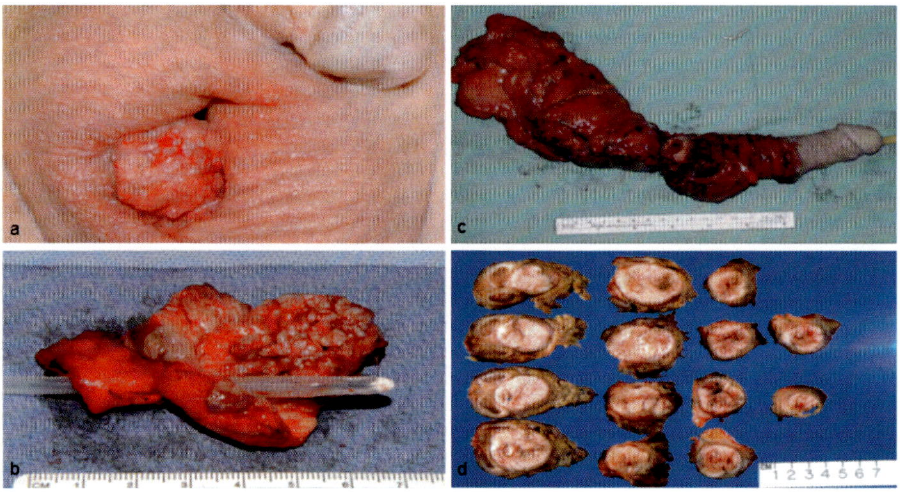

Fig. 13.13 Gross photos—male urethral cancer. (**a**, **b**) In situ and gross photos of a high-grade squamous urethral carcinoma at the orifice of a scrotal urethrostomy. (**c**) Cystoprostatectomy–penectomy–urethrectomy specimen. (**d**) Sections of urethral cancer specimen

urethral carcinoma, which is often associated with extensive local invasion and distant metastasis [25]. Transurethral resection, local excision, or distal urethrectomy and perineal urethrostomy may be acceptable treatment in selected patients with superficial, papillary, or low-grade tumors of the anterior urethra. Long-term disease-free survival has been reported in this setting [26–29]. Partial penectomy with a 2 cm margin is the treatment of choice for tumors infiltrating the corpus spongiosum and localized to the distal half of the penis. Excellent local control after this procedure has been documented [28, 30–34]. If invasive disease extends to or involves the proximal penile urethra, total penectomy is required to obtain an adequate margin of excision. In the largest series to date, a local recurrence rate of 13% was reported after this procedure [30]. Ilioinguinal lymphadenectomy is indicated in the presence of palpable inguinal lymph nodes without evidence of distant metastatic disease.

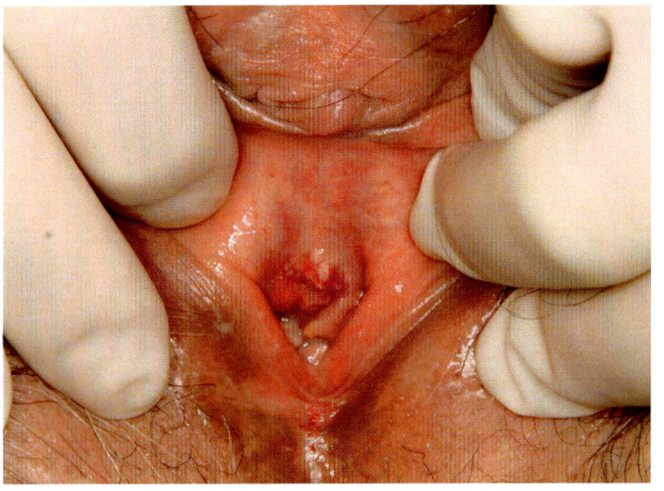

Fig. 13.14 Female urethral cancer

In the bulbomembranous urethra, noninvasive lesions may be treated with transurethral resection or segmental excision of the involved urethral segment with an end-to-end anastomosis. Unfortunately, noninvasive lesions are rare due to the typically late presentation of these patients. Poor survival figures have been recorded for all forms of treatment, but it appears that radical excision offers the best opportunity for long-term disease control and the lowest incidence of local recurrence. Radical cystoprostatectomy, pelvic lymphadenectomy, and total penectomy are usually required. Extending the operation to include in-continuity resection of the pubic rami and the adjacent urogenital diaphragm may improve the margin of resection and local control in some cases [34–38].

In general, radiation therapy has been reserved for patients with early-stage lesions of the anterior urethra who refuse surgery. The long-term results of radiotherapy are difficult to evaluate because few reports are available of patients treated with this modality [39, 40]. A small number of studies have reported the results of neoadjuvant and adjuvant chemotherapy in patients with advanced stage or metastatic disease [41]. The combination of chemotherapy and radiation therapy has shown some success in a small number of patients with localized and metastatic urethral cancer [42, 43]. More commonly, these forms of treatment are combined with surgery in a multimodal approach in patients with advanced disease [8, 28, 44].

Urethral Cancer: Female

Female urethral carcinoma is rare and accounts for approximately 0.02% of all female cancers [45] and less than 1% of cancers in the female genitourinary tract [46]. It is most often diagnosed in the fifth and sixth decades of life [46]. While previous literature had suggested that primary cancers of the urethra were more common in women than in men [47], recent evidence suggests otherwise. A recent survey of the National Cancer Institute Surveillance, Epidemiology, and End Results (SEER) database revealed a 2:1 male-to-female predominance [48].

Clinical Presentation

Clinical presentation is similar to those seen in men, with obstructive voiding complaints, urethral discharge, pain or bleeding, or a urethral mass predominating (Fig. 13.14). While the diagnosis may be made more expeditiously in women owing to a shorter urethra, diagnosis may still often be delayed due to an inability for most women to easily visualize the area or hesitancy to seek medical attention for their symptoms.

Pathogenesis

Several factors are associated with the development of urethral cancer in women, including: chronic irritation, caruncles, polyps, parturition, and HPV or other viral infections [8, 49]. Female urethral diverticula may also predispose the patient to malignant change, with a reported 5% of female urethral carcinomas arising within a diverticulum [50]. A major pitfall from the clinical standpoint is the misinterpretation of urethral carcinoma as a benign caruncle.

Cystoscopic/Clinical Exam Findings

Clinical examination should include a pelvic exam with bimanual palpation, as well as cystoscopy for visualization of the tumor and biopsy for tissue diagnosis. Often, bladder neck involvement can be determined on physical examination alone.

Pathology

According to SEER data, histological subtypes of female urethral cancer are nearly evenly split between urothelial, adenocarcinoma, and squamous cell cancer [48].

Squamous Cell Carcinoma

Squamous cell carcinomas are similar to those described in the male. For HPV-associated urethral carcinomas, patients may have a prior history of or concomitant cervicovulvar dysplasia. Secondary squamous cell carcinoma extending from the uterine cervix is morphologically indistinguishable from a urethral primary. This distinction would depend on clinical/radiographic correlation since HPV testing does not help.

Adenocarcinoma

Approximately 60% of cases are nonclear cell adenocarcinomas similar to those described for males, but 40% are clear cell adenocarcinomas [51–53]. Clear cell adenocarcinoma has many morphologic features similar to those of the uterus and ovary. They are typically characterized by a mixed papillary and tubulocystic growth pattern, but solid patterns may also be seen. Dense stromal hyalinization within papillary cores is common. The epithelial cells often have clear or eosinophilic cytoplasm with a "hobnail" appearance, and nuclear pleomorphism is variable. The architectural growth pattern of clear cell carcinoma may closely mimic nephrogenic adenoma, which is the main differential diagnostic consideration. Primary adenocarcinomas may also arise from the periurethral or Skene's glands. These tumors are characterized by a glandular, papillary, or micropapillary architecture and the tumor cells are either columnar or cuboidal with eosinophilic or clear cytoplasm. In some cases the tumor may be identified with adjacent uninvolved periurethral glands.

Management

The vast majority of women with urethral cancer are symptomatic at the time of diagnosis. Management therefore includes obtaining tissue diagnosis (cystoscopic biopsy) and staging (labwork, exam under anesthesia, computed tomography of the abdomen and pelvis, chest CT). Physical examination, cystoscopy, and occasionally pelvic magnetic resonance imaging (MRI) may help with surgical planning. Given the rarity of female urethral cancer and the heterogeneity of histological subtypes, treatment recommendations are largely based on tumor location and clinical stage. Small, superficial tumors in the distal third of the urethra may be excised without compromising continence. The distal urethra should be excised circumferentially, with a portion of the anterior vaginal wall. While ablative technologies have been described for distal urethral tumors in women, they are not universally accepted [54]. Five-year disease-free survival has been reported up to 71% for distal tumors [55]. Adjuvant radiation for distal T2 tumors often improves survival [28, 56]. Potential complications following partial urethrectomy include incontinence and meatal stenosis, but these complications are usually treatable with subsequent surgical procedures.

Panurethral or proximal tumors require more radical treatment and demonstrate poorer cancer-free survival rates (48% for proximal tumors, 24% for panurethral tumors) [55]. Usually total urethrectomy with anterior pelvic exenteration is performed; however, 5-year survival rates are low after exenteration for proximal urethral tumors [38]. Extent of resection depends on the extent of the tumor, but wide excision (en bloc) of the tumor and surrounding tissue is the rule. This may require vaginectomy, vulvectomy, and/or pubectomy. Due to the poor outcomes demonstrated for monotherapy alone and depending on the pathological subtype, multimodal treatment with radiation and chemotherapy is often considered in these situations.

The female urethra has classically been divided into the anterior (distal third) and posterior (proximal two-thirds) segments. Drainage of the lymphatics from the anterior (distal third) and posterior(proximal two-thirds) segments of the female urethra corresponds to the drainage basins already described for the male anterior and posterior urethra [57]. However, female urethral cancer may be more likely to spread systemically without regional nodal involvement. Therefore, while inguinofemoral lymph node dissection (IFLND) provides important prognostic information for male urethral cancer, it is of little prognostic benefit for female urethral cancer. Despite this, IFLND is recommended for patients with clinically palpable metastatic adenopathy and no evidence of distant disease [58].

Female Urethral Diverticula

Identification of a female urethral diverticulum is a challenging diagnosis and the possibility of a urethral diverticulum is often overlooked in the evaluation of a female urology patient. Although female urethral diverticuli can occur at any age, they are usually diagnosed in the third to fifth decades [59, 60]. The presentation of a woman with a urethral diverticulum may range from asymptomatic to debilitating symptoms. Such a range of presenting symptoms often contributes to a delay in diagnosis. In addition to a variable clinical picture, the increased use of MRI has demonstrated that urethral diverticuli may have a great degree of anatomic variation (Fig. 13.15). Due to underdiagnosis, the historically cited prevalence of 1–6% is likely not an accurate estimation of the true prevalence of female urethral diverticuli [61]. A study conducted by Lorenzo and colleagues examined 140 women who presented to a urologist with lower urinary tract symptoms. Each woman was evaluated with an endorectal coil MRI and 10% of the women were found to have a urethral diverticulum [62].

Clinical Presentation

Classically, the presentation of a urethral diverticulum includes the triad of the "three D's": dysuria, dyspareunia, and postvoid dribbling. These symptoms are neither sensitive nor specific for urethral diverticuli and the majority of patients will not present with the classic triad. While up to 20% of women with a urethral diverticulum are asymptomatic, the majority of patients are symptomatic and most frequently present with irritative lower urinary tract symptoms, pain, and infection [63–66]. In 30–50% of patients, a urethral diverticulum will be associated with recurrent urinary tract infections [64, 67]. In addition to these symptoms, 12–24% of women will experience dyspareunia [63, 64] and 5-32% will complain of postvoid dribbling [64, 67].

Pathogenesis

A urethral diverticulum is an epithelialized cavity that communicates with the urethral lumen and is contained within the periurethral fascia [60]. The majority of urethral diverticuli are acquired; however, there are rare reports of congenital urethral diverticuli, which are thought to be remnants of Gartner's duct cysts. Female urethral diverticuli are commonly found in the distal urethra where the periurethral glands drain. The periurethral glands lie lengthwise along the urethra in a posterolateral position and they are most prominent in the distal two-thirds of the urethra, with the majority of

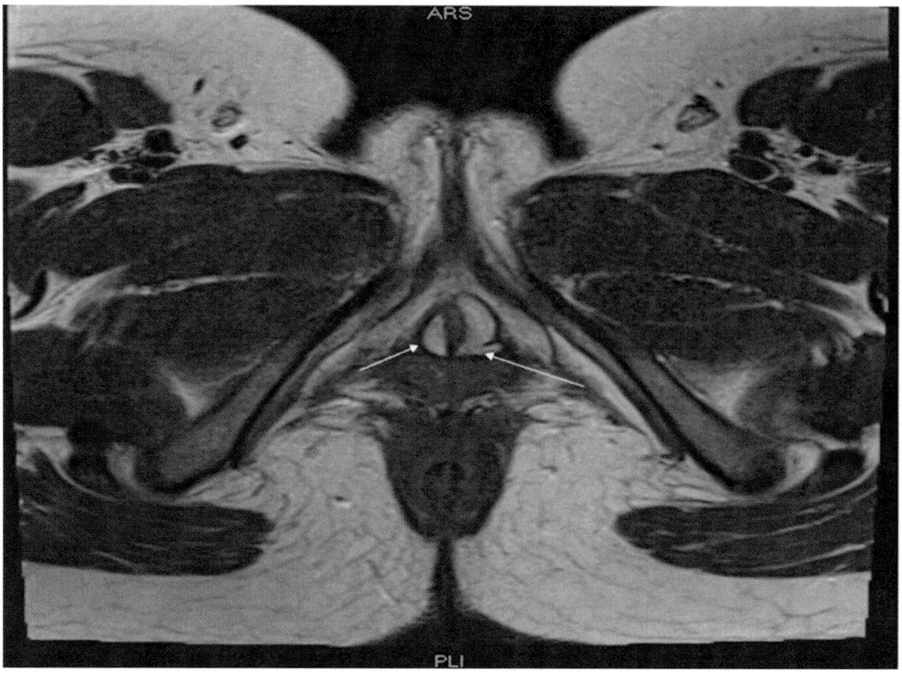

Fig. 13.15 T2-weighted MRI demonstrating classic horseshoe-shaped urethral diverticulum

glands draining into the distal one-third of the urethra. The most widely accepted hypothesis regarding the formation of female urethral diverticuli was first described by Routh in 1890 [68]. According to this hypothesis, repeated infection and subsequent obstruction of the periurethral glands lead to abscess formation. The periurethral abscess then ruptures into the urethral lumen and forms a cavity in communication with the lumen that becomes epithelialized over time [69]. Other possible etiologies include urethral trauma during birth and iatrogenic causes after procedures such as urethral instrumentation or periurethral injections [70]. The periurethral cavity is often connected to the urethral lumen by an ostium or neck. Similar to the variation in symptoms associated with female urethral diverticuli, a range of anatomic variability and complexity also exists.

Clinical Examination/Cystoscopy

The complete evaluation of a female patient who may have a urethral diverticulum includes a thorough history, a genital exam, urine studies in the form of a urinalysis and a urine culture, endoscopic evaluation of the bladder and urethra, and radiologic imaging. The evaluation should also include urodynamic testing if the patient presents with urinary incontinence or voiding dysfunction [71–73]. On physical exam, palpation of the distal anterior vaginal wall may reveal a supple mass with a variable degree of tenderness. Palpation of the distal anterior vaginal wall may also reveal urine or purulent fluid via the meatus when the urethra is “milked.” Physical signs suggestive of a neoplastic process include a firm and fixed mass. A study conducted by Thomas and colleagues determined that 6% of 90 consecutive women who underwent urethral diverticulectomy at a single institution had invasive carcinoma on final pathology [74]. The presence of stagnant urine also leads to the formation of stones in up to 10% of urethral diverticula. Following a thorough physical exam, careful urethroscopy may allow visualization of an ostium.

High-quality imaging is essential as both a diagnostic tool and a key component of preoperative planning. Imaging modalities used to evaluate a patient for a urethral diverticulum include positive pressure urethrography (PPU), voiding cystourethrography (VCUG), ultrasound, and magnetic resonance imaging. Each imaging technique has both advantages and disadvantages and the choice of imaging modality may depend on local availability of imaging, cost, and experience of the radiologist. In the past, VCUG and PPU were the most commonly used studies to detect a urethral diverticulum. VCUG is a widely available imaging technique that can produce high-quality imaging of a urethral diverticulum with a reported sensitivity as high as 65% [75]. PPU, also known as a double balloon urethrogram, utilizes high pressure contrast in the urethra to define urethral anatomy and identify potential communications with periurethral diverticuli. Two studies compared PPU to VCUG and determined that PPU has greater sensitivity [76, 77]. PPU has largely fallen out of favor with the advent of more advanced imaging techniques, which provide better anatomic detail and are easier to administer [78].

MRI provides the greatest anatomic detail and has become the gold standard for the evaluation of female urethral diverticuli. MRI is performed using either an external coil or an endoluminal technique that involves placement of the coil within a body cavity near the tissue of interest. Nietlich and colleagues demonstrated that external coil MRI was more sensitive and had a better negative predictive value compared to PPU [78]. When endovaginal and endorectal techniques were examined, endoluminal MRI was found to be more sensitive and more accurate in its anatomic detail compared to VCUG [79]. T2-weighted series demonstrate increased signal intensity in the urethral diverticulum and this delineation from surrounding tissues provides high resolution multiplanar imaging that can be utilized for surgical planning.

Pathology

Histologic evaluation of urethral diverticula typically shows a saccular invagination of urothelium into the lamina propria or muscularis propria. The surface lining may also show squamous or glandular metaplasia. Diverticula may be associated with benign epithelial lesions that are associated with inflammation, i.e., cystitis cystica et glandularis and nephrogenic adenoma. The incidence of carcinoma arising in the setting of urethral diverticula ranges from 2 to 15%. The carcinomas typically associated with urethral diverticula include adenocarcinoma, squamous cell carcinoma, and urothelial carcinoma. Among women undergoing urethral diverticulectomy and found to have urethral cancer, adenocarcinoma was the predominant histological type. Intestinal metaplasia with dysplasia has also been identified in urethral diverticuli [74].

Management

Both nonsurgical and surgical treatments play a role in the management of urethral diverticuli. A nonsurgical approach with use of suppression-dose antibiotics, anticholinergics, and sitz baths may be appropriate when the patient has a small diverticulum not amenable to surgical excision and minimal to no symptoms. Several surgical techniques have been described for the treatment of urethral diverticuli, including transurethral incision of the diverticulum, marsupialization of the diverticulum into the vagina, and transvaginal excision of the diverticulum with urethral reconstruction as deemed necessary. Transvaginal excision of the diverticulum has become the treatment of choice with a largely uniform technique.

Benign Urethral and Nonurothelial or Squamous Malignant Lesions

A number of other urethral lesions have been described in men and women, usually in the form of case reports, and are rarely encountered. As a general rule, these are found during routine cystoscopy for obstructive voiding complaints. Lesions in men may feel plaque-like and be misdiagnosed as Peyronie's disease, but Peyronie's disease never involves or compromises the urethra. Therefore, patients who are thought to have a ventral Peyronie's plaque but have a lesion involving the urethra or a urethral mass visualized during cystoscopy should undergo biopsy. Some lesions require open excisional biopsy if cystoscopic biopsy fails to acquire enough tissue for a pathological diagnosis to be determined. We favor a midline raphe incision over the tumor with direct dissection down to the mass for lesions in the penile urethra, and a midline perineal approach for bulbar masses that require excisional biopsy. Treatment is driven by etiology and often requires involvement of other medical specialists to treat systemic manifestations of the disease, as with amyloidosis or tuberculosis.

References

1. Lumen N, Hoebeke P, Willemsen P, et al. Etiology of urethral stricture disease in the 21st century. J Urol. 2009;182(3):983–7.
2. Albers P, Fichtner J, Bruhl P, et al. Long term results of internal urethrotomy. J Urol. 1996;156(5):1611–4.
3. Santucci R, Eisenberg L. Uretrotomy has a much lower success rate than previously reported. J Urol. 2010;183(5):1859–62.
4. Xu YM, Qiao Y, Sa YL, et al. Urethral reconstruction using colonic mucosa graft for complex strictures. J Urol. 2009;182(3):1040–3.
5. Barbagli G, Morgia G, Lazzeri M. Dorsal onlay skin graft bulbar urethroplasty: long term follow-up. Eur Urol. 2008;53(3):628–33.
6. Simonato A, Gregori A, Ambruosi C, et al. Lingual mucosal graft urethroplasty for anterior urethral reconstruction. Eur Urol. 2008;54(1):79–85.
7. Webster GD, Ramon J. Repair of pelvic fracture posterior urethral defects using an elaborate perineal approach: experience with 74 cases. J Urol. 1991; 145(4):744–8.
8. Grigsby PW, Herr HW. Urethral tumors. In: Vogelzang N, Scardino PT, Shipley WU, Coffey DS, editors. Comprehensive textbook of genitourinary oncology. 2nd ed. Baltimore: Williams & Wilkins; 2000. p. 1133–40.
9. Dalbagni G, Zhang ZF, Lacombe L, et al. Male urethral carcinoma: analysis of treatment outcome. Urology. 1999;53:1126–32.
10. Weiner JS, Liu ET, Walther PJ. Oncogenic human papillomavirus type 16 is associated with squamous cell cancer of the male urethra. Cancer Res. 1992;52:5018–23.
11. Cupp MR, Reza MS, Goellner JR, et al. Detection of human papillomavirus DNA in primary squamous cell carcinoma of the male urethra. Urology. 1996;48:551–5.
12. Freeman JA, Tarter TA, Esrig D, et al. Urethral recurrence in patients with orthotopic ileal neobladders. J Urol. 1996;156:1615–9.
13. Hassan JM, Cookson MS, Smith Jr JA, et al. Urethral recurrence in patients following orthotopic urinary diversion. J Urol. 2004;172:1338–41.
14. Nieder AM, Sved PD, Gomez P, et al. Urethral recurrence after cystoprostatectomy: implications for urinary diversion and monitoring. Urology. 2004;64:950–4.
15. Varol C, Thalmann GN, Burkhard FC, et al. Treatment of urethral recurrence following radical cystectomy and ileal bladder substitution. J Urol. 2004;172:937–42.
16. Amin MB, Young RH. Primary carcinomas of the urethra. Semin Diagn Pathol. 1997;14(2):147–60.
17. Cheville JC, Dundore PA, Bostwick DG, Lieber MM, Batts KP, Sebo TJ, et al. Transitional cell carcinoma of the prostate: clinicopathologic study of 50 cases. Cancer. 1998;82(4):703–7.
18. Kirkali Z, Canda AE. Superficial urothelial cancer in the prostatic urethra. Sci World J. 2006;6:2603–10.
19. Liedberg F, Chebil G, Mansson W. Urothelial carcinoma in the prostatic urethra and prostate: current controversies. Expert Rev Anticancer Ther. 2007;7(3):383–90.
20. Oliva IV, Smith SL, Chen Z, Osunkoya AO. Urothelial carcinoma of the bladder with transmural and direct prostatic stromal invasion: does extent of stromal invasion significantly impact patient outcome? Hum Pathol. 2011;42(1):51–6.
21. Gogus C, Baltaci S, Orhan D, Yaman O. Clear cell adenocarcinoma of the male urethra. Int J Urol. 2003;10(6):348–9.
22. Miller J, Karnes RJ. Primary clear-cell adenocarcinoma of the proximal female urethra: case report and review of the literature. Clin Genitourin Cancer. 2008;6(2):131–3.
23. Osunkoya AO, Epstein JI. Primary mucin-producing urothelial-type adenocarcinoma of prostate: report of 15 cases. Am J Surg Pathol. 2007;31(9):1323–9.
24. Samaratunga H, Letizia B. Prostatic ductal adenocarcinoma presenting as a urethral polyp: a clinicopathological study of eight cases of a lesion with the potential to be misdiagnosed as a benign prostatic urethral polyp. Pathology. 2007;39(5):476–81.
25. Zeidman EJ, Desmond P, Thompson I. Surgical treatment of carcinoma of the male urethra. Urol Clin North Am. 1992;19:359–72.
26. Mandler JI, Pool TL. Primary carcinoma of the male urethra. J Urol. 1966;96:67–72.
27. Konnak JW. Conservative management of low grade neoplasms of the male urethra: a preliminary report. J Urol. 1980;123:175–7.
28. Gheiler EL, Tefilli MV, Tiguert R, et al. Management of primary urethral cancer. Urology. 1998;52: 487–93.
29. Hakenberg OW, Franke HJ, Froehner M, Wirth MP. The treatment of primary urethral carcinoma—the dilemmas of a rare condition: experience with partial urethrectomy and adjuvant chemotherapy. Onkologie. 2001;24:48–52.
30. Kaplan GW, Bulkley GJ, Grayhack JT. Carcinoma of the male urethra. J Urol. 1967;98:365–71.

31. Ray B, Canto AR, Whitmore Jr WF. Experience with primary carcinoma of the male urethra. J Urol. 1977;117:591–4.
32. Anderson KA, McAninch JW. Primary squamous cell carcinoma of the anterior male urethra. Urology. 1984;23:134–40.
33. Hopkins SC, Nag SK, Soloway MS. Primary carcinoma of the male urethra. Urology. 1984;23:128–33.
34. Dinney CPN, Johnson DE, Swanson DA, et al. Therapy and prognosis for male anterior urethral carcinoma: an update. Urology. 1994;43:506–14.
35. Mackenzie AR, Whitmore Jr WF. Resection of the pubic rami for urologic cancer. J Urol. 1968;100:546–51.
36. Shuttleworth KE, Lloyd-Davies RW. Radical resection for tumors involving the posterior urethra. Br J Urol. 1969;41:739–43.
37. Bracken RB. Exenterative surgery for posterior urethral cancer. Urology. 1982;19:248–51.
38. Klein FA, Whitmore Jr WF, Herr HW, et al. Inferior pubic rami resection with en bloc radical excision for invasive proximal urethral carcinoma. Cancer. 1983;51:1238–42.
39. Raghavaiah NV. Radiotherapy in the treatment of carcinoma of the male urethra. Cancer. 1978;41:1313–6.
40. Forman JD, Lichter AS. The role of radiation therapy in the management of carcinoma of the male and female urethra. Urol Clin North Am. 1992;19:383–9.
41. Scher HI, Yagoda A, Herr HW, et al. Neoadjuvant M-VAC (methotrexate, vinblastine, doxorubicin and cisplatin) for extravesical urinary tract tumors. J Urol. 1988;139:475–7.
42. Licht MR, Klein EA, Bukowski R, et al. Combination radiation and chemotherapy for the treatment of squamous cell carcinoma of the male and female urethra. J Urol. 1995;153:1918–20.
43. Oberfield RA, Zinman LN, Leibenhaut M, et al. Management of invasive squamous cell carcinoma of the bulbomembranous male urethra with coordinated chemo-radiotherapy and genital preservation. Br J Urol. 1996;78:573–8.
44. Johnson DW, Kessler JF, Ferrigni RG, et al. Low dose combined chemotherapy/radiotherapy in the management of locally advanced urethral squamous cell carcinoma. J Urol. 1989;141:615–6.
45. Fagan GE, Hertig AT. Carcinoma of the female urethra; review of the literature; report of eight cases. Obstet Gynecol. 1955;6:1–11.
46. Srinivas V, Khan SA. Female urethral cancer—an overview. Int Urol Nephrol. 1987;19:423–7.
47. Narayan P, Konety B. Surgical treatment of female urethral carcinoma. Urol Clin North Am. 1992;19:373–82.
48. Swartz MA, Porter MP, Lin DW, et al. Incidence of primary urethral carcinoma in the United States. Urology. 2006;68:1164–8.
49. Mevorach RA, Cos LR, di Sant'Agnese PA, Stoler M. Human papillomavirus type 6 in grade I transitional cell carcinoma of the urethra. J Urol. 1990;143:126–8.
50. Rajan N, Tucci P, Mallouh C, Choudhury M. Carcinoma in female urethral diverticulum: case reports and review of management. J Urol. 1993;150:1911–4.
51. Tanabe ET, Mazur MT, Schaeffer AJ. Clear cell adenocarcinoma of the female urethra: clinical and ultrastructural study suggesting a unique neoplasm. Cancer. 1982;49(2):372–8.
52. Young RH, Scully RE. Clear cell adenocarcinoma of the bladder and urethra. A report of three cases and review of the literature. Am J Surg Pathol. 1985;9(11):816–26.
53. Oliva E, Young RH. Clear cell adenocarcinoma of the urethra: a clinicopathologic analysis of 19 cases. Mod Pathol. 1996;9(5):513–20.
54. Staehler G, Chaussy C, Jocham D, Schmiedt E. The use of neodymium-YAG lasers in urology: indications, technique and critical assessment. J Urol. 1985;134:1155–60.
55. Dalbagni G, Zhang ZF, Lacombe L, Herr HW. Female urethral carcinoma: an analysis of treatment outcome and a plea for a standardized management strategy. Br J Urol. 1998;82:835–41.
56. Hahn P, Krepart G, Malaker K. Carcinoma of female urethra. Manitoba experience: 1958–1987. Urology. 1991;37:106–9.
57. Carroll PR, Dixon CM. Surgical anatomy of the male and female urethra. Urol Clin N Am. 1992;19(2):339–46.
58. Sharp DS, Angermeier KW. Surgery of penile and urethral carcinoma in Campbell-Walsh urology. 10th ed. Philadelphia, PA: Elsevier; 2012. p. 948.
59. Burrows LJ, Howden NL, Meyn L, et al. Surgical procedures for urethral diverticula in women in the United States, 1979–1997. Int Urogynecol J Pelvic Floor Dysfunct. 2005;16:158–61.
60. Young GPH, Wahle GR, Raz S. Female urethral diverticulum. In: Raz S, editor. Female urology. Philadelphia, PA: W.B. Saunders; 1996. p. 477–89.
61. Gaston EA, Ferruci J. Calculus formation in a urethral diverticulum in a woman. N Engl J Med. 1939;221:379–83.
62. Lorenzo AJ, Zimmern P, Lemack GE, et al. Endorectal coil magnetic resonance imaging for diagnosis of urethral and periurethral pathologic findings in women. Urology. 2003;61:1129–33.
63. Davis HJ, Telinde RW. Urethral diverticula: an assay of 121 cases. J Urol. 1958;80:34–9.
64. Davis BL, Robinson DG. Diverticula of the female urethra: assay of 120 cases. J Urol. 1970;104:850–3.
65. Leach GE, Schmidbauer H, Hadley HR, et al. Surgical treatment of female urethral diverticulum. Semin Urol. 1986;4:33.
66. Peters III W, Vaughan Jr ED. Urethral diverticulum in the female. Etiologic factors and postoperative results. Obstet Gynecol. 1976;47:549–52.
67. Ganabathi K, Leach GE, Zimmern P, et al. Experience with the management of urethral diverticulum in 63 women. J Urol. 1994;152:1445–52.

68. Routh A. Urethral diverticula. BMJ. 1890;1:361–2.
69. Aspera AM, Rackley RR, Vasavada SP. Contemporary evaluation and management of the female urethral diverticulum. Urol Clin North Am. 2002;29:617–24.
70. Clemens JQ, Bushman W. Urethral diverticulum following transurethral collagen injection. J Urol. 2001;166:626.
71. Reid RE, Gill B, Laor E, et al. Role of urodynamics in management of urethral diverticulum in females. Urology. 1986;28:342–6.
72. Summitt Jr RL, Stovall TG. Urethral diverticula: evaluation by urethral pressure profilometry, cystourethroscopy, and the voiding cystourethrogram. Obstet Gynecol. 1992;80:695–9.
73. Bhatia NN, McCarthy TA, Ostergard DR. Urethral pressure profiles of women with urethral diverticula. Obstet Gynecol. 1981;58:375–8.
74. Thomas AA, Rackley RR, Lee U, et al. Urethral diverticula in 90 female patients: a study with emphasis on neoplastic alterations. J Urol. 2008;180:2463–7.
75. Lee JW, Fynes MM. Female Urethral diverticula. Best Pract Res Clin Obstet Gynaecol. 2005;19:875–93.
76. Jacoby K, Rowbotham RK. Double balloon positive pressure urethrography is a more sensitive test than voiding cystourethrography for diagnosing urethral diverticulum in women. J Urol. 1999;162:2066–9.
77. Wang AC, Wang CR. Radiologic diagnosis and surgical treatment of urethral diverticulum in women. A reappraisal of voiding cystourethrography and positive pressure urethrography. J Reprod Med. 2000;45:377–82.
78. Nietlich JD, Foster Jr HE, Glickman MG, et al. Detection of urethral diverticula in women: comparison of a high resolution fast spin echo technique with double balloon urethrography. J Urol. 1998;159:408–10.
79. Blander DS, Rovner ES, Schnall MD, et al. Endoluminal magnetic resonance imaging in the evaluation of urethral diverticula in women. Urology. 2001;57:660–5.

Part V

Upper Tract Disease

Nonneoplastic and Neoplastic Ureteral and Renal Pelvis Disease

14

Jonathan J. Rhee, Thomas W. Jarrett, and Theodorus H. van der Kwast

Introduction

Although any form of carcinoma identified in the urinary tract may arise in the upper tract, the most common cancer at this site is urothelial carcinoma (UC). The occurrence of upper urinary tract UC is rare, but may occur anywhere from the urothelium of the renal pelvis to the distal ureter (Fig. 14.1). It accounts for approximately 8% of all renal tumors and 5% of all tumors of the urinary tract [1–4]. Its incidence, however, increases among those who are exposed to particular chemicals or who are genetically susceptible. Urothelial carcinoma of the upper urinary tract occurs about three to four times more frequently in the renal pelvis than in the ureter. Bilateral synchronous upper urinary tract UC represents about 3% of the urothelial carcinomas [5]. Although sharing histological and molecular similarities with bladder UC [6, 7], upper tract UC has anatomic differences that may affect disease prognosis.

J.J. Rhee • T.W. Jarrett (✉)
Department of Urology, George Washington University, 2150 Pennsylvania Avenue, NW, Washington, DC 20037, USA
e-mail: tjarrett@mfa.gwu.edu

T.H. van der Kwast
Department of Pathology and Laboratory Medicine, Princess Margaret Hospital, University Health Network, 200 Elizabeth Street, Toronto, ON, Canada, M5G 2C4

Pathogenesis

Epidemiology

Upper urinary tract UC affects 0.7 to 1.1/100,000 individuals [8] and is generally a disease of the elderly, with the mean age of diagnosis in the sixth or seventh decade [8, 9]. The male-to-female incidence ratio is approximately 1.7:1 [8]. Although the frequency of upper urinary tract UC is increasing, it continues to represent only a small percentage of all urothelial carcinomas [8, 10]. This increased incidence is a result of both improved diagnosis in upper urinary tract UC and the more effective treatment of bladder cancer that allows for a longer survival in patients with urinary tract carcinoma. As a consequence, upper urinary tract UC has more time to develop in patients with an initial diagnosis of UC of the lower urinary tract, a phenomenon described as length time bias. Notably, about 80% of upper tract UC occurs in patients with a history of bladder cancer [11].

Risk Factors

Previous Urinary Bladder Cancer

Having a history of bladder cancer is the major risk factor for developing an upper urinary tract UC. The multifocal nature of urinary tract cancer has originally been attributed to the field "cancerization"—a predilection of the entire

D.E. Hansel et al. (eds.), *The Urinary Tract: A Comprehensive Guide to Patient Diagnosis and Management*, DOI 10.1007/978-1-4614-5320-8_14, © Springer Science+Business Media New York 2012

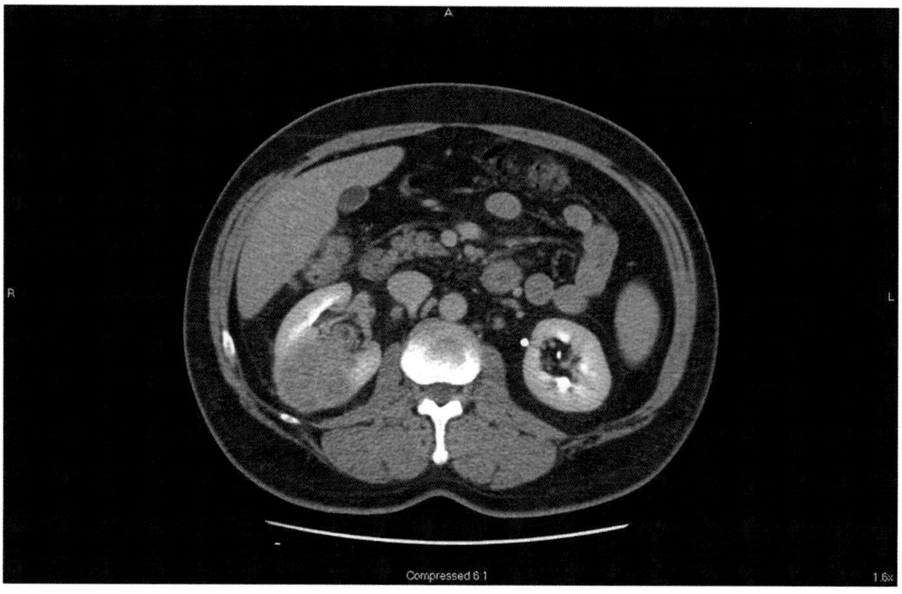

Fig. 14.1 CT scan of a renal pelvic tumor, delay

urothelial lining of the upper and lower urinary tract to develop UC, due to exposure of all parts of the urinary tract to the same carcinogens such as tobacco products and other chemicals (see later). The monoclonality of most multifocal bladder cancers argues against this concept of multifocal de novo bladder carcinogenesis [12]. Instead, it is more commonly believed that implantation of cancer cells shed in the urine and intramucosal spread of cancer cells explain the multifocality of UC. This has been supported by clonality analysis of multifocal bladder tumors by a combination of histopathologic organ mapping, loss of heterozygosity, fluorescence in situ hybridization (FISH), and p53 analyses. Given the frequent association of lower urinary tract UC with upper urinary tract UC, patients with multifocal cancer need to be monitored for the development of an upper urinary tract UC.

Tobacco

Tobacco smoking is an important risk factor for development of UC. Cancer risk increases with both consumption dose and duration of use [13–16]. Smoking exposure is complex and linked to multiple substances that include aromatic amines, like benzopyrene or dimethylbenzanthracene [17]. The aromatic amines are metabolized by the body into *N*-hydroxyalanine, which poses carcinogenic activity. The *N*-hydroxyalanine is modulated by different enzymatic systems (cytochrome P450s including CYP1A1, glutathione *S*-transferases and *N*-acetyl transferases), and any of these enzymatic systems may contain polymorphisms that might explain individual susceptibility to upper urinary tract UC [18]. Exposure to tobacco increases the relative risk of developing upper urinary tract UC to 2.5–7 [15]. Fortunately, the risk for upper urinary tract UC decreases by 60–70% when smoking cessation has been longer than 10 years [13].

Phenacetin

Long-term use of phenacetin has been implicated as a risk factor for upper urinary tract UC [14–16, 19–22]. Nephrotoxicity of phenacetin was first recognized and reported in Sweden in 1961 [23]. There is evidence now that phenacetin indirectly causes carcinogenesis by inducing nephrotoxicity through papillary necrosis, which may promote carcinogenesis or behave as a compounding factor in the presence of chronic irritation, infection, or smoking [24]. The use of phenacetin was abandoned in the 1980s due to the implications of developing upper urinary tract UC [17]. Surprisingly, the average latency period for developing upper urinary tract UC is approximately 22 years [24]. Since the cessation of phenacetin use, the incidence of upper urinary tract UC from this cause is now decreasing [24].

Lynch Syndrome (Hereditary Nonpolyposis Colorectal Cancer Syndrome)

Hereditary nonpolyposis colorectal cancer syndrome (HNPCC), or Lynch syndrome, is a familial cancer syndrome with autosomal dominant inheritance. The main cancers found in families with HNPCC are colorectal carcinomas (63%), but this syndrome also includes extracolonic cancers such as endometrial carcinomas (9%) and upper urinary tract carcinomas (5%). In people with HNPCC the risk of upper tract UC is increased 14–22 times as compared to the general population [5]. The syndrome is caused by germline mutations affecting one or several of the mismatch repair genes (e.g., *hMSH2*, *hMLH1*, *hMSH6*, *hMLH1*). During cellular replication the ensuing mismatch repair defect causes microsatellite repeat replication errors, leading to frameshift mutations in various genes. The frequency of microsatellite instability in upper urinary tract UC varies in the literature between 4 and 26%, depending on the tests used and the characteristics of the investigated population [5]. Immunohistochemistry that reveals the absence of the mismatch repair genes in the nuclei of the tumor cells can help the initial identification of patients with Lynch syndrome among those presenting with an upper urinary tract UC. These patients should be referred for genetic counseling and assessment of family members, who may be at risk for colorectal cancer or an extracolonic cancer manifestation of the syndrome. Urologists should be aware of cancer syndrome, particularly when they encounter a younger patient with upper tract UC. The revised Bethesda criteria (2003) guide clinicians to determine which individuals need testing for microsatellite instability [25].

Balkan Endemic Nephropathy

Balkan endemic nephropathy—first described in the 1950s—is a chronic tubulointerstitial nephropathy with insidious onset that ultimately leads to renal failure [26]. It affects mainly farmers in the plains along the Danube in Bosnia, Herzegovina, Bulgaria, Croatia, Romania, and Serbia [26], who are exposed to degradation products of coal-containing soil. These patients are generally younger, usually present with renal failure, usually have upper urinary tract tumors of lower grade and stage, and have bilateral and/or multiple tumors [27, 28]. The incidence of upper urinary tract UC in the Balkan areas formerly was up to 100 times higher than in the nonendemic areas [27]; however, subsequent reports suggest that the incidence of upper urinary tract UC from the Balkan endemic nephropathy regions of Serbia appears to be decreasing [29, 30]. Unfortunately, though, UC cancer-specific survival rates in the region are decreasing without valid explanation [28].

Aristolochic Acid

End-stage kidney disease has been reported in young women taking weight-loss pills containing Chinese herbs *Stephaniatetrandra* and *Magnolia officinalis* [31]. The pattern of interstitial fibrosis characterized in Chinese herb nephropathy resembles Balkan endemic nephropathy [31–33]. In some instances, it was suspected that aristolochic acid—which has well-established potent carcinogenic properties in animal studies—was inadvertently substituted for tetrandrine when generating extracts [34, 35]. In humans, the metabolites of aristolochic acid (aristolactams) were detected in kidneys that were removed from the patients with Chinese herb nephropathy. In fact, those metabolites were bound to DNA, suggesting a link to carcinogenesis in those patients [36]. Some investigators have shown that these metabolites are directly involved in tumorigenesis [37] and cause development of UC when exposed to them.

Cyclophosphamide

Cyclophosphamide is an alkylating agent and has been used since the 1960s for the treatment of hematologic malignancies and severe manifestations of systemic forms of autoimmune disease. As exposure to cyclophosphamide increases UC risk in a dose- and duration-dependent manner, the prolonged exposure of patients with autoimmune disease to this drug has been associated with an increased risk of urinary tract cancer [38]. A few cases of cyclophosphamide-induced upper urinary tract UC have been reported [39], and one clinical trial has suggested that patients with a history of superficial bladder UC are at increased risk for development of upper urinary tract UC when given a single high dose of cyclophosphamide [40].

Additional Risk Factors

Other risk factors include papillary necrosis, stones, and occupational exposures to petrochemical, plastic materials, coal, asphalt, tar, and thorium-containing contrast media [4, 41].

Prognostic Factors

Tumor stage is the most important prognostic factor [42, 43]; however, location, higher grade, multifocality, and lymphovascular invasion all impact patient survival [44–48]. Importantly, transmural tumor growth (pT3 or pT4) was reported to be less common in distally located tumors (33%) as compared to tumors arising in the midureter (44%), proximal ureter (75%) or renal pelvis (41%). Distally located tumors in the ureter have a much better disease-specific survival (median 53 months) than proximally located ureteric UC (median 16 months) [44]. It is likely that tumors in the distal ureter give earlier rise to clinical symptoms, allowing for their detection before they have reached an advanced stage. There is an ongoing debate as to whether the location of UC within the upper urinary tract is a major prognosticator by itself, independent of stage. According to some studies, renal pelvis UC has a better prognosis than ureteric UC of the same pathological stage [49, 50]; however, one recent large study demonstrated no difference in outcomes following nephroureterectomy between stage-matched patients with tumors of the renal pelvis and the ureter. The latter data would support the current tumor–nodes–metastasis (TNM) staging system, in which renal pelvic and ureteral carcinomas are classified as one integral group of tumors [43].

Lymph node status appears to be another strong prognosticator for disease. The 2-year and 5-year cancer-specific survival rates for nodal involvement after treatment were 26.3% and 15% compared to 95.2% and 85.2% for patients without any nodal involvement [51]. Other independent prognostic factors in upper tract UC for disease-specific survival and disease recurrence are tumor necrosis >10% and tumor architecture that is papillary or sessile [52, 53].

Clinical Presentation

Common symptoms of localized upper urinary tract UC include microscopic or gross hematuria and dysuria. Dysuria may be present especially when the ureteral tumor is located distally and involves the trigone. Patients can also present with flank pain in 10–40% [54]. Pain is usually dull in nature due to gradual obstruction from tumor. However, when hematuria occurs and a blood clot obstructs the ureter, patients may present with acute flank pain. Flank pain does not correlate with locally advanced disease or worse prognosis. Patients with more advanced disease may present with array of constitutional symptoms that include weight loss, anorexia, malaise, abdominal mass, bone pain, fever, anemia, and night sweats.

Upper urinary tract UC spreads by direct extension into the adjacent organs or by lymphatic and hematogenous routes. Common sites for metastases include lung, liver, bone, and regional lymph nodes. The comparatively thin layer of muscularis in the ureter and renal pelvis allows for early penetration and dissemination of tumor (Fig. 14.2a, b) [55]. For renal pelvic UC, the renal parenchyma may serve as a barrier for pT3 tumor and thus may slightly delay dissemination to distant organs (Fig. 14.3a,b). Periureteral tumor extension carries a much higher risk of early tumor dissemination via lymphatic and

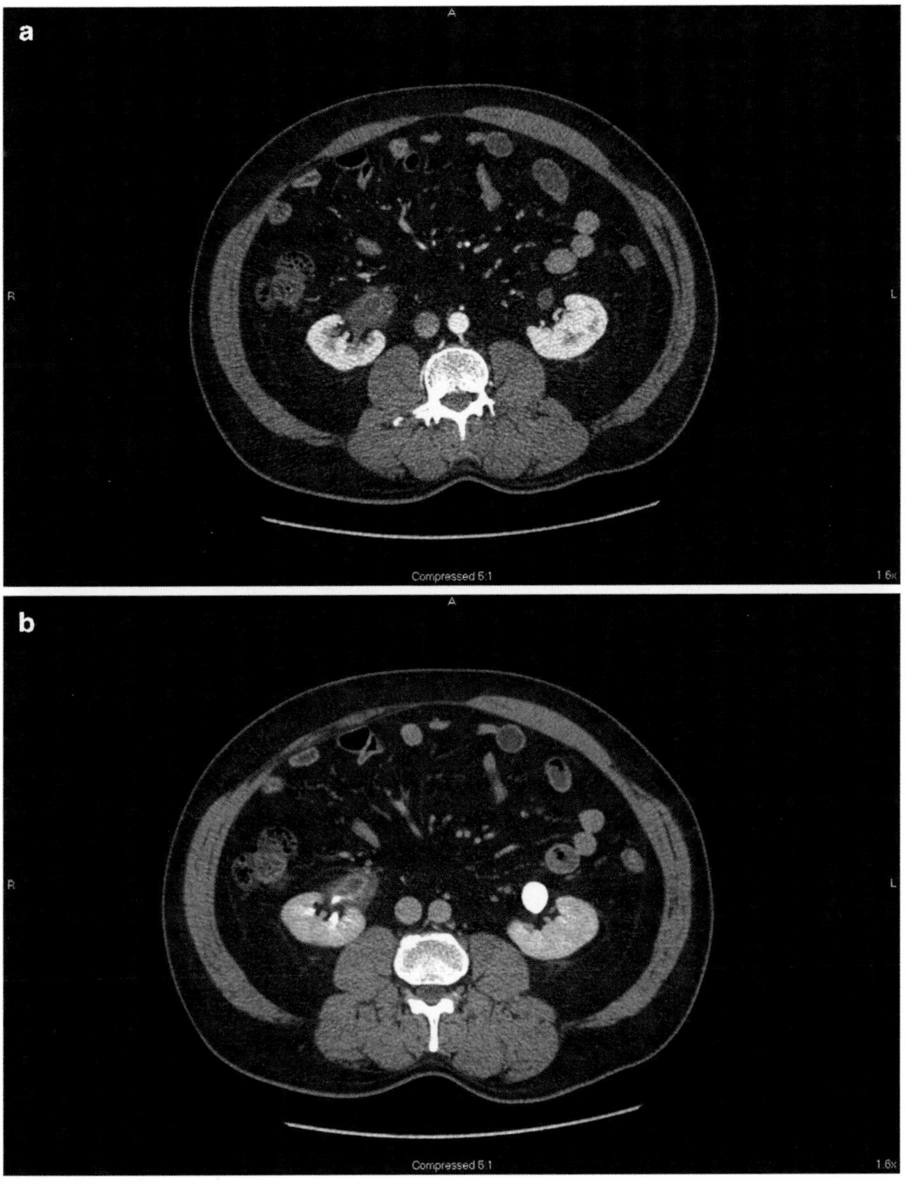

Fig. 14.2 (**a**) CT nephrogram, upper tract. (**b**) CT delay, upper tract

vascular routes (Fig. 14.4). Lymphatic metastases from the renal pelvic and proximal ureteral tumors spread initially to paraaortic and paracaval lymph nodes, whereas distal ureteral tumors tend to spread to pelvic lymph nodes [56–58].

Clinical staging of advanced disease should include chest X-ray, abdominal computed tomography, liver function tests, and possibly nuclear bone scan. All patients should undergo cystoscopy as well.

Clinical Examination

Urine Sample

Cystoscopic ureteral catheterization is required to obtain samples of renal pelvic and ureteral washings or urine. When washings of the upper urinary tract are performed, saline is preferred, as sterile water causes cytolysis of cells that result in disruption of cellular membrane, and makes the specimen interpretation difficult. Washing

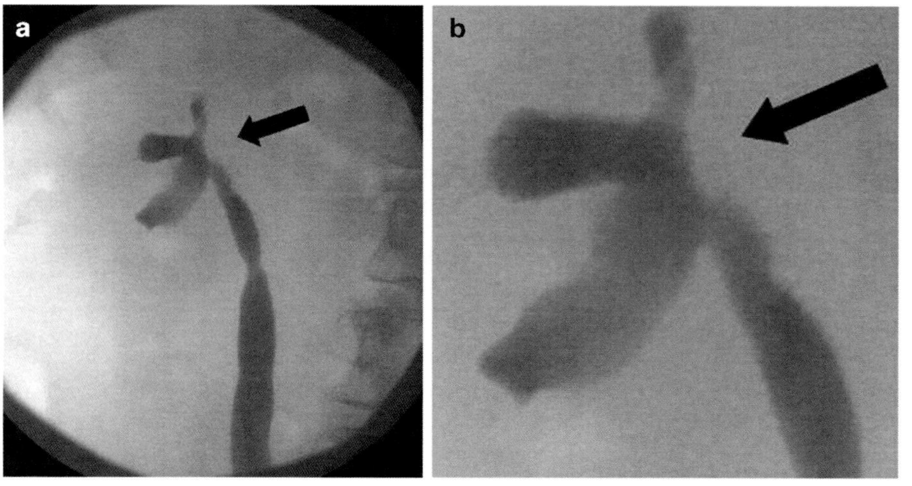

Fig. 14.3 (**a**, **b**) Retrograde filling defect

Fig. 14.4 Ureteral tumor, retrograde

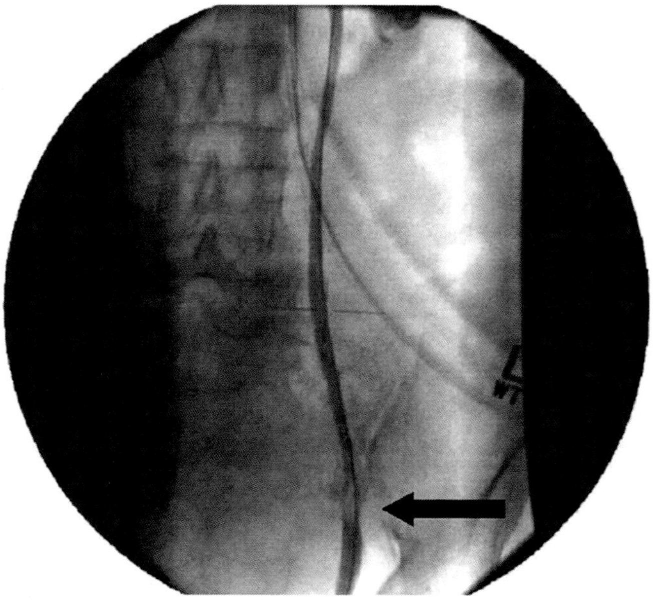

with gentle irrigation, as opposed to passive collection of urine, provides better tissue sampling by releasing loosely attached cells.

Urinary cytology is a valuable diagnostic modality in evaluating patients with suspected upper urinary tract UC. The limitation of urinary cytology as a diagnostic tool is that overall sensitivity is low, especially for detecting low-grade and superficial tumors [59, 60]. This drawback is explained in large part by lack of morphologic criteria for separating well-differentiated low-grade UC from benign urothelial cells [61]. There exists limited literature on the use of urine tests for detection of UC in upper tract urines or washings as a diagnostic or monitoring tool, mainly making use of the cytogenetic aberrations in UC cells. These tests include FISH and microsatellite analysis.

FISH is a cytogenetic technology that is used for analysis of multiple chromosomes. The most commonly used technology for detection of bladder cancer uses the fluorescently labeled DNA

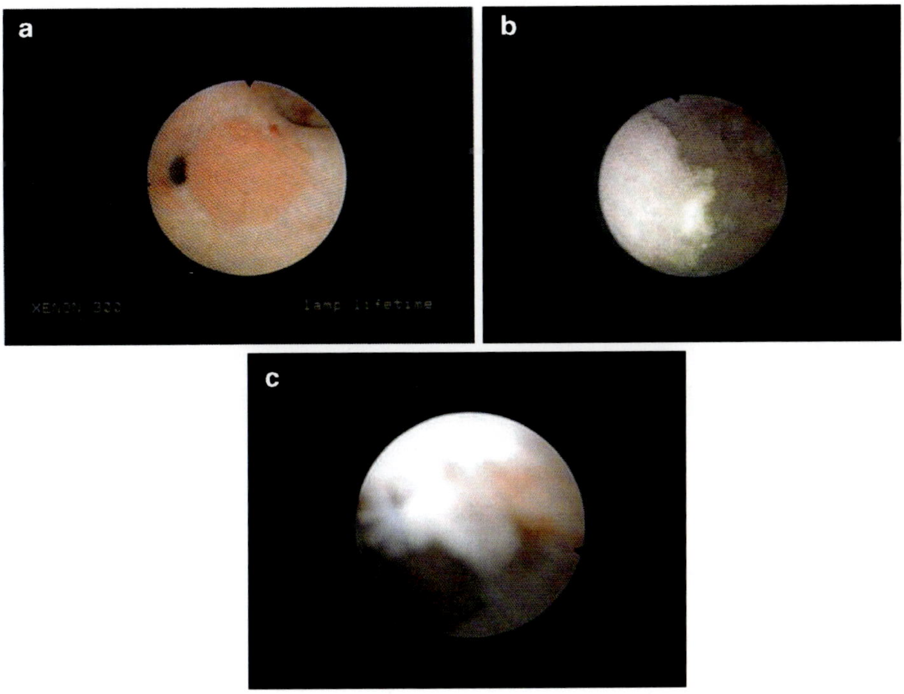

Fig. 14.5 (**a**) Renal pelvic papillary tumor. (**b**, **c**) Ureteroscopic view of a renal pelvic tumor

probes that hybridize to the centromere of chromosomes 3, 7, and 12 as well as the 9p21 locus. Some studies reported the benefit of this FISH analysis on washings of the upper urinary tract, including an increased sensitivity particularly for lower grade UC over cytology, but their sample sizes were small [62, 63]. In patients who underwent a urinary diversion after cystectomy for bladder cancer, FISH performed on ureter washings showed a high sensitivity and a high negative predictive value. However, its positive predictive value was modest, which raised concerns over the cost-effectiveness of this expensive method for follow-up of these patients [64]. Another DNA-based technology to detect UC is microsatellite analysis to demonstrate loss of heterozygosity for selected genetic loci in the cells shed in urine samples. In a randomized clinical trial on the use of microsatellite analysis on voided urine samples for monitoring patients with low-grade UC of the urinary bladder, it was noted that this technique was able to identify all four upper urinary tract recurrences [65]. Since this technique is laborious and costly, its routine use is in monitoring patients for upper tract UC awaits further improvements in its cost-effectiveness.

Biopsy of the Upper Urinary Tract

Improvements in endoscopic technique allow biopsies to be obtained from suspected lesions in the upper urinary tract. The biopsy of upper urinary tract UC may play an important role in the preoperative prediction of the presence of nonorgan-confined UC of the upper urinary tract, with grade, architecture, and location being the strongest predictors [66].

In general, upper tract biopsies are very small, generally with a diameter of a few millimeters. Although usually sufficient for histopathological verification of the disease process and the architecture (papillary, flat, or nonpapillary/sessile), pathological staging is often challenging. Pathological grade is often readily assessed on sampled lesions, although cautery and crush artifact, as well as small sample size, may limit interpretation. For flat lesions of the ureter or renal pelvis, such as carcinoma in situ (Fig. 14.5a, b, c), clinicopathological correlation is required to

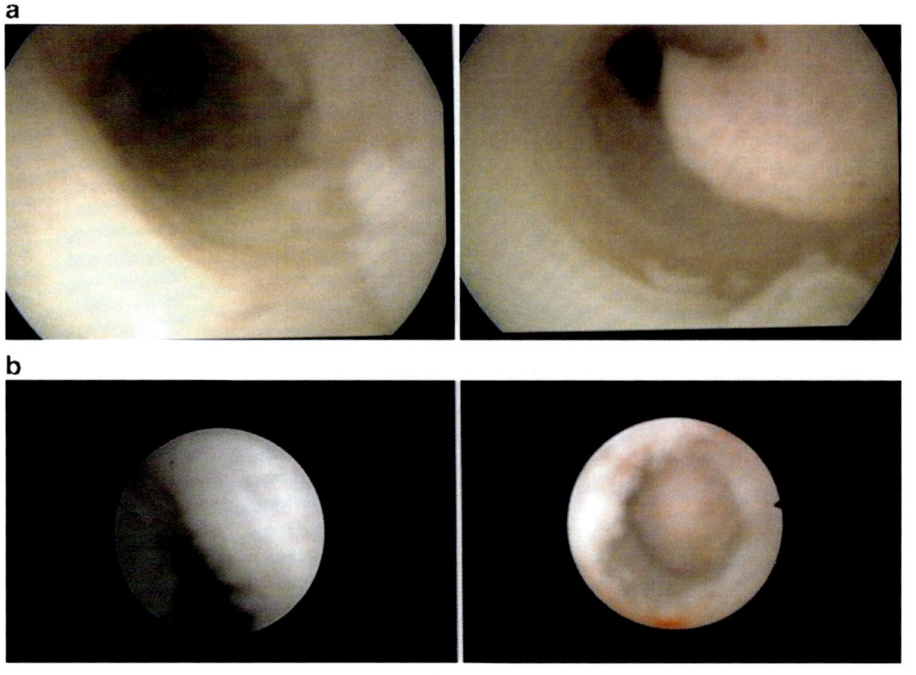

Fig. 14.6 (**a**, **b**) Ureteroscopic views of renal pelvic tumor

determine how representative the biopsy is of the underlying process. Invasion of a high-grade lesion into either the stalk of a papillary lesion or the lesion base may be appreciated in a larger specimen; however, further detailed staging (such as invasion into the muscularis or beyond) is generally not possible on upper tract biopsies due to the lack of subepithelial structures in the majority of biopsies (Fig. 14.6a, b). Finally, a number of lesions may be undergraded or understaged due to limited access to the entire lesion cystoscopically, as well as proposed heterogeneity within the lesion [67]. One recent study suggests that endoscopic biopsies of upper tract lesions may result in undergrading and understaging of urothelial carcinomas in up to 40% of cases [68].

A diagnosis of papillary urothelial neoplasm of unknown malignant potential (PUNLMP) should generally be avoided on small superficial biopsies of the upper urinary tract, as tumor heterogeneity and the presence of invasion may lead to undergrading of the tumor.

Upper tract UC may also be identified on needle biopsy for evaluation of a renal neoplasm. These lesions appear morphologically distinct from all forms of renal cell carcinoma and may be diagnosed directly or with the aid of immunohistochemical stains.

Radiologic Evaluation

Excretory Urography

Traditionally, the diagnosis of upper urinary tract UC had been made with excretory urography. Upper urinary tract UC demonstrates as a filling defect when contrast fills the collecting system. The sensitivity can range from 50 to 80%, which is lower than computed tomography (CT) urography, 88–100% [69, 70] (see next section). The amount of radiation exposed from excretory urography is approximately (7.9 mSv), which is 2.5 less than CT urography (20 mSv) [71].

Any filling defect within the upper urinary tract can be confused with fungal bezoars, clots, papillary necrosis, and so forth [72]. Manifestations of the filling defect can be smooth or irregular. When tumor is irregular, contrast can tract along the crevice of a papillary lesion, creating a "stipple sign" [73]. When tumor obstructs the infundibulum,

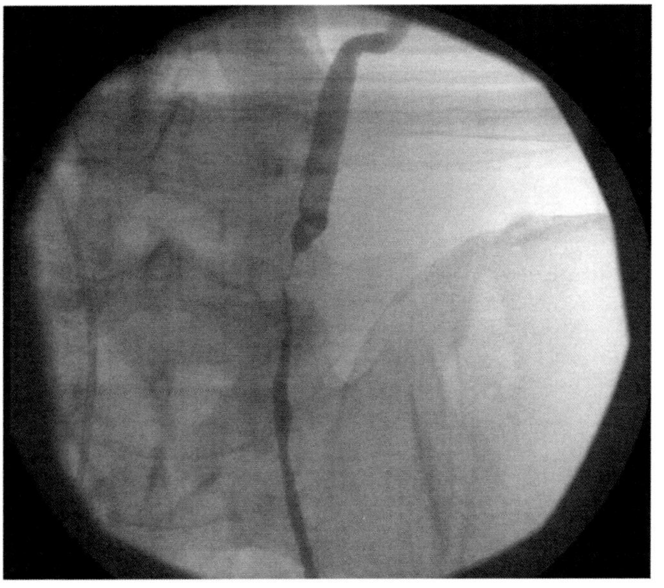

Fig. 14.7 Retrograde stricture

it can create "caliceal amputation" [72]. Moreover, tumors can create a stricture-like lesion that can mimic tuberculosis of the kidney [74]. A major disadvantage of the excretory urography is that a nonfunctioning kidney cannot be assessed since it requires excretion of contrast into the collecting system to create filling defects [72].

Computed Tomography

Computed tomography (CT) urography has replaced excretory urography in evaluating the upper tract urinary system. More sensitive than ultrasonography, it can detect other incidental lesions [69, 75, 76]. CT urography consists of three phases. Initial imaging is performed from the top of the kidney down to the pubic symphysis to exclude nephrolithiasis. Intravenous contrast is administered, and the nephrographic phase is evaluated after 80–140 s. This phase evaluates the renal parenchyma to exclude enhancing renal masses. Lastly, excretory phase is performed 4–8 min after intravenous infusion of contrast. This allows assessment of the collecting system. Any lesion within the upper urinary tract collecting system will manifest as filling defect during the excretory phase of CT urography. Advanced UC of the renal pelvis may extend into the renal parenchyma and distort the architecture of the parenchyma (Fig. 14.7).

Hydronephrosis is a common finding in ureteral tumors, and hydroureter can be seen to the proximal level of obstruction due to tumor. Ureteral wall thickening, luminal narrowing, mass, and/or ureteric fat stranding may be present on CT scan [77]. Figure 14.8a, b demonstrate a CT scan of nephrogram and excretory phases demonstrating stranding around the thickened proximal ureter.

Retrograde Pyelography

Retrograde pyelography is utilized in patients with impaired renal function or intravenous contrast allergy. As with urography, intraluminal filling defect represents a lesion. When infundibulum is involved by the tumor and causes obstruction, as mentioned previously, an "amputated" calyx may be seen. Tumors in the ureter usually present with an "apple core" appearance. A major advantage of retrograde pyelography is that concomitant diagnostic procedures can be performed, such as cystoscopy and ureteroscopy. If an abnormal lesion is encountered, tissue biopsy, cytology, and fulguration can be performed simultaneously.

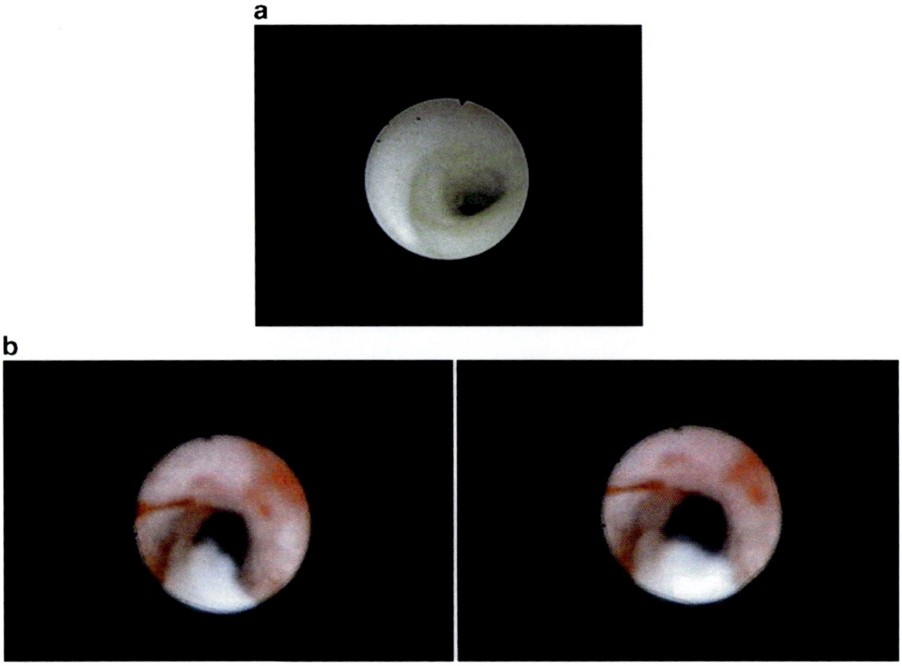

Fig. 14.8 (**a**, **b**) Ureteroscopic view of stricture

Cystoscopic and Ureteroscopic Evaluation

Endoscopic advances have made evaluation of the upper urinary tract more accurate. Modern flexible ureteroscopes are much smaller, and with fiberoptic technology, visualization is significantly enhanced. The superior deflection of the scope allows easy navigation throughout the entire collecting system to locate tumor. Tumors can be localized and biopsied, usually with either a flat wire basket or biopsy forceps. Caution must be practiced during navigation in the collecting system to avoid trauma, since small amounts of bleeding obscure visualization. Accurate staging from ureteroscopic biopsy is usually limited due to small tissue sampling. In order to circumvent this issue, multiple biopsies can be obtained to increase the yield of the tissue sample. Cystoscopy should be performed to exclude bladder cancer when upper urinary tract UC is suspected. When an abnormal lesion is found in the bladder, it should be biopsied and treated.

Pathology of Upper Urinary Tract Lesions

Benign Lesions

Von Brunns nests may be evident in the subepithelial connective tissue of the renal pelvis and the ureters and may rarely raise the differential diagnosis of UC. Another lesion with indolent behavior that occurs in the upper tract is the inverted papilloma [78, 79], which may raise the differential diagnosis of low-grade UC with an inverted growth pattern. In cases where the distinction is challenging due to small biopsy sampling, caution is warranted in the final diagnosis with close follow-up of the patients recommended [78].

Polypoid pyelitis and ureteritis are the upper urinary tract analogues of the more commonly seen polypoid cystitis or papillary cystitis of the bladder. These lesions may mimic low-grade papillary UC, but can be distinguished by the presence of a broad base, the absence of fibrovascular cores, and the presence of edema, fibrosis, and inflammatory cells [80].

Neoplastic Lesions

Urothelial Carcinoma

UC represents more than 95% of the upper urinary tract malignancies, with the same gamut of gross appearances as elsewhere in the urinary tract. The most common tumors include exophytic papillary tumors with or without a prominent inverted growth pattern component, and the nonpapillary, invasive high-grade UC. UC with an inverted growth pattern tends to occur more frequently in the upper urinary tract, and this variant may preclude accurate pathological staging, as it can be difficult to distinguish a true invasion from a mere inverted growth pattern. The latter is defined by discrete, rounded nests of urothelium that often interanastomose and demonstrate a distinct basement membrane. Although invasion may occur in association with an inverted growth pattern, this is characterized by classic features such as irregular nests or individual cells permeating below the basement membrane, paradoxical differentiation, and retraction artifact. The presence of an inverted growth pattern was found to be indicative of microsatellite instability [81].

Large, non-invasive papillary low-grade UC may occur and appears to "fill up" and distend the renal pelvis; these lesions often either lack invasion or have invasion limited to the subepithelial connective tissue. Occasionally, intratubular spread—or spread of tumor cells within the lumen of renal tubules—may occur. This feature in isolation is considered noninvasive; however, it may occur in the presence of invasive carcinoma. In addition to the pure UC and those with squamous and glandular differentiation, all other less common UC variants encountered in the bladder may be found in the upper urinary tract (e.g., micropapillary, nested variant, plasmacytoid variants)[4]. In addition, sarcomatoid carcinomas of the renal pelvis have been reported [82]. Upper tract UC should be graded in a similar way as those of the lower urinary tract, using the World Health Organization (WHO) 2004 grading system. Although the current European Association of Urology (EAU) and American Urological Association (AUA) guidelines also recommend the inclusion of the previous WHO 1973 grading in pathology reporting, as this may add some benefit as an independent prognostic factor for pT1 disease, this practice is generally not followed in the USA due to broad morphological overlap in Grade 2 categorization.

Differential diagnostic problems may especially arise when glandular differentiation of the carcinoma is present. In this scenario, the major differential diagnostic consideration is a collecting duct adenocarcinoma of the kidney, since the latter is localized to the renal pelvis and shows a diffuse and irregular infiltration pattern into the renal parenchyma, similar to high-grade UC with glandular differentiation. A history of bladder cancer, the presence of carcinoma in situ, and the identification of squamous and/or predominantly solid tumor growth are all features that point at a urothelial origin.

Squamous Cell Carcinoma

Pure squamous cell carcinomas of the upper urinary tract are rare, representing less than 5% of upper urinary tract cancers. They are mainly associated with chronic inflammatory conditions, such as nephrolithiasis, and they are mostly found in the renal pelvis. The male-to-female ratio is equal [83]. These lesions are thought to originate from areas of squamous metaplasia, caused by the chronic inflammation. At gross inspection, squamous cell carcinomas are often large, necrotic, and ulcerated, with invasion into the renal parenchyma and the surrounding adipose tissue. A white, flaky appearance may be appreciated due to the presence of keratin formation. Grading is performed using the same criteria as squamous cell carcinomas of other locations, but this has limited prognostic impact. Most renal pelvis squamous cell carcinomas are moderately to poorly differentiated; they are large with extensive infiltration of the renal parenchyma, and as a consequence they have a poor prognosis. Stage for stage, however, the prognosis for pure squamous cell carcinoma of the renal pelvis is similar to that of UC of the same location [83, 84]. If a squamous cell carcinoma of the ureter is encountered in females, the differential diagnosis of infiltrative growth per continuitatem from the cervix must be entertained.

Table 14.1 Pathological staging of invasive carcinoma of the upper tract

T (primary tumor)	
TX	Primary tumor cannot be assessed
T0	No primary tumor
Ta	Papillary noninvasive carcinoma
Tis	Carcinoma in situ
T1	Tumor invades subepithelial connective tissue
T2	Tumor invades the muscularis propria
T3	(Ureter) Tumor invades periureteral fat; (Renal pelvis) Tumor invades beyond muscularis propria into perinephric fat or the renal parenchyma
T4	Tumor invades adjacent organ, or through the kidney into the perinephric fat
N (lymph nodes)	
NX	Regional lymph node cannot be assessed
N0	No regional lymph node metastases
N1	Metastasis to a single lymph node, 2 cm or less in greatest dimension
N2	Metastasis in a single lymph node, more than 2 cm but not more than 5 cm in greatest dimension; or multiple lymph nodes, none more than 5 cm in greatest dimension
N3	Metastasis in a lymph node, more than 5 cm in greatest dimension
M (distant metastasis)	
MX	Distant metastasis cannot be assessed
M0	No distant metastasis
M1	Distant metastasis

Adenocarcinoma

Adenocarcinomas of the upper urinary tract are even rarer than squamous cell carcinoma, and they also occur most often in association with nephrolithiasis. The same morphologic variants as found in the urinary bladder (i.e., signet cell, mucinous, intestinal) have been reported in the upper urinary tract [4]. Clinicopathological correlation and further histopathological workup may be required in order to exclude metastatic adenocarcinoma of the breast, gastrointestinal tract, lungs or gynecologic tract. Multifocality, lack of mucosal involvement, lack of hydronephrosis, and the absence of stones may raise the suspicion of metastatic disease.

Other Neoplasms

Other malignant tumors that may rarely involve the upper urinary tract include small cell carcinoma and leiomyosarcoma. Their behavior is similar as in other body sites [85].

Challenges to Pathological Staging

For pathological staging of upper urinary tract UC, the subepithelial connective tissue, the muscularis, the renal sinus fat/periureteric fat, and renal parenchyma represent the major landmarks, as their involvement by infiltrating cancer determines the actual pathological stage (Table 14.1). Pathological staging of upper urinary tract UC can be challenging for a number of reasons. First, large exophytic renal pelvic tumors have a tendency to display an inverted growth pattern, as discussed previously. Second, the caliber of smooth muscle in the ureter and renal pelvis may be highly variable and may be nearly absent in the calyces and renal sinus, making a distinction between pT1 and pT2 subjective at this site. Finally, poor fixation and processing may also result in artificial retraction artifacts, confounding the establishment of invasiveness.

One mimicker of stromal invasion can be found at the interface between renal pelvis and renal parenchyma, where UC cells of the renal pelvis may propagate along some of the renal collecting ducts, termed "intraductal spread ". In this way, they replace the lining tubular cells of the kidney, but they do not infiltrate the peritubular kidney stroma. This spread of UC cells into the renal tubules does not constitute parenchymal invasion; rather, it represents pTis disease [4]. In particular, large papillary or polypoid masses of the renal pelvis without obvious invasion of surrounding structures as judged from gross inspection require extensive sampling of the pelvicaliceal system, in order to appreciate the presence of invasion, and/or the level of invasion.

Surgical Management

Multiple surgical options are available for managing patients with upper urinary tract UC. Radical nephroureterectomy with bladder cuff excision is the gold standard treatment for upper tract UC. There are different approaches that have been described to manage bladder cuff excision, and it will be discussed in the later portions of the chapter.

Distal ureterectomy with ureteroneocystotomy is an option for bulky distal ureteral tumors that are not amenable to endoscopic treatment. Segmental ureterectomy for proximal ureter or midureter is not recommended unless the tumor is too bulky or renal preservation is absolutely necessary.

Minimally invasive techniques allow alternative treatment options for select patients. It offers reasonable strategy for patients with functional solitary kidney, bilateral upper tract UC, baseline renal insufficiency, and significant comorbid diseases.

Open Radical Nephroureterectomy

Radical nephroureterectomy with bladder cuff excision is considered the gold standard for treating large, high-grade, and invasive upper urinary tract UC [55, 56, 86–89]. Open radical nephroureterectomy can be approached with either a single incision or two separate incisions. When one incision is considered, a thoracoabdominal-type incision or long midline incision can be utilized. Thoracoabdominal incision is started at either the 11th or 12th rib, and then the incision is extended towards the pelvis, either in midline or paramedian. This extension will provide greater exposure of the distal ureter and bladder. The peritoneum may be entered during surgery to achieve better exposure. When the midline incision is used, exposing the retroperitoneum may be limited due to the bowel. However, with adequate retraction, the bowel can be safely packed away from the surgical field. When two separate incisions are utilized, a subcostal or flank incision is made to perform radical nephrectomy; then a Gibson, a low midline, or a Pfannenstiel incision can be made to complete the distal ureterectomy with bladder cuff excision. The urethral catheter is placed on the sterile field to manipulate the bladder during surgery.

The ipsilateral adrenal gland is usually spared because it provides no prognostic benefit when tumor is limited to the kidney. However, when local invasion is discovered, a proper extirpative oncologic principle should be practiced, and adrenalectomy should be performed. The nephrectomy specimen should incorporate Gerota's fascia and perinephric fat.

Distal ureterectomy with bladder cuff is performed and includes the entire ureter, the intramural ureter, and ureteral orifice. The specimen can be removed as "en bloc"; however, the kidney can be removed separately, as it can hinder exposure during surgery. When the specimen is removed separately, caution must be taken so that tumor spillage does not occur. UC has been well recognized for its ability to implant onto the nonurothelial surfaces, especially high-grade urothelial tumors [90]. A closed system is maintained by ties or clips before the ureter is divided. Oftentimes a surgical drain is then placed as well.

Laparoscopic Radical Nephroureterectomy

Laparoscopic radical nephroureterectomy can be performed transperitoneally or retroperitoneally. It can also be performed with hand-assisted transperitoneal or retroperitoneal approaches. The choice of laparoscopic approach depends on a surgeon's experience and comfort level. The retroperitoneal approach involves less bowel manipulation, but this approach limits operative space. The transperitoneal approach offers a larger working space for larger tumors.

To position, the patient is placed slightly rotated at the hip and shoulder with a gel-roll supporting the patient's back. The patient is secured to the table so that the patient can be rotated with table adjustments. The abdomen is insufflated with CO_2 to pressure of 15 mmHg after entry with a Veress needle technique or open technique [91]. After the abdomen is insufflated the remaining three or four trocars are placed under direct vision. An additional 3-mm trocar can be placed at the level of the xiphoid to retract the liver or spleen depending on the side of tumor.

When the transperitoneal approach is performed, the peritoneum is incised along the white line of Toldt to the level of the iliac vessels from the hepatic flexure on the right side and splenic flexure on the left side. The colon is mobilized medially, thus exposing the retroperitoneum. A careful dissection should be performed to prevent duodenal injury in the case of a right-sided tumor and pancreatic injury in the case of a left-sided tumor. The gonadal vessels and ureter are identified. Just medial to the lower pole, a window is created and dissection is carried posteriorly, towards the psoas muscle. Leaving the psoas fascia intact, the plane is further extended posteriorly in a superior and inferior direction, while keeping the lateral attachments of the kidney intact. This method serves to suspend the kidney, thus tenting the renal hilum. A combination of blunt and sharp dissection is performed towards the renal hilum. The artery and vein are dissected and separated, then ligated using a stapler or multiple clips and then divided. It is essential to avoid having clips in between the stapling device because it can lead to catastrophic event by inadequate stapling across the renal hilar vessels. The surgeon should confirm that there are no other accessory arteries before dividing the renal vein, since kidney is an end organ. The superior and lateral attachments of the kidney are then incised. The ipsilateral adrenal gland should be removed when gross evidence of tumor extension from the kidney exists; however, in most cases the ipsilateral adrenal gland can be spared. Ureteral dissection is continued caudally, towards the pelvis. Gonadal vessels are dissected and separated from the ureter. Ideally, the dissection should be performed to the lower level of the iliac vessels when considering an open bladder cuff excision, but if technically feasible, the dissection should continue far distally as possible. When considering a laparoscopic approach to bladder cuff excision, the dissection must continue all the way towards the bladder. At any time, if there is any concern for invasive tumor, the surgical margin should include any abnormally appearing tissue. (Distal ureterectomy and bladder cuff excision will be discussed later in the chapter.)

Distal Uretectomy with Bladder Cuff Excision

Distal ureterectomy with bladder cuff excision can be performed either extravesical or transvesical approach. The extravesical technique can be approached via either Gibson or low midline incision. Dissection is carried out extravesically with a gentle traction of the ureter towards the ureteral orifice. This traction will invert and expose the bladder mucosa along with the ureter, and the specimen is transected allowing adequate margin of the bladder mucosa. The hiatus is closed in two-layer closure as well with absorbable sutures. Special attention should be given not to injure the contralateral ureter and to ensure complete dissection of the intramural portion of the ipsilateral ureter.

Transvesical technique is usually performed with low midline incision. It requires creating an anterior cystotomy. The ipsilateral ureteral orifice is visualized and incised circumferentially along with approximately 1 cm of bladder mucosa. Dissection can be completed either intravesically and/or extravesically. After the excision of distal ureter, the ureteral hiatus and anterior cystotomy are closed in two layers with absorbable sutures.

The Foley catheter is usually left in place for proper drainage for 7–10 days. A pelvic drain is left in place as well.

Transurethral Resection or Incision of Ureteral Orifice (Pluck) Technique

Transurethral resection or incision can be performed to address the intramural ureter, ureteral orifice, and bladder cuff. For this technique, the patient is placed in a dorsal lithotomy position and a resectoscope is inserted into the bladder. First, the bladder is thoroughly inspected for tumor. Either with hook or loop electrode, the ipsilateral orifice is aggressively resected down to perivesical fat [92, 93]. After the intramural ureter is detached, a Foley catheter is inserted and the patient is repositioned for radical nephrectomy. After radical nephrectomy is completed, dissection of ipsilateral ureter is carried down distally, and the ureter is gently pulled for extraction. A clear advantage is that a second incision or extending the incision is not necessary. However, a concern for tumor spillage causing tumor implantation to the nonurothelial surface exists that can predispose a patient to local tumor recurrence. When one adheres to proper surgical principles, the local recurrence is not significantly different from the standard open bladder cuff excision [92], and there is a low complication rate of 2.8% [94]. The ureteral hiatus can be either closed or left alone to heal with proper bladder drainage.

Stripping Technique

For the stripping technique, the ipsilateral ureter is cannulated with a ureteral catheter endoscopically first, and then the nephrectomy is performed. The tip of the ureteral catheter is tied to the top of the ureteral stump. The ureteral catheter is pulled out transurethrally and the distal ureter is intussuscepted. Endoscopic resection through the bladder wall is performed around the everted ureteral orifice and the distal ureter is stripped and removed with a bladder cuff. Giovansili et al. [95] reported 18.7% of failure rate in their series, requiring a Gibson incision. The reasons for failure were retained ureter and inadvertent ureteral transection. However, Geavlete et al. [94] demonstrated a lower complication rate, 7.1%, in their series.

Transvesical Laparoscopic Detachment and Ligation Technique

This technique was described by Gill et al. [96], and it is performed before radical nephrectomy. Two 2-mm trocars are inserted suprapubically through the bladder. A loop ligature is placed around the ureter to maintain a closed system. A Collins knife is positioned cystoscopically and facilitates the dissection around the ureter. The ureter and bladder cuff are dissected and detached, mobilizing approximately 3 cm of the extravesical ureter.

Laparoscopic Ureterectomy

Hattori et al. [97] developed a pure laparoscopic technique for distal ureterectomy with bladder cuff excision. The ipsilateral ureter is ligated distally from the tumor. A stay suture is placed at the anterior bladder wall, and cystotomy is made. The ureteral orifice is visualized and confirmed. A circumferential incision is made around the ureteral orifice, and the distal ureter is mobilized and detached with bladder cuff. The cystotomy is closed with absorbable suture. All specimens in their series had negative surgical margins. Purse-string technique was described by Shoma et al., and it does not require an anterior cystotomy [98]. Intramural ureter is sharply dissected extravesically from the detrusor muscle of the bladder until the ureteral orifice is reached. Then, the detrusor muscle is dissected away from the bladder mucosa for approximately 1 cm around the ureteral orifice. At this point, purse-string suture is placed at the edge of the bladder mucosa, and the bladder cuff is excised.

Kurzer et al. [99] described a combination of hand-assisted with cystoscopic excision of the distal ureter. This technique involves early ligation of the ureter, and utilizes simultaneous transurethral cystoscopic-guided excision of the intramural ureter along with bladder cuff. At completion, a gentle traction is placed on the ureter, extracting the distal ureter. The hiatus is left to heal by secondary intention with bladder drainage. Their results demonstrated no pelvic recurrence during follow-up.

Robotic-Assisted Laparoscopic Distal Ureterectomy

Distal ureterectomy has been performed with the assistance of the da Vinci® Surgical System (Intuitive Surgical, Sunnyvale, CA, USA) [100–102]. Nanigian et al. [102] described their initial series using the da Vinci surgical system with good success. Usually, radical nephrectomy is performed first in a flank position. Then the patient is repositioned in a low dorsal lithotomy position and the da Vinci system is docked. The bladder is clam-shelled in a coronal orientation at the dome, and the distal ureterectomy with bladder cuff excision is performed [102]. Instead of creating an anterior cystotomy, Hu et al. [101] demonstrated an extravesical approach for distal ureterectomy with bladder cuff excision with the da Vinci surgical system.

Segmental Ureterectomy

Segmental ureterectomy is a possible therapeutic choice for noninvasive low-grade tumors of the proximal ureter or midureter that are too large for endoscopic ablation, or for high-grade invasive tumor that requires renal preservation [10].

Open ureterectomy can be approached by Gibson, Pfannenstiel, or flank incision depending on the location of tumor. Ipsilateral ureter is identified and mobilized. Vessel loops are secured proximally and distally from the tumor, and the ureter is ligated with a margin of 1–2 cm. Frozen sections of either ends of the ureter are analyzed for invasive tumor. Kidney and distal ureter are mobilized. Blood supply to the ureter is preserved by leaving adventitia on the ureter, which is critical in preventing ischemic ureteral stricture. Proximal and distal ends of the ureter are spatulated. Tension-free anastomosis is performed with 4–0 absorbable suture, and double-J ureteral stent is placed. A surgical drain is placed as well.

Distal Ureterectomy with Ureteroneocystostomy

Open distal ureterectomy with ureteroneocystostomy is indicated for a distal ureteral tumor. It is recommended for patients whose tumors could not be treated with endoscopic ablation or when renal preservation is a critical objective [1, 10, 103, 104]. The patient is placed in a supine position and Foley catheter is placed on the sterile field. A low midline, Pfannenstiel, or Gibson incision can be utilized. The distal ureter is dissected, and the tumor is identified. A clip is placed proximal to the tumor to avoid tumor spillage. Frozen-section of the proximal margin is sent for analysis. When a short segment of the ureter is excised, ureteroneocystostomy can be performed without manipulating the bladder. However, when a significant length of the ureter is removed due to the size of tumor, either psoas hitch and/or Boari flap should be utilized.

Laparoscopic distal ureterectomy with ureteroneocystostomy can be achieved for the same cohort of patients. In patients with normal contralateral kidney, laparoscopic distal ureterectomy with ureteroneocystostomy can still be recommended for patients with low-grade, unifocal tumor <2 cm without evidence of invasion [105]. Laparoscopic distal ureterectomy with ureteroneocystostomy has been demonstrated to be technically feasible with encouraging outcomes for low-grade distal ureteral tumors [105–108].

Anatomic Distribution of Lymphatic Drainage

Tumors of the renal pelvis and proximal ureter drain into the retroperitoneal lymph nodes and extend further caudally to the external iliac lymph nodes. Tumors of the midureter can involve both the retroperitoneal and pelvic lymph nodes [17]. Tumors of the distal ureter drain predominantly into the pelvic lymph nodes that include external iliac, obturator, and hypogastric regions.

Based on the lymphatic drainage, anatomic boundaries can be offered. Left-sided renal pelvic, upper, or midureteral tumors should, at minimum, encompass the paraaortic, preaortic, and interaortocaval nodes from the renal hilum to aortic bifurcation [109]. Right-sided renal pelvic, upper, or midureteral tumors should include the paracaval, precaval, and interaortocaval nodes from the renal hilum to aortic bifurcation. The mid- or distal ureteral tumors, ipsilateral common iliac, external iliac, obturator, and hypogastric lymphadenectomy should be performed [109].

Patient Selection for Lymphadenectomy

Lower staged tumors are usually present in the distal ureter compared to midureter, proximal ureter, and renal pelvis [109]. This observation can be explained by (1) the tumors in the proximal ureter are less likely to cause symptoms compared to distal ureteral tumors due to greater distensibility of the proximal ureter [109], and (2) the distal ureter consists of three layers of muscle in comparison to the proximal ureter, which has two layers of muscle [110]. Therefore, the proximal ureteral tumors many times present at a more advanced stage than tumors in the distal ureter. Kondo et al. [111] reported 10% of their study cohort had positive lymph node from distal ureteral tumor, and over 40% of their study cohort had positive lymph node from proximal ureteral tumor.

The incidence of nodal disease is associated with primary tumor stage. The lower stage tumors rarely have nodal metastases, and lymphadenectomy may be excluded ≤T1 [111]. However, preoperative staging has limitations that would preclude accurate pathologic staging; consequently, Kundu et al. [109] recommend that all patients should undergo regional lymphadenectomy, since muscle invasion or advanced disease cannot be excluded during nephroureterectomy.

Lymphadenectomy

The role of lymphadenectomy for upper urinary tract transitional cell carcinoma (TCC) is not well defined owing to infrequent disease and variable lymph node dissection templates [109]. The benefit of lymph node dissection is extrapolated from bladder cancer data that when extended pelvic lymph node dissection is performed in conjunction with radical cystectomy, metastatic bladder cancer can be cured in up to 25% of patients [112, 113]. Recent studies suggest that lymphadenectomy at radical nephroureterectomy provides survival benefits in locally advanced upper urinary tract TCC, although the studies comprise small cohorts [45, 111, 114]. To date, there is no large study that definitively demonstrates survival benefit from performing lymphadenectomy at the time of radical nephroureterectomy. The challenges to prove this important issue are due to: (1) no standardization of whether to perform or not to perform a lymph node dissection, (2) various lymph node templates, (3) removal oftentimes of only suspicious nodes, and (4) often lack of therapeutic intent of the lymphadenectomy [109]. It is also compounded by 50% of patients having bladder cancer [115], so mortality rates are influenced by these patients.

Roscigno et al. [116] utilized data from a multicenter cohort and retrospectively evaluated the impact of lymphadenectomy for upper urinary tract UC. Their aim was to determine nodal status impact on cancer-specific survival. Interestingly, they found that in patients with positive nodal disease, there was no association between the number of lymph nodes removed and survival outcome. However, the lymph node density seemed to affect cancer-specific survival [117].

Some argue that there is a clear advantage in performing lymphadenectomy at the time of radical nephroureterectomy since risk stratification can be accomplished by complete staging of upper urinary tract urothelial carcinoma. Lymphadenectomy seems more crucial in patients with pT2–4 disease because lymphatic dissemination is more common than T1 disease [116]. However, it is very difficult to determine muscle invasion at the time of radical nephroureterectomy. Survival benefit of lymphadenectomy is controversial, and further studies are necessary to support cancer-specific survival. Nevertheless, the extent of lymphadenectomy will provide proper staging of disease and identify patients who may benefit from adjuvant chemotherapy.

Endoscopic Management

Endoscopic (percutaneous or ureteroscopic) approaches have been attempted in patients that need renal preservation since the 1980s [118–120]. Tremendous advances in technology have made endourologic management of the upper urinary tract UC possible. For instance, modern ureteroscopes utilize fiberoptic technology that enhances visualization. Smaller caliber ureteroscopes make it safer. Modern flexible ureteroscopes provide a greater ability of deflection to navigate throughout the collecting system safely and to ablate tumor effectively [121–123]. Endourologic management for upper urinary tract UC has made significant strides as a reasonable treatment option with minimal compromise in survival for select patients [124–128].

Patient Selection

Nephron-sparing surgery for the upper urinary tract UC has emerged from the need to treat patients who would otherwise be anephric and require dialysis after nephroureterectomy. This includes patients with (1) an anatomical or functional solitary kidney, (2) renal insufficiency, or (3) bilateral upper urinary tract UC. Moreover, in patients with multiple comorbidities who would not be able to tolerate radical extirpative surgery, endoscopic management serves as a feasible alternative option.

Ureteroscopic Versus Percutaneous Management

Ureteroscopic treatment is a safe option for treating upper urinary tract UC, especially since a closed system is maintained. Patients with small tumors that are easily accessed by a retrograde approach are ideal candidates for ureteroscopic treatment. Complication rates are low, and it is well tolerated by patients.

However, there are limitations to the ureteroscopic approach. For instance, a large tumor or tumor located in the lower pole calyx is often difficult to treat ureteroscopically. The lower pole calyx is difficult to access with a flexible ureteroscope when a laser fiber or bugbee electrode is passed through the working port because it affects the flexible scope's ability to deflect the tip. Irrigation through the flexible ureteroscope becomes limited as well when a laser fiber or bugbee electrode is placed through the working port, and even slight bleeding can obscure visualization. Unfortunately, these limitations can significantly hinder treatment. Moreover, patients who have undergone radical cystectomy with urinary diversion are difficult to access ureteroscopically in a retrograde approach owing to difficulty locating and then cannulating the ureteroenteric anastomosis; thus, often these patients require percutaneous access.

However, even well tolerated by patients, the percutaneous approach tends to have a more significant complication profile. A benefit of the percutaneous approach is that it allows larger scopes, such as nephroscope and/or resectoscope, into the upper urinary tract. Larger scopes provide better irrigation capability and allow superior visualization. The working ports allow larger instruments to pass, thereby providing superior tissue sampling, and hence improved staging of upper urinary tract UC. At completion of a percutaneous treatment, a percutaneous tube is usually left in place for hemostasis and maximal drainage. Later, it can be used to instill *Bacillus Calmette Guerin* (BCG) or to perform subsequent reexaminations. The percutaneous approach is necessary in a certain cohort of patients when limitations of ureteroscopic approach prevent adequate endoscopic management of upper urinary tract UC [129, 130].

Percutaneous Puncture Selection

Principles of obtaining access for percutaneous nephrolithotomy are applied for percutaneous treatment of upper urinary tract UC. As the puncture site moves more medial, the risk of injury to the renal vessels increases and direct puncture into the renal pelvis may occur. Direct puncture into the renal pelvis should be avoided since the posterior branch of the renal artery is in proximity and can cause significant bleeding. In addition, the renal pelvis does not provide stability for the access sheath since there is no parenchymal support, and a large laceration may occur when manipulating the scope during resection.

Location of percutaneous access should be dictated by the location of the tumor. Tumors located in the peripheral calyces are best approached by placing the access in direct line with the tumor and not directly on the tumor [131]. Tumors located in the proximal ureter or renal pelvis may be approached either from the middle calyx or from the upper calyx to access the ureteropelvic junction in a straight path. As with stone disease, more than one access may be required when tumors are located in different calyces.

Techniques of Resection

There are different methods to achieve tumor ablation. Tumors can be resected with monopolar or bipolar loop electrode or they can be ablated with lasers, neodymium (Nd):YAG and/or holmium (Ho):YAG. When a percutaneous approach is utilized, a large access sheath allows the resectoscope with a cutting loop to be introduced into the collecting system. With the standard monopolar or bipolar cutting loop, tumor is electrosurgically resected to the base, and the specimen is extracted. Hemostasis is easily accomplished at the base of the resection by electrocautery. In addition to resection, electrovaporization can be accomplished at 200 W pure cutting current using the monopolar device [132]. Increasing the current creates immediate cell death by direct vaporization and the underlying tissue is desiccated and coagulated [133]. Alternatively, the bipolar device has been utilized for tumor resection since it minimizes the change in serum sodium and other electrolyte abnormalities due to its use of normal saline [134, 135]. With the loop electrode, deep tissue sampling is possible and better tumor staging can be achieved [136].

Tumor ablation can also be accomplished with laser energy. The neodymium (Nd):YAG and holmium (Ho):YAG are two well-established laser systems in urology. The induced effects on soft tissue vary among coagulation, vaporization, and incision depending on contact versus noncontact mode. Both of the lasers on contact mode have the capability to vaporize and incise tissue.

The Nd:YAG laser has been used widely for bladder tumors and upper urinary tract TCC. The Nd:YAG laser fiber is placed in close approximation to tissue, but not in contact, and the laser is activated at around 20–30 W to coagulate the tissue [120]. The distal fiber tip should be directed tangentially in noncontact mode until tissue coagulates. This laser penetrates approximately 5–6 mm in depth of tissue, so that the bulky tumors are ablated much more efficiently. Hence, Nd:YAG laser should never be used circumferentially in the ureter, as it may cause ureteral stricture [137]. As the tissue coagulates, the coagulated portion of the tumor is removed with forceps, which then exposes a deeper portion of the tumor that requires further coagulation. The coagulation and ablation are repeated until the base of the tumor is exposed.

On the other hand, Ho:YAG laser must be in contact with the tumor to coagulate, vaporize, and incise tissue. It has a penetrating depth of 0.5 mm of tissue. The shallow depth of penetration allows for the tissue ablation to be focused and treat lesions that are circumferential. However, it will not coagulate large vessels [138, 139]. Thermal energy that is generated by Ho:YAG laser is highly absorbed by water so that the heat disperses very rapidly. This physical property results in minimal thermal damage to the surrounding tissues [140]. However, one of the drawbacks of Ho:YAG laser is that tumor adheres to the tip of the fiber during ablation, and this often decreases visualization and ablation capacity. This can be minimized by cleaning the fiber tip, but the cleaning process adds to operative time. A gentle flow of irrigation is used to clear tumor debris during the ablative treatment.

Combination of the two lasers can be used during one procedure. The Nd:YAG laser can coagulate majority of the volume of a large tumor, and then the Ho:YAG laser can be employed to ablated remaining tumor tissue [141]. Particular attention should be given to make sure that fiber tip is visible in front of the scope at all times.

BCG Therapy

A mainstay of intravesical treatment for superficial bladder cancer has been the use of BCG [142, 143]. In addition, there are other intravesical chemotherapeutic agents that have been studied and used to treat superficial bladder cancer, but the results have been variable depending on the agent used. To replicate the superficial bladder tumor data with intravesical BCG therapy, the use of intracavitary BCG for upper urinary tract UC was first described by Herr in 1985 [112, 144].

Safety of administration of BCG into the upper urinary tract have been well established [145]. Notwithstanding this fact, some have expressed concerns about systemic BCG infection during infusion. Patients usually present with high fevers, rigor, and malaise. Fortunately, most of the fevers are caused by urinary tract infection and not systemic BCG infection [146]. However, since BCG sepsis can lead to devastating sequelae, there is an absolute need to monitor patients very closely when they present with high fever after receiving intracavitary BCG.

To decrease the risk of systemic BCG infection, the percutaneous tract with a nephrostomy tube is allowed to mature for 1–2 weeks after resection before BCG is instilled [147, 148]. Typically, patients will have a negative urine culture from the percutaneous nephrostomy tube and receive antibiotics prior to BCG instillation. To ensure safety of instillation of BCG, normal saline is infused initially via a percutaneous nephrostomy tube. Infusion is started at a very slow rate, and gradually increased to a rate of approximately 50 mL/h. Normal saline is continued for another hour, monitoring the intrapelvic pressure to maintain pressure of less than 25 cm H_2O. At that point, the BCG is instilled by gravity via percutaneous nephrostomy tube. Instillation should be stopped if the intrapelvic pressure increases to greater than 25 cm H_2O or the patient complains of fever or pain. It is important to monitor intrapelvic pressure because high pressure can lead to pyelovenous backflow of BCG, which can increase the risk of BCG sepsis. BCG is instilled once a week for 6 weeks. When index of suspicion is high after BCG instillation, another nephroscopy can be considered after 2 weeks of completion.

Another method of instilling BCG is a retrograde approach. A straight ureteral catheter is placed into the renal pelvic endoscopically and BCG is instilled into the renal pelvis. Usually, patients are admitted for observation because instrumentation of ureter can cause obstruction from edema, and sepsis can ensue. Alternatively, refluxing double-J stent may be placed endoscopically, and intravesical BCG is then instilled, allowing intravesical BCG to reflux up into the renal pelvis. The amount of intravesical fluid needed to induce reflux ranges from 80 to 250 mL (median of 120 mL) [149]. Cystography should be performed to confirm reflux since double-J stent does not guarantee reflux [150]. Alternatively, ureteral meatotomy can be performed to cause vesicoureteral reflux. After the double-J stent is removed, reflux is confirmed with cystography and volume necessary to cause reflux is recorded. Appropriate volume of BCG can be administered intravesically [151].

Efficacy data of BCG treatment for the upper urinary tract has been mixed, but most of the data show questionable benefit from adjuvant BCG therapy [131, 152]. Hayashida et al. demonstrated a 50% recurrence rate, and showed a 100% mortality rate for patients who recurred [153]. However, Okubo et al. [154] found some long-term benefit with tumor free survival at a median follow-up of 46 months.

Instillation of BCG does not seem to prevent recurrence or progression of the high-grade upper urinary tract UC. However, it may help patients with low grade and stage tumor avoid dialysis and maintain quality of life [155]. One of the major issues with BCG instillation is that it may allow advanced and/or high-grade tumors to progress while the patient is receiving six cycles of BCG therapy. Therefore, some advocate CT scans to monitor lymph nodes or metastatic status during the cycle.

Other adjuvant agents that have been studied include mitomycin C and thiotepa. Keeley and Bagley instilled mitomycin C after ureteroscopic treatment on 19 patients, with 11 of 19 patients tumor-free during their follow-up [156]. Thiotepa had been studied with a poor response rate. Martinez-Pineiro et al. demonstrated a lower recurrence rate for BCG and mitomycin C when compared to thiotepa [125].

Currently, there is no set standard or protocol of adjuvant therapy for upper urinary tract UC. Statistically significant survival benefit has not been demonstrated from a number of studies with small numbers and short follow-up periods. A randomized trial to study efficacy of the adjuvant therapy of the upper urinary tract UC is necessary but will be difficult to achieve.

References

1. Hall MC, Womack S, Sagalowsky AI, Carmody T, Erickstad MD, Roehrborn CG. Prognostic factors, recurrence, and survival in transitional cell carcinoma of the upper urinary tract: a 30-year experience in 252 patients. Urology. 1998;52(4):594–601.
2. Kirkali Z, Tuzel E. Transitional cell carcinoma of the ureter and renal pelvis. Crit Rev Oncol Hematol. 2003;47(2):155–69.
3. Gupta NP, Sharma N, Kumar R. Nuclear matrix protein 22 as adjunct to urine cytology and cystoscopy in follow-up of superficial TCC of urinary bladder. Urology. 2009;73(3):592–6; discussion 596–7. 10.1016/j.urology.2008.04.051.
4. Gupta R, Paner GP, Amin MB. Neoplasms of the upper urinary tract: a review with focus on urothelial carcinoma of the pelvicalyceal system and aspects related to its diagnosis and reporting. Adv Anat Pathol. 2008;15(3):127–39. doi: 10.1097/PAP.0b013e31817145a9.
5. Rouprêt M, Yates DR, Comperat E, Cussenot O. Upper urinary tract urothelial cell carcinomas and other urological malignancies involved in the hereditary nonpolyposis colorectal cancer (lynch syndrome) tumor spectrum. Eur Urol. 2008;54(6):1226–36. Epub 2008 Aug 12. Review.
6. Burger M, van der Aa MN, van Oers JM, Brinkmann A, van der Kwast TH, Steyerberg EC, et al. Prediction of progression of non-muscle-invasive bladder cancer by WHO 1973 and 2004 grading and by FGFR3 mutation status: a prospective study. Eur Urol. 2008;54(4):835–43. Epub 2007 Dec 26.
7. Zhang Z, Furge KA, Yang XJ, Teh BT, Hansel DE. Comparative gene expression profiling analysis of urothelial carcinoma of the renal pelvis and bladder. BMC Med Genomics. 2010;3:58.
8. Munoz JJ, Ellison LM. Upper tract urothelial neoplasms: incidence and survival during the last 2 decades. J Urol. 2000;164(5):1523–5.
9. Olgac S, Mazumdar M, Dalbagni G, Reuter VE. Urothelial carcinoma of the renal pelvis: a clinicopathologic study of 130 cases. Am J Surg Pathol. 2004;28(12):1545–52.
10. Sagalowsky A, Jarrett TW. Management of urothelial tumors of the renal pelvis and ureter. In: Wein AJ, editor. Campbell-Walsh urology, 2. 9th ed. Philadelphia: Saunders; 2007.
11. Sanderson KM, Rouprêt M. Upper urinary tract tumour after radical cystectomy for transitional cell carcinoma of the bladder: an update on the risk factors, surveillance regimens and treatments. BJU Int. 2007;100(1):11–6. Epub 2007 Apr 8. Review.
12. Denzinger S, Mohren K, Knuechel R, Wild PJ, Burger M, Wieland WF, et al. Improved clonality analysis of multifocal bladder tumors by combination of histopathologic organ mapping, loss of heterozygosity, fluorescence in situ hybridization, and p53 analyses. Hum Pathol. 2006;37(2):143–51. Epub 2005 Dec 15.
13. McLaughlin JK, Silverman DT, Hsing AW, et al. Cigarette smoking and cancers of the renal pelvis and ureter. Cancer Res. 1992;52(2):254–7.
14. McCredie M, Stewart JH, Ford JM. Analgesics and tobacco as risk factors for cancer of the ureter and renal pelvis. J Urol. 1983;130(1):28–30.
15. Pommer W, Bronder E, Klimpel A, Helmert U, Greiser E, Molzahn M. Urothelial cancer at different tumour sites: role of smoking and habitual intake of analgesics and laxatives. Results of the Berlin Urothelial Cancer Study. Nephrol Dial Transplant. 1999;14(12):2892–7.
16. Ross RK, Paganini-Hill A, Landolph J, Gerkins V, Henderson BE. Analgesics, cigarette smoking, and other risk factors for cancer of the renal pelvis and ureter. Cancer Res. 1989;49(4):1045–8.
17. Colin P, Koenig P, Ouzzane A, et al. Environmental factors involved in carcinogenesis of urothelial cell carcinomas of the upper urinary tract. BJU Int. 2009;104(10):1436–40. doi:10.1111/j.1464-410X.2009.08838.x.
18. Hung RJ, Boffetta P, Brennan P, et al. GST, NAT, SULT1A1, CYP1B1 genetic polymorphisms, interactions with environmental exposures and bladder cancer risk in a high-risk population. Int J Cancer. 2004;110(4):598–604. doi:10.1002/ijc.20157.
19. McLaughlin JK, Blot WJ, Mandel JS, Schuman LM, Mehl ES, Fraumeni Jr JF. Etiology of cancer of the renal pelvis. J Natl Cancer Inst. 1983;71(2):287–91.

20. McCredie M, Stewart JH, Mahony JF. Is phenacetin responsible for analgesic nephropathy in New South Wales? Clin Nephrol. 1982;17(3):134–40.
21. McCredie M, Ford JM, Taylor JS, Stewart JH. Analgesics and cancer of the renal pelvis in New South Wales. Cancer. 1982;49(12):2617–25.
22. Jensen OM, Knudsen JB, Tomasson H, Sorensen BL. The Copenhagen case–control study of renal pelvis and ureter cancer: role of analgesics. Int J Cancer. 1989;44(6):965–8.
23. Holmang S, Johansson SL. Synchronous bilateral ureteral and renal pelvic carcinomas: incidence, etiology, treatment and outcome. Cancer. 2004;101(4):741–7. doi:10.1002/cncr.20395.
24. Stewart JH, Hobbs JB, McCredie MR. Morphologic evidence that analgesic-induced kidney pathology contributes to the progression of tumors of the renal pelvis. Cancer. 1999;86(8):1576–82.
25. Lynch HT, Boland CR, Rodriguez-Bigas MA, Amos C, Lynch JF, Lynch PM. Who should be sent for genetic testing in hereditary colorectal cancer syndromes? J Clin Oncol. 2007;25(23):3534–42.
26. Stefanovic V, Polenakovic M. Fifty years of research in Balkan endemic nephropathy: where are we now? Nephron Clin Pract. 2009;112(2):c51–6. doi:10.1159/000213081.
27. Petkovic SD. Epidemiology and treatment of renal pelvic and ureteral tumors. J Urol. 1975;114(6):858–65.
28. Dragicevic D, Djokic M, Pekmezovic T, et al. Survival of patients with transitional cell carcinoma of the ureter and renal pelvis in Balkan endemic nephropathy and non-endemic areas of Serbia. BJU Int. 2007;99(6):1357–62. doi:10.1111/j.1464-410X.2007.06793.x.
29. Cukuranovic R, Petrovic B, Cukuranovic Z, Stefanovic V. Balkan endemic nephropathy: a decreasing incidence of the disease. Pathol Biol (Paris). 2000;48(6):558–61.
30. Markovic N, Ignjatovic I, Cukuranovic R, Petrovic B, Kocic B, Stefanovic V. Decreasing incidence of urothelial cancer in a Balkan endemic nephropathy region in Serbia. A surgery based study from 1969 to 1998. Pathol Biol (Paris). 2005;53(1):26–9. doi:10.1016/j.patbio.2004.01.008.
31. Vanherweghem JL, Depierreux M, Tielemans C, et al. Rapidly progressive interstitial renal fibrosis in young women: association with slimming regimen including Chinese herbs. Lancet. 1993;341(8842):387–91.
32. Depierreux M, Van Damme B, Van den Houte K, Van her weghem JL. Pathologic aspects of a newly described nephropathy related to the prolonged use of Chinese herbs. Am J Kidney Dis. 1994;24(2):172–80.
33. Cosyns JP, Jadoul M, Squifflet JP, De Plaen JF, Ferluga D, van Ypersele de Strihou C. Chinese herbs nephropathy: a clue to Balkan endemic nephropathy? Kidney Int. 1994;45(6):1680–8.
34. Vanhaelen M, Vanhaelen-Fastre R, But P, Vanherweghem JL. Identification of aristolochic acid in Chinese herbs. Lancet. 1994;343(8890):174.
35. Chen L, Mei N, Yao L, Chen T. Mutations induced by carcinogenic doses of aristolochic acid in kidney of Big Blue transgenic rats. Toxicol Lett. 2006;165(3):250–6. doi:10.1016/j.toxlet.2006.04.008.
36. Schmeiser HH, Bieler CA, Wiessler M, van Ypersele de Strihou C, Cosyns JP. Detection of DNA adducts formed by aristolochic acid in renal tissue from patients with Chinese herbs nephropathy. Cancer Res. 1996;56(9):2025–8.
37. Nortier JL, Martinez MC, Schmeiser HH, et al. Urothelial carcinoma associated with the use of a Chinese herb (Aristolochia fangchi). N Engl J Med. 2000;342(23):1686–92.
38. Monach PA, Arnold LM, Merkel PA. Incidence and prevention of bladder toxicity from cyclophosphamide in the treatment of rheumatic diseases: a data-driven review. Arthritis Rheum. 2010;62(1):9–21. Review.
39. Shiga Y, Suzuki K, Tsutsumi M, Ishikawa S. Transitional cell carcinoma of the renal pelvis in a patient with cyclophosphamide therapy for malignant lymphoma: a case report and literature review. Hinyokika Kiyo. 2002;48(5):301–5.
40. Volkmer BG, Seidl-Schlick EM, Bach D, Romics I, Kleinschmidt K. As such, cyclophosphamide is contraindicated in patients with a history of UC. Clin Rheumatol. 2005;24:319–23.
41. Jensen OM, Knudsen JB, McLaughlin JK, Sorensen BL. The Copenhagen case–control study of renal pelvis and ureter cancer: role of smoking and occupational exposures. Int J Cancer. 1988;41(4):557–61.
42. Racioppi M, D'Addessi A, Alcini A, Destito A, Alcini E. Clinical review of 100 consecutive surgically treated patients with upper urinary tract transitional tumours. Br J Urol. 1997;80(5):707–11.
43. Raman JD, Ng CK, Scherr DS, Margulis V, Lotan Y, Bensalah K, et al. Impact of tumor location on prognosis for patients with upper tract urothelial carcinoma managed by radical nephroureterectomy. Eur Urol. 2010;57(6):1072–9. Epub 2009 Jul 15.
44. van der Poel HG, Antonini N, van Tinteren H, Horenblas S. Upper urinary tract cancer: location is correlated with prognosis. Eur Urol. 2005;48(3):438–44. doi:10.1016/j.eururo.2005.03.009.
45. Brausi MA, Gavioli M, De LUC G, et al. Retroperitoneal lymph node dissection (RPLD) in conjunction with nephroureterectomy in the treatment of infiltrative transitional cell carcinoma (TCC) of the upper urinary tract: impact on survival. Eur Urol. 2007;52(5):1414–8. doi:10.1016/j.eururo.2007.04.070.
46. Brown GA, Busby JE, Wood CG, et al. Nephroureterectomy for treating upper urinary tract transitional cell carcinoma: time to change the treatment paradigm? BJU Int. 2006;98(6):1176–80. doi:10.1111/j.1464-410X.2006.06524.x.
47. Hong B, Park S, Hong JH, Kim CS, Ro JY, Ahn H. Prognostic value of lymphovascular invasion in transitional cell carcinoma of upper urinary tract. Urology. 2005;65(4):692–6. doi:10.1016/j.urology.2004.11.001.

48. Saito K, Kawakami S, Fujii Y, Sakura M, Masuda H, Kihara K. Lymphovascular invasion is independently associated with poor prognosis in patients with localized upper urinary tract urothelial carcinoma treated surgically. J Urol. 2007;178(6):2291–6; discussion 2296. 10.1016/j.juro.2007.08.019.
49. Guinan P, Vogelzang NJ, Randazzo R, Sener S, Chmiel J, Fremgen A, Sylvester J. Renal pelvic cancer: a review of 611 patients treated in Illinois 1975–1985. Cancer Incidence and End Results Committee. Urology. 1992;40(5):393–9.
50. Park S, Hong B, Kim CS, Ahn H. The impact of tumor location on prognosis of transitional cell carcinoma of the upper urinary tract. J Urol. 2004;171(2 Pt 1):621–5.
51. Kondo T, Nakazawa H, Ito F, Hashimoto Y, Toma H, Tanabe K. Primary site and incidence of lymph node metastases in urothelial carcinoma of upper urinary tract. Urology. 2007;69(2):265–9. doi:10.1016/j.urology.2006.10.014.
52. Remzi M, Haitel A, Margulis V, Karakiewicz P, Montorsi F, Kikuchi E, et al. Tumour architecture is an independent predictor of outcomes after nephroureterectomy: a multi-institutional analysis of 1363 patients. BJU Int. 2009;103(3):307–11. Epub 2008 Oct 16.
53. Zigeuner R, Shariat SF, Margulis V, Karakiewicz PI, Roscigno M, Weizer A, et al. Tumour necrosis is an indicator of aggressive biology in patients with urothelial carcinoma of the upper urinary tract. Eur Urol. 2010;57(4):575–81. Epub 2009 Nov 25.
54. Melamed MR, Reuter VE. Pathology and staging of urothelial tumors of the kidney and ureter. Urol Clin North Am. 1993;20(2):333–47.
55. Cummings KB. Nephroureterectomy: rationale in the management of transitional cell carcinoma of the upper urinary tract. Urol Clin North Am. 1980;7(3):569–78.
56. McCarron JP, Mills C, Vaughn Jr ED. Tumors of the renal pelvis and ureter: current concepts and management. Semin Urol. 1983;1(1):75–81.
57. Mahadevia PS, Karwa GL, Koss LG. Mapping of urothelium in carcinomas of the renal pelvis and ureter. A report of nine cases. Cancer. 1983;51(5):890–7.
58. Jitsukawa S, Nakamura K, Nakayama M, Osawa A, Matsui K. Transitional cell carcinoma of kidney extending into renal vein and inferior vena cava. Urology. 1985;25(3):310–2.
59. Maier U, Simak R, Neuhold N. The clinical value of urinary cytology: 12 years of experience with 615 patients. J Clin Pathol. 1995;48(4):314–7.
60. Konety BR, Getzenberg RH. Urine based markers of urological malignancy. J Urol. 2001;165(2):600–11. doi:10.1097/00005392-200102000-00081.
61. Brown FM. Urine cytology. It is still the gold standard for screening? Urol Clin North Am. 2000;27(1):25–37.
62. Halling KC, Kipp BR. Bladder cancer detection using FISH (UroVysion assay). Adv Anat Pathol. 2008;15(5):279–86. Review.
63. Mian C, Mazzoleni G, Vikoler S, Martini T, Knüchel-Clark R, Zaak D, et al. Fluorescence in situ hybridisation in the diagnosis of upper urinary tract tumours. Eur Urol. 2010;58(2):288–92. Epub 2010 May 5.
64. Fernández MI, Parikh S, Grossman HB, Katz R, Matin SF, Dinney CP, Kamat AM. The role of FISH and cytology in upper urinary tract surveillance after radical cystectomy for bladder cancer. Urol Oncol. 2011. [Epub ahead of print].
65. Van der Aa MN, Zwarthoff EC, Steyerberg EW, Boogaard MW, Nijsen Y, van der Keur KA, et al. Cost-Effectiveness of Follow-Up of Urinary Bladder Cancer trial [CEFUB]. Microsatellite analysis of voided-urine samples for surveillance of low-grade non-muscle-invasive urothelial carcinoma: feasibility and clinical utility in a prospective multicenter study. Eur Urol. 2009;55:659–67.
66. Margulis V, Youssef RF, Karakiewicz PI, Lotan Y, Wood CG, Zigeuner R, et al.; Upper Tract Urothelial Carcinoma Collaborative Group. Preoperative multivariable prognostic model for prediction of nonorgan confined urothelial carcinoma of the upper urinary tract. J Urol. 2010;184(2):453–8. Epub 2010 Jun 17.
67. Cheng L, Neumann RM, Nehra A, Spotts BE, Weaver AL, Bostwick DG. Cancer heterogeneity and its biologic implications in the grading of urothelial carcinoma. Cancer. 2000;88:1663–70.
68. Smith AK, Stephenson AJ, Lane BR, Larson BT, Thomas AA, Gong MC et al. Inadequacy of biopsy for diagnosis of upper tract urothelial carcinoma: implications for conservative management. Urology. 2011;78(1):82–6. Epub 2011 May 7.
69. Wang LJ, Wong YC, Huang CC, Wu CH, Hung SC, Chen HW. Multidetector computerized tomography urography is more accurate than excretory urography for diagnosing transitional cell carcinoma of the upper urinary tract in adults with hematuria. J Urol. 2010;183(1):48–55. doi:10.1016/j.juro.2009.08.144.
70. Jinzaki M, Matsumoto K, Kikuchi E, et al. Comparison of CT urography and excretory urography in the detection and localization of urothelial carcinoma of the upper urinary tract. AJR Am J Roentgenol. 2011;196(5):1102–9. doi:10.2214/AJR.10.5249.
71. Nawfel RD, Judy PF, Schleipman AR, Silverman SG. Patient radiation dose at CT urography and conventional urography. Radiology. 2004;232(1):126–32. doi:10.1148/radiol.2321030222.
72. Browne RF, Meehan CP, Colville J, Power R, Torreggiani WC. Transitional cell carcinoma of the upper urinary tract: spectrum of imaging findings. Radiographics. 2005;25(6):1609–27. doi:10.1148/rg.256045517.
73. Wong-You-Cheong JJ, Wagner BJ, Davis CJ Jr. Transitional cell carcinoma of the urinary tract: radiologic-pathologic correlation. Radiographics. 1998;18(1):123–42; quiz 148.
74. Lee TY, Ko SF, Wan YL, et al. Unusual imaging presentations in renal transitional cell carcinoma. Acta Radiol. 1997;38(6):1015–9.

75. Gray Sears CL, Ward JF, Sears ST, Puckett MF, Kane CJ, Amling CL. Prospective comparison of computerized tomography and excretory urography in the initial evaluation of asymptomatic microhematuria. J Urol. 2002;168(6):2457–60. 10.1097/01.ju.0000036541.52816.98.
76. Lang EK, Macchia RJ, Thomas R, et al. Improved detection of renal pathologic features on multiphasic helical CT compared with IVU in patients presenting with microscopic hematuria. Urology. 2003;61(3):528–32.
77. Caoili EM, Cohan RH, Korobkin M, et al. Urinary tract abnormalities: initial experience with multidetector row CT urography. Radiology. 2002;222(2):353–60.
78. Eiber M, van Oers JM, Zwarthoff EC, van der Kwast TH, Ulrich O, Helpap B, et al. Low frequency of molecular changes and tumor recurrence in inverted papillomas of the urinary tract. Am J Surg Pathol. 2007;31(6):938–46.
79. Darras J, Inderadjaja N, Vossaert P. Synchronous inverted papilloma of bladder and renal pelvis. Urology. 2005;65(4):798.
80. Lane Z, Epstein JI. Polypoid/papillary cystitis: a series of 41 cases misdiagnosed as papillary urothelial neoplasia. Am J Surg Pathol. 2008;32:758–64.
81. Hartmann A, Dietmaier W, Hofstädter F, Burgart LJ, Cheville JC, Blaszyk H. Urothelial carcinoma of the upper urinary tract: inverted growth pattern is predictive of microsatellite instability. Hum Pathol. 2003;34(3):222–7.
82. Lopez-Beltran A, Escudero AL, Cavazzana AO, Spagnoli LG, Vicioso-Recio L. Sarcomatoid transitional cell carcinoma of the renal pelvis. A report of five cases with clinical, pathological, immunohistochemical and DNA ploidy analysis. Pathol Res Pract. 1996;192(12):1218–24.
83. Holmäng S, Lele SM, Johansson SL. Squamous cell carcinoma of the renal pelvis and ureter: incidence, symptoms, treatment and outcome. J Urol. 2007;178(1):51–6. Epub 2007 May 11.
84. Blacher EJ, Johnson DE, Abdul-Karim FW, Ayala AG. Squamous cell carcinoma of renal pelvis. Urology. 1985;25(2):124–6.
85. Gilligan T, Dreicer R. The atypical urothelial cancer patient: management of bladder cancers of non-transitional cell histology and cancers of the ureters and renal pelvis. Semin Oncol. 2007;34:145–53.
86. Babaian RJ, Johnson DE. Primary carcinoma of the ureter. J Urol. 1980;123(3):357–9.
87. Batata M, Grabstald H. Upper urinary tract urothelial tumors. Urol Clin North Am. 1976;3(1):79–86.
88. Skinner DG. Technique of nephroureterectomy with regional lymph node dissection. Urol Clin North Am. 1978;5(1):252–60.
89. Huben RP, Mounzer AM, Murphy GP. Tumor grade and stage as prognostic variables in upper tract urothelial tumors. Cancer. 1988;62(9):2016–20.
90. Abaza R, Keck RW, Selman SH. Intraperitoneal chemotherapy for the prevention of transitional cell carcinoma implantation. J Urol. 2006;175(6):2317–22. doi:10.1016/S0022-5347(06), 00257-6.
91. Hasson HM. Open laparoscopy: a report of 150 cases. J Reprod Med. 1974;12(6):234–8.
92. Li WM, Shen JT, Li CC, et al. Oncologic outcomes following three different approaches to the distal ureter and bladder cuff in nephroureterectomy for primary upper urinary tract urothelial carcinoma. Eur Urol. 2010. 10.1016/j.eururo.2009.12.032.
93. Palou J, Caparros J, Orsola A, Xavier B, Vicente J. Transurethral resection of the intramural ureter as the first step of nephroureterectomy. J Urol. 1995;154(1):43–4.
94. Geavlete P, Georgescu D, Bancu S, Mirciulescu V. Endoscopic ureteral procedures for one-step nephroureterectomy: experience in 100 cases. J Endourol. 2007;21(9):1019–24. doi:10.1089/end.2006.0426.
95. Giovansili B, Peyromaure M, Saighi D, Dayma T, Zerbib M, Debre B. Stripping technique for endoscopic management of distal ureter during nephroureterectomy: experience of 32 procedures. Urology. 2004;64(3):448–52; discussion 452. 10.1016/j.urology.2004.04.080.
96. Gill IS, Soble JJ, Miller SD, Sung GT. A novel technique for management of the en bloc bladder cuff and distal ureter during laparoscopic nephroureterectomy. J Urol. 1999;161(2):430–4.
97. Hattori R, Yoshino Y, Komatsu T, Matsukawa Y, Ono Y, Gotoh M. Pure laparoscopic complete excision of distal ureter with a bladder cuff for upper tract urothelial carcinoma. World J Urol. 2009;27(2):253–8. doi:10.1007/s00345-008-0337-1.
98. Shoma AM. Purse-string technique for laparoscopic excision of a bladder mucosal cuff in patients with transitional cell carcinoma of the upper urinary tract: initial report with intermediate follow-up. BJU Int. 2009;104(10):1505–9. doi:10.1111/j.1464-410X.2009.08598.x.
99. Kurzer E, Leveillee RJ, Bird VG. Combining hand assisted laparoscopic nephroureterectomy with cystoscopic circumferential excision of the distal ureter without primary closure of the bladder cuff--is it safe? J Urol. 2006;175(1):63–7; discussion 67–8. 10.1016/S0022-5347(05)00046-7.
100. Park SY, Jeong W, Ham WS, Kim WT, Rha KH. Initial experience of robotic nephroureterectomy: a hybrid-port technique. BJU Int. 2009;104(11):1718–21. doi:10.1111/j.1464-410X.2009.08671.x.
101. Hu JC, Silletti JP, Williams SB. Initial experience with robot-assisted minimally-invasive nephroureterectomy. J Endourol. 2008;22(4):699–704. doi:10.1089/end.2007.0333.
102. Nanigian DK, Smith W, Ellison LM. Robot-assisted laparoscopic nephroureterectomy. J Endourol. 2006;20(7):463–5; discussion 465–6. 10.1089/end.2006.20.463.

103. Anderstrom C, Johansson SL, Pettersson S, Wahlqvist L. Carcinoma of the ureter: a clinicopathologic study of 49 cases. J Urol. 1989;142(2 Pt 1):280–3.
104. Pagano F. Conservative treatment of lower ureteral tumor: modified ureteroneocystostomy for upper urinary tract endoscopic control. J Urol. 1984;132(3):555–7.
105. Rouppret M, Harmon JD, Sanderson KM, et al. Laparoscopic distal ureterectomy and anastomosis for management of low-risk upper urinary tract transitional cell carcinoma: preliminary results. BJU Int. 2007;99(3):623–7. doi:10.1111/j.1464-410X.2006.06688.x.
106. Basiri A, Karami H, Mehrabi S, Javaherforooshzadeh A. Laparoscopic distal ureterectomy and Boari flap ureteroneocystostomy for a low-grade distal ureteral tumor. Urol J. 2008;5(2):120–2.
107. Gerber E, Dinlenc CZ, Wagner JR. Laparoscopic distal ureterectomy for low grade transitional cell carcinoma. J Urol. 2003;169(6):2295. 10.1097/01.ju.0000060883.54360.cd.
108. Simforoosh N, Mosapour E, Maghsudi R. Laparoscopic ureteral resection and anastomosis for management of low-grade transitional-cell carcinoma. J Endourol. 2005;19(3):287–9. doi:10.1089/end.2005.19.287.
109. Kundu SD, Eggener SE. Retroperitoneal lymph nodes in transitional cell carcinoma of the kidney and ureter. Adv Urol 2009:181927 Epub. 2009:181927. 10.1155/2009/181927.
110. Hanna MK, Jeffs RD, Sturgess JM, Barkin M. Ureteral structure and ultrastructure. Part I. The normal human ureter. J Urol. 1976;116(6):718–24.
111. Kondo T, Nakazawa H, Ito F, Hashimoto Y, Toma H, Tanabe K. Impact of the extent of regional lymphadenectomy on the survival of patients with urothelial carcinoma of the upper urinary tract. J Urol. 2007;178(4 Pt 1):1212–7; discussion 1217. 10.1016/j.juro.2007.05.158.
112. Herr HW, Donat SM. Outcome of patients with grossly node positive bladder cancer after pelvic lymph node dissection and radical cystectomy. J Urol. 2001;165(1):62–4; discussion 64. 10.1097/00005392-200101000-00015.
113. Lerner SP, Skinner DG, Lieskovsky G, et al. The rationale for en bloc pelvic lymph node dissection for bladder cancer patients with nodal metastases: long-term results. J Urol. 1993;149(4):758–64; discussion 764–5.
114. Roscigno M, Cozzarini C, Bertini R, et al. Prognostic value of lymph node dissection in patients with muscle-invasive transitional cell carcinoma of the upper urinary tract. Eur Urol. 2008;53(4):794–802. doi: 10.1016/j.eururo.2008.01.008.
115. Novara G, De Marco V, Gottardo F, et al. Independent predictors of cancer-specific survival in transitional cell carcinoma of the upper urinary tract: multi-institutional dataset from 3 European centers. Cancer. 2007;110(8):1715–22. doi:10.1002/cncr.22970.
116. Roscigno M, Shariat SF, Margulis V, et al. Impact of lymph node dissection on cancer-specific survival in patients with upper tract urothelial carcinoma treated with radical nephroureterectomy. J Urol. 2009;181(6):2482–9. doi:10.1016/j.juro.2009.02.021.
117. Bolenz C, Shariat SF, Fernandez MI, et al. Risk stratification of patients with nodal involvement in upper tract urothelial carcinoma: value of lymph-node density. BJU Int. 2009;103(3):302–6. doi:10.1111/j.1464-410X.2008.07988.x.
118. Zincke H, Neves RJ. Feasibility of conservative surgery for transitional cell cancer of the upper urinary tract. Urol Clin North Am. 1984;11(4):717–24.
119. Orihuela E, Smith AD. Percutaneous treatment of transitional cell carcinoma of the upper urinary tract. Urol Clin North Am. 1988;15(3):425–31.
120. Moore K, Khastgir J, Ghei M. Endoscopic management of upper tract urothelial carcinoma. Adv Urol. 2009:620604 Epub. 2009:620604. 10.1155/2009/620604 .
121. Razvi HA, Chun SS, Denstedt JD, Sales JL. Soft-tissue applications of the holmium:YAG laser in urology. J Endourol. 1995;9(5):387–90.
122. Bagley D, Erhard M. Use of the holmium laser in the upper urinary tract. Tech Urol. 1995;1(1):25–30.
123. Lam JS, Gupta M. Ureteroscopic management of upper tract transitional cell carcinoma. Urol Clin North Am. 2004;31(1):115–28. doi:10.1016/S0094-0143(03), 00099-5.
124. Ziegelbaum M, Novick AC, Streem SB, Montie JE, Pontes JE, Straffon RA. Conservative surgery for transitional cell carcinoma of the renal pelvis. J Urol. 1987;138(5):1146–9.
125. Martinez-Pineiro JA, Garcia Matres MJ, Martinez-Pineiro L. Endourological treatment of upper tract urothelial carcinomas: analysis of a series of 59 tumors. J Urol. 1996;156(2 Pt 1):377–85.
126. Engelmyer EI, Belis JA. Long-term ureteroscopic management of low-grade transitional cell carcinoma of the upper urinary tract. Tech Urol. 1996;2(2):113–6.
127. Elliott DS, Blute ML, Patterson DE, Bergstralh EJ, Segura JW. Long-term follow-up of endoscopically treated upper urinary tract transitional cell carcinoma. Urology. 1996;47(6):819–25. doi:10.1016/S0090-4295(96)00043-X.
128. Sowter SJ, Ilie CP, Efthimiou I, Tolley DA. Endourologic management of patients with upper-tract transitional-cell carcinoma: long-term follow-up in a single center. J Endourol. 2007;21(9):1005–9. doi:10.1089/end.2006.9922.
129. Stewart GD, Tolley DA. What are the oncological risks of minimal access surgery for the treatment of urinary tract cancer? Eur Urol. 2004;46(4):415–20. doi:10.1016/j.eururo.2004.04.030.
130. Roupret M, Traxer O, Tligui M, et al. Upper urinary tract transitional cell carcinoma: recurrence rate after percutaneous endoscopic resection. Eur Urol. 2007;51(3):709–13; discussion 714. 10.1016/j.eururo.2006.07.019.

131. Jarrett TW, Sweetser PM, Weiss GH, Smith AD. Percutaneous management of transitional cell carcinoma of the renal collecting system: 9-year experience. J Urol. 1995;154(5):1629–35.
132. Nakada SY, Clayman RV. Percutaneous electrovaporization of upper tract transitional cell carcinoma in patients with functionally solitary kidneys. Urology. 1995;46(5):751–5. doi:10.1016/S0090-4295(99), 80318-5.
133. Huffman JL, Bagley DH, Lyon ES, Morse MJ, Herr HW, Whitmore Jr WF. Endoscopic diagnosis and treatment of upper-tract urothelial tumors. A preliminary report. Cancer. 1985;55(6):1422–8.
134. Rao PN. Fluid absorption during urological endoscopy. Br J Urol. 1987;60(2):93–9.
135. Chou CH, Chau T, Yang SS, Lin SH. Acute hyponatremia and renal failure following percutaneous nephrolithotomy. Clin Nephrol. 2003;59(3):237–8.
136. Storm DW, Fulmer BR. Case report: percutaneous management of transitional-cell carcinoma of the upper urinary tract using the bipolar resectoscope. J Endourol. 2007;21(9):1011–3. doi:10.1089/end.2006.0415.
137. Grasso M. Ureteroscopic management of upper urinary tract urothelial malignancies. Rev Urol. 2000;2(2):116–21.
138. Schilling A, Bowering R, Keiditsch E. Use of the neodymium-YAG laser in the treatment of ureteral tumors and urethral condylomata acuminata. Clinical experience. Eur Urol. 1986;12 Suppl 1:30–33.
139. Schmeller NT, Hofstetter AG. Laser treatment of ureteral tumors. J Urol. 1989;141(4):840–3.
140. Bader MJ, Sroka R, Gratzke C, et al. Laser therapy for upper urinary tract transitional cell carcinoma: indications and management. Eur Urol. 2008. 10.1016/j.eururo.2008.12.012.
141. Tawfiek ER, Bagley DH. Upper-tract transitional cell carcinoma. Urology. 1997;50(3):321–9. doi:10.1016/S0090-4295(97), 00230-6.
142. Morales A, Eidinger D, Bruce AW. Intracavitary Bacillus Calmette-Guerin in the treatment of superficial bladder tumors 1976. J Urol. 2002;167(2 Pt 2):891–3; discussion 893–5.
143. Lamm DL, Blumenstein BA, Crissman JD, et al. Maintenance bacillus Calmette-Guerin immunotherapy for recurrent TA, T1 and carcinoma in situ transitional cell carcinoma of the bladder: a randomized Southwest Oncology Group Study. J Urol. 2000;163(4):1124–9.
144. Herr HW. Durable response of a carcinoma in situ of the renal pelvis to topical bacillus Calmette-Guerin. J Urol. 1985;134(3):531–2.
145. Bellman GC, Sweetser P, Smith AD. Complications of intracavitary bacillus Calmette-Guerin after percutaneous resection of upper tract transitional cell carcinoma. J Urol. 1994;151(1):13–5.
146. Schnapp DS, Weiss GH, Smith AD. Fever following intracavitary bacillus Calmette-Guerin therapy for upper tract transitional cell carcinoma. J Urol. 1996;156(2 Pt 1):386–8.
147. Liatsikos EN, Dinlenc CZ, Kapoor R, Smith AD. Transitional-cell carcinoma of the renal pelvis: ureteroscopic and percutaneous approach. J Endourol. 2001;15(4):377–83; discussion 397. 10.1089/089277901300189385.
148. Chew BH, Pautler SE, Denstedt JD. Percutaneous management of upper-tract transitional cell carcinoma. J Endourol. 2005;19(6):658–63. doi:10.1089/end.2005.19.658.
149. Irie A, Iwamura M, Kadowaki K, Ohkawa A, Uchida T, Baba S. Intravesical instillation of bacille Calmette-Guerin for carcinoma in situ of the urothelium involving the upper urinary tract using vesicoureteral reflux created by a double-pigtail catheter. Urology. 2002;59(1):53–7.
150. Yossepowitch O, Lifshitz DA, Dekel Y, et al. Assessment of vesicoureteral reflux in patients with self-retaining ureteral stents: implications for upper urinary tract instillation. J Urol. 2005;173(3):890–3. doi:10.1097/01.ju.0000147747.89028.64.
151. Rastinehad AR, Smith AD. Bacillus Calmette-Guerin for upper tract urothelial cancer: is there a role? J Endourol. 2009;23(4):563–8. doi:10.1089/end.2008.0164.
152. Clark PE, Streem SB, Geisinger MA. 13-year experience with percutaneous management of upper tract transitionalcellcarcinoma. J Urol. 1999;161(3):772–5; discussion 775–6.
153. Hayashida Y, Nomata K, Noguchi M, et al. Long-term effects of bacille Calmette-Guerin perfusion therapy for treatment of transitional cell carcinoma in situ of upper urinary tract. Urology. 2004;63(6):1084–8. doi:10.1016/j.urology.2004.01.046.
154. Okubo K, Ichioka K, Terada N, Matsuta Y, Yoshimura K, Arai Y. Intrarenal bacillus Calmette-Guerin therapy for carcinoma in situ of the upper urinary tract: long-term follow-up and natural course in cases of failure. BJU Int. 2001;88(4):343–7.
155. Thalmann GN, Markwalder R, Walter B, Studer UE. Long-term experience with bacillus Calmette-Guerin therapy of upper urinary tract transitional cell carcinoma in patients not eligible for surgery. J Urol. 2002;168(4 Pt 1):1381–5.
156. Keeley Jr FX, Bagley DH. Adjuvant mitomycin C following endoscopic treatment of upper tract transitional cell carcinoma. J Urol. 1997;158(6):2074–7.

Part VI

Chemotherapy and Long-Term Patient Follow-Up

Urothelial Carcinoma: Role of Perioperative Systemic Chemotherapy

15

Jorge A. Garcia, Dale R. Shepard, and Robert Dreicer

Introduction

In the bladder, the vast majority of patients with urothelial carcinoma (UCC) initially present with superficial disease at diagnosis, although approximately one-third will have muscle-invasive disease. Of these, greater than 60% will eventually develop metastatic disease. In 2009, the American Cancer Society estimated that more than 14,000 patients in the USA died as a result of metastatic bladder cancer [1]. Worldwide, surgery and radiation therapy (RT) are considered standard of care for patients with muscle-invasive disease [2,3]. Despite the lack of prospective randomized data comparing surgery to RT in muscle-invasive disease, radical cystectomy, with an extended lymph node dissection and urinary diversion, represents a standard approach at many academic centers in North America. Survival after radical cystectomy is a function of pathologic stage, with several series indicating that patients with pT4 lesions (tumor-penetrating adjacent structures) have a long-term survival rate of 33% compared with 72% for patients with pT2 lesions (tumor invading either the superficial muscularis propria pT2a or the deep muscularis propria pT2b) [4–8]. Similarly, lymph-node involvement at the time of surgery remains a strong predictor of both local and systemic relapses. The 5-year median overall survival after radical cystectomy for patients with lymph node positive disease is less than 30% [7,9].

The high risk for recurrence and death with cystectomy alone (Table 15.1) and the identification of chemotherapeutic agents with activity in advanced urothelial cancer have served as the rationale to evaluate cisplatin-based chemotherapy in the perioperative setting (neoadjuvant and adjuvant) in patients with locally advanced disease in an attempt to minimize risk of recurrence and maximize survival [10,11].

Neoadjuvant Chemotherapy

Despite "curative-intent" local therapy, a relatively high percentage of patients with muscle-invasive disease manifest systemic progression. The potential utility of perioperative chemotherapy is to impact micrometastatic disease. Neoadjuvant chemotherapy has several potential advantages. It has the ability to deliver full-dose effective systemic therapy while the burden of micrometastatic disease is minimal and when the patient's performance status is optimal [12].

J.A. Garcia (✉)
Departments of Solid Tumor Oncology and Urology, Taussig Cancer Institute, Glickman Urological & Kidney Institute, Cleveland Clinic Lerner College of Medicine of CWRU, 9500 Euclid Avenue, R35, Cleveland, OH 44195, USA
e-mail: Garciaj4@ccf.org

D.R. Shepard • R. Dreicer
Department of Solid Tumor Oncology, Taussig Cancer Institute, Cleveland Clinic, 9500 Euclid Avenue, R35, Cleveland, OH 44195, USA
e-mail: shepard@ccf.org; dreicer@ccf.org

D.E. Hansel et al. (eds.), *The Urinary Tract: A Comprehensive Guide to Patient Diagnosis and Management*, DOI 10.1007/978-1-4614-5320-8_15, © Springer Science+Business Media New York 2012

Table 15.1 Pathologic stage and estimated 5-year overall survival with radical cystectomy [4–8]

Pathological stage	Estimated 5-year overall survival (%)
pT1	>80
pT2a/b	72
pT3a	55
pT3b	35
pT4	30
Any pT/N⁺	<30

Patients with UCC often have multiple comorbidities; cisplatin-based chemotherapy can lead to moderate toxicities and recovery after surgery may take longer than expected. Neoadjuvant treatment has also the potential of producing a pathological complete response (pCR) in the primary tumor that has been correlated with disease-free survival and also permits in vivo drug sensitivity testing providing useful information for subsequent therapy [13,14].

A potential disadvantage of the neoadjuvant approach is the discrepancy between initial clinical and actual pathologic staging. This may cause over-treatment (obviated in the adjuvant setting) and provides the patient with insufficient information in terms of prognosis due to incomplete staging. It may also delay the definitive treatment of radical cystectomy by a few months that may be detrimental, especially if the disease is found to be nonresponsive to chemotherapy or if patients experience significant treatment-related adverse events. Lastly, there is the fear of increase perioperative morbidity after chemotherapy. However, there is little evidence to support this as the incidence of surgical complications in patients treated with neoadjuvant chemotherapy appears to be similar to that of patients who were treated with cystectomy alone [15,16]. Several phase II studies conducted during the past two decades demonstrate the feasibility of this approach and provide evidence of antitumor activity with an acceptable toxicity.

Numerous prospective neoadjuvant studies have evaluated the efficacy and safety of cisplatin-based chemotherapy (Table 15.2). Initial trials using single-agent cisplatin failed to demonstrate improvement of outcome [17,18]. Similar studies evaluating the efficacy of neoadjuvant cisplatin-based combination regimens have also failed to show survival benefit. The Nordic Cooperative Bladder Cancer Study Group conducted two randomized studies. Nordic I randomized 311 patients with locally advanced bladder cancer (T1 grade 3, T2–T4a) to neoadjuvant chemotherapy with two cycles of cisplatin and doxorubicin, or no chemotherapy followed by cystectomy and low-dose radiation therapy. Although the initial report suggested a modest improvement in the overall survival of patients receiving chemotherapy, this benefit disappeared after a long-term follow-up (59% vs. 51%; $p=0.1$) [19]. Of interest, however, was a subset of patients with T3–4 disease who appeared to have a greater benefit when compared to those with <T3 disease. A subsequent follow-up study, the Nordic Cystectomy II trial, studied 317 patients with stages T2–T4a, NX, M0 bladder cancer. Patients were randomly assigned to receive either three cycles of cisplatin and methotrexate or no treatment prior to cystectomy and without the use of preoperative radiotherapy. Despite a statistically significant improvement in tumor downstaging (26.4% with chemotherapy vs. 11.5% in the controls, $P=0.001$) at 5 years there was no evident survival advantage [20].

Two additional negative reports were published by the Italian Bladder Tumor Study Group (GISTV). In the first trial, 153 patients were randomized to MVEC (methotrexate, vinblastine, epirubicin, and cisplatin) before cystectomy or cystectomy alone [21]. In the second, Bassi and associates randomly assigned 206 patients to receive either four cycles of neoadjuvant MVAC (methotrexate, vinblastine, doxorubicin, and cisplatin) followed by cystectomy or cystectomy alone [22].

In an effort to define the appropriate timing of chemotherapy (neoadjuvant vs. adjuvant), Millikan and colleagues investigated the activity of neoadjuvant and adjuvant MVAC (two cycles before, and two after radical cystectomy) vs. five cycles of MVAC given exclusively in the adjuvant setting [23]. After randomizing 140 patients with locally advanced disease, there were no significant differences in outcome. Complete

Table 15.2 Selected neoadjuvant trials

Study	N	Treatment arms	Survival (%) 5-year OS or (mOS)	p-value
Neoadjuvant				
Malmstrom nordic I [19]	325	Cis/Doxo→LDXRT/cystectomy	59	NS
		LDXRT/cystectomy alone	51	
Sherif nordic II [20]	317	Cis/MTX→Cystectomy	53	NS
		Cystectomy alone	46	
Cortesi [21] GISTV	171	MVEC→Cystectomy	85	NS
		Cystectomy alone	74	
Bassi [22]	206	MVAC→Cystectomy	55	NS
		Cystectomy alone	53	
Abol-Enein [24]	196	Carbo-MV→Cystectomy	59	$P=0.044$
		Cystectomy alone	41	
Hall [16] MRC/EORTC	976	3×CMV→Cystectomy or XRT	55	$P=0.075$
		Cystectomy or XRT alone	50	
Grossman [15] SWOG-8710	307	3×MVAC→Cystectomy	57	$P=0.06$
		Cystectomy alone	43	

Cis/Doxo cisplatin plus doxorubicin, *LDXRT* low-dose radiation therapy, *Cis/MTX* cisplatin plus methotrexate, *Carbo* carboplatin

pathologic responses (pT0) occurred in 40% of patients receiving two cycles of neoadjuvant MVAC. Toxicity was a major concern in this study, with six treatment-related deaths in each treatment group. At a median follow-up of 6.8 years there was no difference in disease-free survival between the treated groups.

To date, only three contemporary series have demonstrated a survival advantage for patients receiving neoadjuvant chemotherapy prior to local definitive therapy. A relatively small study randomly assigned 196 patients to receive neoadjuvant chemotherapy with two cycles of CMV (cisplatin, methotrexate, and vinblastine) followed by cystectomy or cystectomy alone. The preliminary analysis of this trial suggested an improvement in the 5-year disease-free survival in favor of chemotherapy (62% survived with chemotherapy vs. 42% without, $P=0.013$) [24]. The largest neoadjuvant chemotherapy trial was conducted by the Medical Research Council (MRC) and the European Organization for Research and Treatment of Cancer (EORTC) [25]. More than 970 patients with T2–T4a/N0–NX/M0 bladder cancer were enrolled over 11 years at 126 institutions, making the trial vulnerable to differences in clinical practice between institutions and across treatment eras. The trial was designed to detect a difference in survival of 10% or more at 3 years in favor of cisplatin-based chemotherapy. Patients were randomly assigned to receive either three cycles of neoadjuvant chemotherapy with CMV ($n=491$) or no chemotherapy ($n=485$) before definitive local therapy. Definitive local therapy was selected on the basis of institutional preference and included radical cystectomy, external beam radiotherapy, or preoperative radiation followed by cystectomy. A total of 484 patients underwent cystectomy, 414 received external beam radiotherapy, and 77 patients were treated with combined modality therapy. At the time of the initial report, the median follow-up was 4 years, and by then 485 of the patients had died, the majority (78.6%) from carcinomas secondary to the original transitional cell carcinoma. Mortality from chemotherapy and surgery was 1% and 3.7%, respectively. Neoadjuvant chemotherapy was associated with a higher rate of pCR in primary tumors (32.5% with chemotherapy vs. 12.3% no chemotherapy). The hazard ratio (HR) analysis demonstrated a 15% reduction in the risk of death with the chemotherapy regimen, equating to an absolute 3-year survival difference of 5.5% (95% CI –0.5

to 11.0) $P=0.075$. At a median of 3 years, 55.5% of patients receiving chemotherapy were alive compared with 50% who underwent local therapy alone. At a subsequent follow-up the favorable impact of neoadjuvant chemotherapy on survival was maintained over a median follow-up of 7 years. The overall survival rates at 5 years were 50% with chemotherapy and 44% without, and at 8 years, 43% with chemotherapy and 37% without, respectively [16]. Although significant, the OS improvement observed in the study did not meet the prespecified statistical analysis for the study and thus caution should be used when interpreting these data.

The US Intergroup study led by investigators in the South West Oncology Group (INT-0080-SWOG 8710) evaluated the role of neoadjuvant MVAC plus cystectomy compared with cystectomy alone [15]. Over an 11-year period only 307 patients with T2–T4a/N0/M0 participated in this multi-institutional trial. All patients were stratified by known prognostic factors such as age and clinical and tumor stage. With a median follow-up of 8.4 years, the risk of death was 33% greater for those patients in the cystectomy-alone arm. One hundred seventeen patients survived with 90 deaths with the chemotherapy regimen, and 100 deaths in the surgery-alone group. An intention-to-treat analysis demonstrated a median survival of 46 months in the surgery-alone group (95% CI: 25–60 months) compared with 77 months (95% CI: 55–104 months) for the MVAC-treated patients. Overall survival between the groups was significantly different when a one-sided *t*-test was used, but this difference was lost with a two-sided *t*-test ($p=0.06$). In addition to the improvement in survival, the ability of achieving a pCR was observed in 48 (38%) patients from the cystectomy group. By contrast, only 18 (15%) of patients in the surgery-alone group were pathologically free of disease at the time of cystectomy. More than 85% of patients who achieved a pathological CR were alive at 5 years. Although Grade 3 and 4 toxicity was also common (primarily hematologic and gastrointestinal toxicities), no deaths were attributed to chemotherapy and there appeared to be no increase in rates of postoperative complications.

Interpretation of the results of neoadjuvant studies has been somewhat problematic because of the lack of power and statistical significance observed. Therefore, two large meta-analyses of all known randomized controlled trials of neoadjuvant chemotherapy conducted between 1984 and 2002 were performed. One study included 11 trials with more than 2,600 patients with high-risk bladder cancer, and the observed pooled HR for overall survival was 0.90 (95% CI 0.82–0.99, $p=0.02$). Similarly, the HR for patients receiving only cisplatin-based combinations (8/11 trials) was 0.87 (95% CI 0.78–0.96, $p=0.006$), consistent with an absolute overall survival benefit of 6.5% (95% CI 2–11%) from 50 to 56.5%. This survival benefit was observed irrespective of the type of definitive local treatment administered; however, a pCR was associated with a better outcome [26,27].

Correspondingly, the Advanced Bladder Cancer group conducted a meta-analysis of the existing neoadjuvant literature [28,29]. Eleven randomized controlled trials enrolling 3,005 patients with muscle-invasive (T2–T4a) disease were included in the meta-analysis. Trials employed either cystectomy or radiotherapy as the local definitive therapy, and overall survival from randomization until death was the primary endpoint. Cisplatin-based chemotherapy demonstrated a significant overall survival benefit (HR=0.86, 95% CI 0.77–0.95, $p=0.003$), equivalent to a 5% absolute improvement in survival at 5 years. Similarly, a 9% absolute improvement in the 5-year disease-free survival benefit was observed in those receiving neoadjuvant chemotherapy (HR=0.78 95% CI 0.71–0.86, $p<0.0001$). These analyses must be tempered by the inclusion criteria of each trial, as the vast majority of patients were under 75 years old, less than 5% of patients had an Eastern Cooperative Oncology Group (ECOG) performance status of 2 or greater, and only 3% of patients had glomerular filtration rates less than 59 mL/min.

The use of neoadjuvant cisplatin-based chemotherapy in those patients with concomitant renal insufficiency represents a significant therapeutic dilemma. Renal impairment in patients with UCC is often the result of disease-related

Table 15.3 Selected adjuvant trials

Study	N	Treatment arms	Survival 5-year OS or (mOS)	p-value
Adjuvant				
Skinner [37]	91	Cystectomy → Cisplatin/ doxorubicin/cyclophosphamide Cystectomy	4.25 year 2.41 year	0.099
Stöckle [38] Lehmann [36]	49	Cystectomy → MVAC or MVEC Cystectomy	52 months 20.4 months	0.069
Studer [39]	77	Cystectomy → cisplatin Cystectomy	57% 54%	0.65
Freiha [35]	55	Cystectomy → cisplatin Cystectomy	63 months 36 months	0.32

extrinsic obstruction. Schultz et al. and others have documented that ureteral obstruction is a poor prognostic factor in patients undergoing surgery, radiotherapy, or neoadjuvant chemotherapy for invasive bladder cancer [30,31]. Similarly, various small case series suggest that 16–54% of patients with muscle-invasive bladder cancer have some degree of ureteral obstruction [32,33]. Whether or not carboplatin can be substituted for cisplatin without compromising efficacy remains unclear. Despite the lack of data evaluating carboplatin in the neoadjuvant setting, it is clear from the advanced setting that carboplatin is an inferior agent to cisplatin in urothelial malignancies, and the substitution of carboplatin for cisplatin cannot be recommended for patients able to tolerate cisplatin-based therapy.

Despite the heterogeneous admixture of trials varying in chemotherapy agents and type of local definitive treatment, neoadjuvant chemotherapy should be considered a standard of care.

Adjuvant Chemotherapy

While there is level 1 evidence demonstrating a survival benefit in patients receiving neoadjuvant chemotherapy for locally advanced bladder cancer, the role of adjuvant chemotherapy is far less clear. Proposed advantages to adjuvant chemotherapy compared with neoadjuvant therapy include the ability to obtain proper pathological staging, avoiding delays for definitive local therapy with surgery, and minimizing tumor burden prior to chemotherapy [34]. There is a concern that the time necessary to give neoadjuvant chemotherapy will unnecessarily delay cystectomy or that these patients will develop toxicities from the chemotherapy, which will prevent cystectomy due to changes in performance status. Potential disadvantages of adjuvant chemotherapy compared with neoadjuvant therapy include a delay or inability to receive perioperative chemotherapy due to postoperative complications, an inability to assess tumor response, and an increase in morbidity from the chemotherapy. Most of these concerns are not supported by the data from the neoadjuvant and adjuvant trials.

A number of small randomized trials have attempted to establish a role for adjuvant chemotherapy in patients with muscle-invasive bladder cancer (Table 15.3) [35–39]. The existing trials, however, have significant methodological limitations to their interpretation, and thus benefit of adjuvant chemotherapy in these patients remains unclear. In one of the initial randomized trials, 91 patients with pT3 or pT4 bladder cancer with or without nodal disease and without metastatic disease were randomized to cystectomy followed by observation or four cycles of chemotherapy with cisplatin, doxorubicin, and cyclophosphamide [37]. While this trial demonstrated an increase in time to progression for patients receiving chemotherapy, there was no significant difference in 3-year overall survival. This trial was powered for 75 patients per treatment arm, but randomized

47 patients to observation and 44 patients to chemotherapy. Of these 44 patients assigned to chemotherapy, only 39% received the planned four courses of cisplatin, doxorubicin, and cyclophosphamide, with 25% electing to not get chemotherapy and many patients receiving alternative chemotherapy agents, such as bleomycin, actinomycin, or fluorouracil.

In a second trial, 49 patients with pT3b, pT4a, and/or pN1 or pN2 disease were randomized to either observation (23 patients) or chemotherapy with three cycles of methotrexate, vinblastine, cisplatin, and doxorubicin (MVAC) or methotrexate, vinblastine, cisplatin, and epirubicin (MVEC) with relapse-free survival as the primary endpoint [38]. The trial was stopped early with an interim analysis prior to enrollment of the intended 100 patients showing a significant difference in the number of patients with tumor progression in the control group (82%) compared with the chemotherapy group (27%). As in the previous trial, only 16 of the 26 patients received the intended treatment with 10 patients receiving no chemotherapy. While a subsequent report on the long-term survival of these patients showed a median overall survival of 35.1 months for patients receiving chemotherapy compared with 20.4 months for patients in the control group (HR 1.75; 95% CI 0.95–3.23), it should be noted that the protocol for this trial did not require chemotherapy for patients in the control arm at the time of disease recurrence and only 44% of the patients in this group received further treatment [36].

Adjuvant therapy with single-agent cisplatin was studied in a trial of 80 patients with multifocal, recurrent pT1 UCC or newly diagnosed or recurrent pT2 to pT4a UCC without preoperative evidence for N2 or N3 nodal disease or metastases [39]. Following cystectomy, patients were randomized to 3- to 28-day cycles of cisplatin 30 mg/m^2 daily for 3 days (37 patients) or an untreated control group. At an interim analysis with enrollment of 80 of the anticipated 120 patients, the 5-year survival was 54% in the control group and only 57% in patients receiving adjuvant cisplatin. The study was terminated early due to poor accrual and the inability to show a significant benefit for overall survival.

The benefit of adjuvant CMV was tested in a trial that randomized 55 patients with pT3b or pT4 transitional cell carcinoma with or without positive nodes and without evidence of metastatic disease to either four cycles of chemotherapy or observation with treatment with CMV at the time of recurrence [35]. At a follow-up of approximately 5 years, there was a significant effect on disease progression with a median recurrence in 37 months in patients receiving adjuvant CMV compared with 12 months in patients who did not receive adjuvant therapy ($p=0.01$). Unfortunately, a survival advantage for adjuvant therapy was not shown in this trial. This lack of survival benefit may be due to the use of chemotherapy at recurrence, as suggested by the authors; however the study was underpowered to show a significant difference. The trial was powered to show a 30% difference in survival with enrollment of 40 patients per arm; however, there were only 25 evaluable patients in each arm of this trial.

Despite the lack of any convincing data for the benefit of adjuvant chemotherapy following cystectomy in patients with urothelial cancer and the significant methodological flaws of these trials, the data from these trials were used in a meta-analysis of 491 individual patients enrolled in six randomized trials of local therapy followed by adjuvant chemotherapy compared with local therapy alone [28]. This analysis included the four trials described above, an unpublished trial of 108 patients receiving three cycles of CMEV, and an Italian trial of 93 patients receiving four cycles of cisplatin and methotrexate. While a 9% survival advantage at 3 years is reported, it is also reported that the 283 available events is far short of the 900 events that would be necessary to reliably detect this difference. The use of a meta-analysis also fails to address many of the concerns about the previous trials, such as the inconsistent use of chemotherapy in patients in the control groups at the time of relapse and the use of chemotherapy regimens that were not designated by the protocol.

The failure of the initial clinical trials to show a survival benefit and the continued interest in defining the role of adjuvant chemotherapy as a method for delivering perioperative chemotherapy have led to the development of additional trials with persistent problems with efficacy and accrual despite Cooperative group involvement. A multicenter Italian study of cystectomy followed by adjuvant cisplatin and gemcitabine or cisplatin and gemcitabine at recurrence was studied in 194 patients with pT2 grade 3 or pT3–4, N0–2 patients [40]. At a median follow-up of 32 months, there was no difference in overall survival or disease-free survival and the study was closed due to poor accrual and lack of benefit. Other trial designs that have not recruited well are a protocol by the Spanish Oncology Genito-Urinary Group (SOGUG) randomizing patients to cystectomy followed by either four cycles of adjuvant paclitaxel, cisplatin, and gemcitabine or the same regimen at relapse and a European Organization for the Research and Treatment of Cancer (EORTC) trial that randomized patients to either adjuvant therapy with gemcitabine/cisplatin, MVAC, or high-dose MVAC or one of these regimens at the time of relapse [41,42].

Adjuvant chemotherapy following cystectomy cannot be recommended for most patients and is specifically discouraged by some guidelines, such as those recently updated by the European Association of Urology, but there are patients who may benefit from therapy [43]. For example, not all patients with known muscle-invasive bladder cancer are evaluated by a medical oncologist prior to surgery and offered neoadjuvant chemotherapy. Additionally, due to the difficulties with clinical staging, patients are found to have more extensive disease at the time of surgery. In a retrospective review of 778 patients with transitional cell cancer of the bladder who underwent cystectomy, 40% of patients with nonmuscle-invasive cancer by clinical stage had muscle invasion by pathological stage, and 36% of patients with clinically staged organ confinement were found to have pT3 disease or greater or nodal disease at surgery [44]. A previous series reported a similar discrepancy in clinical staging [45]. These patients who have more extensive disease at the time of surgery may benefit from perioperative chemotherapy, and adjuvant chemotherapy should be considered since they were unable to receive neoadjuvant chemotherapy. The lack of accrual to previous adjuvant trials and the comparative benefits of neoadjuvant therapy in the perioperative setting will make further trials of adjuvant chemotherapy in these patients even more difficult. An alternative to the previous trial designs is consideration of factors that increase the likelihood of benefit for adjuvant therapy with treatment decisions based on factors other than pathological stage. For example, data from 4,462 patients who underwent a cystectomy for bladder cancer without perioperative chemotherapy were recently used to generate a nomogram based on multivariate analysis to determine factors associated with a high risk of death from bladder cancer [46]. Theoretically, enrolling patients at higher risk for death from their bladder cancer into a clinical trial of adjuvant chemotherapy may increase the likelihood that they would benefit from therapy. A recent trial attempted to use p53 mutation by immunohistochemistry, thought to be prognostic for disease recurrence, to decide which patients would receive three cycles of adjuvant MVAC [47]. With enrollment of 499 patients assessed for p53 mutations, 114 were found to have the mutation and randomized. The trial was stopped at an interim safety analysis due to no difference in 5-year relapse-free survival-based p53 status, although 33% of the patients did not receive the three cycles of therapy and 21% received no adjuvant therapy. The ability to use biomarkers to predict which patients are likely to benefit from adjuvant therapy remains unclear. Further trials will be necessary to determine if some patients will benefit from the currently available adjuvant chemotherapy regimens. Until then, adjuvant chemotherapy should only be given in the setting of a clinical trial or after very careful consideration of the benefits.

Perioperative Chemotherapy for Renal Pelvis and Ureteral Cancers

Upper tract cancers occur far less frequently than bladder cancers and represent about 5% of urothelial malignancies, with more than 90% showing urothelial histology. Although randomized trial evidence has demonstrated the potential survival impact of neoadjuvant cisplatin-based chemotherapy in muscle-invasive bladder cancer, whether such benefits can be extrapolated to the setting of upper tract tumors is and will remain unknown, given the relatively small numbers of these neoplasms. Although historically renal pelvis urothelial lesions were felt to be inherently more aggressive than similar lesions in the bladder, there is no evidence of any difference in the response of patients to systemic therapy and the majority of reported clinical trials of advanced urothelial cancer enrolled patients with metastatic UCC, including those of the renal pelvis, ureter, and urethra [48]. Despite the similar potential for systemic failure in patients with high-risk renal pelvis UCC, there are limited data regarding the utility of adjuvant chemotherapy in this setting. A small study conducted by the Hellenic Cooperative Oncology Group prospectively evaluated a cohort of 36 patients exclusively with locally advanced high-risk upper tract UCC who underwent surgery and subsequently received adjuvant paclitaxel and carboplatin. After a median follow-up of 40 months, the investigators reported a 5-year disease-free survival of 42% (95% confidence interval, 15.8–64.6%). The rates of local failure reported were in the range of 30%, with 17% of patients developing distant metastatic disease [49]. Given the lack of data for non-cisplatin-based chemotherapy in the perioperative setting, and the increased risk associated with the administration of cisplatin-based chemotherapy in patients with 1 renal unit, patients at high risk for disease recurrence should have a careful, risk/benefit discussion prior to routine administration of perioperative chemotherapy (Table 15.4).

Table 15.4 Chemotherapy regimens commonly used in the perioperative setting

MVAC chemotherapy (1 cycle = 28 days)		
Drug	Dose (mg/m^2)	Schedule
Methotrexate	30	Days 1, 15, 22
Vinblastine	3	Days 1, 15, 22
Doxorubicin	30	Day 2
Cisplatin	70	Day 2
GC chemotherapy (1 cycle = 28 days)		
Drug	Dose (mg/m^2)	Schedule
Cisplatin	70	Day 1
Gemcitabine	1,000	Days 1, 8, 15

Conclusion

Muscle-invasive UCC of the bladder is an aggressive epithelial neoplasm. Over the past three decades, surgical and radiotherapeutic techniques have been improved, resulting in decreased perioperative and long-term morbidity. Despite these advances, systemic failure of patients undergoing definitive local therapy has remained relatively unchanged, thus reinforcing the need to develop more effective systemic therapies. Neoadjuvantly administered, cisplatin-based multi-agent chemotherapy has been demonstrated to improve survival modestly; however, relatively few patients in the USA receive therapy in this setting.

Although immutable patient factors such as poor renal function or comorbidities make some patients poor candidates for neoadjuvant chemotherapy, lack of understanding of the existing data or problematic patient coordination between urologists and medical oncologists also plays a role. While new and more effective systemic options are developed, maximizing the use of currently available therapeutic options can be and should be an area of emphasis for the urologic oncology community.

References

1. Jemal A, Siegel R, Ward E, et al. Cancer statistics, 2009. CA Cancer J Clin. 2009;59:225–49.
2. Gschwend JE, Fair WR, Vieweg J. Radical cystectomy for invasive bladder cancer: contemporary results and remaining controversies. Eur Urol. 2000;38:121–30.
3. Shipley WU, Winter KA, Kaufman DS, et al. Phase III trial of neoadjuvant chemotherapy in patients with invasive bladder cancer treated with selective bladder preservation by combined radiation therapy and chemotherapy: initial results of Radiation Therapy Oncology Group 89-03. J Clin Oncol. 1998;16:3576–83.
4. Herr HW, Faulkner JR, Grossman HB, et al. Surgical factors influence bladder cancer outcomes: a cooperative group report. J Clin Oncol. 2004;22:2781–9.

5. Madersbacher S, Hochreiter W, Burkhard F, et al. Radical cystectomy for bladder cancer today–a homogeneous series without neoadjuvant therapy. J Clin Oncol. 2003;21:690–6.
6. Shariat SF, Karakiewicz PI, Palapattu GS, et al. Outcomes of radical cystectomy for transitional cell carcinoma of the bladder: a contemporary series from the Bladder Cancer Research Consortium. J Urol. 2006;176:2414–22; discussion 2422.
7. Stein JP, Lieskovsky G, Cote R, et al. Radical cystectomy in the treatment of invasive bladder cancer: long-term results in 1,054 patients. J Clin Oncol. 2001;19:666–75.
8. Tilki D, Svatek RS, Karakiewicz PI, et al. Characteristics and outcomes of patients with pT4 urothelial carcinoma at radical cystectomy: a retrospective international study of 583 patients. J Urol. 2010;183:87–93.
9. Herr HW, Donat SM. Outcome of patients with grossly node positive bladder cancer after pelvic lymph node dissection and radical cystectomy. J Urol. 2001;165:62–4; discussion 64.
10. Herr HW, Dotan Z, Donat SM, et al. Defining optimal therapy for muscle invasive bladder cancer. J Urol. 2007;177:437–43.
11. von der Maase H, Sengelov L, Roberts JT, et al. Long-term survival results of a randomized trial comparing gemcitabine plus cisplatin, with methotrexate, vinblastine, doxorubicin, plus cisplatin in patients with bladder cancer. J Clin Oncol. 2005;23:4602–8.
12. Sternberg CN, Donat SM, Bellmunt J, et al. Chemotherapy for bladder cancer: treatment guidelines for neoadjuvant chemotherapy, bladder preservation, adjuvant chemotherapy, and metastatic cancer. Urology. 2007;69:62–79.
13. Raghavan D, Pearson B, Duval P, et al. Initial intravenous cis-platinum therapy: improved management for invasive high risk bladder cancer? J Urol. 1985;133:399–402.
14. Splinter TA, Scher HI, Denis L, et al. The prognostic value of the pathological response to combination chemotherapy before cystectomy in patients with invasive bladder cancer. European Organization for Research on Treatment of Cancer–Genitourinary Group. J Urol. 1992;147:606–8.
15. Grossman HB, Natale RB, Tangen CM, et al. Neoadjuvant chemotherapy plus cystectomy compared with cystectomy alone for locally advanced bladder cancer. N Engl J Med. 2003;349:859–66.
16. Hall RR. Updated results of a randomized controlled trial of neoadjuvant cisplatin (C), methotrexate (M) and vinblastine (V) chemotherapy for muscle-invasive bladder cancer. Proc Am Soc Clin Oncol. 2002;21:Abst 710.
17. Martinez-Pineiro JA, Gonzalez Martin M, Arocena F, et al. Neoadjuvant cisplatin chemotherapy before radical cystectomy in invasive transitional cell carcinoma of the bladder: a prospective randomized phase III study. J Urol. 1995;153:964–73.
18. Wallace DM, Raghavan D, Kelly KA, et al. Neo-adjuvant (pre-emptive) cisplatin therapy in invasive transitional cell carcinoma of the bladder. Br J Urol. 1991;67:608–15.
19. Malmstrom PU, Rintala E, Wahlqvist R, et al. Five-year followup of a prospective trial of radical cystectomy and neoadjuvant chemotherapy: Nordic Cystectomy Trial I. The Nordic Cooperative Bladder Cancer Study Group. J Urol. 1996;155:1903–6.
20. Sherif A, Rintala E, Mestad O, et al. Neoadjuvant cisplatin-methotrexate chemotherapy for invasive bladder cancer – Nordic cystectomy trial 2. Scand J Urol Nephrol. 2002;36:419–25.
21. Cortesi E. Neoadjuvant treatment for locally advanced bladder cancer: a randomized prospective clinical trial. Proc Am Soc Clin Oncol. 1995;14:Abstr 623.
22. Bassi PF, Pappagallo GL, Sperandio P, et al. Neoadjuvant MVAC chemotherapy of invasive bladder cancer: results of a multicenter phase III trial. J Urol. 1999;161:Abst 264.
23. Millikan R, Dinney C, Swanson D, et al. Integrated therapy for locally advanced bladder cancer: final report of a randomized trial of cystectomy plus adjuvant M-VAC versus cystectomy with both preoperative and postoperative M-VAC. J Clin Oncol. 2001; 19:4005–13.
24. Abol-Enein H, El Makresh M, El Baz M, et al. Neoadjuvant chemotherapy in treatment of invasive transitional bladder cancer: a controlled, prospective randomised study. Br J Urol. 1997;80:49.
25. Neoadjuvant cisplatin, methotrexate, and vinblastine chemotherapy for muscle-invasive bladder cancer: a randomised controlled trial. International collaboration of trialists. Lancet. 1999;354:533–40.
26. Advanced Bladder Cancer Meta-analysis Collaboration. Neoadjuvant chemotherapy in invasive bladder cancer: a systematic review and meta-analysis. Lancet. 2003;361:1927–34.
27. Winquist E, Kirchner TS, Segal R, et al. Neoadjuvant chemotherapy for transitional cell carcinoma of the bladder: a systematic review and meta-analysis. J Urol. 2004;171:561–9.
28. Advanced Bladder Cancer (ABC) Meta-analysis Collaboration. Adjuvant chemotherapy in invasive bladder cancer: a systematic review and meta-analysis of individual patient data Advanced Bladder Cancer (ABC) Meta-analysis Collaboration. Eur Urol. 2005;48:189–99; discussion 199–201.
29. Advanced Bladder Cancer (ABC) Meta-analysis Collaboration. Neoadjuvant chemotherapy in invasive bladder cancer: update of a systematic review and meta-analysis of individual patient data advanced bladder cancer (ABC) meta-analysis collaboration. Eur Urol. 2005;48:202–5; discussion 205–6.
30. Matos T, Cufer T, Cervek J, et al. Prognostic factors in invasive bladder carcinoma treated by combined modality protocol (organ-sparing approach). Int J Radiat Oncol Biol Phys. 2000;46:403–9.
31. Schultz PK, Herr HW, Zhang ZF, et al. Neoadjuvant chemotherapy for invasive bladder cancer: prognostic factors for survival of patients treated with M-VAC with 5-year follow-up. J Clin Oncol. 1994;12:1394–401.

32. Leibovitch I, Ben-Chaim J, Ramon J, et al. The significance of ureteral obstruction in invasive transitional cell carcinoma of the urinary bladder. J Surg Oncol. 1993;52:31–5.
33. Macneil HF, Hall RR, Neal DE, et al. Systemic chemotherapy for urothelial cancer in patients with ureteric obstruction. Br J Urol. 1991;67:169–72.
34. Donat SM. Integrating perioperative chemotherapy into the treatment of muscle-invasive bladder cancer: strategy versus reality. J Natl Compr Canc Netw. 2009;7:40–7.
35. Freiha F, Reese J, Torti FM. A randomized trial of radical cystectomy versus radical cystectomy plus cisplatin, vinblastine and methotrexate chemotherapy for muscle invasive bladder cancer. J Urol. 1996;155: 495–9; discussion 499–500.
36. Lehmann J, Franzaring L, Thuroff J, et al. Complete long-term survival data from a trial of adjuvant chemotherapy vs control after radical cystectomy for locally advanced bladder cancer. BJU Int. 2006;97:42–7.
37. Skinner DG, Daniels JR, Russell CA, Lieskovsky G, Boyd SD, Nichols P, et al. The role of adjuvant chemotherapy following cystectomy for invasive bladder cancer: a prospective comparative trial. J Urol. 1991;145:459–64; discussion 464–7.
38. Stöckle M, Meyenburg W, Wellek S, Voges G, Gertenbach U, Thüroff JW, et al. Advanced bladder cancer (stages pT3b, pT4a, pN1 and pN2): improved survival after radical cystectomy and 3 adjuvant cycles of chemotherapy. Results of a controlled prospective study. J Urol. 1992;148:302–6; discussion 306–7.
39. Studer UE, Bacchi M, Biedermann C, et al. Adjuvant cisplatin chemotherapy following cystectomy for bladder cancer: results of a prospective randomized trial. J Urol. 1994;152:81–4.
40. Cognetti F, Ruggeri EM, Felici A, et al. Adjuvant chemotherapy (AC) with cisplatin + gemcitabine (CG) versus chemotherapy (CT) at relapse (CR) in patients (pts) with muscle-invasive bladder cancer (MIBC) submitted to radical cystectomy (RC). An Italian multicenter randomised phase III trial. J Clin Oncol. 2008;26:Abstr 5023.
41. Cisplatin Plus Gemcitabine With or Without Paclitaxel in Treating Patients With Stage IV Urinary Tract Cancer. 2012. http://clinicaltrials.gov/ct2/show/NCT00022191. Accessed 17 May 2012.
42. Comparison of Immediate and Delayed Adjuvant Chemotherapy in Treating Patients Who Have Undergone a Radical Cystectomy for Stage III or Stage IV Transitional Cell Carcinoma of the Bladder Urothelium. 2012. http://clinicaltrials.gov/ct2/show/NCT00028756. Accessed 17 May 2012.
43. Stenzl A, Cowan NC, De Santis M, et al. The updated EAU guidelines on muscle-invasive and metastatic bladder cancer. Eur Urol. 2009;55:815–25.
44. Shariat SF, Palapattu GS, Karakiewicz PI, et al. Discrepancy between clinical and pathologic stage: impact on prognosis after radical cystectomy. Eur Urol. 2007;51:137–49; discussion 149–51.
45. Dutta SC, Smith Jr JA, Shappell SB, et al. Clinical under staging of high risk nonmuscle invasive urothelial carcinoma treated with radical cystectomy. J Urol. 2001;166:490–3.
46. Vickers AJ, Cronin AM, Kattan MW, et al. Clinical benefits of a multivariate prediction model for bladder cancer: a decision analytic approach. Cancer. 2009;115:5460–9.
47. Stadler WM, Lerner SP, Groshen S, et al. Randomized trial of p53 targeted adjuvant therapy for patients (pts) with organ-confined node-negative urothelial bladder cancer (UBC). J Clin Oncol. 2009;27:15s, Abst 5017.
48. Bajorin DF, Dodd PM, Mazumdar M, et al. Long-term survival in metastatic transitional-cell carcinoma and prognostic factors predicting outcome of therapy. J Clin Oncol. 1999;17:3173–81.
49. Bamias A, Deliveliotis C, Fountzilas G, et al. Adjuvant chemotherapy with paclitaxel and carboplatin in patients with advanced carcinoma of the upper urinary tract: a study by the Hellenic Cooperative Oncology Group. J Clin Oncol. 2004;22:2150–4.

Urine Cytology 16

Stephen S. Raab, Christine N. Booth, and J. Stephen Jones

Total Testing Process

One way to conceptualize urine cytology testing is in terms of a total testing process (TTP), which is a system-based framework for examining all possible interactions and activities that may affect the quality of laboratory tests. The TTP encompasses all components or steps of the cycle from the point of the clinical question to the point of clinical action. For a patient who has urinary tract findings suspicious for cancer (based on clinical history and examination, endoscopic findings, or diagnostic imaging), this cycle traverses from the clinical question of "Does this patient have cancer of the urinary tract?" to the clinical action of cancer treatment and follow-up, if the diagnosis of cancer is rendered. This framework allows for the design and implementation of interventions that may reduce or eliminate errors that adversely affect testing and patient health outcomes. In this regard, the TTP for urine cytology testing is defined by the activities (Fig. 16.1) in three distinct phases that align with clinical workflow internal and external to the pathology laboratory:

1. *Pre-analytic phase*: clinician test selection, test ordering, specimen procurement, patient and specimen identification, and specimen transport
2. *Analytic phase*: specimen processing, preparation, and cytopathologist interpretation
3. *Post-analytic phase*: test results reporting and clinician receipt, clinician interpretation of test results, and clinical action based on interpretation

The utility of the TTP concept lies in the linking together of all testing steps and the crossing of historical boundaries of testing process ownership. Currently, data on the performance and problems of some steps of the TTP for urine cytology are known, but are lacking for other steps.

S.S. Raab (✉)
Department of Pathology, University of Washington School of Medicine, 1959 NE Pacific Street, NE110, Box 356100, Seattle, WA 98195, USA
e-mail: raabss@gmail.com

C.N. Booth
Pathology and Laboratory Medicine Institute, Cleveland Clinic, 9500 Euclid Avenue, L25, Cleveland, OH 44195, USA
e-mail: boothc1@ccf.org

J.S. Jones
Department of Regional Urology, Cleveland Clinic, Glickman Urological Kidney Institute, 9500 Euclid Avenue, Q10-1, Cleveland, OH 44195, USA
e-mail: joness7@ccf.org

The Pre-analytic Phase

Urine Cytology Test Ordering

Urine cytology tests are ordered in the evaluation of three main patient populations:

1. As a screening test in patients who have no signs or symptoms of cancer, but are at higher risk of developing or having a urothelial malignancy

D.E. Hansel et al. (eds.), *The Urinary Tract: A Comprehensive Guide to Patient Diagnosis and Management*, DOI 10.1007/978-1-4614-5320-8_16, © Springer Science+Business Media New York 2012

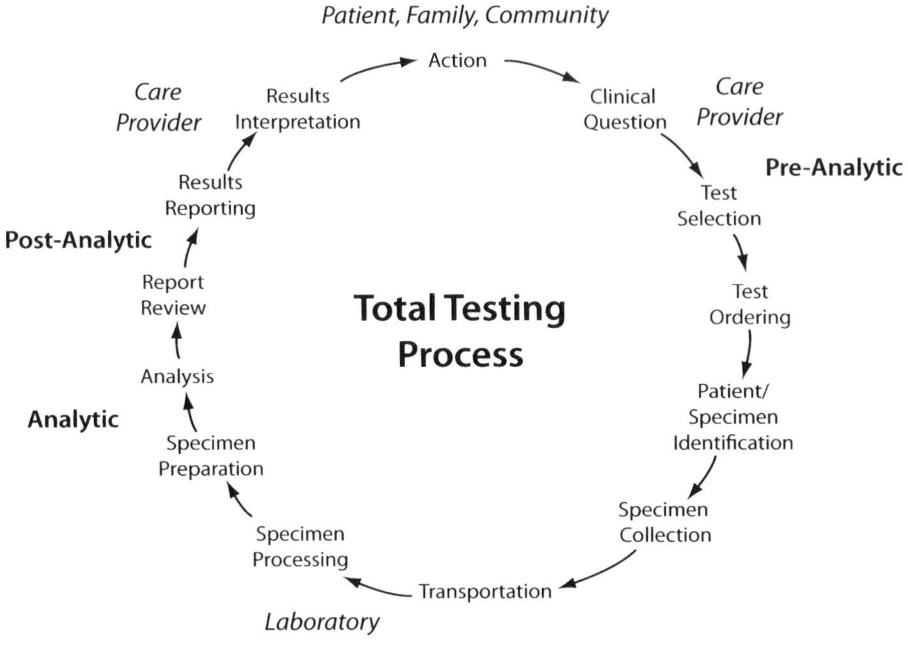

Fig. 16.1 The total testing process. The total testing process (TTP) begins with a clinical question and the care provider and patient. Each larger step in the process is composed of many smaller steps and laboratory medicine is the sum total of all the testing steps. Adapted from Boone J. Presentation at the Institute on Critical Issues in Health Laboratory Practice: Managing for Better Health, September 23–26, 2007. Atlanta, GA: Centers for Disease Control and Prevention

2. As a diagnostic and triage test in patients who have signs and/or symptoms of urinary tract pathology
3. As a surveillance test in patients who have a history of urinary tract malignancy

The frequency with which these tests are ordered depends on geographic region, which in turn depends on patient population and clinician subspecialty and expertise. An accurate description of the patient history that includes a reason for the test order (e.g., screening, diagnostic, or surveillance) is important for the cytopathology laboratory, as different mimics are seen in different patient populations.

In patients who have had high levels of exposure to known bladder carcinogens or who work in industries with high risks of exposure, urine cytology testing may be used as the initial screening test for early bladder cancer detection.

The most common use of urine cytology is as a diagnostic and triage test for patients who have signs (such as hematuria) or symptoms (such as painful urination) of cancer. Urine cytology diagnoses are used in conjunction with history, physical examination, and other testing results to triage patients with different follow-up management protocols.

The frequency of obtaining urine cytology specimens as part of an overall surveillance protocol for patients who have been previously diagnosed with urothelial cancer varies. Some urologists procure a urine specimen at every surveillance cystoscopic examination visit. For example, following the diagnosis of a low-grade urothelial carcinoma, a urine specimen may be obtained at 3 months, 9 months, and then yearly. Following the diagnosis of a high-grade urothelial carcinoma, a urine specimen may be obtained every 3 months for a year for surveillance and then yearly following negative results. Any suspicious or malignant urine cytology diagnosis with a normal cystoscopic examination will usually result in repeat imaging, if it has not been performed recently, and performing bladder and prostatic urethral biopsies (in men).

Urine Samples: Specimen Procurement and Transport

Urine cytology specimens are classified as either voided or instrumented. This distinction is important as the cytological appearance of cancers and the diagnostic pitfalls are often unique for these two specimen types.

This binary separation of urine specimens follows the classic cytological separation into those specimens obtained through a normal cellular shedding mechanism (voiding) and those collected by scraping or forcible discharge (instrumentation), the first being of low cellularity, unless the patient has urothelial disease, and the second being more cellular. An exception to this rule is a urine specimen procured post-cystoscopic examination. The cytological findings in these voided urines are essentially the same as in instrumented urines.

A final type of urine specimen is the "conduit" specimen, procured in a patient who had a cystectomy with a conduit constructed from other body tissues, such as the ileum. The conduit connects the upper urinary tract to a body outlet. As clinicians obtain conduit specimens to track disease in the upper tract (renal pelvises, calyces, or ureters), the cells of interest are the urothelial cells, which tend to be few in number compared to the numerous intestinal cells. Urine from patients with urinary neobladders is affected likewise.

Voided Urine Specimens

Voided specimens (also known as clean catch specimens) are the most common specimens examined in most cytology laboratories. A random specimen (and not an early morning specimen) is recommended to limit cellular degeneration caused by hyper concentrated urine that has remained in the bladder for prolonged periods at night, which is a source of diagnostic error. As previously mentioned, voided urine specimens tend to be of low cellularity, *unless* the patient has:

1. A high-grade urothelial cell carcinoma of the bladder (in some cases)
2. An irritative lesion, such as lithiasis or infection
3. A contaminated urine, most frequently procured from a woman, in which the predominant component is non-urinary tract cells

Voided urines are superior to instrumented urines in detecting malignancies of the urethra based on the fact that urine in the bladder has not been exposed to the lesion that would source the cells, whereas voiding may capture cells from the urethral lesion.

Instrumented Urine Specimens

Instrumented urine specimens are further divided into three types, which are procured through a catheter or after an instrument (such as a cystoscope) is introduced into the urinary tract. Instrumented specimens include catheterized urines, bladder washings, brushings, and upper urinary tract urines obtained by ureteric catheterization. Instrumented urine specimens are superior to voided urine specimens in detecting malignancies of the bladder and upper tract.

Catheterized Specimens

Catheterized specimens are collected for a variety of reasons, such as the work-up of patients who may have a urinary tract infection, determining the cause of hematuria, or for urothelial cancer screening in patients who have an in-dwelling catheter.

Washing Specimens

A washing may be performed of any part of the urinary tract, although the most common location of a washing specimen is of the bladder. Washing specimens may be directed or undirected and in a washing procedure, a solution (e.g., electrolytic or saline) is injected into the cavity of interest and then withdrawn. Washing specimens are often performed as a method for examining a large area for cancer. Washings are the most sensitive cytological method for urothelial cancer detection. Upper tract specimens often are a type of washing specimen, but often are discussed separately because the cytological findings of the upper tract differ from that of the bladder, the upper tract consisting of the renal collecting ducts, pelvis, and ureters.

Table 16.1 Failures in the pre-analytic phase of urine cytology testing

Inappropriate test ordering
Procurement of a poor-quality sample
Poor preservation prior to transport
Specimen mix-up
Specimens loss or destruction during transport
Lack of clinical information on urine requisition form

Brushing Specimens

A brushing is performed under cystoscopic guidance of a specific area of concern. Brushing may be performed on any portion of the urinary tract and may be collected in conjunction with a washing. The brushing specimen is either placed directly on a slide and smeared or placed into a fixative and processed similar to other urine specimens.

Testing Failures and Quality in the Pre-analytic Phase

Root cause analysis has shown a variety of failures in different steps of the pre-analytic testing phase (Table 16.1). For example, using the Eindhoven method of root cause analysis, failures in obtaining a quality sample are secondary to inappropriate protocols, faulty techniques or equipment, practitioner inexperience, and patient-related factors. Several causes of error may be identified in an individual patient case, and errors are often compounded through the testing cycle.

Cytological–histological correlation is a commonly used root cause analytic method to identify causes of error in patients who have both a urine specimen for cytological analysis and a simultaneous or follow-up biopsy for histological analysis. In the correlation process, the diagnoses of the two specimens are compared and non-correlating specimens are reviewed to determine if the source of error was secondary to failures in the diagnostic interpretation steps or the steps prior to interpretation (e.g., sampling error, or a failure in the procurement or processing steps).

In examining errors detected through correlation of urine and bladder biopsy specimens, 60% of non-correlating cases were caused by a sampling failure. Most of these errors were classified as a false negative and methods to decrease sampling error will be discussed later. More than 12% of testing failures were secondary to sampling or interpretation defects in the cystoscopic examination tissue procurement and/or interpretation steps following an appropriately interpreted urine specimen. Thus, the correlation method may be used to identify problems in the larger testing cycle involving the follow-up steps of cystoscopic examination.

Forty-nine percent of urine/biopsy testing failures led to some degree of patient harm, generally consisting of additional diagnostic testing (either procurement of a repeat urine or biopsy) to establish the diagnosis, delays in treatment, or unnecessary cystoscopic examination.

The Analytic Phase

Specimen Handling

Specimen Accessioning and Processing

The analytic phase begins when a urine specimen arrives in the cytopathology laboratory. Laboratory technical staff members accession the specimen, which involves assigning a unique laboratory identification number. In urine specimen laboratory processing, a variety of methods are used to create microscopic slides. These processing methods include centrifugation, filter, smear, and cell block techniques. In the last decade, technologies that create monolayer urine preparations have become widespread. In the last steps of processing, the microscopic slides are stained and the preferential stain for most cytopathologists is the Papanicolaou stain, which highlights both nuclear and cytoplasmic characteristics. Some cytopathologists use additional stains for interpretation, such as a modified Wright-Giemsa stain.

Processing and staining methods are critical for specimen quality, and there is a general lack of study on optimal processing methods, as processing is non-standardized across laboratories. As noted previously, sampling failures identified by the correlation process include failures in processing.

Table 16.2 Failures in the analytic phase of urine cytology testing

Failures
Accessioning phase
Specimen mix-up
Specimen loss
Processing phase
Specimen mix-up
Specimen loss
Poor preparation
Poor staining
Poor cover slipping
Cytotechnologist screening phase
Failure to locate malignant cells
Incorrect diagnosis rendered
Pathologist interpretation phase
Specimen mix-up
Failure to locate malignant cells
Incorrect diagnosis rendered
Incorrect report created

Errors that occur in the accessioning and processing phases as well as other analytic phases are shown in Table 16.2.

Cytotechnologist Screening

In many laboratories, cytotechnologists screen urine slides to identify cells that are the most suggestive of cancer or other lesions. These slides are then passed to cytopathologists who make a final diagnostic determination, often based on the cytotechnologist's opinion and examination of the most worrisome areas marked. The process of screening involves the careful observation of every portion of the slide. In non-gynecologic pathology, this practice is largely based on expert opinion—careful observation by an individual trained in the screening process adds value by decreasing the false-negative fraction of missing pre-neoplastic lesions and cancers. In some laboratories, cytotechnologists are not used for this practice.

Diagnostic Interpretation

Diagnostic interpretation is a complex cognitive task performed by cytopathologists.

Table 16.3 Diagnostic categories in urine cytology

Categories
Tier 1. Specimen adequacy
Adequacy for evaluation
Adequacy for evaluation, but limited by:
Low cellularity, obscuring material, blood, etc.
Unsatisfactory for evaluation
Tier 2. Assessment of cancer risk
Benign
Atypical
Suspicious
Malignant/neoplastic
Tier 3. Classification of disease processes
Benign
No abnormalities observed
Reactive processes (specify):
Inflammation, lithiasis, infection (bacterial, viral, fungal, tuberculosis)
Chemotherapy, radiation therapy, malakoplakia
Malignant/neoplastic
Urothelial carcinoma
Low-grade urothelial carcinoma
High-grade urothelial carcinoma
Squamous cell carcinoma
Adenocarcinoma
Small cell carcinoma
Renal cell carcinoma (upper tract)
Malignant lymphoma
Metastasis

Diagnostic Categories

For each patient specimen, a cytopathologist renders a diagnostic interpretation using a three-tier diagnostic categorical system (Table 16.3):

1. An assessment of specimen adequacy and quality
2. An assessment of cancer risk in adequate specimens
3. A classification of specific neoplastic and non-neoplastic diseases in some adequate specimens

In the United States, there is a lack of standardization on how these three tiers are used.

Tier 1. Specimen Adequacy

An adequate specimen is critical for determining if cancer is present. The assessment of adequacy is based on the number of cells present and the absence of limiting factors, such as obscuring blood. Yet, criteria for urine specimen adequacy

Table 16.4 Likelihood ratios for the diagnoses of low- and high-grade urothelial carcinoma in urine specimens

	Urine diagnoses for urothelial carcinoma				
Specimen and cancer grade	Benign	Atypical	Suspicious	Malignant	Total cases
Voided, high grade	0.384	1.116	5.294	4.080	271
Voided, low grade	0.738	1.855	1.611	0.439	235
Instrumented, high grade	0.162	1.050	3.150	5.250	103
Upper tract, high grade	0.400	0.800	∞	∞	18
Instrumented, low grade	0.538	1.400	2.000	2.500	84
Upper tract, low grade	0.400	0.800	-	∞	13

are not standardized for different specimen types and preparation methods. Many cytopathologists do not formally grade adequacy, especially in voided urine specimens.

As the cells present in voided urine specimens are obtained through the sloughing of epithelial layers of the entire urinary tract, the number of cells present in any given sample depends on the disease process. Thus, voided urine specimens may be highly cellular in conditions in which cellular sloughing is common, such as high-grade malignancies and inflammatory or reactive conditions. More commonly, they tend to be of low cellularity. Most voided urine specimens contain at least a few urothelial, inflammatory cells, and/or acellular components such as crystals or debris. Instrumented urine specimens generally show higher cellularity.

Tier 2. Cancer Risk

Cytopathologists traditionally use a four categorical scale (benign, atypical, suspicious, and malignant) to denote risk of neoplasia in urine specimens. Cytopathologists and clinicians have not standardized clinical management recommendations for these diagnostic categories. The frequency of use of specific diagnostic categories depends on factors such as patient population, specimen type, specimen quality, and cytopathologist experience. In voided urine specimens, the atypical rate may be as high as 20%, and in instrumented urine specimens the atypical rate may be even higher.

The likelihood ratio of a diagnostic category may be used to calculate the posttest probability of malignancy from the pretest probability of malignancy. Table 16.4 shows the likelihood ratio of urine specimen diagnostic categories depending on the specimen type and grade (low or high) of urothelial carcinoma for a university-based practice. For high-grade urothelial cancer and voided specimens, the diagnosis of benign cytologic findings lowers the probability of cancer and the diagnoses of atypical, suspicious, and malignancy confer an increasing risk of cancer. Based on the practices at both authors' institutions, the atypical diagnosis only slightly increases the risk of a high-grade urothelial cancer.

These authors also showed that individual cytopathologist likelihood ratios exhibit considerable variability for the diagnosis of atypical (in estimating the posttest probability of high-grade cancer) and for almost all categories of atypical and higher for estimating the posttest probability of low-grade cancer. These data indicate that the use of non-definitive categories (atypical and suspicious) is non-standardized. Knowing the expertise of individual cytopathologists is critical in assessing the cancer risk associated with specific diagnoses.

Tier 3. Disease Classification

Cytopathologists classify both non-neoplastic and neoplastic diseases on urine specimens in the categories shown in Table 16.3. Learning the cytomorphologic criteria of these diseases forms the basis of urine cytology apprenticeship training. Summaries of these disease criteria and photomicrographs of the "classical presentations" are presented below. The challenge in actual cytopathology practice is in accurately classifying the myriad of patient specimens that are not classical in presentation. Some of the cognitive biases that lead to errors in diagnostic interpretation will be discussed, including the inappropriate use of heuristics.

Sensitivity and Specificity of Disease Classification and Risk Assessments

By far, the most common malignancy encountered in urine cytology specimens is urothelial carcinoma, although other primary and secondary malignancies have been well described in the literature. Reports of urine diagnostic accuracy generally are descriptive of urothelial carcinoma detection, as the detection of other malignancies is rare in comparison.

For diagnostic purposes, cytopathologists separate urothelial neoplasia into high- and low-grade cancers, and this two-category system is a means to report the degree of tumor differentiation and to correlate findings with World Health Organization (WHO) histology categories [1]. Criteria describing these malignancies will be discussed later.

Urine cytology sensitivity and specificity depend on specimen type. Although urine cytology generally is regarded as sensitive for high-grade urothelial cancer, controversy is high regarding the sensitivity of urine cytology for low-grade urothelial carcinoma. Furthermore, recent reports have shown diminishing sensitivity compared to historical controls.

Koss et al. reported that the sensitivity of voided urine for the diagnosis of high-grade urothelial carcinoma was 94.2%. The sensitivity increased as the number of voided urine specimens increased, with 79% of cancers detected on the first specimen, 14% on the second specimen, and 7% on the third specimen. Other authors have confirmed this high level of sensitivity. Monolayer preparation methods detect high-grade lesions at a similar percentage, although indeterminate rates may initially rise after implementation. Several recent reports have failed to live up to historical findings. Halling reported that published urine cytology series after 1990 actually identified only 11, 31, and 60% of grades 1, 2, and 3 tumors, respectively [2]. More recently, cytology found only 10.3% of all cancers in a recent large study of patients under bladder cancer surveillance, and only 19.4% of high-grade lesions [3]. In other words, cytology missed the overwhelming majority of cancers, high-grade or not. The level of specificity of voided urine cytology for high-grade urothelial carcinoma depends on how indeterminate diagnoses are assessed. The false-positive rate of a definitive diagnosis of high-grade urothelial carcinoma is very low. The use of cystoscopic examination and biopsy also has its limits, as definitive high-grade urothelial carcinomas may be diagnosed on urine specimens but not be seen on cystoscopic examination or biopsied. For example, during investigation of fluorescence cystoscopy, detection was improved for carcinoma in situ (CIS) (95% vs. 68%) and papillary tumors (96% vs. 85%), demonstrating the reality that malignancy often exists that is too small to be identified by endoscopic recognition alone [4].

Table 16.5 shows the sensitivity and specificity of single urine cytology using strict histological follow-up as the gold standard. Of patients who had an indeterminate voided urine diagnosis (atypical or suspicious), 40% had follow-up of a high-grade urothelial carcinoma; only 26% of patients had a benign lesion. These data indicate that indeterminate diagnoses have a moderate to high risk of cancer.

The sensitivity of bladder wash specimens for the diagnosis of high-grade urothelial carcinoma is higher than that seen in voided urine specimens.

For low-grade urothelial cancer, the reported sensitivity (based on making a definitively malignant diagnosis) in bladder wash specimens in the literature ranges from 0 to 73%. Some cytopathologists will never make an outright diagnosis of low-grade urothelial carcinoma. However, for some experienced cytopathologists, the diagnostic sensitivity is over 50%. Based on the same follow-up study listed previously, 67% (14 of 21) patients had a diagnosis of atypical, suspicious, or malignant and a low-grade urothelial carcinoma on follow-up.

The literature is virtually unanimous that the outright diagnosis of a low-grade urothelial carcinoma is exceedingly difficult to make on a

Table 16.5 Sensitivity and specificity of voided, instrumented lower tract, and upper tract urine cytology

Atypical urine diagnoses considered negative				
	Low grade	High grade		
Specimen type	Sensitivity (%)	Sensitivity (%)	Specificity (%)	
Voided urine	8.9	49.2	89.0	
Instrumented lower tract urine	33.3	65.0	85.7	
Upper tract urine	40.0	40.0	100	
Atypical urine diagnoses considered positive				
	Low grade	High grade		
Specimen type	Sensitivity (%)	Sensitivity (%)	Specificity (%)	
Voided urine	51.1	74.6	66.2	
Instrumented lower tract urine	66.7	90.0	61.9	
Upper tract urine	80.0	80.0	50.0	
	Low grade		High grade	
Atypical urine diagnoses considered negative	Sensitivity (%)	Specificity (%)	Sensitivity (%)	Specificity (%)
Primary diagnosis voided urine	9.7	97.7	45.2	97.7
Surveillance voided urine	8.5	76.3	51.2	76.3
Primary diagnosis instrumented urine	25.0	96.8	57.1	96.8
Surveillance instrumented urine	35.3	75.0	66.7	75.0
	Low grade		High grade	
Atypical urine diagnoses considered positive	Sensitivity (%)	Specificity (%)	Sensitivity (%)	Specificity (%)
Primary diagnosis voided urine	32.3	73.3	66.7	73.3
Surveillance voided urine	61.0	55.9	78.6	55.9
Primary diagnosis instrumented urine	50.0	71.0	100	71.0
Surveillance instrumented urine	70.6	53.1	87.9	53.1

voided urine specimen. However, one study showed that 48% of biopsy-proven low-grade urothelial carcinomas had a voided urine diagnosis of atypical or suspicious. In this study, 11% of all institutional voided urine cases had an indeterminate diagnosis, as the vast majority of patients did not have histology follow-up. These data indicate that indeterminate diagnoses raise the posttest probability of low-grade cancer, even in voided urine specimens.

Cytomorphological Criteria of Benign and Neoplastic Lesions

"Normal" Urine Specimens

Normal urine specimens are obtained in patients without urinary tract disease and display cells that lack pre-neoplastic, neoplastic, or reactive changes. Completely normal urine specimens are obtained in some patients who undergo screening and in some patients who undergo cystoscopic examination and do not have disease.

Voided urine specimens may contain a variety of cell types from different regions of the urinary tract lined by urothelial cells, squamous cells, and glandular cells. Instrumented and ileal conduit specimens are usually more cellular.

Cellular Components

Urothelial Cells

Urothelium is divided into three cell layers: superficial, intermediate, and basal/parabasal. Superficial urothelial cells are large and also known as umbrella cells. These cells may normally be multinucleated although they generally contain from one to three nuclei. The cytoplasmic borders are well defined and the cytoplasm is finely granular. The intermediate cell layer is variable in thickness and the cells are cuboidal and smaller than superficial cells. The basal/parabasal cell layer also is a single layer in thickness and the cells are in similar shape but slightly smaller compared to intermediate urothelial cells.

Table 16.6 Sources of glandular cells in urine specimens

Normal lining
Cystitis glandularis
Periurethral glands
Prostate
Kidney
Seminal vesicle
Epididymis
Vas deferens
Female genital tract
Nephrogenic adenoma
Adenocarcinoma
Urothelial carcinoma with adenocarcinomatous differentiation

Squamous Cells

Portions of both the male and female urothelial tract are normally lined by squamous epithelium. In women, the urinary tract squamous cells are often confused with benign squamous cell contaminant from the gynecological tract. The presence of bacteria associated with squames, in the absence of reactive changes and inflammation, is usually a sign that the squamous cells are not of urinary tract origin.

Glandular Cells

Glandular cells have a number of sources (Table 16.6). Glandular cells exhibit oval, basally placed nuclei with finely granular blue to green cytoplasm. Glandular cells may normally display cytoplasmic vacuolation or cilia. Glandular cells may differentiate from the urothelial lining. Glandular epithelium also may arise as a response to chronic irritation. Mucous-secreting glands are normally found in the spongy portion of the male urethra and in the female urethra; hence these cells may be shed in voided urine specimens.

Malignancy and Its Pitfalls

Urothelial Cancer

Cytopathologists use different cytomorphologic criteria to diagnose low-grade and high-grade urothelial carcinoma. Low-grade cancer diagnostic criteria describe features of a well-differentiated carcinoma and high-grade cancer diagnostic criteria describe features of a moderately or poorly differentiated carcinoma. Quite understandably, the diagnosis of a low-grade cancer is far more difficult and some cytopathologists argue that it is impossible. As noted previously, the diagnosis of both high- and low-grade cancers depends on several factors, one of which is individual expertise. Prior to interpreting cancer risks associated with cytopathologic reports, it is important that clinicians know whether individual cytopathologists use the diagnostic category of low-grade urothelial carcinoma.

The histopathologic correlates of the cytopathologic diagnosis of high-grade urothelial carcinoma includes in situ, some grade 2 papillary, and most invasive carcinomas. The histopathologic correlates of the cytopathologic diagnosis of low-grade urothelial carcinoma include grade 1 papillary carcinoma and other low-grade entities, such as papillary urothelial neoplasm of low malignant potential (PUNLMP).

The concept of urothelial dysplasia is poorly captured in the cytology binary grading system. The histologic diagnoses of high-grade urothelial dysplasia and CIS are classified as high-grade urothelial carcinoma in the cytologic system. The histologic diagnosis of low-grade urothelial dysplasia does not have a cytologic counterpart, and can be regarded as benign.

The indeterminate diagnoses of atypical and suspicious may be used to describe either high- or low-grade carcinomas in which definitive cytopathologic criteria are absent. In the following sections, we describe the cytopathologic features of both high-grade and low-grade urothelial carcinoma and report the mimics of each of these entities.

High-Grade Urothelial Carcinoma

The main mimics of high-grade urothelial carcinoma are cellular degeneration, treatment effect (systemic or local chemotherapy, such as Bacillus Calmette-Guérin therapy, or radiation therapy), lithiasis, and infections, including human polyoma virus. The diagnostic criteria for cancer tend to be seen in combination. Classic examples of high-grade urothelial carcinoma are shown in Figs. 16.2, 16.3, and 16.4, and mimics are shown in Figs. 16.5, 16.6, 16.7, 16.8, and 16.9.

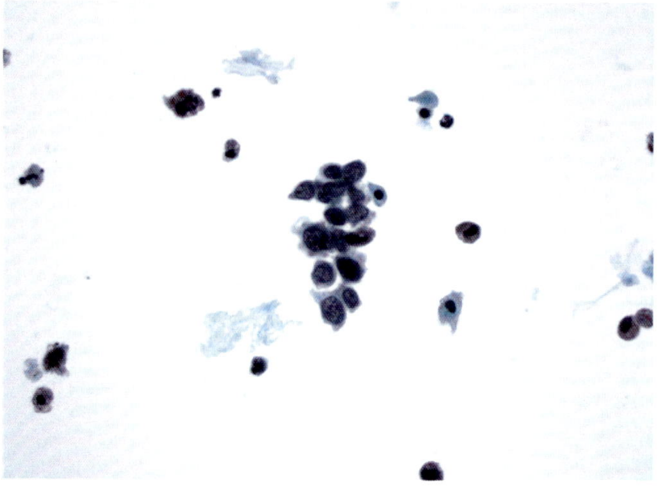

Fig. 16.2 Urine, voided: high-grade urothelial carcinoma. The malignant urothelial cells vary in size and shape and exhibit variable degrees of degeneration. Not the coarse, dark chromatin and high nuclear:cytoplasmic ratios (Papanicolaou X HP)

Fig. 16.3 Urine, voided: high-grade urothelial carcinoma. The malignant urothelial cells contain a thin rim of homogeneous cytoplasm. There is an absence of cytoplasmic vacuoles (Papanicolaou X HP)

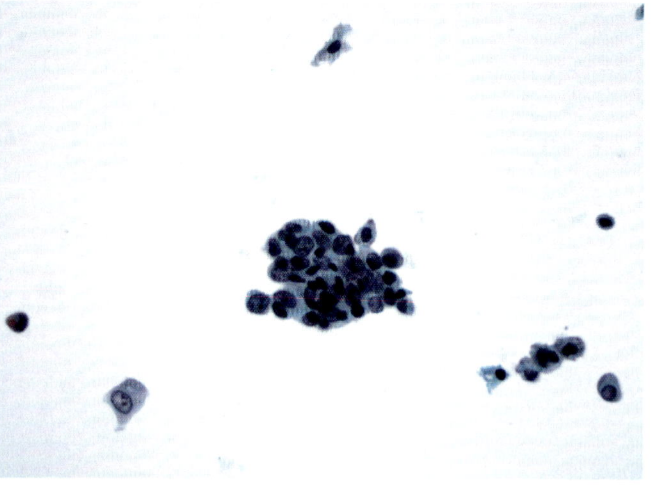

Fig. 16.4 Urine, voided: high-grade urothelial carcinoma. The malignant cell nuclei are large and the nuclear membranes are irregular. The nuclear membranes show focal thickening. Several of the nuclei show multiple prominent nucleoli (Papanicolaou X HP)

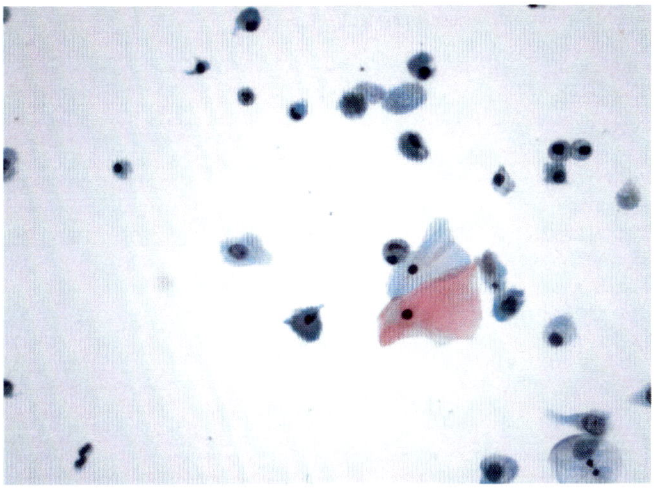

Fig. 16.5 Urine, voided: degeneration. Numerous single degenerated urothelial cells contain hyperchromatic nuclei and irregular nuclear membranes. These cells contain a moderate amount of cytoplasm and lack the high nuclear:cytoplasmic ratio of high-grade urothelial carcinoma cells. Background squamous cells are hardier and show fewer degenerative features (Papanicolaou X HP)

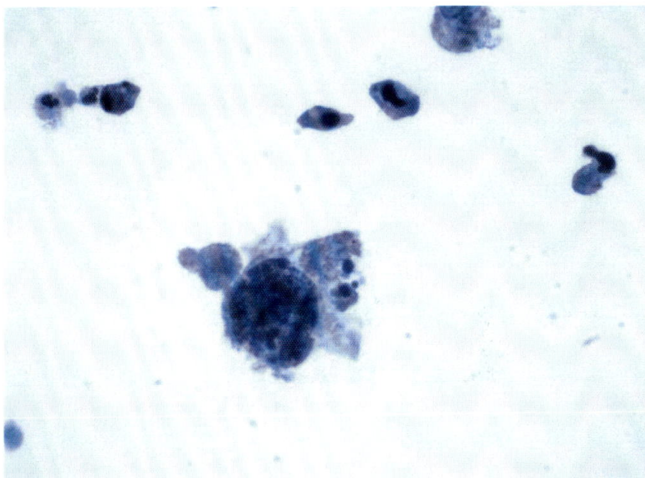

Fig. 16.6 Urine, voided: chemotherapy effect. The urothelial cell shows nuclear enlargement, slight hyperchromasia, and nuclear membrane irregularities. The nuclear membrane is not markedly thickened and the nuclear hyperchromasia is less than that seen in a high-grade urothelial carcinoma. This patient was receiving systemic chemotherapy for leukemia (Papanicolaou X HP)

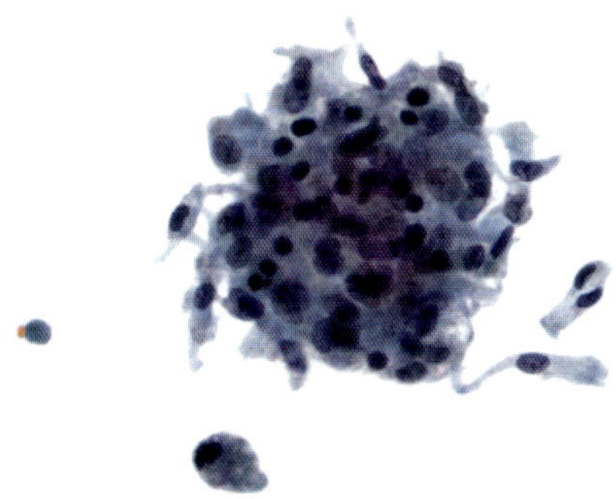

Fig. 16.7 Urine, bladder washing: Bacillus Calmette-Guérin therapy effect. Histiocytes and granulomas in latter stage therapy may be seen in instrumented urine specimens. Numerous histiocytes are admixed with small, round lymphocytes in this granuloma (Papanicolaou X HP)

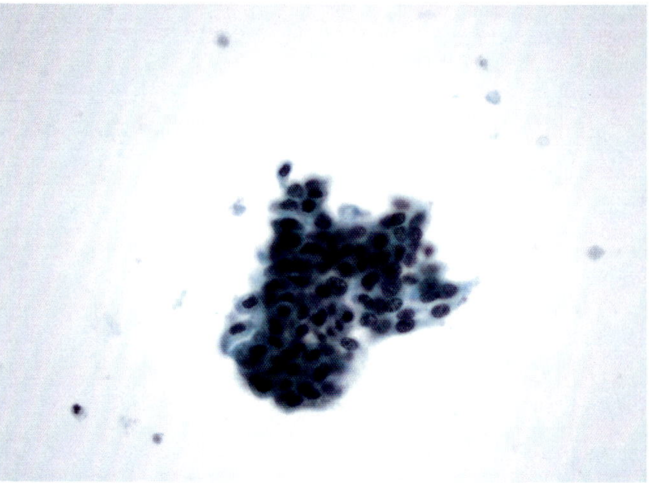

Fig. 16.8 Urine, ureter washing: lithiasis. In lithiasis, marked acute inflammation, squamous metaplasia, and reactive squamous cells may be seen. The urothelial cells often have slightly hyperchromatic nuclei (Papanicolaou X HP)

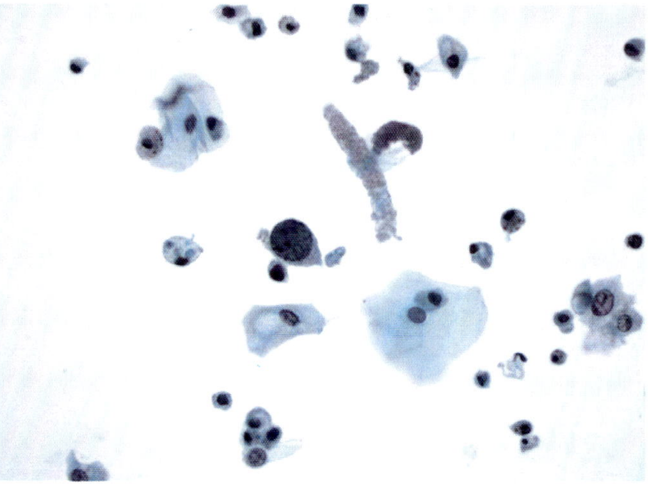

Fig. 16.9 Urine, voided: human polyomavirus. The human polyomavirus infected urothelial cell shows an eccentrically placed nucleus. The cell has the appearance of a comet with a cytoplasmic tail (Papanicolaou X HP)

The definitive diagnosis of urothelial carcinoma depends on several factors, including number of tumor cells present in the specimen and specimen quality. Voided urine specimens tend to have fewer cells and exhibit more cellular degeneration compared to instrumented urine specimens, which may contain larger groups of malignant cells.

In upper tract urine specimens, the benign urothelial cells show larger nuclei with higher nuclear-to-cytoplasmic ratios and more prominent nuclear membrane irregularities, compared to bladder washing specimens. However, the diagnosis of a high-grade urothelial carcinoma generally is relatively straightforward in a high-quality specimen.

The challenge in diagnostic interpretation lies in making a definitive diagnosis if only a few malignant (or atypical) cells are present or if the specimen is of low quality, such as exhibiting extensive degeneration or obscuring material (e.g., blood, debris, lubricant). In these cases, non-definitive diagnoses may be rendered, depending on other factors such as cytopatholo-

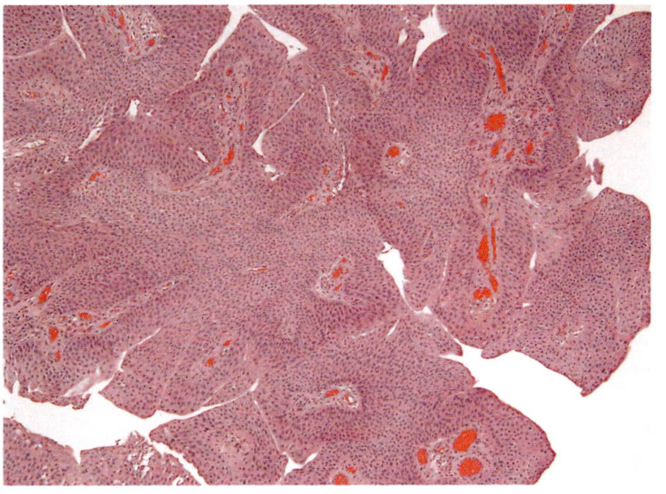

Fig. 16.10 Histology: low-grade urothelial carcinoma. Numerous fibrovascular cores are surrounded by well-differentiated neoplastic cells. The malignant cells have abundant cytoplasm with monotonous round to oval nuclei (H&E X LP)

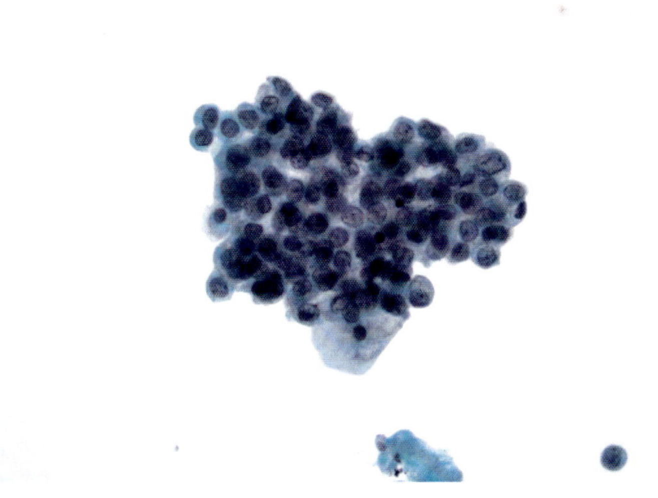

Fig. 16.11 Urine, bladder washing: low-grade urothelial carcinoma. A cluster of low-grade carcinoma cells lies inferior to a squamous epithelial cell. The low-grade carcinoma cells have high nuclear to cytoplasmic ratios, slightly thickened nuclear membranes, and finely granular chromatin. The cytoplasm is difficult to see, but is metaplastic and non-vacuolated (Papanicolaou X HP)

gist experience or patient history. Improvement efforts to increase tumor cellularity and specimen quality have involved preparing additional slides, using additional methods of preparation, and collecting additional specimens.

Low-Grade Urothelial Carcinoma

As has been mentioned previously, the diagnosis of low-grade urothelial carcinoma is controversial, and most published criteria are based on case series of instrumented specimens. Classic examples of low-grade urothelial carcinoma are shown in Figs. 16.10, 16.11, and 16.12, and mimics are shown in Figs. 16.13, 16.14, and 16.15. The main mimics are instrumentation artifact and a variety of reactive conditions.

As low-grade cancers are well differentiated, they cytologically appear very similar to normal urothelium. Thus, the criteria for diagnosis essentially are those of slight changes in nuclear and cytoplasmic features, which must be observed in the absence of stimuli that cause reactive changes. In other words, the presence of inflammation or more pronounced cytologic changes limit the ability to make a definitive diagnosis.

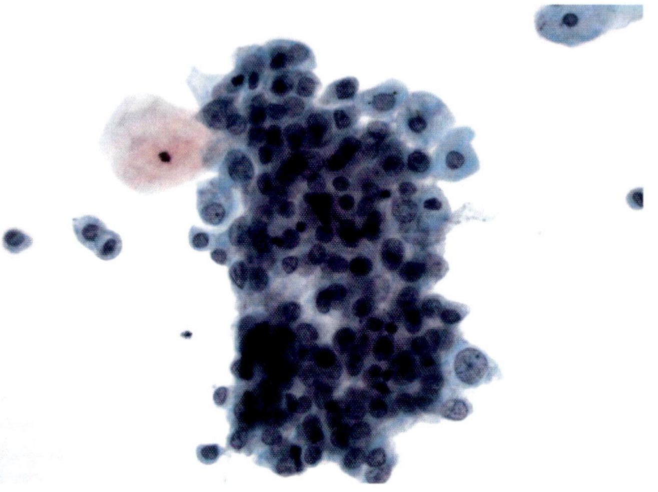

Fig. 16.12 Urine, bladder washing: low-grade urothelial carcinoma. A cluster of cells of low-grade urothelial carcinoma shows densely homogeneous cytoplasm. The nuclear:cytoplasmic ratio is only slightly enlarged and some nuclear membranes are irregular in contour (Papanicolaou X HP)

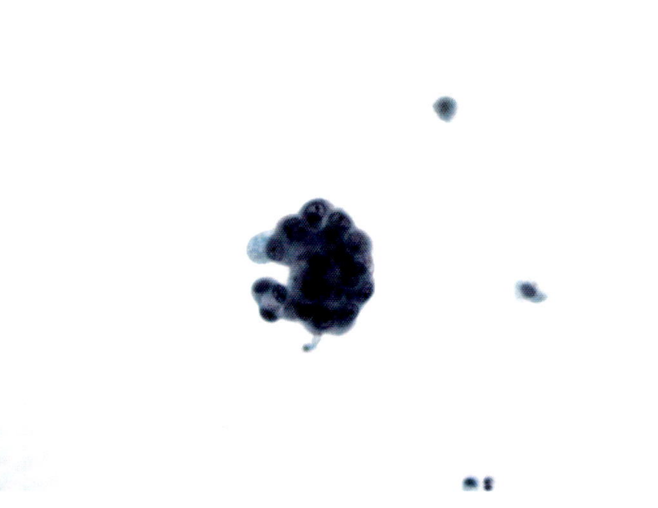

Fig. 16.13 Urine, voided: reactive urothelial cells. Although these urothelial cells show nuclear hyperchromasia, increased nuclear:cytoplasmic ratios, and nuclear membrane irregularities, the presence of cytoplasmic vacuolization indicates a reactive process (Papanicolaou X HP)

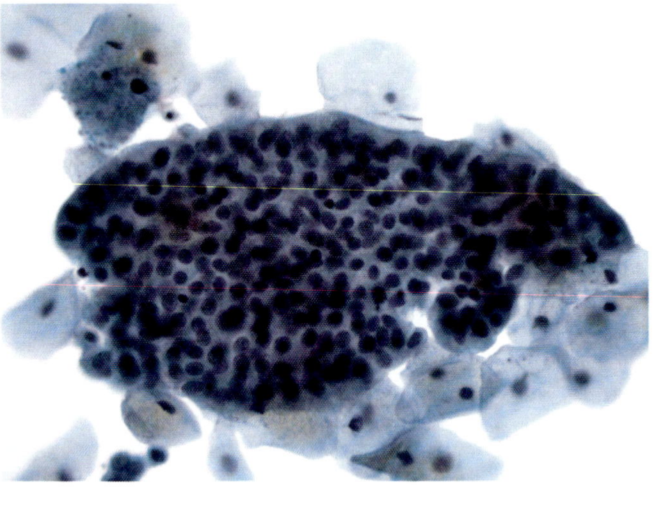

Fig. 16.14 Urine, bladder washing: instrumentation artifact. Large groups of benign urothelial cells often are dislodged with instrumentation. In this group, superficial urothelial cells overly numerous intermediate urothelial cells. The urothelial cells are crowded but do not exhibit significant atypia (Papanicolaou X HP)

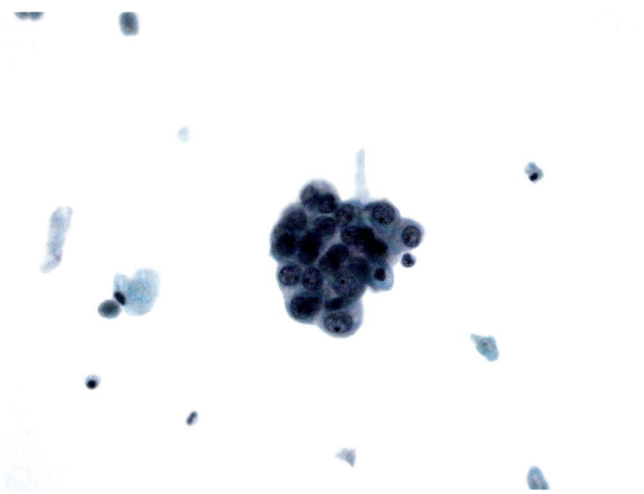

Fig. 16.15 Urine, voided: reactive findings. The urothelial cells show vacuolated cytoplasm and low nuclear:cytoplasmic ratios with conspicuous nucleoli and fine nuclear membranes. The patient has a history of lithiasis (Papanicolaou X HP)

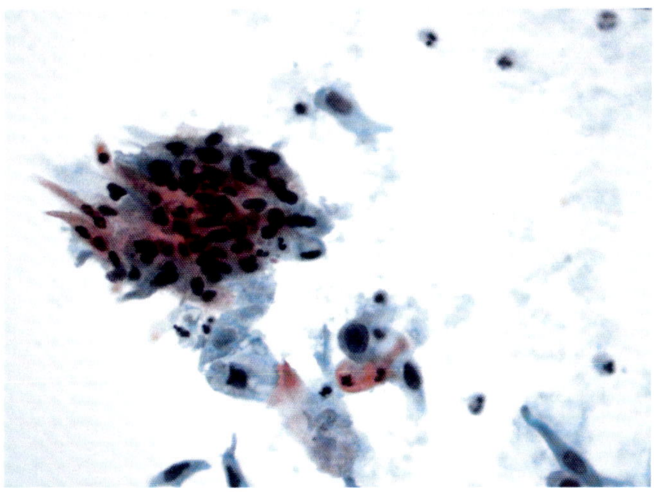

Fig. 16.16 Urine, voided: squamous cell carcinoma. The malignant cells show keratinizing and non-keratinizing features. The malignant keratinized cells show either small, hyperchromatic nuclei or enlarged nuclei with irregular cytoplasmic shapes (Papanicolaou X HP)

Deshpande and McKee reported that cytological criteria more indicative of low-grade urothelial carcinoma on voided specimens were increased specimen cellularity, cell clusters, and nuclear membrane irregularities. These authors reported that pseudoclusters are difficult to distinguish from true cell clusters on monolayer preparations, limiting interpretation.

Other Malignancies

Non-urothelial malignancies are diagnosed with considerable less frequency. Examples of these malignancies are shown in Figs. 16.16, 16.17, 16.18, and 16.19.

Ancillary Testing

In the last decade the United States Federal Drug Administration approved biomarker assays specific for the detection of bladder cancer. These assays include (1) assays for urine proteins (proteomic) such as NMP22, BTA stat, and BTA TRAK; (2) immunocytochemical

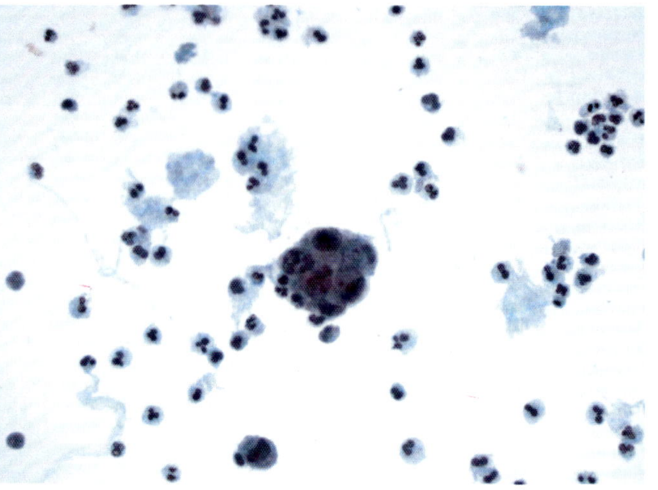

Fig. 16.17 Urine, voided: adenocarcinoma. The malignant cells form three-dimensional clusters with cytoplasmic vacuolization in a background of inflammation. Many of the malignant cells display a prominent nucleolus (Papanicolaou X HP)

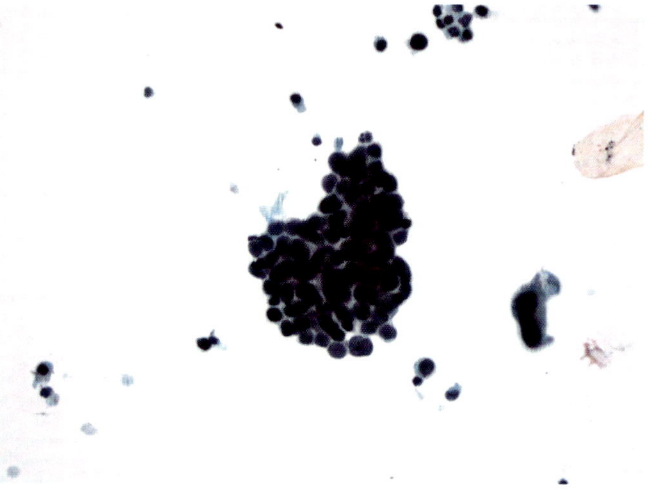

Fig. 16.18 Urine, voided: small cell carcinoma. Single malignant cells and a large central cluster of malignant cells are present. The malignant cells have granular chromatin and high nuclear to cytoplasmic ratios (Papanicolaou X HP)

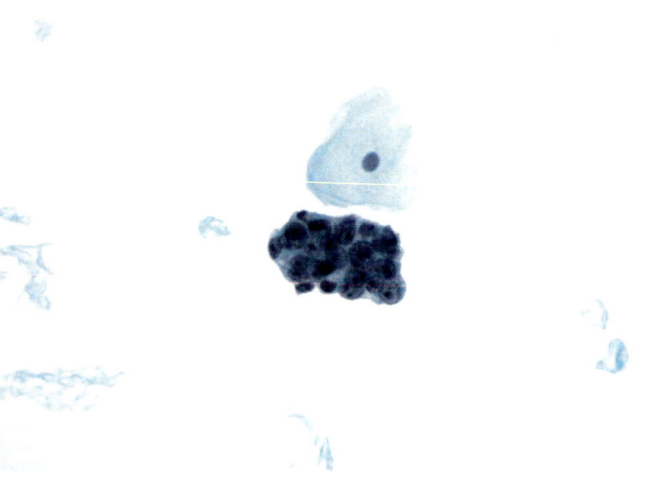

Fig. 16.19 Urine, voided: prostatic adenocarcinoma. In this prostatic adenocarcinoma, the nuclei contain prominent nucleoli (Papanicolaou X HP)

Table 16.7 Sensitivity and specificity of urinary markers

Test	Marker	Sensitivity (%)	Specificity (%)
Fibrin degradation product (FDP)	Fibrin degradation product	78–91	75–90
ImmunoCyt	High molecular weight carcinoembryonic antigen and mucins	70–95	70–85
UroVysion	Chromosomal probes	69–75	82–85
Bladder tumor antigen (BTA) stat	Human complement factor H-related protein	60–70	50–75
Bladder tumor antigen (BTA) TRAK	Human complement factor H-related protein	60–70	50–75
Nuclear matrix proteins (NMP) 22	Nuclear matrix apparatus proteins	60–75	70–85

assays such as ImmunoCyt; and (3) fluorescence in situ hybridization (FISH). The development of these assays has reflected the remarkable advances in proteomics and genomics. Lam and Nabi wrote that the ideal biomarker should be able to replace cystoscopic examination and be cost effective: in the current environment, existing protein or molecular biomarkers have not met this challenge.

The sensitivity and specificity of currently available biomarkers is shown in Table 16.7. The utility of biomarkers generally is assessed by comparing the sensitivity and specificity with urine cytology. For example, the UroVysion test (Abbott Molecular, Abbott Park, IL, USA) relies on chromosomal alterations associated with bladder cancer by the use of fluorescent probes to centromeres on chromosomes 3, 7, 17, and recognition of deletion of 9p21. The protocol for test performance is both labor-intensive and operator dependent, requiring expertise of the person who counts and examines the slides. In a meta-analysis of diagnostic accuracy, Hadjdinjak reported that excluding Ta tumors, the sensitivity for UroVysion and cytology was 86% and 61%, respectively. Differences in test performance disappeared when non-muscle-invasive cases were excluded from the analysis. Hajdinjak concluded that cytology results were highly specific, although a negative cytology result did not meaningfully change the posttest probability of urothelial cancer. UroVysion results did not provide conclusive evidence of the presence or absence of cancer, but both positive and negative results altered the posttest probability of malignancy.

A number of genetic markers have been studied to determine their role in bladder cancer development and progression. These markers include tumor-suppressor genes (e.g., p53), cell cycle regulators (e.g., Ki-67), protooncogenes and oncogenes (e.g., c-myc or EGFR), and cell adhesion molecules (E-cadherin). Some of these markers have potential prognostic value for cancer recurrence, progression, and survival.

Epigenetics is the study of inherited reversible changes in gene function or other cell phenotypes that occur without any change in DNA sequence. An epigenetic mechanism for long-term silencing of gene expression is DNA methylation. Molecular diagnosis may allow for the detection of some epigenetic events that occur early in the disease process. Methylation analysis in urine is being studied for cancer detection and prognosis. Promotor hypermethylation occurs in bladder cancer and methylation-specific polymerase chain reaction is being used to detect specific methylation markers in the urine. Lastly, gene-expression analysis using microarray technology is currently being studied as an approach to determine the biological behavior of bladder cancer, including tumor growth, progression, and metastatic potential. In the future, these research efforts may alter ancillary testing in urine cytology specimens.

The Post-analytic Phase

Clinical utilization of urine cytology results should be based on diagnostic findings and the clinical scenario. The scenarios can be broken into patients with and without history of urothelial malignancy, and findings can be categorized as benign, suspicious, and malignant.

Patients with findings such as hematuria or refractory irritative voiding symptoms suggesting malignancy but no history of urothelial malignancy will usually not require repeat investigation if initial evaluation by cystoscopy, upper tract imaging with computed tomography (CT) urography, and urinary cytology fail to identify abnormalities. We regard cytology findings of benign or atypia to carry no implications of future malignancy, and these should not drive further testing. However, cytology findings suspicious for unrecognized malignancy merit meticulous investigation and careful surveillance involving repeat testing in no more than 3 months. A low threshold to perform bilateral ureteronephroscopy, combined with random bladder biopsies and prostatic urethral biopsy, is in order, and based on the high positive predictive value we regard these as almost mandatory if the cytologic diagnosis identifies malignancy that is not otherwise known and addressed.

Patients with known bladder malignancy concurrent to positive cytological diagnosis are managed per the urologists' routine to address the known malignancy. A European Organisation for Research and Treatment of Cancer (EORTC) retrospective review found that only 10% of random biopsies were positive (3.5% CIS) and concluded such biopsies were not routinely warranted [5]. However, Fujimoto prospectively evaluated the role of random biopsies of normal-appearing urothelium and found cancer in only 8 of 100 biopsies, 5 of which were CIS. Notably, their random biopsies were positive primarily in the setting of positive cytology, so positive cytology in the setting of suspected low-grade tumor is a reasonable indication for random bladder biopsies [6].

The final related setting involves patients under surveillance for bladder cancer recurrence. Based on low negative predictive values, normal readings should not greatly affect treatment algorithms. However, a positive reading in the absence of recognized recurrence merits meticulous investigation as described previously for the same situation in patients without history of bladder cancer. Furthermore, consideration of fluorescence is reasonable in either setting.

Conclusion

Urine cytology provides insight into the likelihood of urothelial cancer. Negative readings are of limited value, but positive readings should be regarded as signifying the presence of malignancy until proven otherwise. Even then, careful surveillance to assure that misdiagnosis has not occurred is in order. Direct collaboration between pathologist and urologist can be highly beneficial to identify cases where more careful investigation is necessary.

References

1. Epstein JI, Amin MB, Reuter VR, Mostofi FK. The World Health Organization/International Society of Urological Pathology consensus classification of urothelial (transitional cell) neoplasms of the urinary bladder. Bladder Consensus Conference Committee. Am J Surg Pathol. 1998;22:1435–48.
2. Halling K, King W, Sokolova I, et al. A comparison of cytology and fluorescence in situ hybridization for the detection of urothelial carcinoma. J Urol. 2000; 164:1768–75.
3. Grossman HB, Messing E, Soloway M, Tomera K, Katz G, Berger Y, et al. Surveillance for recurrent bladder cancer using a point-of-care proteomic assay. JAMA. 2006;295(3):299–305.
4. Jocham D, Witjes F, Wagner S, et al. Improved detection and treatment of bladder cancer using hexaminolevulinate imaging: a prospective, phase III multicenter study. J Urol. 2005;174:862–6.
5. van der Meijden AP, Oosterlinck W, Brausi M, et al. Significance of bladder biopsies in Ta, T1 bladder tumors: a report from the EORTC Genito-Urinary Tract Cancer Cooperative Group EORTC-GU Group Superficial Bladder Committee. Eur Urol. 1999;35: 267–71.
6. Fujimoto N, Haradas S, Terado M, et al. Multiple biopsies of normal looking urothelium in patients with superficial bladder cancer: are they necessary? Int J Urol. 2003;10:631–5.

17 Pathology–Endoscopy Correlations of Bladder, Urachal, and Urethral Lesions

Gregory T. MacLennan, William A. Larchian, Liang Cheng, Donald R. Bodner, Brent M. Hardin, Howard B. Goldman, Edward E. Cherullo, and Lee E. Ponsky

Introduction

Through experience, urologists learn to recognize endoscopic abnormalities and—in the great majority of cases—they are able to predict with considerable accuracy the final pathological diagnosis. In this chapter, we present a number of endoscopic images and illustrate the pathological findings that correlate with these images. In many instances, the pathological images are derived from the exact endoscopic case shown. Although this chapter is by no means an exhaustive treatise on the spectrum of pathological conditions of the urinary tract, we hope the reader finds the correlations interesting and informative.

Bladder

Normal Urothelium

The normal urothelial lining has been discussed in detail in Chap. 1. On cystoscopy, the bladder wall appears white-gray in color, with thin vessels apparent below the luminal surface (Fig. 17.1a). On histology, this appearance correlates with a normal urothelial thickness of 4–7

G.T. MacLennan (✉)
Department of Pathology, University Hospitals Case Medical Center, Case Western Reserve University, 2085 Adelbert Road, Cleveland, OH 44106, USA
e-mail: gtm2@case.edu

W.A. Larchian
Department of Urology, Case Western Reserve University School of Medicine, 11000 Euclid Avenue, Cleveland, OH 44106, USA
e-mail: william.larchian@uhhospitals.org

L. Cheng
Indiana University School of Medicine, 350 West 11th Street, Rm 4010, Indianapolis, IN 46202, USA
e-mail: lcheng@iupui.edu

D.R. Bodner
Department of Urology, UH Case Western Medical Center, Case Western Reserve University, 11100 Euclid Avenue, Suite L84, Cleveland, OH 44115, USA
e-mail: donald.bodner@uhhospitals.org

B.M. Hardin
University of Tennessee Graduate School of Medicine, 1924 Alcoa Highway, Knoxville, TN 37920, USA

H.B. Goldman
Cleveland Clinic, Glickman Urological Kidney Institute, 9500 Euclid Avenue, Q10, Cleveland, OH 44195, USA
e-mail: goldmah@ccf.org

E.E. Cherullo
Department of Urology, UH Case Western Medical Center, 11100 Euclid Avenue #4500, Cleveland, OH 44106, USA
e-mail: edward.cherullo@uhhospitals.org

L.E. Ponsky
University Hospitals Case Medical Center, Urology Institute, 11100 Euclid Avenue, Cleveland, OH 44106, USA
e-mail: lee.ponsky@uhhospitals.org

D.E. Hansel et al. (eds.), *The Urinary Tract: A Comprehensive Guide to Patient Diagnosis and Management*, DOI 10.1007/978-1-4614-5320-8_17, © Springer Science+Business Media New York 2012

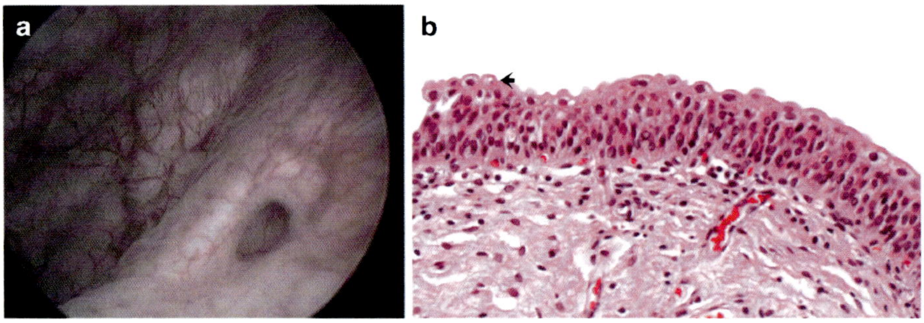

Fig. 17.1 Normal urothelium. (**a**) Normal ureteral orifice and normal bladder mucosa. (**b**) Normal urothelium and underlying lamina propria in the bladder. The *arrow* indicates a layer of umbrella cells at the surface

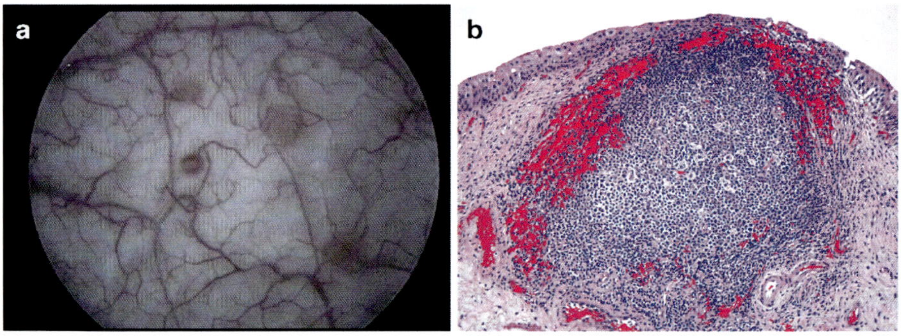

Fig. 17.2 Follicular cystitis. (**a**) Multiple discrete small mucosal irregularities are present. They do not significantly obscure the vasculature beneath them. (**b**) Lamina propria contains lymphoid follicles oftentimes with a germinal center

cell layers, consisting of pale to pink urothelial cells lined by a surface layer of umbrella cells (Fig. 17.1b). Normal urothelial cells show centrally located nuclei with dispersed chromatin and inconspicuous nucleoli; in contrast, umbrella cells may demonstrate more overt atypia and may be multinucleated. Underlying the urothelium is the lamina propria, muscularis propria (detrusor muscle), and perivesical fat, respectively.

Follicular Cystitis

Follicular cystitis is an associated finding in up to 40% of bladder cancer patients and in about 35% of patients with recurrent urinary infection. Endoscopically, the bladder mucosa appears studded with tiny pink, white, or gray nodules (Fig. 17.2a). Microscopically, the lamina propria contains lymphoid follicles that usually contain germinal centers (Fig. 17.2b).

Cystitis Cystica Et Glandularis

This benign condition is characterized by cystically dilated nests of urothelium below the luminal surface that may appear as localized or florid cystic dilations of the urothelial surface (Fig. 17.3a). Microscopically, these lesions demonstrate a benign histology and often show characteristic eosinophilic secretions (Fig. 17.3b). Although considered one entity, cystitis glandularis has been distinguished by the presence of columnar cells and/or goblet cells that are supported by urothelial cells. Cystitis cystica et glandularis is very common and may be considered within the spectrum of normal bladder.

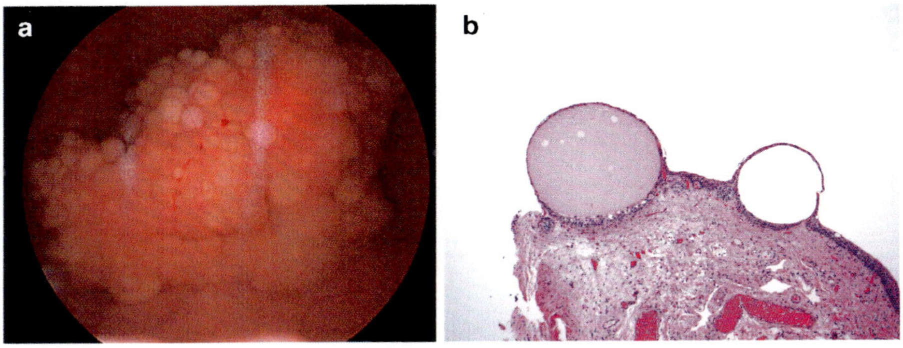

Fig. 17.3 Cystitis cystica. (**a**) The mucosal surface is studded with innumerable bleb-like lesions that appear to contain straw-colored fluid. The remainder of the mucosa looks normal. (**b**) Normal urothelial cells often with eosinophilic secretions. The lumens of some cells are lined by taller columnar-type cells, consistent with cystitis glandularis of the typical type. The cystic spaces lined by goblet cells comprise cystitis glandularis of the intestinal type, also sometimes designated intestinal metaplasia

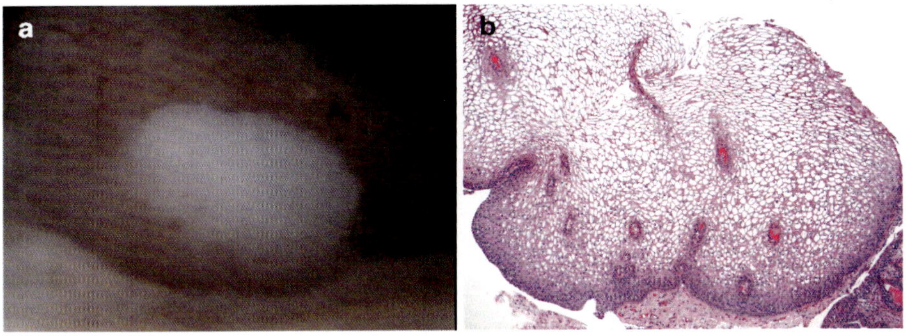

Fig. 17.4 Squamous metaplasia. (**a**) Lesions tend to have a *white* color and are elevated. (**b**) Cells are lined by squamous epithelium, rather than urothelium and do not have atypia. This example does not have surface keratin

Squamous Metaplasia

Squamous metaplasia is a common finding in patients suffering from severe chronic cystitis. Squamous metaplasia appears endoscopically as a gray-white patch or nodule, and is most often located distally in the bladder (Fig. 17.4a). On histology, the lesions consist of layers of squamous epithelium, lacking cytologic atypia (Fig. 17.4b), with or without an overlying layer of keratin.

Melanosis

Melanosis is a descriptive term for the presence of dark brown or brown-black tissue pigmentation due to melanin deposition. Fewer than a dozen cases of melanosis of bladder mucosa have been reported. At cystoscopy, the bladder mucosa exhibits multiple widespread areas of black or dark brown discoloration, without any particular site predilection (Fig. 17.5a). Microscopically, aggregates of black or dark brown granules are evident in the lamina propria and sometimes also in urothelial cells (Fig. 17.5b).

Amyloidosis

Amyloidosis encompasses a heterogeneous group of diseases in which soluble proteins aggregate and accumulate extracellularly in a single organ

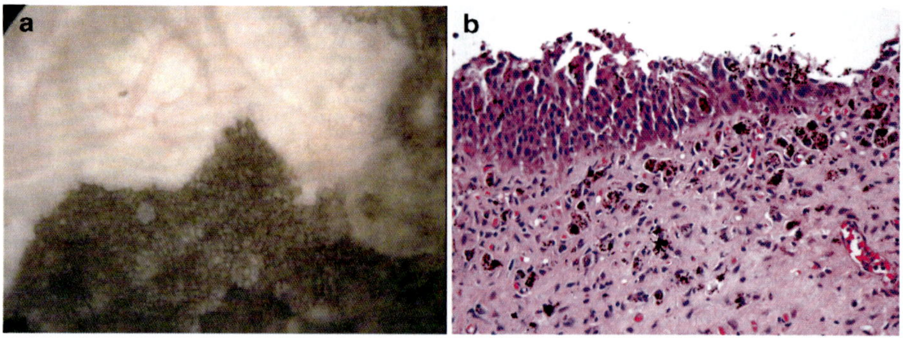

Fig. 17.5 Melanosis of the bladder. (**a**) Large areas of *brownish/black* discoloration represent sites of melanosis. (**b**) Microscopically, abundant minute *brown/black* granules are seen in the lamina propria and within surface urothelial cells

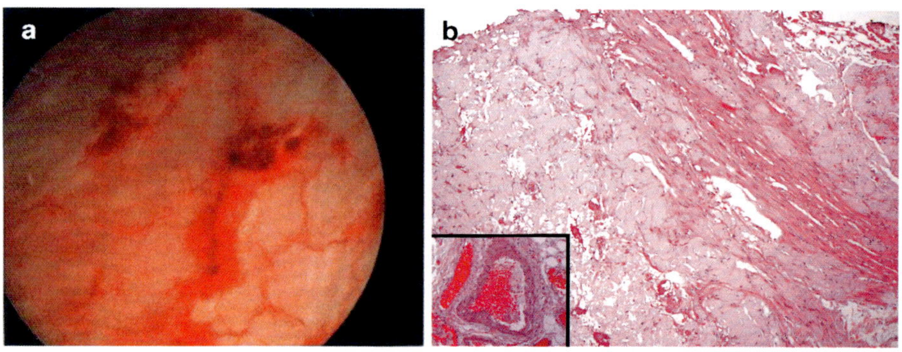

Fig. 17.6 Amyloidosis of the bladder. (**a**) Histologically, deposits of acellular eosinophilic material in the lamina propria are seen and surround and separate the fibers of detrusor muscle. (**b**) *Inset*: A blood vessel from a separate section in this case is normal

(localized) or in multiple sites (systemic). It is designated by internists and pathologists as primary amyloidosis if associated with a plasma cell dyscrasia, and as secondary amyloidosis if coupled with a chronic systemic inflammatory disorder. On endoscopy, amyloidosis varies from multiple yellow plaques or nodules studding the bladder lining to solitary or multiple ulcerated polypoid masses, or to diffuse irregular thickening of the bladder wall (Fig. 17.6a). Histologically, primary and secondary bladder amyloidosis exhibit somewhat different features. Primary amyloidosis typically shows extensive deposits of acellular, eosinophilic material in the lamina propria as well as in the detrusor muscle (Fig. 17.6b). In contrast, the amyloid depositions in cases of secondary bladder involvement by systemic amyloidosis tend to accumulate preferentially within mural blood vessels, perhaps accounting for the propensity for massive bleeding in some of these cases. The diagnosis of amyloidosis is facilitated by the fact that amyloid shows positive histochemical staining for Congo red stain and exhibits a characteristic "apple green" birefringence when viewed on polarized microscopy.

Schistosomiasis

Schistosomiasis is endemic to Eastern Africa, the Middle East, and Western Asia. The species

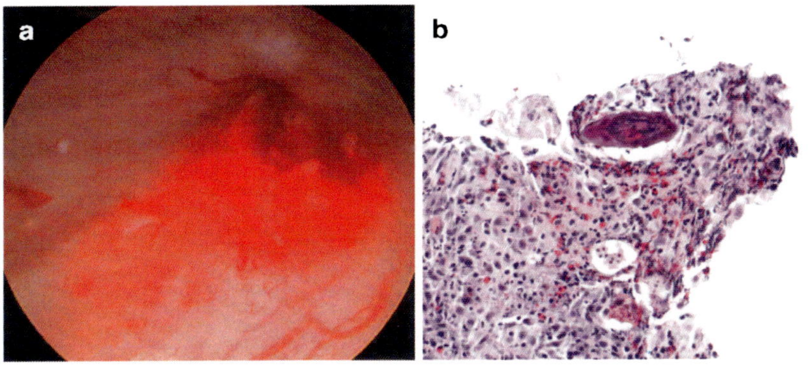

Fig. 17.7 Schistosomiasis of the bladder. (**a**) Cystoscopy reveals a hyperemic and irregularly polypoid lesions. (**b**) Histologic foreign-body reaction with granulomatous inflammation and eosinophils is shown. A calcified *S. haematobium* egg is illustrated. Figures reprinted with permission from Hardin et al. [1]

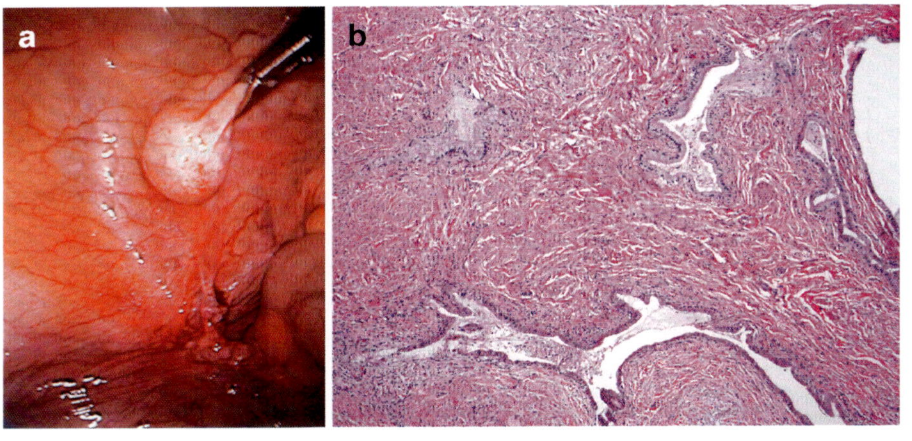

Fig. 17.8 Endocervicosis of bladder. (**a**) This nodular lesion may occur anywhere in the bladder. Image courtesy of Raymond Onders, MD. (**b**) Irregular glands, some containing *pale blue* wispy mucin, are randomly interspersed between detrusor muscle bundles. The glands are lined by a single layer of columnar cells that lack cytologic atypia and mitotic activity and have abundant pale cytoplasm

S. haematobium is capable of living part of its life cycle in humans and gains access by penetrating the skin of a person standing in fresh water, then migrates to the urogenital tract, especially the bladder, and eventually matures into adult worms. The mature worms lay eggs in the bladder wall that cause mucosal edema, hyperemia, and urothelial ulceration, forming reddened plaques near the ureteral orifices and on the trigone (Fig. 17.7a). Foreign-body granulomatous inflammation with giant cells, and often abundant eosinophils (Fig. 17.7b), is initiated by the dead calcified eggs that may appear endoscopically as "sandy patches."

Endocervicosis

This rare Mullerian lesion involves the bladder infrequently, with most patients between 30 and 50 years of age. The common complaints are irritative bladder symptoms, lower abdominal pain, and/or hematuria. A history of previous caesarian section is common in these patients. Lesions may involve any level of the bladder wall and are evident as mural nodules at cystoscopy or laparoscopy (Fig. 17.8a). Histologically, the nodules are composed of mucin-containing glandular structures of variable shape and size, mainly involving the muscularis propria and/or outer bladder wall,

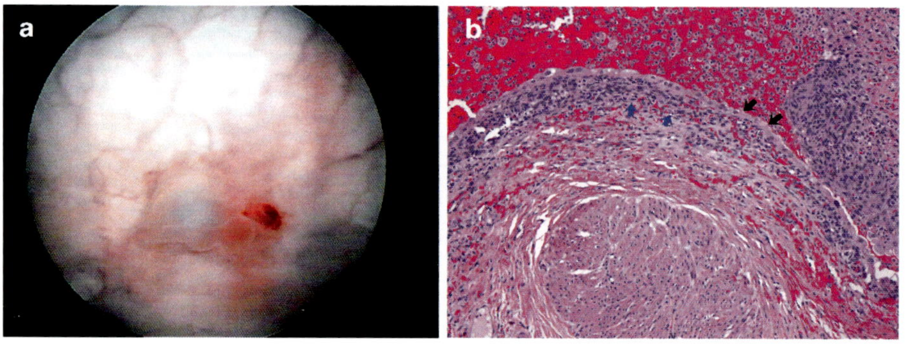

Fig. 17.9 Endometriosis of bladder. (**a**) A typical congested vascular mucosal nodule. (**b**) A blood-filled space is enclosed by endometrial tissue: a layer of endometrial epithelial cells (*black arrows*), under which is a layer of small dark endometrial stromal cells (*blue arrows*). A thick bundle of detrusor muscle is seen at *bottom*

and lined by a single layer of columnar or flat cuboidal cells (Fig. 17.8b). The glands appear remarkably similar to the normal histology of the uterine endocervix.

Endometriosis

Endometriosis is defined as the presence of endometrial glands and stroma outside the confines of the endometrial cavity and uterine musculature. About 12% of women between the ages of 25 and 40 are affected by endometriosis; of these, about 1–2% have endometriosis involving the urinary tract, with frequency of bladder, ureter, and kidney involvement of 40:5:1, respectively. Endoscopically, endometriosis may appear as blue, red, black, or brown nodules; the mucosa overlying the nodules may be normal or ulcerated (Fig. 17.9a). Microscopically, the lesions consist of glandular spaces lined by endometrial epithelium and surrounded by a variable amount of endometrial stroma (Fig. 17.9b).

Nephrogenic Adenoma

Nephrogenic adenoma is a reactive mucosal lesion that most often occurs in the bladder, but may also occur in the renal pelvis, ureter, or urethra. In most patients, its presence can be attributed to an initiating factor such as trauma, calculus disease, infection, or recent genitourinary surgery. On endoscopy, lesions may be single or multiple, polypoid, sessile, or papillary (Fig. 17.10a). Although usually less than 1 cm in diameter, a lesion can be over 4 cm in greatest dimension. Tubular, cystic, papillary, or polypoid structures are common, and cells may occasionally be arranged as small solid sheets (Fig. 17.10b). The cells are generally uniform and cytologically benign, with virtually no mitotic activity, but hobnail cells and cells with clear cytoplasm may be noted focally.

Flat Urothelial Carcinoma In Situ

Flat urothelial carcinoma in situ (CIS) is an intraepithelial carcinoma that may occur de novo or in the setting of a background high-grade papillary or invasive urothelial carcinoma. Patients with CIS are typically men over 50 years old, with hematuria, irritative voiding symptoms, and/or bladder pain of a severity suggestive of interstitial cystitis. Cystoscopy may show areas of velvety mucosal erythema (Fig. 17.11a); however, the mucosa may appear entirely unremarkable endoscopically. Urothelial involvement is commonly multifocal. Microscopically, CIS is characterized by flat, disordered proliferation of urothelial cells with severe cytologic atypia

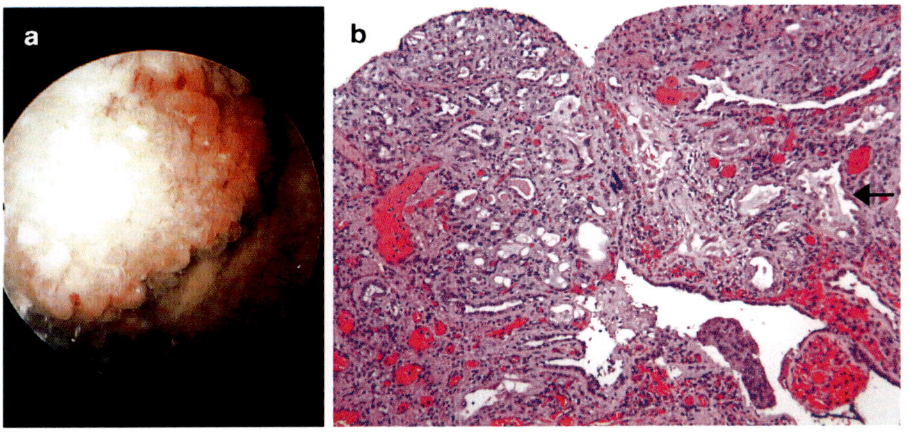

Fig. 17.10 Nephrogenic adenoma. (**a**) A papillary/polypoid lesion typical of nephrogenic adenoma. (**b**) The stroma is occupied by numerous small tubular structures lined by epithelial cells, some of which show hobnail morphology (*arrow at right*). Some tubules contain wispy pale blue mucinous material. Scattered inflammatory cells are present in the stroma

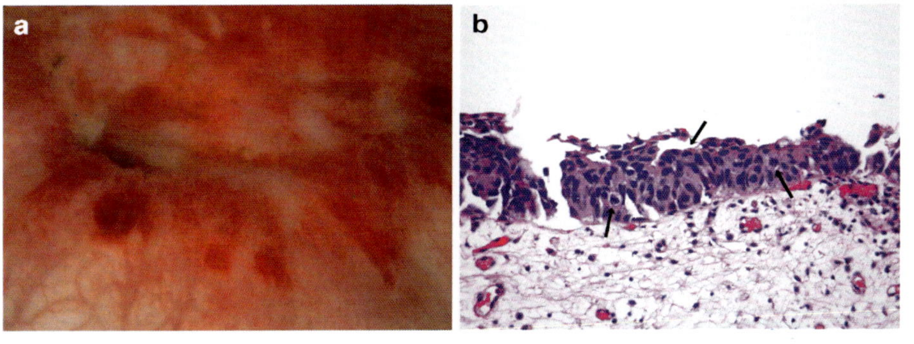

Fig. 17.11 Flat urothelial carcinoma in situ. (**a**) The urothelium may appear normal but many times may have an erythematous and slightly edematous appearance. Image courtesy of Allan Seftel, MD. (**b**) A disordered proliferation of malignant urothelial cells that exhibit a high nuclear/cytoplasmic ratio, nuclear pleomorphism, irregular nuclear contours, and nuclear hyperchromasia is seen. Cellular polarity is lost. Mitotic figures (*arrows*) are abundant, and are not basally located

(Fig. 17.11b). The tumor cells show marked architectural disorganization with loss of cell polarity and cohesiveness, and are typically large and pleomorphic with moderate to abundant cytoplasm, although they are sometimes small with a high nucleus-to-cytoplasmic ratio. Tumor cell nuclei exhibit coarse clumped chromatin and often have prominent and sometimes multiple nucleoli. Mitotic figures are frequent and sometimes atypical and may be found in any level of the urothelium.

Papillary Urothelial Neoplasm of Low Malignant Potential

Papillary urothelial neoplasm of low malignant potential (PUNLMP) is a low-grade urothelial tumor that occurs predominantly in males with a mean age of 65 years. Cystoscopically, PUNLMP is typically 1–2 cm in greatest dimension and located on the bladder lateral wall or near the ureteric orifices (Fig. 17.12a). Its cystoscopic appearance has been likened to that of "seaweed

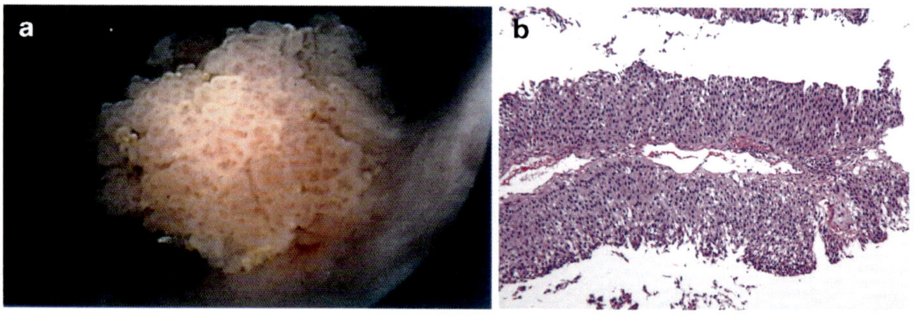

Fig. 17.12 (**a**) Papillary urothelial neoplasm of low malignant potential (PUNLMP). (**b**) Tumor cells have a low nuclear/cytoplasmic ratio and their nuclei are of uniform size and shape. Mitotic figures are absent or rare

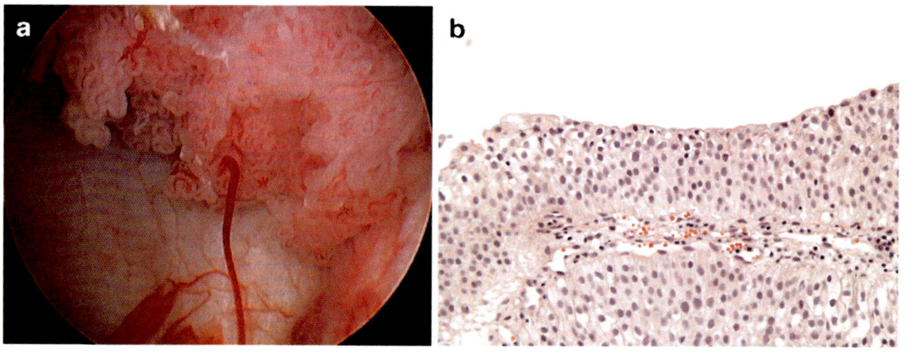

Fig. 17.13 Low-grade papillary urothelial carcinoma. (**a**) These lesions are universally papillary and exophytic. (**b**) Cell nuclei are moderately variable in size and shape with some nuclei being hyperchromatic and some having one or more distinct nucleoli. Mitotic figures are readily found

in the ocean." Microscopically, it has a papillary architecture lined by a markedly thickened urothelial lining that is otherwise normal in appearance (Fig. 17.12b). Mitotic figures are infrequent, and, if present, they are usually found only in the basal layer.

Low-Grade Papillary Urothelial Carcinoma

Low-grade papillary urothelial carcinoma occurs predominantly in males, with a male:female ratio of 3:1 and a mean age of 70 years (range 28–90 years). Most patients present with some form of hematuria. Although most have a single tumor in the posterior or lateral bladder wall, 22% of patients with low-grade papillary urothelial carcinoma have two or more tumors. Cystoscopically, papillary architecture is readily apparent (Fig. 17.13a). Microscopically, low-grade papillary urothelial carcinoma is composed of papillary fronds lined by multiple layers of urothelial cells with mild to moderate architectural and cytologic atypia; a characteristic finding is the presence of enlarged, hyperchromatic nuclei (Fig. 17.13b). Mitotic figures may be identified and can be found at any level of the urothelium.

High-Grade Papillary Urothelial Carcinoma

Patients with high-grade papillary urothelial carcinoma frequently present with hematuria. Endoscopically, these cancers may be papillary, sessile and nodular, or ulcerative (Fig. 17.14a). Tumors may be solitary or multiple. In high-grade

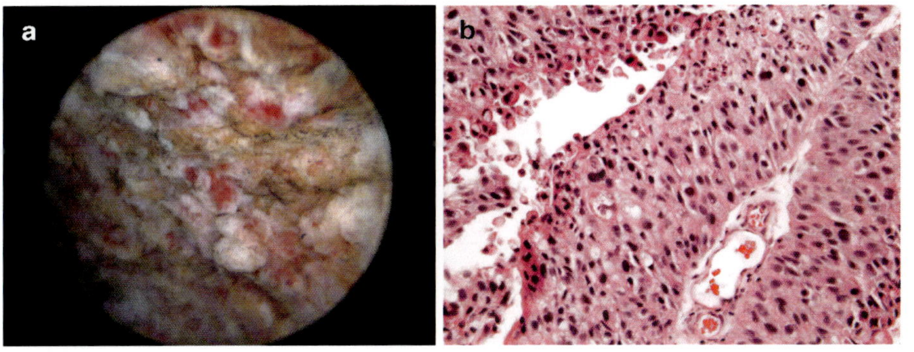

Fig. 17.14 High-grade urothelial carcinoma. (**a**) The lesion is erythematous, nodular, and highly irregular. Image courtesy of Benjamin Canales, MD. (**b**) Histological examination reveals marked cellular atypia, with complete loss of cellular orientation. Nuclei are large and hyperchromatic, and many have prominent nucleoli. Tumor cells have high nuclear/cytoplasmic ratios, and vary considerably in shape and size. Abundant mitotic figures are present

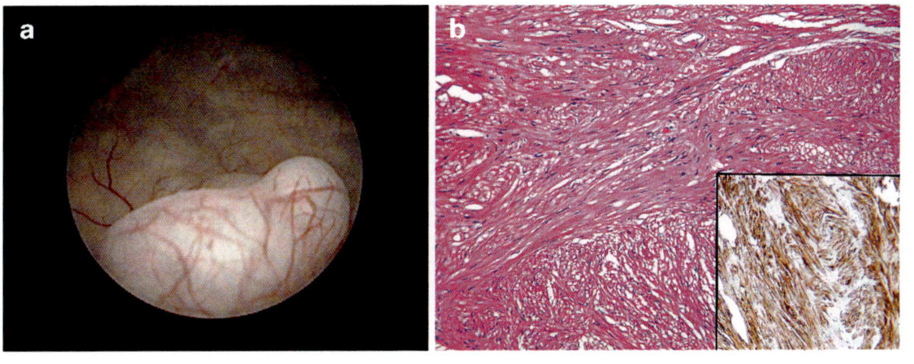

Fig. 17.15 Leiomyoma of the bladder. (**a**) Cystoscopy reveals a mural mass covered by normal mucosa. (**b**) Intersecting fascicles of spindle cells, morphologically suggestive of smooth muscle bundles, are seen. There is a lack of nuclear atypia, necrosis, and mitotic activity but abundant eosinophilic cytoplasm. Tumor cells show positive immunostaining for desmin, a smooth muscle marker (*inset*)

urothelial carcinomas, the tumor cells show profound loss of polarity and marked cytologic atypia (Fig. 17.14b); prominent nucleoli and numerous mitotic figures—often atypical—are usually present.

Leiomyoma of the Bladder

Leiomyomas are benign tumors of smooth muscle origin. Although bladder leiomyoma is uncommon—and accounts for less than 1% of bladder tumors—it is the most common benign soft tissue neoplasm of the bladder. Its occurrence in the bladder may be related to hormonal influences and thus the great majority of bladder leiomyomas arise in women in the third through sixth decades of life, with an average patient age of 44 years. Bladder leiomyomas are most commonly found within the bladder, but may also be extravesical or intramural. Cystoscopy discloses a mural mass with normal overlying mucosa (Fig. 17.15a). Bladder leiomyomas range in size from a few millimeters to as large as 30 cm, weighing up to 9 kg. Microscopically, leiomyomas are composed of fascicles of smooth muscle cells with moderate to abundant eosinophilic cytoplasm (Fig. 17.15b). Their nuclei are oval to cigar-shaped, centrally located, blunt-ended, and devoid of significant atypical features such as hyperchromasia,

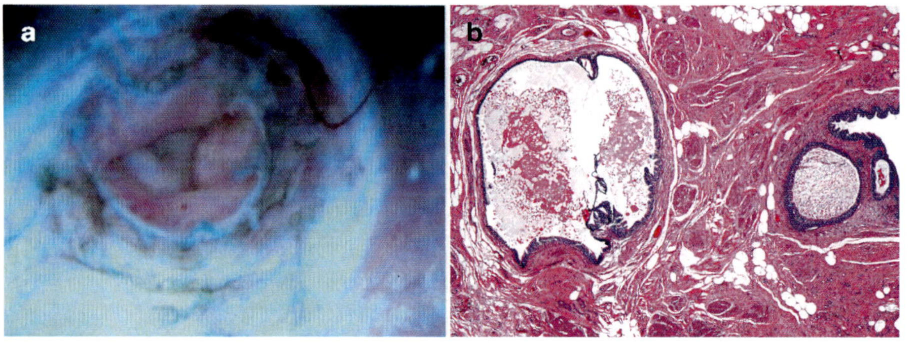

Fig. 17.16 Urachal cyst. (**a**) Located in the dome of the bladder, the mucosa overlying a urachal cyst is normal. The bladder tissue overlying the cyst has been resected in this figure. Photo courtesy of Tom Leininger, M.D. (**b**) These cystic structures are lined by flat cuboidal or columnar epithelium

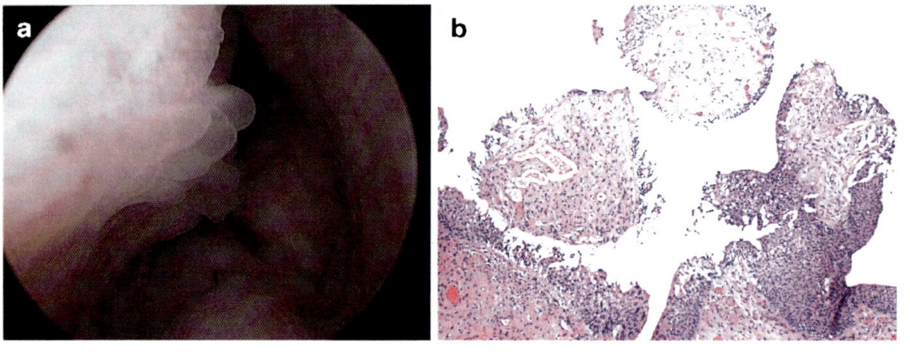

Fig. 17.17 Polypoid urethritis. (**a**) Often presenting with hematuria, these polypoid lesions may occur as solitary or multiple lesions. (**b**) Microscopic evaluation reveals edematous stroma infiltrated by acute and chronic inflammatory cells and prominent blood vessels

pleomorphism, or individual cell necrosis, and demonstrate minimal mitotic activity.

Urachal Lesions

Urachal Cyst

In early fetal life, the urachus connects the apex of the bladder to the allantois, located at the umbilicus. Failure of obliteration of the urachus, which usually occurs by the fourth month in utero, results in a number of malformations that may be complicated by abdominal pain, chronic drainage from the umbilicus, infection, abscess formation, or stone formation. Urachal cysts are classified as juxtaumbilical, intermediate, juxtavesical, giant, or multiple. Endoscopically within the bladder, a urachal cyst is evident as a mural nodule in the dome or posterior wall of the bladder, with normal overlying mucosa (Fig. 17.16a). Microscopically, urachal cysts are lined by flattened epithelium that may be cuboidal, columnar, or of urothelial type (Fig. 17.16b).

Urethra

Polypoid Urethritis

Polypoid urethritis is a nonneoplastic condition that is often reactive in nature. It is usually noted incidentally during cystoscopy as single or multiple polypoid or papillary growths in the prostatic

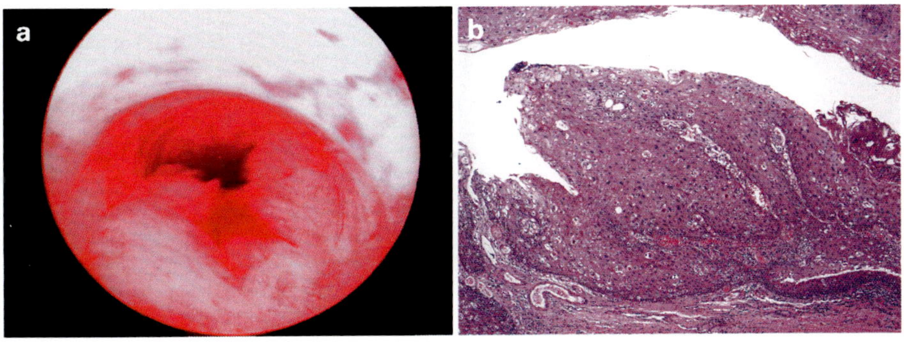

Fig. 17.18 Urethral condyloma. (**a**) Occurring as solitary or multiple lesions, condyloma appears as whitish, raised mucosal lesions. (**b**) The squamous epithelium is proliferative and thickened but shows delayed maturation. The nuclei of the squamous cells are hyperchromatic and irregular in shape and size (koilocytic atypia), and many have clear perinuclear halos

urethra near the verumontanum in males or at the bladder neck in females (Fig. 17.17a). Histologically, the polypoid protrusions are the result of edematous stroma containing prominent blood vessels and chronic inflammatory cells that bulges up into the bladder lumen (Fig. 17.17b). The urothelial lining may show ulceration, metaplastic changes, or other findings such as urethritis cystica.

Urethral Condyloma

This lesion, which is estimated to account for up to 30% of male urethral lesions, is caused by human papillomavirus and is sexually transmitted. Endoscopically, lesions appear as solitary or multiple white papillomatous mucosal excrescences (Fig. 17.18a). Histologically, condylomata consist of flat or papillary hyperplastic squamous epithelium, with nuclear features collectively called "koilocytic atypia"—eccentrically placed hyperchromatic nuclei with irregular nuclear outlines and cytoplasmic retraction artifact that produces a perinuclear halo effect (Fig. 17.18b).

Benign Prostatic Hyperplasia

Nodular hyperplasia or benign prostatic hyperplasia (BPH) consists of overgrowth of prostatic glandular epithelium and fibromuscular stroma of the transition zone and periurethral area. Three pathologic changes are involved in its genesis: nodule formation, diffuse enlargement of the transition zone and periurethral tissue, and enlargement of nodules. In relatively younger men, diffuse enlargement predominates, whereas in older men, epithelial proliferation and expansile growth of existing nodules predominate. The proportion of epithelium to stroma increases as obstructive symptoms become more severe. The endoscopic findings are familiar to urologists: encroachment of prostatic tissue upon the prostatic urethra by enlarged lobes of prostatic tissue that may also project into the bladder lumen.

On gross inspection, nodular hyperplasia consists of variably sized nodules that are soft or firm, rubbery, and yellow-gray, and bulge from the cut surface upon transection. Prostatic calculi and zones of infarction may be present. Histologically, nodular hyperplasia is composed of varying proportions of epithelium and stroma that is comprised of fibrous connective tissue and smooth muscle.

Ureter

Ureterocele

This is a congenital distal ureteral dilatation that protrudes into the bladder lumen and occasion-

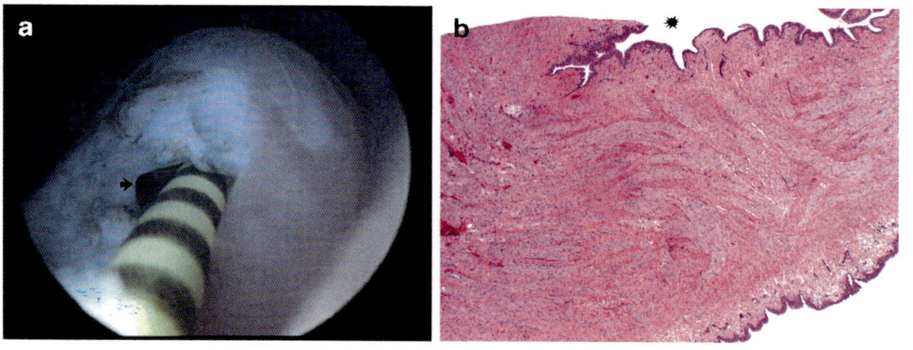

Fig. 17.19 Ureterocele. (**a**) A large submucosal lesion is visualized as it protrudes into the vesical cavity with normal overlying mucosa. *Arrow* indicates the left ureteral orifice. (**b**) Although little muscle may be present, this example reveals thick musculature. The ureteral lumen is at *top center*, indicated by the *starburst* symbol; the bladder lumen is at *bottom right*

ally into the urethra (Fig. 17.19a). It typically involves the upper pole ureter of a duplex system and rarely occurs in a single ureter. More than two-thirds of ureteroceles are accompanied by segmental dysplasia of the upper pole of the kidney. The mucosa overlying the bulging ureterocele appears normal endoscopically. Microscopic evaluation of the ureterocele wall may reveal muscular hypertrophy, muscular atrophy, or absence of musculature (Fig. 17.19b).

Bibliography

1. MacLennan GT, Cheng L. Atlas of genitourinary pathology. London, UK: Springer; 2011.
2. Hardin BM, White WM, Clark CT, MacLennan GT. Urinary tract schistosomiasis. J Urol. 2010;184(5):2136–7.

Molecular Pathogenesis of Bladder Cancer

18

Luigi Marchionni and Dan Theodorescu

Introduction

The most common variant of bladder cancer in Western countries is urothelial carcinoma (UCC), formerly known as "transitional cell carcinoma," which has significant health costs and morbidity [1,2]. This neoplasm has two distinct clinical presentations: approximately 30% of UCs are muscle-invasive (MIUC), while the remainder present with nonmuscle-invasive disease (NMIUC). These are not mere pathological distinctions, but rather two distinct clinical entities, which show different outcomes and are therefore treated differently. For instance, NMIUC (corresponding to stages Ta, Tis, and T1) is generally treated by endoscopic transurethral tumor resection, which may be followed by intravesical immunotherapy or chemotherapy. This approach generally results in good outcomes, with 85% 10-year disease-specific survival for Ta, and 70% for T1 stage disease [3]. On the contrary, patients with MIUC are generally treated with radical cystectomy and bilateral pelvic iliac lymphadenectomy, which can be preceded or followed by chemotherapy [4]. In spite of this more aggressive treatment, however, approximately half of the patients in this group will experience treatment failure within 2 years [4].

It is notable that these two clinical–pathological presentations not only require alternative diagnostic and therapeutic management, but also represent two different disease entities, which are mediated by specific and distinct underlying molecular mechanisms, and therefore call for the development and use of distinct sets of prognostic and predictive molecular biomarkers. For this reason, we will summarize the current knowledge on the molecular pathogenesis of the two forms of UC separately.

Molecular Pathogenesis of Nonmuscle-invasive Urothelial Carcinoma

Over the past several years, a growing body of evidence on the molecular mechanisms underlying the pathogenesis of nonmuscle-invasive urothelial carcinoma (NMIUC) has been obtained from the analysis of in vivo and in vitro models, as well as from clinical specimens. Overall, such studies have identified a number of gain-of-function mutations in genes within defined signaling pathways, as well as loss of specific tumor-suppressor genes. Such data

L. Marchionni (✉)
Department of Oncology, Johns Hopkins University School of Medicine, 1550 Orleans Street, The Koch Cancer Research Building, Suite 1M52, Baltimore, MD 21231, USA
e-mail: marchion@jhu.edu

D. Theodorescu
University of Colorado Cancer Center, Consortium Comprehensive Cancer Center, 13001 E. 17th Pl. MS #F-434, Aurora, CO 80045, USA
e-mail: dan.theodorescu@ucdenver.edu

D.E. Hansel et al. (eds.), *The Urinary Tract: A Comprehensive Guide to Patient Diagnosis and Management*, DOI 10.1007/978-1-4614-5320-8_18, © Springer Science+Business Media New York 2012

clearly implicated a prominent pathogenic role for the activation of tyrosine kinase receptors, such as the fibroblast growth factor receptor FGFR3, the *HRAS* oncogene, and downstream mitotic pathways [5,6], as well as alterations involving chromosome 9. A better understanding of such molecular changes in the context of NMIUC pathogenesis is of paramount relevance, since many of the proteins involved in these biological processes and signaling pathways may represent novel therapeutic targets.

Role of *HRAS* in Urothelial Cancer

HRAS is a proto-oncogene belonging to the Ras GTPase family. Activation of Ras proteins can be elicited by physiologic stimuli or through mutation. Once activated, these proteins signal to downstream pathway effectors involved in survival, cell growth, differentiation, and migration [7]. These downstream pathways include PI3 kinase [8], RalGEF [9], and the Raf-MAP kinase [10].

The mutant form of the *HRAS* oncogene was identified and cloned in 1982 from the T24 cancer cell line, which was originally obtained from a high-grade papillary urothelial carcinoma [11–13]. In subsequent years, *HRAS* has been demonstrated to be the most commonly mutated RAS family oncogene in UCC [14–16], and a number of distinct point mutations have been identified, with those occurring at codons 12, 13, and 61 being the most frequent in bladder cancer [17–20]. Interestingly, such mutations determine the production of mutant proteins that lack the capability of hydrolyzing GTP to GDP, and that therefore are constitutively active and capable of transforming NIH 3T3 fibroblasts [12,21]. Over the years, a number of other additional activating mutations of the *HRAS*, *NRAS*, and *KRAS* genes have been also documented [22], with rates between 15 and 30%, depending on the relative composition of NMIUC and MIUC of the cohorts that were studied [23,24].

Despite the early identification of *HRAS*, the complete characterization of the role of *HRAS* mutation in UCC has proven complex, with a number of functional and epidemiologic studies showing conflicting results. It was initially thought that *HRAS* overexpression and its mutation were linked to invasive UCC. One early study reported that *HRAS*-mediated transformation of the NMIUC cell line RT4 could modify the cellular phenotype, making it more similar to that of cell lines derived from UCC of higher grade and stage [25]. Similarly, another report showed that high-grade UCCs were overrepresented in a subset of 30 neoplasms carrying a specific *HRAS* mutation out of a total of 67 tumors analyzed [23], and lower *HRAS* expression levels were demonstrated in the T24 cell line as compared to its highly tumorigenic counterpart T24T [26]. In contrast to such findings, the evaluation of a larger cohort of 152 bladder tumors showed that the presence of *HRAS* mutations was not associated with either grade or stage [27], and another study on a cohort of 100 patients showed that *HRAS* mutations, as identified from DNA analysis in urine specimens, were better at identifying low-grade UCC (47%) than cytology alone (16%) [28].

The causal role of the *Ras* oncogene in the pathogenesis of NMIUC was definitively established by the specific expression of *HRAS* in the urothelium of transgenic mice. In this study, Zhang and colleagues used a urothelial-specific uroplakin promoter to drive the expression of mutant *HRAS* in the bladder of transgenic mice [29]. This investigation revealed that low copy numbers of mutant *HRAS* were sufficient to cause the development of urothelial hyperplasia, followed by the onset of superficial papillary tumors [29].

Moreover, this group also demonstrated that high copy numbers of mutated *HRAS* induced urothelial hyperplasia, followed by accelerated onset of superficial tumors. It is notable that none of these tumors showed progression to invasive carcinoma in the 26-month follow-up interval—equivalent to the entire lifespan of a normal mouse. The same group also found that the formation of superficial papillary tumors mediated by *HRAS* was independent of the loss of function of the protein encoded by the *TP53* gene, a prominent tumor-suppressor that is mutated in most human cancers and is frequently deleted or mutated in the majority of invasive UCCs [30]. Specifically, mice expressing an activated form of *HRAS* were bred with mice harboring either a dominant-negative *TP53* protein or a *TP53* knockout. The progeny derived from the former cross exhibited urothelial hyperplasia and dysplasia, while only the mice obtained from the latter cross developed superficial papillary UCC of either low or high grade [30].

Finally, a more recent study by Mo and colleagues demonstrated that mutant *HRAS* dosage is responsible for the progression to papillary UCC [31]. In this study, it was reported that mice homozygous for the mutant-activated form of *HRAS* showed early onset of superficial tumors, while the development of superficial papillary tumors was not observed in heterozygous mice, independent of the mutational status of other potential tumor-suppressor genes [31]. Taken together, these findings clearly implied that activating mutations in *HRAS* are important in the development of superficial bladder tumor oncogenesis.

The Role of the Fibroblast Growth Factor Receptor 3 in NMIUC

Upstream of the H-Ras protein, a number of receptor tyrosine kinases have been implicated in urothelial pathogenesis. The activation of these receptors leads to a cascade of cellular phosphorylation events, which result in the recruitment of members of the son of sevenless protein family, which ultimately cause the conversion of the Ras protein to its active GTP-bound state [32]. Recently, significant emphasis has been placed on the role played by fibroblast growth factor receptor 3 (FGFR3).

FGFR3 represents a tyrosine kinase receptor with two distinct splice variants that show differential expression in specific cell compartments: the FGFR3c variant is expressed in mesenchymal cells, whereas the FGFR3b variant is expressed in epithelial cells [33]. Prior to its proposed role in UCC, specific point germline mutations occurring in the *FGFR3* gene were linked to a number of human autosomal dominant syndromes, including achondroplasia, thanatophoric dysplasia, and hypochondroplasia [34–40]. The involvement of FGFR3 in human cancer was first demonstrated when *FGFR3* germline mutations identified in thanatophoric dysplasia were also found as somatic mutations in 3 out of 12 cervical carcinomas and in 9 out of 26 UCCs [41]. In later studies, it was also demonstrated that such *FGFR3* mutations characteristic of UCC, also occur (although at lower rates) in multiple myeloma and cervical carcinomas, and that they are in practice never found in cancers occurring in other tissue types and organs such as lung, rectum, colon, stomach, esophagus, prostate, ovary, breast, brain, and kidney [42,43].

FGFR3 mutations have been shown to cause its constitutive activation, ultimately leading to continuous downstream intracellular signaling, especially via the Ras signaling pathway [44,45]. One study showed that FGFR3 interacts with a number of adaptor proteins, such as GRB2 and Sos, to modulate Ras signaling through Raf-1 [46], while another study demonstrated that the transformation of NIH 3T3 fibroblasts induced by constitutively active *FGFR3* mutants was accompanied the activation of the Ras-MAPK and PIK3 signaling pathways [47]. The role of FGFR3 and Ras pathways in urothelial carcinogenesis is especially compelling in that *HRAS* and *FGFR3* mutations appear to be mutually exclusive in UCC, therefore strongly suggesting that these events are the phenocopy of one another and are functionally equivalent [24]. Taken together, all of these findings implicate *FGFR3* as an oncogene in UCC that likely acts through the Ras-MAPK signaling pathway.

Given the clear association of *FGFR3* gene mutations with the pathogenesis of human bladder cancer, a number of studies have investigated the clinical relevance of these mutations. One study identified *FGFR3* mutations in 37 of 50 pTa tumors analyzed (74%), whereas pTis, pT1, and pT2-4 lesions demonstrated mutations in 0, 21, and 16% of cases, respectively [48]. Furthermore, when these cancers were stratified by grade, *FGFR3* mutations proved to be more frequent in grade 1 than in grade 2 or 3 tumors [48]. Similarly,

Van Rhijn and colleagues identified *FGFR3* somatic mutations in 34 out of 53 pTa grade 1 and 2 ("low" grade) bladder cancers, whereas no grade 3 ("high" grade) tumors showed *FGFR3* mutations [49]. This inverse correlation between grade/stage of bladder cancer and *FGFR3* mutation was further validated in a larger cohort of 81 patients [50], as well as in other studies [51], suggesting that FGFR3 is probably not involved in the progression to high stage/grade UCC. Since *FGFR3* mutations should be retained if such progression were to occur, it also indicates that low-grade pTa lesions are likely not the precursor of more aggressive forms of UCC.

Finally, given this inverse correlation, a number of studies have tried to ascertain the predictive role of *FGFR3* mutations in patients with low stage/grade bladder cancer. In one study [49] it was noted that only 7 of 34 patients with mutant *FGFR3* developed recurrent tumors within a year, as compared to 14 out of 23 patients with wild-type *FGFR3*. In another study it was then found that *FGFR3* mutational status was a better predictor of recurrence rate, progression, and disease-specific survival than pathologic grade [52]. A later study in a large cohort of 772 patients, which included TaG1, TaG2, TaG3, and T1G3, demonstrated an overall reduced disease recurrence for patient with tumors harboring *FGFR3* mutations, but an increased risk for the TaG1 subgroup, suggesting that a different genetic pathway could be at play in this subgroup of NMIUC [53]. A parallel finding was obtained from another cohort of 221 patients where *FGFR3* mutational status proved to be associated with a decreased risk of progression in low-grade disease as compared to high-grade disease [54]. Finally, another study failed to find any association between *FGFR3* mutational status and disease recurrence or survival in T1G3 tumors [55].

Several investigators have used immunohistochemistry to further delineate the role of FGFR3 in other forms of low-grade urothelial disease, such as in papillary urothelial neoplasm of low malignant potential (PUNLMP). Strong staining for FGFR3 was present in the vast majority of nonrecurrent PUNLMPs (80.5%) as compared to weaker staining in recurrent PUNLMP (56.4%), thus implying that the expression of the FGGR3 protein may help define nonrecurring low-stage and grade urothelial neoplasia [56].

Collectively this evidence indicates that the role of FGFR3 is less relevant in NMIUC of higher grade, especially the T1G3 subset of tumors, in which other molecular alterations, such as *TP53* mutational status, might play a prominent role.

The Role of Genomic Alterations Involving Chromosome 9 in NMIUC

Genomic alterations involving chromosomes are commonly found in cancers and include both gene amplification and/or loss of heterozygosity (LOH). In NMIUC, the most frequent and common chromosomal alteration is LOH of chromosome 9, which is evident in the earliest stages of disease. Allelic loss of the long arm of chromosome 9 (9q) has been identified in a large proportion of bladder cancers and appears to be independent of tumor grade [57,58]. In addition, an analysis of 252 bladder specimens showed that 50% of pTa cases harbored LOH on either 9p or 9q, possibly implying that such genomic regions harbor tumor-suppressor loci relevant to the early development of urothelial cancers [59]. Further mapping at a higher resolution was later obtained, implicating the genomic region that spans from 9q34.1 to 9p12, and leading to the identification of the specific tumor-suppressor genes that are lost upon such chromosomal alterations [60–65].

Chromosome 9q

A refined analysis of the genes present on chromosome 9q and their role in NMIUC has been difficult, given the lower frequency at which alterations of such regions are found. A study by Knowles and colleagues first identified a common partial deletion of 9q in 5 out of 70 cases [60], which was later shown to encompass the *Tuberous Sclerosis 1* gene (*TSC1*) [66], a candidate tumor-suppressor gene silenced in tuberous sclerosis hamartomas [67]. Follow-up analysis of these somatic mutations revealed that 90% of them are specific to bladder cancer, with distinct alterations in the amino acid encoding portions of the gene [68] and associated TSC1 protein localization defects [69].

Another study of 4 bladder cancers with chromosome 9q34 LOH and *TSC1* inactivating mutations showed lower expression the of cyclin-dependent kinase inhibitor protein p27, suggesting a possible cross-talk in UCC between TSC1 and p27 [70]. The same group also identified relatively frequent LOH involving 9q32-q33 [71]. This region was later found to harbor the DCB1 (previously known as DBCCR1) gene, a potential tumor-suppressor whose expression was undetectable in 5 out of 10 bladder cancer cell lines evaluated. Furthermore frequent hypermethylation of the DCB1 gene promoter was also identified, which could also play a role in pathogenesis of the UCC, even in the absence of genomic deletion [72].

Finally, additional frequent deletions were found in two other chromosome 9 regions, 9q22.3 and 9q31 [65,73]. The deletions found in the 9q22.3 locus encompass the *multiple self-healing squamous epithelioma* (*MSSE*) and *patched* (*PTCH*) genes, which are involved in the development of skin tumors. However, a study by Thievessen and colleagues [74] has suggested that Hedgehog pathway activation through loss of PTCH1 function is rare or absent in UCCs, thus leaving the relevance of these mutations unresolved.

Chromosome 9p

Genomic alterations of chromosome 9p have been well characterized in bladder cancer, and their relevance in the molecular pathogenesis of NMIUC is well established [75]. Among these, the most important alterations occur in two well-known negative regulators of the cell-cycle *p16* and *p15* (respectively also known as *CDKN2/INK4A* and *INK4B*). The proteins encoded by these two tumor-suppressor genes inhibit the activity of the cyclin D/cyclin dependent kinase 4 (CDK4) complex [76,77], which catalyzes hyperphosphorylation and subsequent inactivation of the RB protein, ablating its repressive effect on progression from the G1 to S phase of the cell-cycle [78,79].

A study by El-baz and colleagues has documented hemizygous and homozygous deletions and sequence mutations involving the *p16* gene in UCC, although at a lower frequency when compared to squamous cell carcinomas of the bladder [80]. Similarly another group has identified significant methylation of the *p16* gene promoter region in 12 out of 18 UCCs, suggesting that methylation of this gene may be responsible for its functional inactivation [81]. Frequent homozygous and hemizygous deletions of both the *p15* and *p16* genes have subsequently been reported in UCC [82], including homozygous *p15* and *p16* deletions in 13 human bladder cancer cell lines [83] and decreased expression of the p15 transcript in NMIUC [84]. These findings point to a key role for the chromosome 9p21 region locus in squamous and urothelial bladder cancers, through its encoded *p15* and *p16* tumor-suppressor genes.

Prognostic Significance of LOH on Chromosome 9 on Recurrence

Given the clear implication and association of chromosome 9 in the pathogenesis of NMIUC, a number of studies addressed its prognostic value. One study identified LOH of chromosome 9 in only 12% of nonrecurrent UCCs as compared to 54% of recurrent cases [85]. When stratified by the specific genomic region involved, however, a significant association with tumor recurrence was shown only for *TSC1* LOH. A later study showed that LOH of the *p16* gene region on chromosome 9p21 was not statistically associated with recurrence-free interval in NMIUC [86]. In contrast, a third study showed an opposite result, with *p16* loss associated with a shorter recurrence-free interval in 33 out of 56 low-grade UCCs [87]. Finally, the *DCB1* locus on 9q32-33 has also been implicated in bladder cancer, with LOH of this locus in adjacent normal urothelium correlated with tumor recurrence in NMIUC [89]. *DCB1* LOH in bladder cancer cells did not appear to impact outcomes.

Overall this body of evidence suggests that events of LOH at chromosome 9q have greater prognostic value than those occurring at chromosome 9p, and that further investigations—perhaps using higher resolution methods now becoming available (i.e., copy number variation analysis by microarray analysis and high-throughput sequencing) on larger cohorts—are still needed to fully ascertain their potential use as prognostic factors for recurrence in NMIUC.

Microarray Studies

Over the past 15 years, the analysis of gene expression by DNA microarray has had a significant impact on human cancer research. This technique evaluates expression levels of thousands of transcripts at once, providing a high-throughput "snapshot" of genomic programs operating in a cell or tissue of interest, which can be then compared across distinct individuals or conditions. A number of gene expression studies have been performed in UCC with the purpose of identifying biomarkers for classification, diagnosis, and prognosis.

One early study [90] analyzed the gene expression profiles associated with a number of different bladder cancer cell lines derived from UCCs of different grade, stage, and histology. The invasive tumor-derived cell lines grouped in accordance with their alteration of the p53 and RB pathways, which are hallmarks of invasive tumors [30,47]. This analysis identified three relevant genes—*E-cadherin*, *Moesin*, and *Zyxin*—further investigated by tissue microarray analysis (TMA) showing that Moesin expression was significantly associated with overall survival [90].

In a second landmark study, Dyrskjøt and colleagues analyzed normal urothelium and 40 bladder cancers of various stages and grades to identify a gene expression classifier capable of discriminating the analyzed tumors. This group used the gene expression data set to develop a 32-gene classifier capable of correctly classifying 84% of stage Ta, 50% of stage T1, and 74% of stage T2 and above tumors in an independent cohort of 68 patients. An interesting finding from this study was that the misclassified Ta tumors showed a significantly increased progression rate. This finding was used to construct a 26-gene progression classifier for Ta cancers, which was later proved to correctly classify 75% of NMIUC in follow-up studies [91].

A similar approach was used by another group for the classification of NMIUC versus MIUC [92] with similar results. Also in this study it was possible to apply gene expression data to identify a subgroup of early-stage tumors with gene expression profiles resembling those of invasive lesions. Immunohistochemical analysis was used to validate a number of the identified targets, including p21, p33ING1, and neuropilin-2. This analysis confirmed that these proteins were significantly correlated with tumor stage and grade, although only p33ING1 proved to be associated with overall survival [92]. Finally, the analysis of 67 bladder cancers enabled the identification of 225 genes correlated to bladder cancer stage [93] and the development of a classifier for progression based on ten. Cathepsin E was ultimately validated as a biomarker for papillary growth on a large cohort of more than 700 bladder cancers based on this study [93].

These early studies demonstrated that distinct gene expression profiles are associated with non-invasive and invasive bladder cancers, and that the NMIUC that appears to be similar at the molecular level to the invasive tumors are more likely to recur and/or progress [91]. Following these early studies, several groups have further identified prognostic gene expression signatures in superficial bladder cancer. Examples of such studies include the identification of a subset of genes differentially expressed between *FGFR3*- and *TP53*-mutated tumors [94], a new 45-gene classifier that showed a significant concordance between the actual and the predicted progression ($P<0.03$; [95]), and a 20-gene, 52-gene, and 88-gene progression predictors that showed highly significant concordance between predicted and actual pathologic stage ($P<0.0001$) across patients from several different countries [96]. The latter study confirmed the observation that NMIUC misclassified as MIUC showed shorter disease-specific survival. Furthermore a 40% cumulative probability of progression was found for the patients classified as progressors versus less than 15% for the patients predicted as nonprogressors ($P<0.001$), which appeared to be independent of standard clinical parameters such as stage, grade, age, sex, and intravesical treatment. While very promising, the performance characteristics of such molecular signatures would likely have to improve further before they could become clinically useful.

A recent meta-analysis used a set of published gene expression profiling data sets to develop a progression classifier for NMIUC [98]. This 96-gene classifier was then implemented into a quantitative RT-PCR-based assay, which was applied to an independent set of 107 patients, that included 11 benign cases, 54 progressors, and 42 superficial nonprogressors. Of 96 genes analyzed, 57 proved to be significantly associated with muscle invasion, and were therefore used to stratify Ta and T1 tumors into low- or high-risk progression groups. The tumors that were classified at high progression risk showed a higher rate of progression at 2 years than those classified at low progression risk (45% vs. 12%, $P<0.004$). Similar results were also obtained in the T1 stage group (22% of progression for low-risk patients as opposed to 61% for high-risk ones, $P<0.03$).

Finally, based on the success of tissue-based approaches, a recent study using a 14-gene classifier was used for the detection and classification of bladder cancer in the urine, with a combination of CDC2 and HOXA13 able to stratify tumors by stage [99].

The Role of Immune Response in NMIUC

Bacillus Calmette-Guérin (BCG) is currently used to reduce the recurrence rate and risk of progression in superficial bladder cancer. The success of BCG in many patients underscores the crucial role of inflammatory responses in the treatment of UCC, which includes the secretion of cytokines and activation of lymphocytes and macrophages. The antitumor activity of BCG is largely mediated by a nonspecific immunological response initiated by immunocompetent cells that follows the interaction of BCG with the bladder wall and its internalization in urothelial cells [101,102]. The activation of this response is mediated by both professional antigen-presenting cells (APCs), like dendritic cells and macrophages, and urothelial carcinoma cells, which have acquired antigen-presenting properties and can therefore present to CD4+ T-helper lymphocytes the antigen in the context of MHC class II molecules. Following the activation of the immune system associated with intravesical BCG instillation, a number of cytokines are produced, including tumor necrosis factor alpha (TNF), inteferon gamma (IFNG), interleukin-1 (IL-1), IL-2, IL-6, IL-8, IL-12, and IL-18. This activation also results in the recruitment of cytotoxic effector cells, including cytotoxic T lymphocytes, natural killer cells, lymphokine-activated killer cells, and macrophage-activated killer cells, which mediates antitumor effects [103].

The type of inflammatory cell associated with BCG treatment has been shown to impact patient prognosis. One study by Ayari and colleagues suggested that a high level of infiltration by CD83 positive tumor-infiltrating dendritic cells and CD68 positive tumor-associated macrophages is associated with a decreased response to BCG treatment [104]. This finding further underscores the need for larger studies that evaluate the role of the immune response in UCC treatment.

Molecular Pathogenesis of Muscle-Invasive Urothelial Carcinoma

Muscle-invasive urothelial carcinomas (MIUCs) are distinct from NMIUC at the pathologic, molecular, and prognostic level. Despite advances in treatment, few patients with metastatic urothelial cancer survive 5 years [105]. The depth of invasion into the muscularis propria has been correlated with lymphatic and hematogenous invasion, as well as with subsequent metastatic dissemination of the disease to the regional lymph nodes or to distant organs [106]. MIUC is also often accompanied by local invasion of the adjacent tissue, in particular the prostate and prostatic urethra [106], and the extent of the local invasion, as well as the presence of lymph node metastases, directly impacts survival after cystectomy

[106]. Nodal metastases are most commonly found in the pelvic lymph nodes, especially in the external iliac (65%) and obturator (74%) nodes, while the internal iliac lymph nodes are involved in about 20% of patients [106]. Distant metastases to the liver, lung, bone, and adrenal glands are also common [107–109].

Given the aggressive nature and the poor outcome associated with MIUC, research into the molecular mechanisms underlying invasion and metastatic spread of UCC has been a major focus of molecular investigation.

Deregulation of p53 Pathways in MIUC

Among the most relevant molecular alterations associated with MIUC is the loss of function of the p53 protein, usually through mutation of one allele on chromosome 17p13.1, and deletion of the remaining one [96]. The p53 protein is encoded by the *TP53* tumor-suppressor gene [110] and impacts cell-cycle progression from the G1 to the S phase through the transcriptional activation of the WAF1/CIP1 and the expression of the p21 protein [111]. As nuclear immunohistochemical staining for the p53 protein accompanies *TP53* mutation and loss of protein function, this technique has been therefore frequently used for the identification of p53-mutant UCC. Nuclear p53 appears to be an independent predictor of mortality in invasive tumors, independent of tumor stage, grade, and lymph node status [110–119], and it is significantly correlated with tumor grade and stage [120–124]. Finally, although promising as prognostic marker, nuclear p53 immunostaining cannot identify homozygous deletions of both *TP53* alleles or detect *TP53* gene silencing by promoter hypermethylation [125]. As such, immunohistochemical analysis is therefore not a sensitive test for loss of p53 function in cancer cells.

Role of Retinoblastoma (Rb) Pathway Deregulation in MIUC

A number of genomic deletions in bladder cancer have been identified in the 13q14 chromosomal region, which harbors the *RB* tumor-suppressor gene [126]. Altered expression of this gene has been correlated with survival of MIUC patients [113,127,128], with a better prognosis associated with normal Rb and p53 protein expression in T1 tumors [129]. Finally, it has also been reported that the combination of multiple cell-cycle regulatory proteins, like pRb, p53, and p21waf1/CIP1, can improve independent prediction of UCC outcome [130] compared with commonly used clinico-pathologic parameters.

Other Signaling Pathways

Epidermal Growth Factor Receptor

Higher expression levels of Epidermal Growth Factor Receptor (EGFR) have been shown to positively correlate in UCC with higher stage and grade, as well as disease recurrence [131–133]. One study has also shown that increased expression of the protein encoded by the *ERBB2* gene, which is a member of the epidermal growth factor (EGF) receptor family of receptor tyrosine kinases, has prognostic value in patients with recurrent progressive UCC [134]. However, other studies have shown that EGFR expression did not predict survival in patients with invasive disease, which might imply that EGFR could be associated with the transition to invasive forms of the disease [135]. It should also be noted that the increased EGFR expression in UCC in general is not mediated by gene amplification, which occurs late in tumor progression, and that therefore other functional mechanisms must be at play to mediate such EGFR increase [136].

Fibroblast Growth Factors and Their Receptors

Among the fibroblast growth factor (FGF) family members, two in particular have been implicated in bladder cancer pathogenesis: FGF1 (also referred to as "acidic," aFGF), and FGF2 (also known as "basic," bFGF). Both of these factors are found in the extracellular matrix (ECM), complexed with heparan sulfates. During ECM degradation associated with cancer progression, both types of FGFs are released by the action of several proteases [137,138]. These two proteins may determine a more aggressive course of disease, and their evaluation by immunohistochemical staining may identify cancers likely to progress [137,138]. In support of this, increased expression of FGF2 was documented in carcinoma in situ (CIS) specimens [137,139–141].

There is also evidence for involvement in UCC of the cognate receptors for FGFs, with a specific role in signaling within the epithelial and mesenchymal tissue compartments [143]. For instance, the transcript for the FGFR2IIIb variant is present in all normal urothelial cells (with the exception of the superficial umbrella layer), whereas low levels of FGFR2IIIc are usually present in the stromal compartment [144]. Loss of FGFR2IIIb expression has been associated with poor prognosis in UCC, and in nude mice the re-expression of this receptor in the human T24 bladder cancer cell line has shown to reduce the proliferation rate and tumor growth [144–146].

Vascular Endothelial Growth Factors and Their Receptors

The vascular endothelial growth factor (VEGF) family encompasses five members: VEGFA, VEGFB, VEGFC, VEGFD, and placental growth factor (PGF). In humans, VEGFA mediates angiogenesis, signaling through its two tyrosine kinase receptors, VEGFR1 and VEGFR2 (respectively also known as FLT1 and KDR), while PGF and VEGFB activate only FLT1 [147]. It has been shown that the activation of FLT1 upon binding of VEGFA and PGF recruits bone marrow-derived macrophages to inflammatory and cancer tissues, thus enhancing pathological angiogenesis. Finally, FLT4, also known as VEGFR3, is expressed in endothelial cells of the lymphatic system, regulating lymphangiogenesis upon activation by VEGFC and D, which are indeed overexpressed in cancers that preferentially metastasize to lymph nodes [147].

High levels of VEGF transcripts were identified in patients with T1 UCC of low or intermediate grade and were associated with recurrence and progression [148]. Increased VEGFA immunostaining has been associated with increased tumor stage, while serum VEGF proved to be positively correlated with the presence of CIS, increased grade, increased stage, vascular invasion, and the presence of metastatic disease [149–151]. Interestingly, the T24 bladder tumor cell line has an autocrine VEGF mitogenic signaling loop, with expression of both VEGFA and its receptor KDR [152].

Finally, a study on 286 tumors by TMA revealed that IHC staining with VEGFD was associated with stage and metastasis to regional lymph nodes, while it was negatively correlated with disease-free interval. It has been shown that the expression of VEGFR3 in high-grade tumors was associated with a shorter disease-free survival, and the expression of VEGFR3 and VEGFD has proven to be an independent predictor of tumor stage and lymph node metastasis in multivariate analysis. In the same studies, matched primary tumors and the corresponding metastases were compared, and the expression of VEGFR3 and VEGFD proved significantly higher in primary cancers [153,154].

Transforming Growth Factor-Beta Family

The transforming growth factor (TGF)-beta family of proteins includes TGF-beta 1 through 5, inhibin, activin, and the Müllerian inhibitory substance [155]. Overall, TGF-beta proteins act as proliferation inhibitors through phosphorylation and inhibition of the Rb protein [156]. A number of studies have investigated the expression of these proteins in the bladder with somewhat contrasting results. One study showed higher TGF-beta 1 and 2 transcripts in indolent rather than aggressive UCCs [156], while another study reported higher TGF-beta in UCC versus normal urothelial cells [157].

TGF-beta family members have strong angiogenic activity and higher concentrations of TGF-beta 1 have been found in the serum of patients with invasive tumors compared to patients with NMIUC [158,159]. Moreover, increased TGF-beta 1 expression is associated with advanced pathological stage and risk of disease progression [160]. However, contrasting findings have been reported, including the association of reduced TGF-beta receptors with worsened cancer stage, grade, progression, and survival [160–163].

In conclusion, conflicting evidence about the role of TGF-beta signaling in UCC may be due to the complex cross-talk between distinct compartments in the tumor and its microenvironment and further investigation is needed. A plausible explanation for this is that—similar to its role in other cancers—TGF-beta might exert a dual role in UCC: preventing cancer formation and progression in early tumorigenesis and promoting progression late in the course of disease [164].

Rho Family GTPases and Their Regulators

The proteins of the Rho family of GTPases are small monomeric guanine nucleotide-binding proteins related to RAS that regulate a number of cellular signaling pathways involved in cell adhesion and motility, cell migration, cell-cycle progression, cell survival, and epithelial to mesenchymal transition (EMT) [165–167]. The activity of these proteins is tightly regulated by guanine nucleotide exchange factors (GEFs) that stimulate the exchange of GDP to GTP, as well as by GTPase activator proteins (GAPs), which stimulate GTP hydrolysis [168]. Accordingly, the Rho/ROCK pathway has been implicated in the development of metastases and bladder cancer invasion, and significantly higher expression levels of ROCK, RhoA, and RhoC proteins were shown in primary cancers and lymph node metastases as compared to normal specimens. In contrast, RhoB expression was inversely correlated to stage and grade [167]. Among the regulators of this pathway, a relevant role has been shown for the Rho GDP dissociation inhibitor 2 protein (RhoGDI2, also known as Ly-GDI or D4-GDI), which is highly expressed in the normal genitourinary tract epithelium [169]. It has been reported that reduced RhoGDI2 expression correlates with the metastatic activity of human bladder cancer lines [170,171] and that RhoGDI2 works as a metastasis suppressor gene in a novel bladder cancer animal model [172]. Multivariate analysis supports the finding that RhoGDI2 is an independent prognostic factor that is negatively associated with UCC recurrence after radical cystectomy [171].

E-Cadherin and Epithelial to Mesenchymal Transition in Urothelial Cancer

E-cadherin is a calcium-dependent cell adhesion protein that maintains normal urothelial integrity and impermeability to urine [137,173]. The loss of E-cadherin activity has been implicated in UCC progression and invasion through both genetic and epigenetic mechanisms [137]. E-cadherin gene silencing by promoter methylation has been shown to be associated with poor prognosis and progression in UCC [174,175] and E-cadherin LOH and promoter hypermethylation have been significantly correlated with tumor grade [176].

E-cadherin immunostaining has been performed, with protein levels inversely correlated with muscle invasion, lymph node metastasis [90,177–179], tumor stage and grade [180,181], recurrence [182], and survival at 5 years [173,183]. Overall, immunohistochemical evaluation of E-cadherin either alone or in combination with other adhesion proteins can be used as a predictor of disease progression in patients treated by cystectomy [183–185]. Loss of E-cadherin appears to be accompanied by the concomitant expression of another adhesion protein, N-cadherin, which is usually not expressed in normal urothelium. Interestingly N-cadherin expression appears to be correlated with invasion, since it arises in pT1 UC, and increases in muscle-invasive cancers. Multivariate analyses have shown that N-cadherin immunostaining is an independent prognostic marker for progression to invasive UCC [186].

Finally, abnormal expression of E-cadherin and beta-catenin has been associated with high stage and grade disease and with poor patient survival [187], and higher plasma and urine E-cadherin levels have been shown in patients with UCC as compared to healthy individuals. Preoperative soluble E-cadherin proved to be an independent predictor of lymph node metastases and disease progression [161,188].

Based on these findings, studies using an NBT-II nitrosamine-induced rat bladder cancer cell line have shown that reduced E-cadherin expression, downstream AKT signaling, and nuclear factor kappa B (NFKB) activation are coordinately mediated by the induction of the ectodermal transcriptional repressor Snail, which is known to control EMT [189]. More recently, the basic helix-loop-helix transcription factor TWIST1 has been proposed to mediate UCC metastatic progression, since its expression was significantly higher in cancer compared to normal tissue. In the same study, it was also shown that TWIST1 expression was negatively correlated with E-cadherin expression and was higher in the metastases compared to matched primary tumors [190]. These findings were further confirmed in an independent study on 70 bladder cancers, in which TWIST1 proved to be negatively correlated with E-cadherin, positively associated with tumor stage and grade, and shorter progression-free survival [191].

Cell Adhesion, Integrins, and Tumor–Stroma Interactions in Urothelial Cancer

In the basal layer of normal urothelium, alpha 6/beta 4 is the most commonly expressed integrin heterodimer. Altered alpha 6/beta 4 expression has been reported as an early event UCC carcinogenesis, with CIS lesions exhibiting reduced levels of the beta 4 subunit and concomitant preferential expression of the alpha 6 beta 1 heterodimer expression [192]. Accordingly, immunostaining for alpha 6 beta 4 integrin has shown a prognostic value in relation to invasion and the establishment of metastatic disease [193,194]. The relevance of integrin signaling in UCC is further underscored by the role of alpha 5 beta 1 integrin in the cellular response to immunotherapy with BCG therapy [195,196].

A number of studies have addressed the role of alterations of basement membrane (BM) proteins in UCC. Invasive and metastatic bladder tumors exhibit aberrant glycosylation of the Sialosyl-Lewis X epitope (SLeX), which can increase tumor cell adhesion to E-selectin and was correlated with metastases and shorter 5 year survival [197]. Alteration of BM proteins including laminin and type IV collagen has also been investigated [137]. For instance, type IV collagen alterations have been correlated with poor survival in high stage UCC, while laminin alterations have been correlated with metastatic disease [198]. Furthermore, levels of additional BM proteins, such as laminin, fibronectin, and elastase, are significantly higher in cancer specimens as compared to normal urothelium, and laminin levels in the urine and serum have been shown to be valuable for the diagnosis of invasive UCC [137]. Unlike other laminin subtypes, laminin 5 appears to be downregulated during UCC progression through promoter methylation. By analyzing bladder tumors, bladder washes, and urine, it has been shown that promoter methylation is responsible for laminin-5 silencing, and that methylation frequency could distinguish NMIUC from invasive tumors and was significantly correlated with a number of poor prognosis parameters, such as tumor stage and grade, and muscle invasion [199].

The establishment of an invasive phenotype is also accompanied by alterations involving the extracellular matrix (ECM). In tumor tissues, for instance, it has been shown that the degradation of stromal derived hyaluronic acid by cancer cell-derived hyaluronidase 1 (HYAL1) can induce angiogenesis by releasing angiogenic hyaluronic acid fragments, which in turn can be measured in the urine of high-grade bladder cancer patients [200–202]. Moreover, it has also been shown that urinary hyaluronic acid correlates with matched tissue levels, functions as diagnostic biomarker [200,201,203,204], and predicts treatment failure and UCC recurrence when analysis of transmembrane hyaluronic acid synthase 1 gene (HAS1) is performed [205,206]. Hyaluronic acid can regulate cell migration, adhesion, and proliferation through its interaction with the CD44 receptor, which is a member of a family of transmembrane glycoproteins that has been shown to be involved in cell–cell and cell–matrix interaction and to play a relevant role in tumor metastasis [207]. In UCC, progressive loss of CD44 has been correlated with advanced stage, although its value as an independent prognostic marker is still unclear [137,208–212].

A role for Thrombospondin-1 (TSP1) has also been proposed in UCC tumor suppression. Expression of this endogenous constituent of the

ECM inhibits tumor neovascularization and therefore has tumor-suppressor functions [151,213]. By immunohistochemical analysis, TSP1 levels were inversely correlated with stage [151], vascular density [214], and survival rate at 5 years, suggesting that it could be a useful prognostic biomarker [214].

Other Determinants of Progression and Metastasis in UC

CD24, a glycosyl phosphatidyl inositol-linked surface protein, has been shown to be highly expressed in bladder and other cancers, and its loss of function proved to be associated with apoptosis, decreased anchorage-independent growth and cell proliferation [215]. CD24 immunostaining in bladder cancer demonstrated that CD24 expression is significantly associated with shorter disease-free survival [215]. Similar findings were also obtained in a second study where low CD24 immunostaining was present in the cytoplasm of normal luminal cells, while higher CD24 levels were detected in NMIUC, which further increased with stromal and muscle invasion [216].

Several cytokines and inflammatory mediators have been linked to urothelial cancer pathogenesis. For instance, higher interleukin-8 (IL-8) expression has been demonstrated in MIUC and in CIS as compared to NMIUC [150,217], and cyclooxygenase-2 (COX2) has been shown to be expressed at high levels in invasive UCC, but undetectable in normal bladder urothelium [218]. The expression of COX2 has also been associated with increased angiogenesis, increased recurrence risk, and shorter disease-specific mortality [218–221].

In a number of cancers, endothelins (ETs) have been implicated in autocrine and paracrine signaling loops and associated with aberrant proliferation, formation of new blood vessels, escape from apoptosis, invasion, and metastases. Endothelin 1 expression is inversely correlated to that of RhoGDI2 [165], and two studies have demonstrated aberrant expression of ETs signaling components in the vast majority of bladder cancer samples when compared to expression in normal urothelial cells [220,222]. In particular, expression of the endothelin B receptor (ETBR) was associated with a favorable prognosis [222], and suppression of ETBR in UCC could be explained by promoter hypermethylation. Accordingly, methylation frequency of the ETBR promoter proved to be correlated with tumor stage and grade, and was inversely associated with UCC aggressiveness [220].

Finally, the presence of tumor-infiltrating cells—cytotoxic T lymphocytes (TILs) in particular—has been shown to be associated with favorable outcomes in a number of tumor types. Local immune responses mediated by cytotoxic lymphocytes (CD8 positive T cells) may play a role in cancer cell eradication through the recognition of cancer-associated antigens in the context of MHC class I molecules. To this end it has been recently shown that the presence of CD8 positive T cells infiltrating MIUC, along with the expression of MHC class I antigen and CTAG1B cancer/testis antigen 1B (also known as NY-ESO-1 tumor antigen), is associated with favorable clinical outcome. This finding speaks to relevance of tumor microenvironment, and further studies in the field will assist establishing novel prognostic indicators in MIUC.

Microarray Studies of Survival Outcomes in MIUC

In the clinical management of MIUC, the prediction of metastatic recurrence and therapy response are among the most relevant questions. Similar to what has been described for superficial urothelial cancer, gene expression profiling has also been widely adopted to address these issues in MIUC. Modlich and colleagues [223] identified a group of genes differentially expressed between MIUC with different prognoses. One group of these genes encoded for proteins related to cell–cell adhesion, transcription, and cell-cycle regulation, while another group encoded for proteins involved in cell proliferation and growth [223].

Another report identified a gene expression signature associated with poor prognosis in invasive bladder cancers [224] by profiling 52 normal bladder samples, 33 superficial cancers, and 72 invasive cancers. This group was able to identify a signature of 100 genes capable of predicting disease outcome with 90% accuracy, and a larger one, comprising 174 genes, that was significantly associated with disease-specific clinical outcome and with lymph node status (both $P < 0.0001$) [225]. In another study, the same group used antibody arrays and analyzed the serum of bladder cancer patients [226]. By this approach, they compared serum samples between 37 bladder cancer patients and 58 controls, proving that serum protein profiles could distinguish normal controls from bladder cancer patients with 89.2% sensitivity and 96.5% specificity. They further evaluated whether this subset of antibodies provided prognostic information among the 37 cancer patients, identifying two distinct groups of patients with different overall survival ($P = 0.05$) [226].

Gene expression analysis has also been used to predict the response to chemotherapy in order to distinguish patients who are going to benefit from this additional therapy. One early study has shown that gene expression can be used to build predictive models of the response to a single drug, as well as to combination regimens [227]. In this study, baseline gene expression profiles from a panel of 40 bladder cancer cell lines were used to develop chemotherapy response prediction models, which showed highly significant concordance with empirically assessed responses [227].

In another study by Takata and colleagues, gene expression was measured in 27 invasive bladder cancer biopsies prior to treatment with neoadjuvant methotrexate vinblastine, adriamycin, and cisplatin (MVAC) chemotherapy [228]. The authors identified a set of 50 genes that significantly differed between 14 responders and 13 non-responders. A further refinement of this signature was obtained using a subset of the patients as a training set, enabling the development of a 14-gene MVAC response predictor that could correctly classify 8 out of 9 samples from the test set. The same investigators have subsequently validated their predictive signature on 22 additional patients [229], showing that their gene expression signature could correctly predict MVAC response in 19 out of 22 cases with approximately 100% sensitivity and 73% specificity. Moreover, in this independent cohort the negative predictive value of the assay proved to be approximately 100%, with 8 out of 8 nonresponders identified, while the positive predictive value was around 79% [229].

Finally, Als and colleagues analyzed gene expression in 30 patients with locally advanced or metastatic bladder cancer [230], identifying 55 genes that proved to be expressed at lower levels in patients with longer survival. In this study the authors failed to observe any difference in terms of gene expression between patients treated with different chemotherapy regimens. Two of the genes that discriminate patients by their survival Emmprin and Survivin—were further investigated by immunostaining, showing that they were significantly associated with overall survival ($P \leq 0.001$). The investigators also documented different response rates to chemotherapy based on Emmprin and Survivin staining, with double positive tumors exhibiting a response rate of 27%, and double negative tumors exhibiting a response rate of 82%, with an odds ratio in double negative tumors of 11.9 (95% CI, 3.2–42.3) [230].

Overall this evidence emphasizes the fact that the use of gene expression for prognostication and prediction in invasive bladder cancer is promising and further investigation in larger cohort is required.

References

1. Botteman MF, Pashos CL, Redaelli A, Laskin B, Hauser R. The health economics of bladder cancer: a comprehensive review of the published literature. Pharmacoeconomics. 2003;21(18):1315–30.
2. Jemal A, Siegel R, Ward E, Hao Y, Xu J, Thun MJ. Cancer Statistics, 2009. CA Cancer J Clin. 2009;59(4):225–49.
3. Dalbagni G. The management of superficial bladder cancer. Nat Clin Pract Urol. 2007;4(5):254–60.

4. Ghoneim MA, Abol-Enein H. Management of muscle-invasive bladder cancer: an update. Nat Clin Pract Urol. 2008;5(9):501–8.
5. Wu XR. Urothelial tumorigenesis: a tale of divergent pathways. Nat Rev. 2005;5(9):713–25.
6. Lopez-Beltran A, Cheng L, Mazzucchelli R, et al. Morphological and molecular profiles and pathways in bladder neoplasms. Anticancer Res. 2008;28(5B):2893–900.
7. Downward J, Targeting RAS. signalling pathways in cancer therapy. Nat Rev Cancer. 2003;3(1):11–22.
8. Jiang B, Liu L, George FVW, George K. Chapter 2 PI3K/PTEN signaling in angiogenesis and tumorigenesis. Advances in cancer research. New York: Academic; 2009. p. 19–65.
9. Rusanescu G, Gotoh T, Tian X, Feig LA. Regulation of Ras signaling specificity by protein kinase C. Mol Cell Biol. 2001;21(8):2650–8.
10. Herrera R, Sebolt-Leopold JS. Unraveling the complexities of the Raf/MAP kinase pathway for pharmacological intervention. Trends Mol Med. 2002;8(4):S27–31.
11. Santos E, Tronick SR, Aaronson SA, Pulciani S, Barbacid M. T24 human bladder carcinoma oncogene is an activated form of the normal human homologue of BALB- and Harvey-MSV transforming genes. Nature. 1982;298(5872):343–7.
12. Reddy EP, Reynolds RK, Santos E, Barbacid M. A point mutation is responsible for the acquisition of transforming properties by the T24 human bladder carcinoma oncogene. Nature. 1982;300(5888):149–52.
13. McBride OW, Swan DC, Santos E, Barbacid M, Tronick SR, Aaronson SA. Localization of the normal allele of T24 human bladder carcinoma oncogene to chromosome 11. Nature. 1982;300(5894):773–4.
14. Feinberg AP, Vogelstein B, Droller MJ, Baylin SB, Nelkin BD. Mutation affecting the 12th amino acid of the c-Ha-ras oncogene product occurs infrequently in human cancer. Science. 1983;220(4602):1175–7.
15. Fujita J, Srivastava SK, Kraus MH, Rhim JS, Tronick SR, Aaronson SA. Frequency of molecular alterations affecting ras protooncogenes in human urinary tract tumors. Proc Natl Acad Sci USA. 1985; 82(11):3849–53.
16. Fujita J, Yoshida O, Yuasa Y, Rhim JS, Hatanaka M, Aaronson SA. Ha-ras oncogenes are activated by somatic alterations in human urinary tract tumours. Nature. 1984;309(5967):464–6.
17. Boulalas I, Zaravinos A, Karyotis I, Delakas D, Spandidos DA. Activation of RAS family genes in urothelial carcinoma. J Urol. 2009;181(5):2312–9.
18. Joyce AD, D'Emilia JC, Steele Jr G, Libertino JA, Silverman ML, Summerhayes IC. Detection of altered H-ras proteins in human tumors using western blot analysis. Lab Invest. 1989;61(2):212–8.
19. Saito S, Hata M, Fukuyama R, et al. Screening of H-ras gene point mutations in 50 cases of bladder carcinoma. Int J Urol. 1997;4(2):178–85.
20. Visvanathan KV, Pocock RD, Summerhayes IC. Preferential and novel activation of H-ras in human bladder carcinomas. Oncogene Res. 1988;3(1): 77–86.
21. Tabin CJ, Bradley SM, Bargmann CI, et al. Mechanism of activation of a human oncogene. Nature. 1982;300(5888):143–9.
22. Oxford G, Theodorescu D. The role of Ras superfamily proteins in bladder cancer progression. J Urol. 2003;170(5):1987–93.
23. Czerniak B, Cohen GL, Etkind P, et al. Concurrent mutations of coding and regulatory sequences of the Ha-ras gene in urinary bladder carcinomas. Hum Pathol. 1992;23(11):1199–204.
24. Jebar AH, Hurst CD, Tomlinson DC, Johnston C, Taylor CF, Knowles MA. FGFR3 and Ras gene mutations are mutually exclusive genetic events in urothelial cell carcinoma. Oncogene. 2005;24(33): 5218–25.
25. Theodorescu D, Cornil I, Fernandez BJ, Kerbel RS. Overexpression of normal and mutated forms of HRAS induces orthotopic bladder invasion in a human transitional cell carcinoma. Proc Natl Acad Sci USA. 1990;87(22):9047–51.
26. John JG, Wendy LG, Michael AH, Dan T. Genetic and phenotypic changes associated with the acquisition of tumorigenicity in human bladder cancer. Genes Chromosomes Cancer. 2000;27(3):252–63.
27. Knowles MA, Williamson M. Mutation of H-ras is infrequent in bladder cancer: confirmation by single-strand conformation polymorphism analysis, designed restriction fragment length polymorphisms, and direct sequencing. Cancer Res. 1993;53(1):133–9.
28. Fitzgerald JM, Ramchurren N, Rieger K, et al. Identification of H-ras mutations in urine sediments complements cytology in the detection of bladder tumors. J Natl Cancer Inst. 1995;87(2):129–33.
29. Zhang ZT, Pak J, Huang HY, et al. Role of Ha-ras activation in superficial papillary pathway of urothelial tumor formation. Oncogene. 2001;20(16): 1973–80.
30. Gao J, Huang H-Y, Pak J, et al. p53 deficiency provokes urothelial proliferation and synergizes with activated Ha-ras in promoting urothelial tumorigenesis. Oncogene. 2004;23(3):687–96.
31. Mo L, Zheng X, Huang H-Y, et al. Hyperactivation of Ha-ras oncogene, but not Ink4a/Arf deficiency, triggers bladder tumorigenesis. J Clin Invest. 2007;117(2):314–25.
32. Pasin E, Josephson DY, Mitra AP, Cote RJ, Stein JP. Superficial bladder cancer: an update on etiology, molecular development, classification, and natural history. Rev Urol. 2008;10(1):31–43.
33. Murgue B, Tsunekawa S, Rosenberg I, de Beaumont M, Podolsky DK. Identification of a novel variant form of fibroblast growth factor receptor 3 (FGFR3 IIIb) in human colonic epithelium. Cancer Res. 1994;54(19):5206–11.
34. Rousseau F, Bonaventure J, Legeai-Mallet L, et al. Mutations in the gene encoding fibroblast growth

factor receptor-3 in achondroplasia. Nature. 1994; 371(6494):252–4.
35. Shiang R, Thompson LM, Zhu YZ, et al. Mutations in the transmembrane domain of FGFR3 cause the most common genetic form of dwarfism, achondroplasia. Cell. 1994;78(2):335–42.
36. Bonaventure J, Rousseau F, Legeai-Mallet L, Le Merrer M, Munnich A, Maroteaux P. Common mutations in the gene encoding fibroblast growth factor receptor 3 account for achondroplasia, hypochondroplasia and thanatophoric dysplasia. Acta Paediatr Suppl. 1996;417:33–8.
37. Bonaventure J, Rousseau F, Legeai-Mallet L, Le Merrer M, Munnich A, Maroteaux P. Common mutations in the fibroblast growth factor receptor 3 (FGFR 3) gene account for achondroplasia, hypochondroplasia, and thanatophoric dwarfism. Am J Med Genet. 1996;63(1):148–54.
38. Tavormina PL, Shiang R, Thompson LM, et al. Thanatophoric dysplasia (types I and II) caused by distinct mutations in fibroblast growth factor receptor 3. Nat Genet. 1995;9(3):321–8.
39. Bellus GA, McIntosh I, Smith EA, et al. A recurrent mutation in the tyrosine kinase domain of fibroblast growth factor receptor 3 causes hypochondroplasia. Nat Genet. 1995;10(3):357–9.
40. Tavormina PL, Rimoin DL, Cohn DH, Zhu YZ, Shiang R, Wasmuth JJ. Another mutation that results in the substitution of an unpaired cysteine residue in the extracellular domain of FGFR3 in thanatophoric dysplasia type I. Hum Mol Genet. 1995;4(11):2175–7.
41. Cappellen D, De Oliveira C, Ricol D, et al. Frequent activating mutations of FGFR3 in human bladder and cervix carcinomas. Nat Genet. 1999;23(1):18–20.
42. Karoui M, Hofmann-Radvanyi H, Zimmermann U, et al. No evidence of somatic FGFR3 mutation in various types of carcinoma. Oncogene. 2001;20(36):5059–61.
43. Sibley K, Stern P, Knowles MA. Frequency of fibroblast growth factor receptor 3 mutations in sporadic tumours. Oncogene. 2001;20(32):4416–8.
44. Naski MC, Wang Q, Xu J, Ornitz DM. Graded activation of fibroblast growth factor receptor 3 by mutations causing achondroplasia and thanatophoric dysplasia. Nat Genet. 1996;13(2):233–7.
45. Webster MK, Donoghue DJ. FGFR activation in skeletal disorders: too much of a good thing. Trends Genet. 1997;13(5):178–82.
46. Kanai M, Göke M, Tsunekawa S, Podolsky DK. Signal transduction pathway of human fibroblast growth factor receptor 3. J Biol Chem. 1997; 272(10):6621–8.
47. Agazie YM, Movilla N, Ischenko I, Hayman MJ. The phosphotyrosine phosphatase SHP2 is a critical mediator of transformation induced by the oncogenic fibroblast growth factor receptor 3. Oncogene. 2003;22(44):6909–18.
48. Billerey C, Chopin D, Aubriot-Lorton M-H, et al. Frequent FGFR3 mutations in papillary non-invasive bladder (pTa) tumors. Am J Pathol. 2001;158(6): 1955–9.
49. van Rhijn BWG, Lurkin I, Radvanyi F, Kirkels WJ, van der Kwast TH, Zwarthoff EC. The fibroblast growth factor receptor 3 (FGFR3) mutation is a strong indicator of superficial bladder cancer with low recurrence rate. Cancer Res. 2001;61(4): 1265–8.
50. Takahiro K, Hideaki S, Toya O, Kouji A, Hiroshi K, Yoshikatsu E. The incidence of thanatophoric dysplasia mutations in FGFR3 gene is higher in low-grade or superficial bladder carcinomas. Cancer. 2001;92(10):2555–61.
51. van Rhijn BW, Montironi R, Zwarthoff EC, Jöbsis AC, van der Kwast TH. Frequent FGFR3 mutations in urothelial papilloma. J Pathol. 2002;198(2): 245–51.
52. van Rhijn BWG, Vis AN, van der Kwast TH, et al. Molecular grading of urothelial cell carcinoma with fibroblast growth factor receptor 3 and MIB-1 is superior to pathologic grade for the prediction of clinical outcome. J Clin Oncol. 2003;21(10): 1912–21.
53. Hernandez S, Lopez-Knowles E, Lloreta J, et al. Prospective study of FGFR3 mutations as a prognostic factor in nonmuscle invasive urothelial bladder carcinomas. J Clin Oncol. 2006;24(22):3664–71.
54. Burger M, van der Aa MNM, van Oers JMM, et al. Prediction of progression of non-muscle-invasive bladder cancer by WHO 1973 and 2004 grading and by FGFR3 mutation status: a prospective study. Eur Urol. 2008;54(4):835–44.
55. Hernandez S, Lopez-Knowles E, Lloreta J, et al. FGFR3 and Tp53 mutations in T1G3 transitional bladder carcinomas: independent distribution and lack of association with prognosis. Clin Cancer Res. 2005;11(15):5444–50.
56. Francesca B, Alfredo S, Roberta M, et al. Strong immunohistochemical expression of fibroblast growth factor receptor 3, superficial staining pattern of cytokeratin 20, and low proliferative activity define those papillary urothelial neoplasms of low malignant potential that do not recur. Cancer. 2008;112(3):636–44.
57. Olumi AF, Tsai YC, Nichols PW, et al. Allelic loss of chromosome 17p distinguishes high grade from low grade transitional cell carcinomas of the bladder. Cancer Res. 1990;50(21):7081–3.
58. Tsai YC, Nichols PW, Hiti AL, Williams Z, Skinner DG, Jones PA. Allelic losses of chromosomes 9, 11, and 17 in human bladder cancer. Cancer Res. 1990;50(1):44–7.
59. Cairns P, Shaw ME, Knowles MA. Initiation of bladder cancer may involve deletion of a tumour-suppressor gene on chromosome 9. Oncogene. 1993; 8(4):1083–5.
60. Habuchi T, Devlin J, Elder PA, Knowles MA. Detailed deletion mapping of chromosome 9q in bladder cancer: evidence for two tumour suppressor loci. Oncogene. 1995;11(8):1671–4.

61. Keen AJ, Knowles MA. Definition of two regions of deletion on chromosome 9 in carcinoma of the bladder. Oncogene. 1994;9(7):2083–8.
62. Linnenbach AJ, Pressler LB, Seng BA, Kimmel BS, Tomaszewski JE, Malkowicz SB. Characterization of chromosome 9 deletions in transitional cell carcinoma by microsatellite assay. Hum Mol Genet. 1993;2(9):1407–11.
63. Miyao N, Tsai YC, Lerner SP, et al. Role of chromosome 9 in human bladder cancer. Cancer Res. 1993;53(17):4066–70.
64. Orlow I, Lianes P, Lacombe L, Dalbagni G, Reuter VE, Cordon-Cardo C. Chromosome 9 allelic losses and microsatellite alterations in human bladder tumors. Cancer Res. 1994;54(11):2848–51.
65. Simoneau AR, Spruck 3rd CH, Gonzalez-Zulueta M, et al. Evidence for two tumor suppressor loci associated with proximal chromosome 9p to q and distal chromosome 9q in bladder cancer and the initial screening for GAS1 and PTC mutations. Cancer Res. 1996;56(21):5039–43.
66. Hornigold N, Devlin J, Davies AM, Aveyard JS, Habuchi T, Knowles MA. Mutation of the 9q34 gene TSC1 in sporadic bladder cancer. Oncogene. 1999;18(16):2567–61.
67. van Slegtenhorst M, de Hoogt R, Hermans C, et al. Identification of the tuberous sclerosis gene TSC1 on chromosome 9q34. Science. 1997;277(5327):805–8.
68. Knowles MA, Habuchi T, Kennedy W, Cuthbert-Heavens D. Mutation spectrum of the 9q34 tuberous sclerosis gene TSC1 in transitional cell carcinoma of the bladder. Cancer Res. 2003;63(22):7652–6.
69. Pymar LS, Platt FM, Askham JM, Morrison EE, Knowles MA. Bladder tumour-derived somatic TSC1 missense mutations cause loss of function via distinct mechanisms. Hum Mol Genet. 2008; 17(13):2006–17.
70. Adachi H, Igawa M, Shiina H, Urakami S, Shigeno K, Hino O. Human bladder tumors with 2-hit mutations of tumor suppressor gene TSC1 and decreased expression of p27. J Urol. 2003;170(2 Pt 1):601–4.
71. Habuchi T, Yoshida O, Knowles MA. A novel candidate tumour suppressor locus at 9q32-33 in bladder cancer: localization of the candidate region within a single 840 kb YAC. Hum Mol Genet. 1997; 6(6):913–9.
72. Habuchi T, Luscombe M, Elder PA, Knowles MA. Structure and methylation-based silencing of a gene (DBCCR1) within a candidate bladder cancer tumor suppressor region at 9q32-q33. Genomics. 1998; 48(3):277–88.
73. Simoneau M, Aboulkassim TO, LaRue H, Rousseau F, Fradet Y. Four tumor suppressor loci on chromosome 9q in bladder cancer: evidence for two novel candidate regions at 9q22.3 and 9q31. Oncogene. 1999;18(1):157–63.
74. Thievessen I, Wolter M, Prior A, Seifert HH, Schulz WA. Hedgehog signaling in normal urothelial cells and in urothelial carcinoma cell lines. J Cell Physiol. 2005;203(2):372–7.
75. Sonny LJ, Samuel MC. Epidemiology and etiology of bladder cancer. Semin Surg Oncol. 1997;13(5): 291–8.
76. Serrano M, Hannon GJ, Beach D. A new regulatory motif in cell-cycle control causing specific inhibition of cyclin D/CDK4. Nature. 1993;366(6546):704–7.
77. Hannon GJ, Beach D. p15INK4B is a potential effector of TGF-beta-induced cell cycle arrest. Nature. 1994;371(6494):257–61.
78. Schulze A, Zerfass K, Spitkovsky D, Henglein B, Jansen-Dürr P. Activation of the E2F transcription factor by cyclin D1 is blocked by p16INK4, the product of the putative tumor suppressor gene MTS1. Oncogene. 1994;9(12):3475–82.
79. Johnson DG. Regulation of E2F-1 gene expression by p130 (Rb2) and D-type cyclin kinase activity. Oncogene. 1995;11(9):1685–92.
80. Gonzalez-Zulueta M, Shibata A, Ohneseit PF, et al. High frequency of chromosome 9p allelic loss and CDKN2 tumor suppressor gene alterations in squamous cell carcinoma of the bladder. J Natl Cancer Inst. 1995;87(18):1383–93.
81. Gonzalez-Zulueta M, Bender CM, Yang AS, et al. Methylation of the 5' CpG island of the p16/CDKN2 tumor suppressor gene in normal and transformed human tissues correlates with gene silencing. Cancer Res. 1995;55(20):4531–5.
82. Orlow I, Lacombe L, Hannon GJ, et al. Deletion of the p16 and p15 genes in human bladder tumors. J Natl Cancer Inst. 1995;87(20):1524–9.
83. Southgate J, Proffitt J, Roberts P, Smith B, Selby P. Loss of cyclin-dependent kinase inhibitor genes and chromosome 9 karyotypic abnormalities in human bladder cancer cell lines. Br J Cancer. 1995;72(5): 1214–8.
84. Le Frere-Belda MA, Cappellen D, Daher A, et al. p15INK4b in bladder carcinomas: decreased expression in superficial tumours. Br J Cancer. 2001;85(10): 1515–21.
85. Joanne E, Pamela D, James JG, Amanda DW, Kenneth MG, John MSB. Identification of loci associated with putative recurrence genes in transitional cell carcinoma of the urinary bladder. J Pathol. 2002;196(4):380–5.
86. Friedrich MG, Blind C, Milde-Langosch K, et al. Frequent p16/MTS1 inactivation in early stages of urothelial carcinoma of the bladder is not associated with tumor recurrence. Eur Urol. 2001;40(5):518–24.
87. Riccardo B, Tommaso C, Gabriella N, Lucia Roberta G, Gianna B, Maurizio Dal C. Loss of P16 expression and chromosome 9p21 LOH in predicting outcome of patients affected by superficial bladder cancer. J Surg Res. 2007;143(2):422–7.
88. Bartlett JM, Watters AD, Ballantyne SA, Going JJ, Grigor KM, Cooke TG. Is chromosome 9 loss a marker of disease recurrence in transitional cell carcinoma of the urinary bladder? Br J Cancer. 1998;77(12):2193–8.
89. Lopez-Beltran A, Alvarez-Kindelan J, Luque RJ, et al. Loss of heterozygosity at 9q32-33 (DBC1

locus) in primary non-invasive papillary urothelial neoplasm of low malignant potential and low-grade urothelial carcinoma of the bladder and their associated normal urothelium. J Pathol. 2008;215(3):263–72.

90. Sanchez-Carbayo M, Socci ND, Charytonowicz E, et al. Molecular profiling of bladder cancer using cDNA microarrays: defining histogenesis and biological phenotypes. Cancer Res. 2002;62(23):6973–80.
91. Dyrskjot L, Thykjaer T, Kruhoffer M, et al. Identifying distinct classes of bladder carcinoma using microarrays. Nat Genet. 2003;33(1):90–6.
92. Sanchez-Carbayo M, Socci ND, Lozano JJ, et al. Gene discovery in bladder cancer progression using cDNA microarrays. Am J Pathol. 2003;163(2):505–16.
93. Wild PJ, Herr A, Wissmann C, et al. Gene expression profiling of progressive papillary noninvasive carcinomas of the urinary bladder. Clin Cancer Res. 2005;11(12):4415–29.
94. Lindgren D, Liedberg F, Andersson A, et al. Molecular characterization of early-stage bladder carcinomas by expression profiles, FGFR3 mutation status, and loss of 9q. Oncogene. 2006;25(18):2685–96.
95. Dyrskjot L, Zieger K, Kruhoffer M, et al. A molecular signature in superficial bladder carcinoma predicts clinical outcome. Clin Cancer Res. 2005;11(11):4029–36.
96. Dyrskjot L, Zieger K, Real FX, et al. Gene expression signatures predict outcome in non-muscle-invasive bladder carcinoma: a multicenter validation study. Clin Cancer Res. 2007;13(12):3545–51.
97. Dyrskjot L, Kruhoffer M, Thykjaer T, et al. Gene expression in the urinary bladder: a common carcinoma in situ gene expression signature exists disregarding histopathological classification. Cancer Res. 2004;64(11):4040–8.
98. Wang R, Morris DS, Tomlins SA, et al. Development of a multiplex quantitative PCR signature to predict progression in non-muscle-invasive bladder cancer. Cancer Res. 2009;69(9):3810–8.
99. Holyoake A, O'Sullivan P, Pollock R, et al. Development of a multiplex RNA urine test for the detection and stratification of transitional cell carcinoma of the bladder. Clin Cancer Res. 2008;14(3):742–9.
100. Fan C, Oh DS, Wessels L, et al. Concordance among gene-expression-based predictors for breast cancer. N Engl J Med. 2006;355(6):560–9.
101. Alexandroff AB, Jackson AM, O'Donnell MA, James K. BCG immunotherapy of bladder cancer: 20 years on. Lancet. 1999;353(9165):1689–94.
102. Bevers RF, Kurth KH, Schamhart DH. Role of urothelial cells in BCG immunotherapy for superficial bladder cancer. Br J Cancer. 2004;91(4):607–12.
103. Kawashima T, Norose Y, Watanabe Y, et al. Cutting edge: major CD8 T cell response to live bacillus Calmette-Guerin is mediated by CD1 molecules. J Immunol. 2003;170(11):5345–8.
104. Ayari C, LaRue H, Hovington H, et al. Bladder tumor infiltrating mature dendritic cells and macrophages as predictors of response to bacillus Calmette-Guerin immunotherapy. Eur Urol. 2009;55(6):1386–95.
105. Jemal A, Siegel R, Ward E, et al. Cancer Statistics, 2008. CA Cancer J Clin 2008.
106. Messing EM. Urothelial tumors of the bladder. In: Wein A, Kavoussi L, Novick A, Partin A, Peters C, editors. Campbell-Walsh urology. 9th ed. Philadelphia: Saunders Elsevier; 2007.
107. Babaian RJ, Johnson DE, Llamas L, Ayala AG. Metastases from transitional cell carcinoma of urinary bladder. Urology. 1980;16(2):142–4.
108. Goldman SM, Fajardo AA, Naraval RC, Madewell JE. Metastatic transitional cell carcinoma from the bladder: radiographic manifestions. AJR Am J Roentgenol. 1979;132(3):419–25.
109. Sengelov L, Kamby C, von der Maase H. Pattern of metastases in relation to characteristics of primary tumor and treatment in patients with disseminated urothelial carcinoma. J Urol. 1996;155(1):111–4.
110. Mitra AP, Datar RH, Cote RJ. Molecular pathways in invasive bladder cancer: new insights into mechanisms, progression, and target identification. J Clin Oncol. 2006;24(35):5552–64.
111. Mitra AP, Birkhahn M, Cote RJ. p53 and retinoblastoma pathways in bladder cancer. World J Urol. 2007;25(6):563–71.
112. Spruck III CH, Ohneseit PF, Gonzalez-Zulueta M, et al. Two molecular pathways to transitional cell carcinoma of the bladder. Cancer Res. 1994;54(3):784–8.
113. Ioachim E, Charchanti A, Stavropoulos NE, Skopelitou A, Athanassiou ED, Agnantis NJ. Immunohistochemical expression of retinoblastoma gene product (Rb), p53 protein, MDM2, c-erbB-2, HLA-DR and proliferation indices in human urinary bladder carcinoma. Histol Histopathol. 2000;15(3):721–7.
114. Peyromaure M, Ravery V. Prognostic value of p53 overexpression in bladder tumors treated with Bacillus Calmette-Guerin. Exp Rev Anticancer Ther. 2002;2(6):667–70.
115. Stavropoulos NE, Filiadis I, Ioachim E, et al. Prognostic significance of p53, bcl-2 and Ki-67 in high risk superficial bladder cancer. Anticancer Res. 2002;22(6B):3759–64.
116. Sarkis AS, Bajorin DF, Reuter VE, et al. Prognostic value of p53 nuclear overexpression in patients with invasive bladder cancer treated with neoadjuvant MVAC. J Clin Oncol. 1995;13(6):1384–90.
117. Sarkis AS, Dalbagni G, Cordon-Cardo C, et al. Nuclear overexpression of p53 protein in transitional cell bladder carcinoma: a marker for disease progression. J Natl Cancer Inst. 1993;85(1):53–9.
118. Esrig D, Elmajian D, Groshen S, et al. Accumulation of nuclear p53 and tumor progression in bladder cancer. N England J Med. 1994;331(19):1259–64.

119. Esrig D, Spruck 3rd CH, Nichols PW, et al. p53 nuclear protein accumulation correlates with mutations in the p53 gene, tumor grade, and stage in bladder cancer. Am J Pathol. 1993;143(5):1389–97.
120. Fujimoto K, Yamada Y, Okajima E, et al. Frequent association of p53 gene mutation in invasive bladder cancer. Cancer Res. 1992;52(6):1393–8.
121. Matsuyama H, Pan Y, Mahdy EA, et al. p53 deletion as a genetic marker in urothelial tumor by fluorescence in situ hybridization. Cancer Res. 1994;54(23):6057–60.
122. Moch H, Sauter G, Moore D, Mihatsch MJ, Gudat F, Waldman F. p53 and erbB-2 protein overexpression are associated with early invasion and metastasis in bladder cancer. Virchows Arch A Pathol Anat Histopathol. 1993;423(5):329–34.
123. Soini Y, Turpeenniemi-Hujanen T, Kamel D, et al. p53 immunohistochemistry in transitional cell carcinoma and dysplasia of the urinary bladder correlates with disease progression. Br J Cancer. 1993;68(5): 1029–35.
124. Yamamoto S, Masui T, Murai T, et al. Frequent mutations of the p53 gene and infrequent H- and K-ras mutations in urinary bladder carcinomas of NON/Shi mice treated with N-butyl-N-(4-hydroxybutyl)nitrosamine. Carcinogenesis. 1995; 16(10):2363–8.
125. Thomas CY, Theodorescu D. Molecular markers of prognosis and novel therapeutic strategies for urothelial cell carcinomas. World J Urol. 2006;24(5):565–78.
126. Cairns P, Proctor AJ, Knowles MA. Loss of heterozygosity at the RB locus is frequent and correlates with muscle invasion in bladder carcinoma. Oncogene. 1991;6(12):2305–9.
127. Cordon-Cardo C, Sheinfeld J, Dalbagni G. Genetic studies and molecular markers of bladder cancer. Semin Surg Oncol. 1997;13(5):319–27.
128. Cordon-Cardo C, Wartinger D, Petrylak D, et al. Altered expression of the retinoblastoma gene product: prognostic indicator in bladder cancer. J Natl Cancer Inst. 1992;84(16):1251–6.
129. Grossman HB, Liebert M, Antelo M, et al. p53 and RB expression predict progression in T1 bladder cancer. Clin Cancer Res. 1998;4(4):829–34.
130. Shariat SF, Tokunaga H, Zhou J, et al. p53, p21, pRB, and p16 expression predict clinical outcome in cystectomy with bladder cancer. J Clin Oncol. 2004;22(6):1014–24.
131. Gorgoulis VG, Barbatis C, Poulias I, Karameris AM. Molecular and immunohistochemical evaluation of epidermal growth factor receptor and c-erb-B-2 gene product in transitional cell carcinomas of the urinary bladder: a study in Greek patients. Mod Pathol. 1995;8(7):758–64.
132. Lipponen P, Eskelinen M. Expression of epidermal growth factor receptor in bladder cancer as related to established prognostic factors, oncoprotein (c-erbB-2, p53) expression and long-term prognosis. Br J Cancer. 1994;69(6):1120–5.
133. Chow NH, Liu HS, Lee EI, et al. Significance of urinary epidermal growth factor and its receptor expression in human bladder cancer. Anticancer Res. 1997;17(2B):1293–6.
134. Ravery V, Grignon D, Angulo J, et al. Evaluation of epidermal growth factor receptor, transforming growth factor alpha, epidermal growth factor and c-erbB2 in the progression of invasive bladder cancer. Urol Res. 1997;25(1):9–17.
135. Nguyen PL, Swanson PE, Jaszcz W, et al. Expression of epidermal growth factor receptor in invasive transitional cell carcinoma of the urinary bladder. A multivariate survival analysis. Am J Clin Pathol. 1994;101(2):166–76.
136. Sauter G, Haley J, Chew K, et al. Epidermal-growth-factor-receptor expression is associated with rapid tumor proliferation in bladder cancer. Int J Cancer. 1994;57(4):508–14.
137. Gontero P, Banisadr S, Frea B, Brausi M. Metastasis markers in bladder cancer: a review of the literature and clinical considerations. Eur Urol. 2004;46(3): 296–311.
138. Knowles MA. Molecular subtypes of bladder cancer: Jekyll and Hyde or chalk and cheese? Carcinogenesis. 2006;27(3):361–73.
139. Miyake H, Hara I, Gohji K, Yoshimura K, Arakawa S, Kamidono S. Expression of basic fibroblast growth factor is associated with resistance to cisplatin in a human bladder cancer cell line. Cancer Lett. 1998;123(2):121–6.
140. Miyake H, Yoshimura K, Hara I, Eto H, Arakawa S, Kamidono S. Basic fibroblast growth factor regulates matrix metalloproteinases production and in vitro invasiveness in human bladder cancer cell lines. J Urol. 1997;157(6):2351–5.
141. Munro NP, Knowles MA. Fibroblast growth factors and their receptors in transitional cell carcinoma. J Urol. 2003;169(2):675–82.
142. Thomas-Mudge RJ, Okada-Ban M, Vandenbroucke F, et al. Nuclear FGF-2 facilitates cell survival in vitro and during establishment of metastases. Oncogene. 2004;23(27):4771–9.
143. Ornitz DM, Itoh N. Fibroblast growth factors. Genome Biol 2001;2(3):Reviews 3005.
144. Ricol D, Cappellen D, El Marjou A, et al. Tumour suppressive properties of fibroblast growth factor receptor 2-IIIb in human bladder cancer. Oncogene. 1999;18(51):7234–43.
145. Bernard-Pierrot I, Brams A, Dunois-Larde C, et al. Oncogenic properties of the mutated forms of fibroblast growth factor receptor 3b. Carcinogenesis. 2006;27(4):740–7.
146. Bernard-Pierrot I, Ricol D, Cassidy A, et al. Inhibition of human bladder tumour cell growth by fibroblast growth factor receptor 2b is independent of its kinase activity. Involvement of the carboxy-terminal region of the receptor. Oncogene. 2004;23(57):9201–11.
147. Shibuya M. Vascular endothelial growth factor-dependent and -independent regulation of angiogenesis. BMB Rep. 2008;41(4):278–86.

148. Crew JP, O'Brien T, Bradburn M, et al. Vascular endothelial growth factor is a predictor of relapse and stage progression in superficial bladder cancer. Cancer Res. 1997;57(23):5281–5.
149. Bouck N, Campbell S. Anti-cancer dividends from captopril and other inhibitors of angiogenesis. J Nephrol. 1998;11(1):3–4.
150. Campbell CL, Savarese DM, Quesenberry PJ, Savarese TM. Expression of multiple angiogenic cytokines in cultured normal human prostate epithelial cells: predominance of vascular endothelial growth factor. Int J Cancer. 1999;80(6):868–74.
151. Campbell SC, Volpert OV, Ivanovich M, Bouck NP. Molecular mediators of angiogenesis in bladder cancer. Cancer Res. 1998;58(6):1298–304.
152. Wu W, Shu X, Hovsepyan H, Mosteller RD, Broek D. VEGF receptor expression and signaling in human bladder tumors. Oncogene. 2003;22(22):3361–70.
153. Herrmann E, Eltze E, Bierer S, et al. VEGF-C, VEGF-D and Flt-4 in transitional bladder cancer: relationships to clinicopathological parameters and long-term survival. Anticancer Res. 2007;27(5A):3127–33.
154. Herrmann E, Eltze E, Kopke T, et al. New markers for pharmacological targeting in bladder cancer with lymph node metastasis. Aktuelle Urol. 2007;38(5):392–7.
155. Sporn MB, Roberts AB. Transforming growth factor-beta. Multiple actions and potential clinical applications. JAMA. 1989;262(7):938–41.
156. Coombs LM, Pigott DA, Eydmann ME, Proctor AJ, Knowles MA. Reduced expression of TGF beta is associated with advanced disease in transitional cell carcinoma. Br J Cancer. 1993;67(3):578–84.
157. Miyamoto H, Kubota Y, Shuin T, Torigoe S, Dobashi Y, Hosaka M. Expression of transforming growth factor-beta 1 in human bladder cancer. Cancer. 1995;75(10):2565–70.
158. Eder IE, Stenzl A, Hobisch A, Cronauer MV, Bartsch G, Klocker H. Transforming growth factors-beta 1 and beta 2 in serum and urine from patients with bladder carcinoma. J Urol. 1996;156(3):953–7.
159. Eder IE, Stenzl A, Hobisch A, Cronauer MV, Bartsch G, Klocker H. Expression of transforming growth factors beta-1, beta 2 and beta 3 in human bladder carcinomas. Br J Cancer. 1997;75(12):1753–60.
160. Kim JH, Shariat SF, Kim IY, et al. Predictive value of expression of transforming growth factor-beta(1) and its receptors in transitional cell carcinoma of the urinary bladder. Cancer. 2001;92(6):1475–83.
161. Matsumoto K, Shariat SF, Casella R, Wheeler TM, Slawin KM, Lerner SP. Preoperative plasma soluble E-cadherin predicts metastases to lymph nodes and prognosis in patients undergoing radical cystectomy. J Urol. 2003;170(6 Pt 1):2248–52.
162. Shariat SF, Casella R, Monoski MA, Sulser T, Gasser TC, Lerner SP. The addition of urinary urokinase-type plasminogen activator to urinary nuclear matrix protein 22 and cytology improves the detection of bladder cancer. J Urol. 2003;170(6 Pt 1):2244–7.
163. Shariat SF, Matsumoto K, Kim J, et al. Correlation of cyclooxygenase-2 expression with molecular markers, pathological features and clinical outcome of transitional cell carcinoma of the bladder. J Urol. 2003;170(3):985–9.
164. Wieser R. The transforming growth factor-beta signaling pathway in tumorigenesis. Curr Opin Oncol. 2001;13(1):70–7.
165. Titus B, Frierson Jr HF, Conaway M, et al. Endothelin axis is a target of the lung metastasis suppressor gene RhoGDI2. Cancer Res. 2005;65(16):7320–7.
166. Ellenbroek SI, Collard JG. Rho GTPases: functions and association with cancer. Clin Exp Metastasis. 2007;24(8):657–72.
167. Kamai T, Tsujii T, Arai K, et al. Significant association of Rho/ROCK pathway with invasion and metastasis of bladder cancer. Clin Cancer Res. 2003;9(7):2632–41.
168. Nitz MD, Harding MA, Theodorescu D. Invasion and metastasis models for studying RhoGDI2 in bladder cancer. Methods Enzymol. 2008;439:219–33.
169. Theodorescu D. Molecular biology of invasive and metastatic urothelial cancer. In: Lerner S, Schoenberg M, Sternberg C, editors. Textbook of bladder cancer. New York: Taylor & Francis; 2006. p. 147–56.
170. Seraj MJ, Harding MA, Gildea JJ, Welch DR, Theodorescu D. The relationship of BRMS1 and RhoGDI2 gene expression to metastatic potential in lineage related human bladder cancer cell lines. Clin Exp Metastasis. 2000;18(6):519–25.
171. Theodorescu D, Sapinoso LM, Conaway MR, Oxford G, Hampton GM, Frierson Jr HF. Reduced expression of metastasis suppressor RhoGDI2 is associated with decreased survival for patients with bladder cancer. Clin Cancer Res. 2004;10(11):3800–6.
172. Gildea JJ, Seraj MJ, Oxford G, et al. RhoGDI2 is an invasion and metastasis suppressor gene in human cancer. Cancer Res. 2002;62(22):6418–23.
173. Thiery JP. Epithelial-mesenchymal transitions in tumour progression. Nat Rev Cancer. 2002;2(6):442–54.
174. Bornman DM, Mathew S, Alsruhe J, Herman JG, Gabrielson E. Methylation of the E-cadherin gene in bladder neoplasia and in normal urothelial epithelium from elderly individuals. Am J Pathol. 2001;159(3):831–5.
175. Dhawan D, Hamdy FC, Rehman I, et al. Evidence for the early onset of aberrant promoter methylation in urothelial carcinoma. J Pathol. 2006;209(3):336–43.
176. Horikawa Y, Sugano K, Shigyo M, et al. Hypermethylation of an E-cadherin (CDH1) promoter region in high grade transitional cell carcinoma of the bladder comprising carcinoma in situ. J Urol. 2003;169(4):1541–5.
177. Nakopoulou L, Zervas A, Gakiopoulou-Givalou H, et al. Prognostic value of E-cadherin, beta-catenin, P120ctn in patients with transitional cell bladder cancer. Anticancer Res. 2000;20(6B):4571–8.

178. Sun W, Herrera GA. E-cadherin expression in urothelial carcinoma in situ, superficial papillary transitional cell carcinoma, and invasive transitional cell carcinoma. Hum Pathol. 2002;33(10): 996–1000.
179. Sun W, Herrera GA. E-cadherin expression in invasive urothelial carcinoma. Ann Diagn Pathol. 2004;8(1):17–22.
180. Imao T, Koshida K, Endo Y, Uchibayashi T, Sasaki T, Namiki M. Dominant role of E-cadherin in the progression of bladder cancer. J Urol. 1999;161(2):692–8.
181. Syrigos KN, Krausz T, Waxman J, et al. E-cadherin expression in bladder cancer using formalin-fixed, paraffin-embedded tissues: correlation with histopathological grade, tumour stage and survival. Int J Cancer. 1995;64(6):367–70.
182. Mahnken A, Kausch I, Feller AC, Kruger S. E-cadherin immunoreactivity correlates with recurrence and progression of minimally invasive transitional cell carcinomas of the urinary bladder. Oncol Rep. 2005;14(4):1065–70.
183. Shariat SF, Pahlavan S, Baseman AG, et al. E-cadherin expression predicts clinical outcome in carcinoma in situ of the urinary bladder. Urology. 2001;57(1):60–5.
184. Byrne RR, Shariat SF, Brown R, et al. E-cadherin immunostaining of bladder transitional cell carcinoma, carcinoma in situ and lymph node metastases with long-term followup. J Urol. 2001;165(5): 1473–9.
185. Rao J, Seligson D, Visapaa H, et al. Tissue microarray analysis of cytoskeletal actin-associated biomarkers gelsolin and E-cadherin in urothelial carcinoma. Cancer. 2002;95(6):1247–57.
186. Rieger-Christ KM, Lee P, Zagha R, et al. Novel expression of N-cadherin elicits in vitro bladder cell invasion via the Akt signaling pathway. Oncogene. 2004;23(27):4745–53.
187. Clairotte A, Lascombe I, Fauconnet S, et al. Expression of E-cadherin and alpha-, beta-, gamma-catenins in patients with bladder cancer: identification of gamma-catenin as a new prognostic marker of neoplastic progression in T1 superficial urothelial tumors. Am J Clin Pathol. 2006;125(1):119–26.
188. Shariat SF, Matsumoto K, Casella R, Jian W, Lerner SP. Urinary levels of soluble e-cadherin in the detection of transitional cell carcinoma of the urinary bladder. Eur Urol. 2005;48(1):69–76.
189. Julien S, Puig I, Caretti E, et al. Activation of NF-kappaB by Akt upregulates Snail expression and induces epithelium mesenchyme transition. Oncogene. 2007;26(53):7445–56.
190. Zhang Z, Xie D, Li X, et al. Significance of TWIST expression and its association with E-cadherin in bladder cancer. Hum Pathol. 2007;38(4):598–606.
191. Fondrevelle ME, Kantelip B, Reiter RE, et al. The expression of Twist has an impact on survival in human bladder cancer and is influenced by the smoking status. Urol Oncol. 2009;27(3):268–76.
192. Harabayashi T, Kanai Y, Yamada T, et al. Reduction of integrin beta4 and enhanced migration on laminin in association with intraepithelial spreading of urinary bladder carcinomas. J Urol. 1999;161(4): 1364–71.
193. Grossman HB, Lee C, Bromberg J, Liebert M. Expression of the alpha6beta4 integrin provides prognostic information in bladder cancer. Oncol Rep. 2000;7(1):13–6.
194. Liebert M, Gebhardt D, Wood C, et al. Urothelial differentiation and bladder cancer. Adv Exp Med Biol. 1999;462:437–48.
195. Chen F, Zhang G, Iwamoto Y, See WA. Bacillus Calmette-Guerin initiates intracellular signaling in a transitional carcinoma cell line by cross-linking alpha 5 beta 1 integrin. J Urol. 2003;170(2 Pt 1): 605–10.
196. Kausch I, Ardelt P, Bohle A, Ratliff TL. Immune gene therapy in urology. Curr Urol Rep. 2002; 3(1):82–9.
197. Numahata K, Satoh M, Handa K, et al. Sialosyl-Le(x) expression defines invasive and metastatic properties of bladder carcinoma. Cancer. 2002; 94(3):673–85.
198. Al-Sukhun S, Hussain M. Molecular biology of transitional cell carcinoma. Crit Rev Oncol Hematol. 2003;47(2):181–93.
199. Sathyanarayana UG, Maruyama R, Padar A, et al. Molecular detection of noninvasive and invasive bladder tumor tissues and exfoliated cells by aberrant promoter methylation of laminin-5 encoding genes. Cancer Res. 2004;64(4):1425–30.
200. Lokeshwar VB, Obek C, Pham HT, et al. Urinary hyaluronic acid and hyaluronidase: markers for bladder cancer detection and evaluation of grade. J Urol. 2000;163(1):348–56.
201. Lokeshwar VB, Selzer MG. Differences in hyaluronic acid-mediated functions and signaling in arterial, microvessel, and vein-derived human endothelial cells. J Biol Chem. 2000;275(36):27641–9.
202. Lokeshwar VB, Obek C, Soloway MS, Block NL. Tumor-associated hyaluronic acid: a new sensitive and specific urine marker for bladder cancer. Cancer Res. 1997;57(4):773–7.
203. Lokeshwar VB, Block NL. HA-HAase urine test. A sensitive and specific method for detecting bladder cancer and evaluating its grade. Urol Clin North Am. 2000;27(1):53–61.
204. Lokeshwar VB, Selzer MG. Urinary bladder tumor markers. Urol Oncol. 2006;24(6):528–37.
205. Kuncova J, Urban M, Mandys V. Expression of CD44s and CD44v6 in transitional cell carcinomas of the urinary bladder: comparison with tumour grade, proliferative activity and p53 immunoreactivity of tumour cells. APMIS. 2007;115(11):1194–205.
206. Muramaki M, Miyake H, Kamidono S, Hara I. Over expression of CD44V8-10 in human bladder cancer cells decreases their interaction with hyaluronic acid and potentiates their malignant progression. J Urol. 2004;171(1):426–30.

207. Naor D, Sionov RV, Ish-Shalom D. CD44: structure, function, and association with the malignant process. Adv Cancer Res. 1997;71:241–319.
208. Garcia del Muro X, Torregrosa A, Munoz J, et al. Prognostic value of the expression of E-cadherin and beta-catenin in bladder cancer. Eur J Cancer. 2000;36(3):357–62.
209. Hong RL, Pu YS, Chu JS, Lee WJ, Chen YC, Wu CW. Correlation of expression of CD44 isoforms and E-cadherin with differentiation in human urothelial cell lines and transitional cell carcinoma. Cancer Lett. 1995;89(1):81–7.
210. Hong RL, Pu YS, Hsieh TS, Chu JS, Lee WJ. Expressions of E-cadherin and exon v6-containing isoforms of CD44 and their prognostic values in human transitional cell carcinoma. J Urol. 1995;153(6):2025–8.
211. Lipponen P, Aaltoma S, Kosma VM, Ala-Opas M, Eskelinen M. Expression of CD44 standard and variant-v6 proteins in transitional cell bladder tumours and their relation to prognosis during a long-term follow-up. J Pathol. 1998;186(2):157–64.
212. Sugino T, Gorham H, Yoshida K, et al. Progressive loss of CD44 gene expression in invasive bladder cancer. Am J Pathol. 1996;149(3):873–82.
213. Ioachim E, Michael MC, Salmas M, et al. Thrombospondin-1 expression in urothelial carcinoma: prognostic significance and association with p53 alterations, tumour angiogenesis and extracellular matrix components. BMC Cancer. 2006;6:140.
214. Goddard JC, Sutton CD, Jones JL, O'Byrne KJ, Kockelbergh RC. Reduced thrombospondin-1 at presentation predicts disease progression in superficial bladder cancer. Eur Urol. 2002;42(5): 464–8.
215. Smith SC, Oxford G, Wu Z, et al. The metastasis-associated gene CD24 is regulated by Ral GTPase and is a mediator of cell proliferation and survival in human cancer. Cancer Res. 2006;66(4):1917–22.
216. Choi YL, Lee SH, Kwon GY, et al. Overexpression of CD24: association with invasiveness in urothelial carcinoma of the bladder. Arch Pathol Lab Med. 2007;131(2):275–81.
217. Black PC, Dinney CP. Bladder cancer angiogenesis and metastasis–translation from murine model to clinical trial. Cancer Metastasis Rev. 2007;26(3–4): 623–34.
218. Margulis V, Shariat SF, Ashfaq R, et al. Expression of cyclooxygenase-2 in normal urothelium, and superficial and advanced transitional cell carcinoma of bladder. J Urol. 2007;177(3):1163–8.
219. Hammam OA, Aziz AA, Roshdy MS, Abdel Hadi AM. Possible role of cyclooxygenase-2 in schistosomal and non-schistosomal-associated bladder cancer. Medscape J Med. 2008;10(3):60.
220. Yates DR, Rehman I, Abbod MF, et al. Promoter hypermethylation identifies progression risk in bladder cancer. Clin Cancer Res. 2007;13(7):2046–53.
221. Zu X, Tang Z, Li Y, Gao N, Ding J, Qi L. Vascular endothelial growth factor-C expression in bladder transitional cell cancer and its relationship to lymph node metastasis. BJU Int. 2006;98(5):1090–3.
222. Wulfing C, Eltze E, Piechota H, et al. Expression of endothelin-1 and endothelin-A and -B receptors in invasive bladder cancer. Oncol Rep. 2005;13(2): 223–8.
223. Modlich O, Prisack HB, Pitschke G, et al. Identifying superficial, muscle-invasive, and metastasizing transitional cell carcinoma of the bladder: use of cDNA array analysis of gene expression profiles. Clin Cancer Res. 2004;10(10):3410–21.
224. Sanchez-Carbayo M, Socci ND, Lozano J, Saint F, Cordon-Cardo C. Defining molecular profiles of poor outcome in patients with invasive bladder cancer using oligonucleotide microarrays. J Clin Oncol. 2006;24(5):778–89.
225. Stein JP, Lieskovsky G, Cote R, et al. Radical cystectomy in the treatment of invasive bladder cancer: long-term results in 1,054 patients. J Clin Oncol. 2001;19(3):666–75.
226. Sanchez-Carbayo M, Socci ND, Lozano JJ, Haab BB, Cordon-Cardo C. Profiling bladder cancer using targeted antibody arrays. Am J Pathol. 2006;168(1): 93–103.
227. Havaleshko DM, Cho H, Conaway M, et al. Prediction of drug combination chemosensitivity in human bladder cancer. Mol Cancer Ther. 2007; 6(2):578–86.
228. Takata R, Katagiri T, Kanehira M, et al. Predicting response to methotrexate, vinblastine, doxorubicin, and cisplatin neoadjuvant chemotherapy for bladder cancers through genome-wide gene expression profiling. Clin Cancer Res. 2005;11(7):2625–36.
229. Takata R, Katagiri T, Kanehira M, et al. Validation study of the prediction system for clinical response of M-VAC neoadjuvant chemotherapy. Cancer Sci. 2007;98(1):113–7.
230. Als AB, Dyrskjot L, von der Maase H, et al. Emmprin and survivin predict response and survival following cisplatin-containing chemotherapy in patients with advanced bladder cancer. Clin Cancer Res. 2007;13(15 Pt 1):4407–14.

Index

D.E. Hansel et al. (eds.), *The Urinary Tract: A Comprehensive Guide to Patient Diagnosis and Management*, DOI 10.1007/978-1-4614-5320-8,

C

V

W

13-135

Printed by Publishers' Graphics LLC
SO20130208.08.01.34